W9-AZM-113

Ethnicity and Medical Care

Ethnicity and Medical Care

Edited by

ALAN HARWOOD

(cf)

A Commonwealth Fund Book
HARVARD UNIVERSITY PRESS
Cambridge, Massachusetts, and London, England
1981

Library of Congress Cataloging in Publication Data

Main entry under title:

Ethnicity and medical care.

  "A Commonwealth Fund book."
  Includes index.
    1. Minorities—Medical care—United States.
2. Medical anthropology—United States.
3. Ethnology—United States. 4. Ethnicity.
I. Harwood, Alan. [DNLM: 1. Ethnic groups—
United States. 2. Delivery of health care—
United States. 3. Professional—Patient relations.
WA300 E85]
RA448.4.E83   362.1   80–19339
ISBN 0–674–26865–2

Contributors

KATHERINE GOULD-MARTIN

Senior Lecturer
Department of Anthropology
University of Southern
California

ALAN HARWOOD

Professor of Anthropology
University of Massachusetts,
Boston

JOHN P. HOMIAK

Department of Anthropology
Brandeis University

JACQUELYNE JOHNSON JACKSON

Associate Professor of Medical
Sociology
Department of Psychiatry
Duke University Medical Center

STEPHEN J. KUNITZ

Associate Professor of
Preventive, Family, and
Rehabilitation Medicine
University of Rochester
School of Medicine

MICHEL S. LAGUERRE

Assistant Professor of
Anthropology
Department of
Afro-American Studies
University of California at
Berkeley

JERROLD E. LEVY

Professor of Anthropology
University of Arizona

CHORSWANG NGIN

Department of Anthropology
University of California at Davis

ANTOINETTE T. RAGUCCI   *Associate Professor of Medical-Surgical Nursing*

Frances Payne Bolton School of Nursing
Case Western Reserve University

JANET M. SCHREIBER   *Associate Professor of Anthropology*
University of Texas
School of Public Health
at Houston

Acknowledgments

THIS VOLUME WAS supported by a grant-in-aid from the Commonwealth Fund, and I am particularly grateful to Dr. Reginald H. Fitz for his advice and assistance during my association with the Fund. I would also like to thank the University of Massachusetts at Boston for granting me research leave for working on the book.

In seeing the manuscript through to completion, a number of people have provided invaluable assistance. Marcia Sorcinelli acted as research assistant, typist, and general factotum from the inception of the project, and her reliability, support, and efficiency greatly eased the burdens of editorship. Bibliographic assistance was provided by Robert Jordan, Nancy Knittle, and Susan LoGuidice. In addition to the various people who at my request read chapters in draft form and whose assistance is acknowledged in the relevant chapters, I would like to thank Dr. H. Jack Geiger and Dr. Cornelius L. Hopper for their helpful comments. I particularly want to thank Dr. Benjamin Siegel, friend and physician, who was always willing to explain to this outsider an arcane word or rite of the medical profession. His help has enhanced the value of the book for health professionals.

A number of people at Harvard University Press made important contributions. William Bennett encouraged me to develop my plans for the volume, and Mary Ellen Arkin enhanced the readability of the manuscript through her careful editing.

Not least among those who made this book possible are my family—Judy, Seth, and Jessica. For their gifts of time and patience I am most appreciative, and for Judy's practical wisdom I am always indebted.

Finally, I thank my fellow contributors. A multiauthor volume is always something of a feat, but to have all the contributors follow the same outline and still emerge at the conclusion on cordial terms is evidence of their good sense, fair-mindedness, and downright hard work. I am very grateful to them.

A.H.

Contents

Tables

Ethnicity and Medical Care

Introduction

ALAN HARWOOD

PEOPLE WHO HAVE BEEN RAISED in an ethnic collectivity—that is, a group with common origins, a sense of identity, and shared standards for behavior—often acquire from that experience not only basic concepts and attitudes toward health and illness but also fundamental styles of interpersonal behavior and concerns about the world. The effects of this enculturation carry over into health-care situations and also become an important influence on personal activities devoted to health maintenance and disease prevention. Ethnic differences are therefore of practical concern in treatment situations when patients and providers of care come from different ethnic backgrounds—that is, when the providers are likely to be unaware of the culturally derived expectations and views of their patients. In such circumstances, health personnel may be unable to respond appropriately to the personal needs of patients for information, reassurance, and effective treatment (Gillum and Barsky 1974; Eisenberg 1977a).

Ethnic subcultural differences between patients and providers may be further complicated by additional subcultural orientations prevalent among members of the health-care professions today.[1] With the growth and development of the scientific and technical aspects of medical care in recent decades, the health-care professions have become increasingly specialized and even subspecialized. Moreover, health care has come to focus more and more on the treatment of abnormalities in the structure and function of body organs and systems, with a resulting neglect of concern with patients' experiences of these abnormalities. In the jargon of the day, the health-care professions, by and large, treat *disease* rather than *illness*. Although this approach has been highly successful in reducing and controlling the prevalence of many diseases, its effects have not been entirely salutary and have produced a disjunction between what is important to patients and what is important to providers in health care. With the growing professional focus on subspecialization and on disease, providing personalized and supportive treatment has become a diminishing part of the professional conception of adequate health care, while it still remains a central concern of laymen.

For health-care professionals who wish to narrow this disjunction and who seek to treat illness as well as disease among their patients of varying ethnic backgrounds, this book brings together material from a wide variety of sources on the health beliefs and practices of seven American ethnic groups: urban blacks, Chinese, Haitians, Italians, Mexicans, Navajos, and Puerto Ricans. To set the stage for the chapters on these groups, the remainder of this introduction examines the nature of ethnicity in this country and its relationship to health behavior and health care, concluding with some general suggestions to health-care professionals as to how the data in this book can be used to provide more personalized, culturally relevant care to patients of different ethnic backgrounds. This theme is pursued further in Chapter 8, where data on the seven groups is used to develop general guidelines for providing health care to members of American ethnic groups. Thus health-care professionals whose patients come from groups not specifically surveyed in this book may nevertheless enhance their ability to treat their patients by reading both this introduction and the concluding chapter.

The Phenomenon of Ethnicity in Contemporary United States Society

The concept of ethnicity has undergone a great deal of rethinking among social scientists in recent years (see, for example, Barth 1969; Schermerhorn 1970; A. Cohen 1974b; Isajiw 1974; van den Berghe 1974; Bennett 1975; De Vos and Romanucci-Ross 1975; Glazer and Moynihan 1975b; R. Cohen 1978). Thus, before we can profitably look at the relationship between ethnicity and medical care, it is necessary to review some of this recent thinking to sharpen our conception of the phenomenon and its various manifestations in our society.

The sociologist R. A. Schermerhorn has provided a definition of ethnic group which serves as a good starting point for discussion. According to Schermerhorn, "An ethnic group is . . . a collectivity within a larger society having real or putative common ancestry, memories of a shared historical past, and a cultural focus on one or more symbolic elements defined as the epitome of their peoplehood. Examples of such symbolic elements are: kinship patterns, physical contiguity (as in localism or sectionalism), religious affiliation, language or dialect forms, tribal affiliation, nationality, phenotypical features, or any combination of these. A necessary accompaniment is some consciousness of kind among members of the group" (1978:12). This definition highlights three fundamental aspects of ethnicity as the basis for forming either collectivities or groups.[2]

1. *Ethnicity establishes social ties by reference to common origins.* These origins can refer to derivation from the same geographical locale, to mutual historical experiences, or to a shared cultural heritage. The common origins may be real and verifiable or putative and assumed, but the definitional emphasis is always "transgenerational" (Parsons 1975:57).

2. *Ethnicity also implies that the people of a particular collectivity or group share at least some learned standards for behavior—that is, symbols or social norms that shape the thought and behavior of individual members.* Some of these shared standards or cultural traits may determine behavior in many social contexts, such as language, sex roles, or family communication patterns, while others, such as food preferences or the celebration of certain holidays, circumscribe behavior only superficially, though they may nevertheless carry strong emotional weight. The degree to which standards or symbols are in fact shared within the group may also vary with such factors as social class, region, and generation.

3. *Ethnic collectivities or groups participate with one another in a larger social system.* Indeed, it is the larger sociocultural system that sometimes defines the component ethnic categories. For example, late nineteenth century immigrants from northern Italy had little cultural or political identification with southern Italians or Sicilians, yet they were all included in a single category "Italian" by the American system of ethnic classification (Glazer and Moynihan 1963:183–184). In such cases the symbols and behavioral standards that have served to differentiate ethnic collectivities in one geographic context may become deemphasized or reinterpreted, and other standards (some preexisting, some developed in the new social context) come to mark the emergent, joint category.

Participation in a larger social system also means that ethnic groups often occupy different positions of power. Members of one ethnic group may function as the guardians of the dominant value system, incumbents of most governmental offices, and dispensers of rewards, whereas others, from "minority" ethnic groups, function in few of these roles and may even, in cases of the most oppressed groups, be systematically barred from them. This situation has certainly been true of interethnic relations in the United States, where white Anglo-Saxon Protestants have dominated political and economic institutions, and later immigrants have moved on arrival into the lower rungs of the social hierarchy (Hannerz 1974:46, 61–62).

"Behavioral" and "Ideological" Ethnicity

Ethnicity, in short, defines collectivities on the basis of both common origins and shared symbols and standards for behavior (culture), and these collectivities interact within a larger social system. Applying this concept to the contemporary American scene, sociologists and anthropologists have observed two somewhat different kinds of ethnic manifestations, both of which, however, display the three basic characteristics of ethnic collectivities discussed above. These two phenomena have been variously referred to as the "old" and the "new" ethnicity (Novak 1972, 1977), "behavioral" and "ideological" ethnicity (Stein and Hill 1977:14), or a contrast between "cultural groups" and true "ethnic groups" (Patterson 1975:305–310). The fundamental differences between these two manifestations of ethnicity in this country are (1) the degree to which members of ethnic categories in fact share cultural standards, and (2) the range of social situations in which their ethnic identity is expressed.

With behavioral ethnicity, distinctive values, beliefs, behavioral norms, and languages or distinctive dialects are learned by members of the ethnic category during the process of socialization, and these distinctive cultural standards serve as the basis for interaction within the group and, in addition, influence not only interactions with members of other ethnic groups but also participation in mainstream social institutions. Behavioral ethnicity is manifested in this country primarily by first- and second-generation residents (Gordon 1964) and by ethnic minorities with a history of systematic exclusion from mainstream educational institutions and positions of political power—most notably blacks, Hispanics, and Native Americans.

Ideological ethnicity, on the other hand, is based largely on customs that are neither central to a person's social life nor necessarily learned from early socialization—for example, special food preferences, the celebration of certain holidays, or the use of certain dialectal turns of phrase or words from an ancestral language in speaking English. These cultural traits are merely symbols of the earlier immigrant subculture (Gans 1979) or, in the words of the anthropologist David Schneider, "marks of identity . . . symbols empty of elaborate social distinctions" (quoted in Parsons 1975:65). Indeed, advocates for this form of ethnic expression often stress the need to create in "new" ethnics a conscious awareness of a "deeper" ethnic culture which is presumed to exist only in latent or unconscious form (Novak 1977:35–36).

Because of the relatively fragmentary and situational nature of ideological ethnicity, it is more voluntaristic than the behavioral type. People whose ancestry encompasses a number of different ethnic backgrounds can choose to identify with one or another collectivity by displaying appropriate markers and appearing at relevant celebrations. This voluntaristic quality of ideological ethnicity is further related to its most salient characteristic: namely, that ideologically defined ethnic collectivities operate in the larger social system primarily as interest groups (Glazer and Moynihan 1963). They are, in other words, "invisible organizations" which have materialized at a particular moment in American history to advance certain political and economic interests (A. Cohen 1974a:90). Drawn largely from third- and fourth-generation whites, who in most situations behave indistinguishably from others of the same class and regional background as themselves, ideological ethnics today are "renovating" their cultural heritages and emphasizing their cultural autonomy in order to gain material advantages in the larger social system.[3]

Behavioral and ideological ethnicity might best be viewed not as mutually exclusive manifestations of the ethnic phenomenon, but as "the two extreme ends of a continuum" (A. Cohen 1974a:93). Thus some ethnic collectivities may for various reasons maintain more "social content" to their common identity than others (in other words, they may exhibit more behaviors that are normatively regulated and passed on intergenerationally), while other collectivities may rely more on Schneider's so-called empty symbols for providing a consciousness of kind. In addition, ethnic collectivities may have some members (primarily first-generation Americans) for whom ethnic identity is predominantly behavioral and other members for whom it is primarily ideological (that is, people who display ethnic markers and otherwise manifest their ethnicity in restricted social contexts, often through ethnically based interest groups).

Ethnicity and Social Class in the United States

Though analytically separable, ethnic and class phenomena are in reality closely interrelated in the United States, as in any stratified society (van den Berghe 1976:244; R. Cohen 1978:391–395). Within the larger American social system, some ethnic groups are to a significant degree confined to lower-class positions because of barriers to both power and economic resources that are built into the status system by informal and, to some extent still, legal norms. Individual mobility in the class system is also limited for members of these groups. Although the reasons for these political and economic barriers may be explained differently by social scientists of various theoretical persuasions,[4] few would deny that blacks, Native Americans, and Hispanics in the United States disproportionately occupy the lowest strata of the class system and have historically been restrained within these strata by legal and economic means. It is also true that since immigrant nationalities have tended to enter the American labor market as unskilled workers, those who have most clearly displayed behavioral ethnicity have also been socioeconomically of the lower class (Hannerz 1974:46–48, 61–62).

In short, the American social system has in various ways caused ethnic and class statuses to be closely interrelated and at times inseparable. Therefore, one cannot explain statistically common behavioral patterns among members of any one ethnic collectivity totally by ethnic factors. It is only by comparative analysis of specific variables either across ethnic groups or across classes, with the correlative factor held constant, that the implications of these two sociocultural factors for behavior and belief can be assessed. Unfortunately, most of the available data on health beliefs and behaviors do not permit this type of fine-grained, controlled comparison. The best we have been able to do in this volume is to indicate, where the data exist, the effects of class differences within each ethnic group.

Ethnicity, Health Beliefs, and Health Behavior

Health beliefs and behavior comprise a wide range of knowledge and activities, including techniques for health maintenance, standards for recognizing and evaluating symptoms, estimates of the seriousness of various conditions and of one's susceptibility to them, familiarity with biomedical disease categories, information about therapeutic resources (both medication and personnel) and how to obtain them, ways of interacting with health professionals (how to give a history, describe the problem, request specific services, and so on), and adherence to therapeutic regimens. A great many factors go into determining what any individual believes and how he behaves with regard to these various health practices, and different factors are more determinative of some practices than others (Rosenstock 1966; Douglass 1971; Becker and Maiman 1975; Hershey, Luft, and Gianaris 1975).

Of the many factors determining health belief and behavior, ethnicity (both behavioral and ideological) has been shown to be particularly relevant to certain of the components enumerated above, although it has admittedly been difficult to separate out the influence of related variables, such as socioeconomic class and acculturation, in studying its effects.

Relationships between Ethnicity and Health Behavior

DISEASE RATES   Ethnic collectivities have been observed to vary in rates of morbidity and mortality for different diseases. Statistical summaries and comparative studies involving blacks (Shiloh and Selavan 1974; Williams 1974), Chinese Americans (King 1975), Jews (Shiloh and Selavan 1973), Mexican Americans (Bullough and Bullough 1972;

Quesada and Heller 1977:94–95), Navajos (McDermott et al. 1960), and Puerto Ricans (Alers 1978), for example, all reveal important differentials. Whether these differentials can be attributed to biases in vital statistics, which derive in part from the unequal access of various ethnic groups to treatment; to nonbehavioral factors, such as genetic predisposition; to shared risk factors (largely due to class membership), such as poverty, poor nutrition, or exposure to different pathogenic agents; or, in fact, to ethnically patterned, pathogenic cultural standards or behaviors is often moot. Distinguishing which of these causes are determinative for particular diseases is a matter for research, though unfortunately little of it has been done. Ethnic differences in disease rates serve, nevertheless, as an important ecological background against which to view differing health beliefs and behaviors.

HEALTH MAINTENANCE AND HOME TREATMENT   Comparative studies have shown that ethnic subcultures differ both in their conceptions of well-being and in their health maintenance practices (see, for example, Bullough and Bullough 1972; Spicer 1977b; Weidman 1978). In addition, studies of specific ethnic enclaves report health-care practices within the home that differ across these collectivities (Padilla 1958; Clark 1959; Everett 1971; Hill 1973; Hand 1976). A knowledge of these differing home health practices is especially useful for understanding the increasingly important social-medical issues of prevention and self-care. Although ethnic home health practices also affect the usage of both mainstream and nonmainstream sources of medicine, their principal significance lies in shedding light on the large proportion of illness episodes in this country that never reach the biomedical profession for treatment (Zola 1972a).

ILLNESS BEHAVIOR   The term "illness behavior" refers to the ways in which "symptoms are differentially perceived, evaluated, and acted upon (or not acted upon) by different kinds of people and in different social situations" (Mechanic 1968:116). Several pioneer studies document the importance of ethnicity as a determinant of observed differences in this aspect of health behavior (Zborowski 1952, on pain perception among Irish, Italians, Jews, and Yankees; Suchman 1964, 1965a, 1966, on the degree to which the cohesiveness and exclusivity of different ethnic groups influence illness behavior; Zola 1964, on differential "triggers" to seeking medical care among Italian, Irish, and Anglo-Saxon workers). In addition to these comparative investigations, many studies of individual ethnic groups have also shown culturally distinctive ways in which symptoms are evaluated and acted upon (Adair and Deuschle 1970, for the Navajo;

Clark 1959, Weaver 1970, for Mexican Americans; Gaw 1975, for Chinese Americans; and Garrison 1977, for Puerto Ricans).

Although many studies that relate ethnicity and illness behavior have failed to pay sufficient attention to intervening variables and intraethnic variation, a recent review of the data has nevertheless concluded that "cultural and social conditioning play an important though not exclusive role in patterns of illness behavior, and that ethnic memberships, peer pressures, and age-sex role learning to some extent influence attitudes towards risks and towards the significance of common threats" (Mechanic 1972:208).

UTILIZATION PATTERNS   Although utilization of mainstream medical services is determined in multiple ways, with both class factors and the organization of the delivery system itself playing significant parts (Antonovsky 1972; Andersen and Newman 1973), ethnic factors have nevertheless been shown to relate to utilization in at least three ways.

First, direct evidence of ethnic preferences in the source of mainstream medical care has been provided by several studies (see, for example, Solon 1966, comparing Jews and non-Jewish whites; Berkanovic and Reeder 1973, comparing blacks, Mexican Americans, and whites of high and low income.)

Second, many ethnic collectivities support alternative providers of health care, who may be used prior to, in conjunction with, or following mainstream services. *Curanderos* and other lay practitioners among Mexican Americans (Rubel 1966; Kiev 1968), *espiritistas* and *santiguadores* among Puerto Ricans (Garrison 1977; Harwood 1977), singers among the Navajo (Luce 1971), herbalists and other curers among Chinese Americans (Hessler et al. 1975), bonesetters among French Canadians (Lacourcière 1976), *remède-mans* among Louisiana Cajuns (Brandon 1976), and various healers among urban blacks (Snow 1978) are just a few of the ethnic curers who have recently been described in the literature. For members of many ethnic groups, the range of options available for treating illness thus extends considerably beyond establishment and even "marginal" providers (chiropractors or osteopaths). Consequently, investigations of health-service utilization must be much more broadly framed for these groups (see Scott 1974 and Weidman 1978 for results of one such broadly defined comparative ethnic study in Miami, Florida).

A third way in which ethnicity relates to utilization is indirectly through ethnic residential segregation, a phenomenon that is still found in many United States cities and their environs (Lieberson 1963; Kantrowitz 1973; Kain 1975). In view of the much-observed tendency for people to use medical services that are convenient to their residences, ethnic residential clustering tends to produce patient populations in hospitals, clinics, or private practices composed preponderantly of specific local ethnic groups. This ethnic weighting of patient populations affects the delivery of services in a number of ways: for example, the services may have to be modified to accommodate to ethnic epidemiological patterns and behavioral styles; or health-care institutions may hire more employees from the ethnic category of users in response to organized pressure from local ethnic groups.

CONCEPTS OF DISEASE AND ILLNESS   Ethnic background has been shown to influence people's concepts of disease and illness in three ways. First, ethnic groups exhibit varying degrees of knowledge about biomedical categories of disease (Samora, Saunders, and Larson 1961; Suchman 1964; Jenkins 1966; Plaja, Cohen, and Samora 1968). Second, ethnic groups may also differ in the ways in which symptoms are classified into illness categories, the most obvious manifestation of this phenomenon being the "culture-specific syndrome"—for example, *susto* among Mexican Americans (Rubel 1964), the evil eye among various circum-Mediterranean groups (Maloney 1976), Arctic hysteria among Eskimos (Foulkes 1972), or *hattement de coeur* among Haitian Americans (Weidman 1976:345–346). Finally, ethnicity has been shown to correlate with conceptions about the causes of disease and illness, such as "hot"/"cold" theories among Hispanics (Harwood 1971; Kay 1977), etiological ideas about God's punishment or possession by the Devil among Southern blacks (Snow 1977), or *gaz* and blood perturbations among Haitian Americans (Weidman 1978). It is important to point out that ethnically influenced concepts of disease and illness in turn affect other aspects of health behavior, such as the evaluation of symptoms, utilization of non-mainstream medical services, and compliance with treatment regimens.

INTERACTIONS WITH MAINSTREAM HEALTH PROFESSIONALS AND ORGANIZATIONS   Behavioral ethnicity often entails general styles of interaction, attitudes toward authority figures, sex-role allocations, and ways of expressing emotion and asking for help which are carried over into health-care situations. These general sociocultural factors influence people's interactions with health professionals, as well as their overall reactions to hospitals, clinics, and private practitioners. For example, the Latin preference for a personalistic style of interaction often conflicts with the value of efficiency and the de facto impersonality embodied in much mainstream medical care (Center for Human Resources Planning and Development et al. 1977); and culturally based patterns of interaction between blacks and whites intrude in doctor-patient interactions involving members of these two racial groups (Harrison and Harrison 1971).

In addition to exhibiting these general interactional styles that carry over into medical contexts, ethnic collectivities have also been shown to behave differently specifically as patients—that is, in the ways they present symptoms (Leighton and Kennedy 1959; Zola 1966), their expectations of physician behavior (Zborowski 1952, 1969; Shaw 1958:67; Quesada and Heller 1977:98), their understanding of terms used in patient-physician interviews (Samora, Saunders, and Larson 1961), and their responses to diagnoses and treatment regimens (Berle 1958; Harwood 1971; Snow 1974).

To the extent that these general and specific ethnic characteristics create barriers to communication and empathy between patients and practitioners, the technical equality and effectiveness of biomedical care suffer.

ETHNIC INTEREST GROUPS AND MEDICAL DELIVERY   The effects of ideological ethnicity on the health-care delivery system have been felt most strongly in the areas of personnel and consumer management, as one would expect. As a result of pressure from ethnic groups, both Affirmative Action measures and training subsidies for members of ethnic minorities have moderately increased the numbers of health professionals and (more typically) paraprofessionals who identify as ethnics. Moreover, the development of federally funded neighborhood health centers has tended to give ethnic interest groups a voice in managing health-care facilities (Lewis 1976:203). To the extent that these ethnic health workers and members of community boards have real responsibility for managing health care, the goals of health-care providers and ethnic consumers can be more readily negotiated and meshed within the delivery system.

Intraethnic Variation in Health Behavior

Though the foregoing review leaves little doubt that ethnic factors play a role in a wide range of health behaviors, we must nevertheless recognize that much of the social science and medical literature relating ethnicity and health is noticeably deficient in its treatment of intraethnic variation in both beliefs and behavior. Since ethnic collectivities comprise people who not only may conceive of their ethnicity somewhat differently but also may behave quite differently in various contexts, it is important for both theoretical and practical reasons to analyze such intraethnic variation with regard to health care.

A major theoretical contribution provided by an analysis of intraethnic variation is to illuminate intervening variables between ethnicity and health behavior. Even though there are numerous correlations between these two variables, it is often impossible to know which aspect of an ethnic subculture more specifically determines particular health behaviors. Several studies of health behavior have examined intraethnic variation to discover intervening variables in this way; some of these studies will be reviewed in the following section.

From a practical standpoint, an appreciation of intraethnic diversity serves to mitigate the tendency of health professionals and others in this society to stereotype members of ethnic groups. In contrast to a stereotype, an accurate description of the culture and behavior of members of an ethnic group ideally provides an assessment of the range of behavior and cultural standards observed within the collectivity and the factors that tend to predict the observed variation. The practical importance of such a description for health professionals would be to increase their ability to identify accurately those patients within an ethnic category whose relations with the mainstream medical system are most affected by culturally patterned beliefs and behaviors.

Unfortunately, too few of the health descriptions of ethnic groups contain sufficient information on intraethnic diversity to provide indicators of the health behavior of individual patients as accurately as one would wish. There are, however, a number of general predictors of this variation that apply across ethnic collectivities.

GENERAL SOURCES OF INTRAETHNIC VARIATION   Though regional cultural differences within each ethnic group's country of origin remain a significant cause of intraethnic variation among immigrants, the principal sources of intraethnic variation across generations are acculturation to the norms of the dominant WASP ethnic group and class differentiation within each ethnic collectivity—two different, though related, phenomena (Gordon 1964; Hannerz 1974:46, 60–72). Although these two variables have been extensively studied in relation to ethnic factors in the political arena (Dahl 1961; Litt 1970; Krickus 1976) as well as in economic contexts (Pelling 1960; Glazer and Moynihan 1963; Foner 1974), their relationship to ethnic factors in the health sphere has been generally neglected. This neglect has been due in part to a tendency among researchers to view the determinants of health behavior *either* in economic *or* in cultural terms, with the result that only one or the other set of variables has been isolated for study. In part, too, the deficiency stems from generalizing to a whole ethnic group from samples that are largely undifferentiated with regard to class (for example, clinic patients) or, conversely, from treating socioeconomically heterogeneous ethnic samples as though they were homogeneous.

Notwithstanding these general deficiencies of the health-care literature, several large-scale surveys (Suchman 1964; Guttmacher and Elinson 1971; Berkanovic and Reeder 1973; Greenblum 1974) have permitted the analysis of class and ethnic relationships in health behavior, although the survey method itself undeniably introduces biases because of the differing responses of various ethnic groups and classes to the interview situation (Denzin 1970:123–143). A review of these studies, as well as of research that focuses on ethnic variation within a single socioeconomic class (for example, Zola 1964; Olendzki 1974), reveals that although ethnic differences diminish among members of the upper socioeconomic classes (as measured by income, education, occupation, or any combination of these factors), they do not entirely disappear. The health behaviors for which this persistence of ethnic differences has been observed across class lines include certain aspects of utilization practices (see Solon 1966 and Roth 1969, before Medicaid; Berkanovic and Reeder 1973 and Olendzki 1974, after Medicaid); conceptions of mental illness (Guttmacher and Elinson 1971); and such "health orientations" as knowledge about disease, skepticism about medical care, and willingness to assume a dependent role when ill (Suchman 1964; Greenblum 1974).

Looked at from the clinician's point of view—that is, of having to predict variations in health beliefs and behavior within ethnic groups—these data indicate that the more educated, more affluent, and occupationally advantaged members of ethnic categories tend to differ in their health beliefs and behavior from the less educated, less affluent, and occupationally disadvantaged members of the same ethnic category. Furthermore, the health beliefs and behaviors of members of higher socioeconomic classes tend to be more similar across ethnic groups than the behaviors of lower socioeconomic groups. In other words, people of lower socioeconomic status tend to display behavioral ethnicity in health matters to a greater degree than do those of higher socioeconomic standing.

Few studies of intraethnic variation in health behavior go beyond an analysis of the effects of demographic variables of the kind discussed above. An exception is the somewhat problematic but still classic study by Suchman (1964). Suchman showed that although ethnicity and social class independently influence such health orientations as knowledge about disease, faith in mainstream medical care, and reluctance to assume a dependent role when ill, social organizational factors within the ethnic group itself are most directly determinative of these orientations. The factor that specifically predicts these health orientations is the degree of homogeneity and closeness of interpersonal relationships within the group. Thus, the more homogeneous and close-knit social relationships are for individuals within any ethnic group, the less biomedically oriented their health attitudes are likely to be.

SUMMARY   Both social class and involvement in a close-knit ethnic network are thus factors that help in general to predict variations in health behavior within ethnic groups. The clinician should use this information much as he would any epidemiological generalization: first to match the individual patient with the general predictor, and then to perform the appropriate test (or tests) to see whether in fact the patient fits the pattern. Obviously with these variables the "tests" performed are observational or verbal rather than physiochemical. For example, discussions with patients about their involvement and dependence on kin and friends within the ethnic group would serve to reveal their adherence to ethnic health orientations and probably behaviors as well.

Selection of Ethnic Collectivities

In choosing ethnic collectivities for coverage in this volume, I attempted to include those for which cultural beliefs and practices demonstrably and significantly influence the medical care of substantial numbers of members. I therefore drew up a preliminary list of American ethnic collectivities that meet at least one of the following two criteria.

1. The group should be among those with the highest rates of immigration during the last 15-year period for which data were available at the time (1962–1976). This criterion was introduced to ensure the inclusion of ethnic groups that contain large numbers of first-generation members and presumably, therefore, people unacculturated to prevailing WASP or American norms of health belief or behavior. According to the annual reports of the Immigration and Naturalization Service, the following eight countries yielded the highest numbers of immigrants during the period under consideration: Mexico, Canada, Italy, Cuba, Great Britain, Germany, the West Indies, and the Philippines (in that order). Although Puerto Rican immigration is technically an internal migration, Puerto Rico was also included in this category for selection purposes.

2. The group should possess a distinctive health subculture and behaviors, as demonstrated by recent, competent research. By this criterion, the following kinds of ethnic categories were covered: (a) collectivities for whom recent immigration is not relevant but for whom economic and social discrimination have played a role in the preservation or development of distinctive patterns of health belief and behavior (in particular, Native Americans and U.S.-born blacks); and (b) collectivities that have well-known, distinctive health beliefs and behaviors, although they do not qualify for inclusion as one of the largest immigrant populations (criterion 1). The latter collectivities, as well as specific Native American groups, nevertheless had to represent a sufficiently large population to warrant inclusion in a publication designed for national distribution. Thus the groups included under this latter criterion were Chinese, Haitians, and among Native Americans, the three most populous groups— Navajo, Cherokee, and Apache (in that order).

These criteria obviously produced a list that specifically selected for collectivities in which a significant proportion of members manifested behavioral ethnicity. If ideological ethnicity was also relevant to the medical care of the group, it could of course be dealt with as well. But the bulk of medical-care issues relating to ethnicity were considered to be behavioral in nature—that is, stemming from cultural standards and behaviors that influenced utilization and interaction in medical-care settings.

Once the list of ethnic categories was assembled using these criteria, an effort was made to locate social scientists to contribute chapters for each group. Each contributor was expected to have carried out recent research among the ethnic group and to have had experience in health-care settings so that he might be able to draw out the implications of the data in a manner most useful to clinicians.

Among the ethnic groups from countries that have provided large numbers of immigrants in the past 15 years (criterion 1), no health-oriented research has been done, as far as I was able to ascertain, specifically with Canadians, Germans, or the British; and only fragmentary information is available on Anglo-speaking West Indians (Weidman 1978, on Bahamians in Miami) and Filipinos (McKenzie 1974; McKenzie and Chrisman 1977). This situation reflects several biases in American social science research. In general, little social research tends to be done among ethnic groups that have cultural backgrounds similar to the dominant Anglo-Saxon group and therefore rank high in the stratification system (Lavender and Forsyth 1976). (This pattern of research prevails even when these groups present interesting problems for investigation in the area of health—for example, changes in health status and medical practices that doubtless occur for Britains and Canadians in moving from a socialized to a fee-for-service system of medical care.) The lack of major research among Filipinos in this country would seem to reflect, in part, the same bias against studying upper-status groups, since a significant proportion of Philippine immigrants consists of wealthy professionals (many, in fact, are nurses and doctors). On the other hand, the paucity of health-oriented research specifically on English-speaking West Indians in this country relates to the tendency in sampling, pointed out by Jackson in Chapter 1, to merge West Indians with U.S.-born blacks—a manifestation, I believe, of the American cultural bias toward treating all blacks as a homogeneous underclass.

Of the remaining collectivities selected by the two criteria stipulated above, I was unsuccessful for various reasons in securing contributors for chapters on Cherokees, Cubans, and Apaches, although recent and relatively extensive research has been done on these last two groups.[5] Thus, of the original ethnic categories selected, urban blacks, Chinese, Haitians, Italians, Mexicans, Navajos, and Puerto Ricans are represented in this volume.

This selection of ethnic groups is obviously and significantly biased toward "oppressed minorities," to use Mullings's term (1978)—that is, groups that have experienced and in most cases continue to experience overt, structural discrimination in the American social system. This biased selection derives mainly from two factors. First, the correlation mentioned earlier between behavioral ethnicity and lower-class status in the United States has meant that by specifically selecting groups with high proportions of "behavioral ethnics," I have ipso facto selected oppressed minorities. Second, the tendency of American social science research to study ethnic minorities in preference to dominant ethnic groups has perforce carried over to health behaviors and thus affected the contents of this book.

The lower-class bias in the ethnic coverage of this book raises a critical issue: how can a volume like this, with an approach that focuses primarily on effective communication and understanding between receivers and deliverers of health care, be justified when the most pressing health issues of most of the populations covered in the book derive in large part from their depressed economic, social, and political situations? In response, I must point out that despite the dominant orientation of this volume, it still provides important information on the structural bases of many of the health and medical-care problems of the ethnic groups described. This information may be used in working on a societal level toward solutions of problems of economic and social inequality in health care, the only way fundamental issues of inequality can be resolved.

What this volume assumes, however, is that medical care, regardless of the degree of class equality or inequality in the society, always involves interactions between lay seekers after health or well-being and practitioners with specialized and therefore somewhat esoteric knowledge. As a result of these differences in perspective and training, the parties to these interactions hold presuppositions, concepts, and goals that are not necessarily congruous. The information provided in this book is therefore aimed toward increasing the range of common understandings between practitioners, on the one hand, and patients and their associates, on the other, in order to improve communication in medical interactions and thereby make them more effective and more humane. For, as Mechanic has observed, "failures in communication and empathy not only harm a vital function of medical care [to ameliorate distress and to provide support and relief from pain and discomfort], but also diminish the opportunities for technical quality and effectiveness" (1976:11).

Organization of the Book

In putting together this volume, I have addressed two somewhat different audiences. As mentioned at the outset, the book is designed primarily for physicians, nurses, social workers, and other providers and

C. Current population and geographic distribution in the United States.
D. Demographic information—age structure, income distribution, education.

II. Evaluation of the Existing Data.
A. Population whose medical practices have been studied—socioeconomic status, region of origin in the mother country and of settlement in the United States, length of time in the United States.
B. Interpretation problems caused by the nature of the data base.
C. Intraethnic diversity in medical practices because of differences in socioeconomic status, generation, region of origin or settlement, religion, or education. (This section provides general evidence for internal variation and the major factors that produce it; specific influences of intraethnic diversity on medical care are covered in other sections.)

III. Epidemiological Characteristics.
A. Biases in or cautions concerning available data.
B. Prevalence of major diseases (biomedically defined) and mortality and morbidity statistics, emphasizing diseases with high prevalence within the group; those diseases, usually genetic, that are particular to the group; and those that carry strong emotional impact.

IV. Concepts of Disease and Illness.
A. Description of the major nosological and etiological concepts used by the group, as derived from both popular and biomedical sources. (The practical implications of these concepts are discussed in later sections.) Popular concepts include both older ("folk") traditions and concepts promulgated in the mass media (see Spicer 1977a:5–6). Biomedical concepts are presumably congruent with those of biomedical professionals and are disseminated either by physicians or by professional organizations, such as the American Cancer Society. How concepts from these sources interdigitate and merge.
B. Social contexts in which nosology and etiology are discussed.
C. How these concepts are learned.
D. Intraethnic variation in concepts.

V. Becoming Ill.
A. Perception and evaluation of symptoms (see Mechanic 1969: 195).
1. Extent to which popular and biomedical concepts are used to interpret symptoms.

2. Tolerance for symptoms and its correlates, such as sex or family role.

3. Persons with whom symptoms are discussed for further clarification.

VI. Coping with Illness outside the Mainstream Medical System.

A. In the home and family.

1. Family role responsibilities for care of illness.

2. Illnesses, diseases, and symptoms most often treated at home and treatments used (home remedies, tonics, over-the-counter drugs, borrowed prescription drugs).

3. Extent to which family members are relieved of role responsibilities before a professional is consulted.

B. Lay consultation and referral.

1. Patterns of consultation within the ill person's family and personal network to identify and label the illness, recommend treatment, and refer to sources of care outside the home.

2. Persons most likely to be influential in these consultations.

3. Particular patterns in seeking care (delay in consulting an outside source, for example) of persons of certain family or occupational status.

C. Nonmainstream medical care outside the home.

1. Alternatives people of the ethnic group consider when they decide to go outside the home for medical care, the sequence in which they turn to these alternatives, and the factors that influence their choices. Use of multiple sources of care.

2. Particular forms of care outside the mainstream of American medicine (for example, spiritists, herbalists, root workers, bone-setters) in terms of theories of disease and illness, types of treatment, prevalence of the form of care, and problems or benefits associated with it from the point of view of mainstream medicine.

VII. Encounters with Mainstream Medical Practitioners.

A. Settings in which mainstream medical care occurs.

B. Expectations in the medical encounter.

1. What people of the ethnic group want from a doctor or nurse.

2. Circumstances under which patients of the ethnic group want to know the diagnosis, generally and in terminal illness.

C. Issues of deference and demeanor and norms of interaction with those of different sex, age, or authority that may influence encounters with medical personnel.

D. Influence of nosological and etiological concepts on reactions to medical diagnosis.

VIII. Adherence to Biomedical Treatment.

    A. Available hard data on adherence to medical treatment.

    B. Specific subcultural, familial, interactional, or other factors that influence adherence or nonadherence.

    C. Dietary patterns that may influence adherence to dietary restrictions.

IX. Recovery, Rehabilitation, and Death.

    A. Patterns of coping with chronic and terminal illness and death.

    B. Rituals associated with resumption of normal roles.

    C. Cultural or socioeconomic factors that may lead to nonrecovery or malingering.

X. Any additional issues that are not readily encompassed in the preceding categories. Summary statement.

Each chapter includes a review of the published data and, in some cases, previously unpublished data on each of the preceding subjects, along with discussions of their implications for health care. Most practical recommendations to health-care professionals are contained within the section of each chapter covering a particular topic.

Practical Applications of the Data

Although the contributors to this volume feel they are providing information that can potentially improve the quality of care for the ethnic groups they are writing about, each of them is also aware of major social-structural barriers to the actual application of this information. These barriers primarily include those of class and professionalism, which stem from the embeddedness of health-care institutions in the larger American social system. For the encompassing system exerts economic pressures and social constraints on people interacting in health-care situations that make the kinds of concerns described in this volume difficult to put into practice.

Yet it is also true that many of the health-care issues raised in this book can be handled on an interpersonal level. For this reason, they may be more likely to be implemented than issues that can be remedied only by a national commitment of funds or by major social changes. Obviously, to improve the quality of health services to ethnic minorities, efforts at both the interpersonal and sociopolitical levels are necessary. A personal commitment by health-care personnel to improve face-to-face interactions in health-care situations can make a significant contribution toward greater patient satisfaction and more effective medical care. To assist in this endeavor, the following sections discuss general areas in which the information contained in this volume can be used by both clinicians and health planners.

Dealing with Class and Professional Barriers to the Realization of Ethnically Appropriate Health Care

I shall begin by examining some of the barriers that stand in the way of delivering ethnically appropriate health services and discussing how this book may help weaken these barriers to some extent for the individual clinician. The barriers I speak of here stem, it must be understood, not for the most part from group or individual ill will or from actions deliberately taken to withhold quality medical services from ethnic groups; they are in many cases unintended consequences of certain cultural assumptions or of certain group actions, which may even at the same time have clearly beneficial consequences. The two main sources of difficulty in implementing ethnically appropriate health services would seem to derive from professional and class orientations.

Much has been written about the ways in which the fundamentally biomedical outlook of health care in this country precludes or severely inhibits treatment of the personal and social concerns that patients and their families bring into treatment situations. By focusing mainly on the biological phenomenon of "disease"—"deviations from the norm of measurable biological (somatic) variables" (Engel 1977:130)—the biomedical orientation virtually excludes a concern with "illness"—that is, the cultural, social, and psychological (phenomenological) construction of the problem by the patient, his family, other relatives, and associates (Fabrega 1972; Kleinman 1973; Eisenberg 1977b). In general, biomedical professionals are ill equipped by training to probe and deal with this latter aspect of their patients' problems, a deficiency that becomes all the more acute when patients and health-care workers come from different cultures or subcultures.

Another way in which the biomedical perspective makes it difficult to provide appropriate health services to ethnic groups arises from its interpretation of disease primarily as "person-centered, temporally bounded, and discontinuous" (Fabrega 1974:198). This view, "with its emphasis on boundedness and separation . . . promotes a discrete and segmental approach to medical care that requires an episodic focus and encourages the practice of fees for service and a concentration on salient and describable deviations" (Fabrega 1974:199). In short, a biologically oriented perspective on disease, whatever its benefits, inhibits an appreciation of the cultural, social, and environmental aspects of deviations in somatic variables, particularly those that are apparent only on long-term observation or in non-crisis situations.

In addition to these difficulties engendered by the biological orientation of medical care, several specific concomitants of professionalism also inhibit treatment of the phenomenological aspects of illness episodes. These professional influences relate, as well, to the class structure of American society. For physicians, public health officials (also mostly physicians), and researchers—all occupationally, educationally, and usually economically in the upper ranks of the status hierarchy—perform the function in this society of establishing what phenomena are considered to be diseases, of deciding what the causes of particular diseases are, of diagnosing and treating cases of disease, and of certifying their remission or termination (Fabrega 1976:309–311). This authority accorded professional standards of health and medical care in this culture, supported by the ascendency of health professionals in the class system, contributes to making a patient's own experience of his illness seem incorrect, irrelevant, and inferior.

The extent to which the patient's percepts and concepts are considered insignificant compared with those of high-status biomedical professionals is plainly illustrated in much of the language ordinarily and unthinkingly used to describe the "delivery" of health care in this culture (Weidman 1976:346–347, 1978:829–830). Thus professionals speak, for example, of "providers" and "recipients" of care, of "target populations," and of "compliance" with medical "orders"—all phrases which imply that the patient is simply a passive receiver of the ontological categories and technical knowledge of the health professional, an "empty vessel" awaiting the "new wine of [biomedical] information" and technology (Polgar 1963:411). As Weidman has observed:

> In every way, the health institution is viewed as acting upon, impinging upon, or being introduced into communities or specific population groups to inject something into their lives that they do not already have. While this may be a laudable undertaking in the interest of sharing the specific health-related strengths of the orthodox system, the problem lies in the unicultural [i.e., biomedical] focus underlying such efforts. Reality is perceived in terms of introducing *something* where *nothing* of significance existed before. The acknowledgment that individuals and communities have *something* already, such as their own health cultural traditions, is not required by the concepts in current use by orthodox providers of health care. (1978:829; italics in original)

Thus, before the sociocultural data presented in this book can be applied, this culturally conditioned predisposition for health professionals to depreciate or even deny the patient's view, simply because they are unaware of the effect on patients of their professional and class positions, must be managed in some way. This may be partly accomplished by professionals' becoming more aware of both their inherent biases and the overweening influence of the biomedical model in medical-care situations.

This book can help clinicians in the process of moving outside their own subculture by providing descriptions of other people's viewpoints on issues of health and medical care. How different ethnic groups handle illness episodes can become a model with which the clinician can compare and contrast his own construction of these phenomena and thereby gain some insights into the ways in which a professional view highlights certain aspects of the situation and ignores others. By this process the clinician may come to comprehend more fully the particular concerns, articulated by other cultural groups, that fall outside the purview of the biomedical model and thereby reassess the limitations and strengths of a biomedical perspective on treating health problems. For, until a clinician is conscious of his own biases in approaching an illness episode, he is unlikely to attend to the views of laymen or to comprehend their importance not only in the joint enterprise of healing and curing but also in the more long-term, non-episodic processes of health maintenance.

Eliciting the Patient's Model of the Problem and Treating the Illness

The cultural traditions of most ethnic groups tend to view illness episodes in both a psychosomatic and an ecological framework That is, in many ethnic subcultures both psychological stresses, worry, and strained interpersonal relations, on the one hand, and unfavorable environmental and living conditions, on the other, figure importantly among the multiple etiological factors that are used to interpret and understand illness. This perspective contrasts with the predominant clinical focus on the biological (physiochemical) parameters of the situation.

In other ways, too, the cultural patterns of ethnic groups structure illness and treatment situations differently from professional perceptions. As the following chapters will show, concepts of how the body functions may differ from professional views, the range of etiological agents thought to cause biological deviations from the norm may diverge, expectations concerning the proper mode of interacting with a professional may vary, evaluations of the seriousness of particular symptoms or diseases may be divergent, and so forth.

Because these differing kinds of cultural concepts and behavioral standards influence patients' participation in and reactions to treatment situations, they need to be made overt in patient-practitioner encounters. Eliciting the patient's model of his problem in a nonjudgmental fashion can serve both to improve the quality of biomedical care and to satisfy the expectations with which he has sought medical attention (Kleinman 1975, 1978; Kleinman, Eisenberg, and Good 1978). (Obviously, not all discrepancies between the patient's and the clinician's models of the problem will arise from cultural differences. Psychological and social factors will also be relevant—for example, the patient's general level of anxiety, age, occupation, marital status.)

Kleinman, Eisenberg, and Good have outlined procedures for eliciting the patient's model of his illness (1978:256–257), and the reader may find it helpful to consult them.[6] The present volume can further contribute to this important clinical task in the following ways:

1. The health-care worker can read chapters on the particular ethnic groups he is most likely to see in treatment in order to provide a general cultural and social background on the group. Assuming that intraethnic variation and its sources are understood, this general background can help the clinician in eliciting the patient's model of the problem by focusing on questions that are likely to concern members of the particular ethnic group.
2. Familiarity with patients' sociocultural backgrounds will alert the clinician in advance to possible sources of discrepancy between biomedical and ethnic models of sickness. This foreknowledge can help the clinician in eliciting any discrepancy promptly and in devising alternative ways of resolving it.
3. When therapy management problems occur with a "behavioral ethnic," the book can serve as a reference to suggest possible sources for the problem, which can then be explored with the patient.
4. By suggesting resources available within the patient's sociocultural milieu, the book may also assist in finding care for those aspects of an illness episode that the clinician considers to be beyond his competence.

In short, this volume provides sociocultural information on various ethnic groups that may be used to guide questioning on illness issues in health care; to anticipate the culture shock, cognitive discrepancies, or dissatisfactions that members of various ethnic groups may experience in medical-care situations; and to suggest to the clinician or health planner resources within different ethnic milieus that may be used to support the individual or family with a health problem.

Making Medical Treatment More Conformable with the Patient's Life-style

Disease or illness, as perceived by a patient, is just one part of his entire life. Diagnosis and cure compete with many other goals, activities, pleasures, and duties that make up a person's total life experience. This fact often becomes obscured for health-care professionals, who tend to see people at a point when disease has either totally or significantly inhibited the performance of valued or even essential life activities. The focal concern with disease which patients manifest at these points in their lives (and which health-care professionals manifest by occupational choice) is not typically sustained in ordinary social life (and indeed, there are strong social deterrents for maintaining such a focus).

Thus, outside the critical phase, chronic disease and its treatment become just one part of the everyday life of the patient. As a consequence, it behooves the health-care professional to know as much about the lifestyle of a patient as possible, in order to design treatment interventions that will stand the greatest chance of integration into that life-syle (see Gillum and Barsky 1974). For example, if a medication is prescribed to be taken three times a day with meals, and the patient regularly eats only two meals a day, then that treatment intervention is unlikely to be implemented.

Part of every patient's life-style is determined by his cultural background, and part of many Americans' cultural backgrounds derives from their ethnic heritage. Food preferences, meal patterns, caretaking responsibilities, pain responses, and so on, as we have observed earlier, are likely to be influenced by socialization and enculturation in an ethnic group. The ethnic descriptions in this book should therefore alert the clinician to aspects of patients' life-styles that are ethnically influenced and that must be taken into account in planning not only therapeutic but also preventive interventions that are likely to be adopted.

Improving the Articulation between Mainstream and Nonmainstream Sources of Health Care

It has been estimated that between 70 and 90 percent of all illness episodes are treated outside mainstream medical facilities, either at home or by alternative healers (Zola 1972a). Yet the ways in which laymen treat illness, the ways in which self-care really works, have rarely been studied. From available ethnographic and community studies, however, we know that various ethnic groups emphasize different forms of home treatment and support different kinds of alternative healers, as discussed earlier.

Apart from the general features of ethnic life-styles mentioned in the previous section, specific knowledge of lay treatment practices can be useful to both clinicians and health planners, particularly in dealing with chronic diseases, when the patient and family ultimately become responsible for care and management of the disease. How people self-prescribe and take non-professionally-prescribed medications, as well as what activities they see as important to health maintenance, constitute fundamental patterns of self care which must serve as the basis for devising therapeutic modifications, instead of the typical "canned" therapeutic approach which attempts to introduce new behaviors as though no prior health-care habits existed. In other words, information on already existing habits of self-medication and health maintenance (some of which are ethnically determined) can be used to develop treatment plans for people with chronic diseases which will be more likely to be followed, since they conform with preexisting health habits. In the clinical setting, a knowledge of what kinds of symptoms people from different ethnic groups attend to most can also help in educating patients with chronic conditions about signs of relapse or of adverse drug reactions.

For health planners, an awareness of nonmainstream sources of treatment (healers, herbalists, *curanderos,* spiritists, acupuncturists, and so on) may also help in devising better ways of articulating the biomedical and lay spheres of care so that people can move appropriately between them and take advantage of the particular strengths and functions of each. Various methods of articulating the biomedical and lay spheres have been suggested, and some of them have already been implemented, though usually only in pilot fashion. Among the suggested methods for redefining the relationship between biomedical and lay caretakers have been the following: (1) establishing mechanisms for regular consultation and referral between existing health-care providers in the two spheres (see, for example, Pattison 1973; Lauer 1974; Ruiz 1976; Ruiz and Langrod 1976); (2) creating a new role or profession, that of the bicultural, bilingual "culture broker" (Weidman 1976:350–352, 1978: 848–855), whose knowledge of both systems would permit a certain objectivity in acting as troubleshooter and "transcultural" interpreter for both patients and health-care professionals; (3) training more biomedical professionals from ethnic minorities who, because of their early socialization, would be aware of cultural issues in health behavior; and (4) "medicalizing" some lay functions by redefining the roles of existing health professionals (for example, nurses, psychiatrists, social workers) to include some support and treatment services now provided in the lay sphere.

Although little information is available to evaluate the relative effectiveness of each of these modes of articulating the biomedical and lay spheres of care, it is probable that different health problems demand different degrees or kinds of articulation between the two systems and therefore that an array of different modes may be necessary. (For example, psychiatric problems seem to lend themselves to mutual referral and consultation between existing health-care providers.) In any event, the information contained in this volume on the kinds of nonmainstream practitioners that members of various ethnic groups consult, as well as the kinds of problems for which these practitioners provide assistance, constitutes fundamental data for examining the interface between the biomedical and lay spheres of care.

A Concluding Caveat

I began this introduction by saying that the information contained in this volume could help health professionals deliver more personalized, culturally appropriate care to members of various American ethnic groups. However, it is also true that the information can, instead of increasing the degree of personalization of care, be used as a screen to obscure the individual patient. This situation can occur if the health-care provider treats the information stereotypically and acts as if all members of an ethnic category must behave and believe in the same fashion. Although all contributors have attempted to mitigate this problem by discussing intraethnic variation and trying to specify predictors of this variation for the groups they describe, stereotypical thinking is still a possibility. In order to sensitize health-care workers to this problem further and to help reduce misapplication of the data, I have attempted in this introduction to indicate how complex a phenomenon ethnicity is. The degree to which the information contained in the following chapters can serve the needs of patients, however, depends on the ability and willingness of each health-care provider to apply his expanded knowledge of ethnic health beliefs and practices with due attention to the needs of the individual patient.

Notes

1. By "culture" anthropologists and other social scientists generally mean the standards for behavior that one acquires as a member of a social group. These standards include percepts, concepts, beliefs, and values that help individuals to order and thereby give meaning to their experience of both social relationships and the physical world. In analyzing complex societies, many social scientists have found it useful to distinguish between a "culture" and a "subculture." This distinction is based on the *range* of behaviors that are constrained by a set of shared standards. That is, a culture may be seen as a set of broad-ranging guidelines that are widely shared and that structure phenomena and events in a variety of contexts from the cradle to the grave. A subculture, on the other hand, pertains only to those standards that are operative when a person is acting in a particular social capacity or group. For example, occupations and ethnic groups develop their own subcultures standards for what exists, what goals are to be valued, how one should behave —which are relevant when one is acting either on the job or as a member of the ethnic group but which are largely irrelevant outside those contexts. The medical profession is an excellent example of such a subculture, with its concepts for what exists in the world, as represented by the technical language and focal concerns of physicians when seeing patients; its valued goals, embodied partly in the Hippocratic oath; and its standards for how one should behave as a physician, incorporated into various professional and legal codes. In short, a subculture is a partial "blueprint" for behavior that helps to guide people acting in certain specific social capacities or in certain groups.

2. Although the usual term for referring to ethnic aggregates is "groups," this word generally implies more structured relationships among members than may in fact exist in all cases. The term "collectivity" is more neutral, since it does not suggest the degree to which roles are institutionalized among members; it will be used in preference during the following discussion. In some

instances where the more colloquial term "ethnic group" is appropriate, it will be used, however. The term "ethnic category," which will also be used on occasion, is more neutral still, implying simply that members possess certain common attributes, without suggesting that they interact with one another at all. See also Kunstadter (1978) for a discussion of distinctions between ethnic group, ethnic identity, and ethnic category.

3. Although I have chosen to adopt Stein and Hill's terms for these two expressions of ethnicity, I do not subscribe to their interpretation of ideological ethnicity as somehow bogus or "dime-store" (1977:22). Nor do I agree with their view that it is "diagnostic of developmental arrest and regression" (1977: 8). Instead, like A. Cohen (1974a:93), I see these two manifestations of ethnicity as a continuum in which people with reputed common origins utilize certain cultural standards to structure social relationships in a larger social system; but in the case of behavioral ethnicity, the collectivities tend over time to lose their cultural distinctiveness, while in the case of ideological ethnicity, they are in the process of emphasizing it.

4. In recent years two major theoretical frameworks have been used to analyze the institutionalized barriers to power and economic resources placed before different American ethnic groups. Perlo (1975) and Mullings (1978), focusing their analysis mainly on blacks, exemplify the Marxian view in seeing the barriers as erected mainly by the profit motive typical of American capitalists, who have wanted to ensure for themselves maximum gains from the labor of immigrant groups. On the other hand, Glazer and Moynihan (1975a: 12–18), influenced by Dahrendorf, hold that the class positions of different ethnic groups are founded on their differential ability, given their own intragroup norms, to embody the norms promulgated by the dominant segment of the population, however the position of the latter has been attained.

5. Extensive data on Cuban health beliefs and practices were collected as part of the Health Ecology Project, a comparative study of five ethnic groups in Miami, Florida. Some of these data have been analyzed and made accessible (see, for example, Halifax and Weidman 1973; Scott 1974, 1975; Weidman 1978), but for the most part the Cuban material remains unavailable. The findings that have been discussed indicate, however, that Cuban health and medical practices, in Miami at any rate, are strongly influenced by the establishment of private "clinics" staffed by Cuban physicians.

White Mountain Apaches have been studied in the past decade by Michael Everett, who has written on medical decision making (1971). Although Cherokee medical beliefs and practices were described in the literature in the early 1960s (Fogelson 1961; Kilpatrick and Kilpatrick 1964), little medically oriented research on this group has been published in the past decade.

6. Most helpful to the clinician are the following eight questions which Kleinman, Eisenberg, and Good suggest as being instrumental for eliciting the patient's model of illness (1978:256). I have reworded questions (4) and (5) to bring them into greater accord with the expectations of certain ethnic groups. That is, for members of ethnic groups that generally expect physicians to be the ultimate experts on diagnosis and treatment (because of the many years of training they have undergone and the high fees they command),

asking the patient about such matters suggests an abrogation of professional responsibility. I suspect that even the rephrased questions will strike some patients as inappropriate.

1. What do you think has caused your problem?
2. Why do you think it started when it did?
3. What do you think your sickness does to you? How does it work?
4. How bad [severe] do you think your illness is? Do you think it will last a long time, or will it be better soon in your opinion?
5. What kind of treatment would you like to have?
6. What are the most important results you hope to get from treatment?
7. What are the chief problems your illness has caused you?
8. What do you fear most about your sickness?

References

ADAIR, JOHN, and KURT DEUSCHLE. 1970. *The People's Health.* New York: Appleton-Century-Crofts.

ALERS, JOSE OSCAR. 1978. *Puerto Ricans and Health: Findings from New York City.* Hispanic Research Monograph Series, Fordham University, Monograph no. 1.

ANDERSEN, RONALD, and J. F. NEWMAN. 1973. Societal and Individual Determinants of Medical Care Utilization in the United States. *Milbank Memorial Fund Quarterly* 51:95–124.

ANTONOVSKY, AARON. 1972. A Model to Explain Visits to the Doctor: With Specific Reference to the Case of Israel. *Journal of Health and Social Behavior* 13:446–454.

BARTH, FREDRIK, ed. 1969. *Ethnic Groups and Boundaries.* Boston: Little, Brown.

BECKER, MARSHALL H., and LOIS A. MAIMAN. 1975. Sociobehavioral Determinants of Compliance with Health and Medical Care Recommendations. *Medical Care* 13:10–24.

BENNETT, JOHN W., ed. 1975. *The New Ethnicity: Perspectives from Ethnology.* 1973 Proceedings of the American Ethnological Society. St. Paul, Minn.: West.

BERKANOVIC, EMIL, and LEO G. REEDER. 1973. Ethnic, Economic, and Social Psychological Factors in the Source of Medical Care. *Social Problems* 21:246–259.

BERLE, BEATRICE. 1958. *80 Puerto Rican Families in New York City: Health and Disease Studied in Context.* New York: Columbia University Press. (Reprinted 1975, Arno Press.)

BRANDON, ELIZABETH. 1976. Folk Medicine in Louisiana. In *American Folk Medicine: A Symposium,* ed. Wayland D. Hand. Berkeley: University of California Press.

BULLOUGH, BONNIE, and VERN L. BULLOUGH. 1972. *Poverty, Ethnic Identity, and Health Care.* New York: Appleton-Century-Crofts.

CENTER FOR HUMAN RESOURCES PLANNING AND DEVELOPMENT, et al. 1977. The Americans: Boricuas. Multimedia training manual. Human Resources Development Trust, B.C.P.O. Box 3006, East Orange, N.J. 07019.

CHRISMAN, NOEL J. 1977. The Health Seeking Process: An Approach to the Natural History of Illness. *Culture, Medicine and Psychiatry* 1:351–377.

CLARK, MARGARET. 1959. *Health in the Mexican-American Culture.* Berkeley: University of California Press.

COHEN, ABNER. 1974a. *Two-Dimensional Man: An Essay on the Anthropology of Power and Symbolism in Complex Society.* Berkeley: University of California Press.

COHEN, ABNER, ed. 1974b. *Urban Ethnicity.* London: Tavistock.

COHEN, RONALD. 1978. Ethnicity: Problem and Focus in Anthropology. *Annual Review of Anthropology* 7:379–403.

DAHL, ROBERT A. 1961. *Who Governs? Democracy and Power in an American City.* New Haven: Yale University Press.

DENZIN, NORMAN K. 1970. *The Research Act: A Theoretical Introduction to Sociological Methods.* Chicago: Aldine.

DE VOS, GEORGE, and LOLA ROMANUCCI-ROSS, eds. 1975. *Ethnic Identity: Cultural Continuities and Change.* Palo Alto, Calif.: Mayfield.

DOUGLASS, CHESTER W. 1971. A Social-Psychological View of Health Behavior for Health-Services Research. *Health Services Research* 6:6–14.

EISENBERG, LEON. 1977a. The Search for Care. *Daedalus* 106:235–246.

————. 1977b. Disease and Illness: Distinctions between Professional and Popular Ideas of Sickness. *Culture, Medicine and Psychiatry* 1:9–23.

ENGEL, GEORGE L. 1977. The Need for a New Medical Model: A Challenge for Biomedicine. *Science* 196:129–136.

EVERETT, MICHAEL W. 1971. White Mountain Apache Medical Decision-Making. In *Apachean Culture, History and Ethnology.* Anthropological Papers of the University of Arizona, no. 21. Tucson: University of Arizona Press.

FABREGA, HORACIO, JR. 1972. Concepts of Disease: Logical Features and Social Implications. *Perspectives in Biology and Medicine* 15:583–616.

————. 1974. *Disease and Social Behavior: An Interdisciplinary Perspective.* Cambridge, Mass.: MIT Press.

————. 1976. Toward a Theory of Human Disease. *The Journal of Nervous and Mental Disease* 162:299–312.

FOGELSON, RAYMOND. 1961. Change, Persistence, and Accommodation in Cherokee Medico-magical Beliefs. In *Symposium on Cherokee and Iroquois Culture,* ed. William Fenton and John Gulick. Washington, D.C.: U.S. Government Printing Office.

FONER, PHILIP S. 1974. *Organized Labor and the Black Worker, 1916–1973.* New York: Praeger.

FOULKES, EDWARD F. 1972. *The Arctic Hysterias of the North Alaskan Eskimo.* American Anthropological Association, Anthropological Studies, no. 10.

GANS, HERBERT J. 1979. Symbolic Ethnicity: The Future of Ethnic Groups and Cultures in America. In *On the Making of Americans: Essays in Honor of David Riesman,* ed. Herbert J. Gans et al. Philadelphia: University of Pennsylvania Press.

GARRISON, VIVIAN. 1977. Doctor, *Espiritista,* or Psychiatrist: Health-Seeking Behavior in a Puerto Rican Neighborhood of New York City. *Medical Anthropology* 1.2:65–180.

GAW, ALBERT C. 1975. An Integrated Approach in the Delivery of Health Care to the Chinese Community in America: The Boston Experience. In *Medicine in Chinese Cultures: Comparative Studies of Health Care in Chinese and Other Societies,* ed. Arthur Kleinman et al. Washington, D.C.: Department of Health, Education and Welfare. DHEW Publication No. (NIH) 75–653.

GILLUM, RICHARD F., and ARTHUR J. BARSKY. 1974. Diagnosis and Management of Patient Noncompliance. *Journal of the American Medical Association* 228:1563–1567.

GLAZER, NATHAN, and DANIEL P. MOYNIHAN. 1963. *Beyond the Melting Pot: The Negroes, Puerto Ricans, Jews, Italians, and Irish of New York City.* Cambridge, Mass.: MIT Press.

———. 1975a. Introduction. In *Ethnicity: Theory and Experience,* ed. Nathan Glazer and Daniel P. Moynihan. Cambridge, Mass.: Harvard University Press.

GLAZER, NATHAN, and DANIEL P. MOYNIHAN, eds. 1975b. *Ethnicity: Theory and Experience.* Cambridge, Mass.: Harvard University Press.

GORDON, MILTON M. 1964. *Assimilation in American Life: The Role of Race, Religion, and National Origins.* New York: Oxford University Press.

GREENBLUM, JOSEPH. 1974. Medical and Health Orientations of American Jews: A Case of Diminishing Distinctiveness. *Social Science and Medicine* 8:127–134.

GUTTMACHER, SALLY, and JACK ELINSON. 1971. Ethno-Religious Variation in Perceptions of Illness: The Use of Illness as an Explanation for Deviant Behavior. *Social Science and Medicine* 5:117–125.

HALIFAX, JOAN, and HAZEL H. WEIDMAN. 1973. Religion as a Mediating Institution in Acculturation: The Case of Santeria in Greater Miami. In *Religious Systems and Psychotherapy,* ed. Richard H. Cox. Springfield, Ill.: Thomas.

HAND, WAYLAND D., ed. 1976. *American Folk Medicine: A Symposium.* Berkeley: University of California Press.

HANNERZ, ULF. 1974. Ethnicity and Opportunity in Urban America. In *Urban Ethnicity,* ed. Abner Cohen. London: Tavistock.

HARRISON, IRA, and DIANA S. HARRISON. 1971. The Black Family Experience and Health Behavior. In *Health and the Family,* ed. Charles Crawford. New York: Macmillan.

HARWOOD, ALAN. 1971. The Hot-Cold Theory of Disease: Implications for Treatment of Puerto Rican Patients. *Journal of the American Medical Association* 216:1153–1158.

———. 1977. *Rx: Spiritist as Needed. A Study of a Puerto Rican Community Mental Health Resource.* New York: Wiley.

HERSHEY, JOHN C., HAROLD S. LUFT, and JOAN M GIANARIS. 1975. Making Sense Out of Utilization Data. *Medical Care* 13:838–854.

HESSLER, RICHARD M., et al. 1975. Intraethnic Diversity: Health Care of the Chinese-Americans. *Human Organization* 34:253–262.

HILL, CAROLE E.   1973.   Black Healing Practices in the Rural South. *Journal of Popular Culture* 6:829–853.

ISAJIW, WSEVOLOD W.   1974.   Definitions of Ethnicity. *Ethnicity* 1:111–124.

JENKINS, C. DAVID.   1966.   Group Differences in Perception: A Study of Community Beliefs and Feelings about Tuberculosis. *American Journal of Sociology* 71:417–429.

KAIN, JOHN F.   1975.   Race, Ethnicity, and Residential Location. In *Urban Planning: Policy Analysis and Administration*, Discussion Paper D75–3, Department of City and Regional Planning, Harvard University.

KANTROWITZ, NATHAN.   1973.   *Ethnic and Racial Segregation in the New York Metropolis: Residential Patterns among White Ethnic Groups, Blacks, and Puerto Ricans.* New York: Praeger.

KAY, MARGARITA ARTSCHWAGER.   1977.   Health and Illness in a Mexican American Barrio. In *Ethnic Medicine in the Southwest,* ed. Edward H. Spicer. Tucson: University of Arizona Press.

KIEV, ARI.   1968.   *Curanderismo: Mexican American Folk Psychiatry.* New York: The Free Press.

KILPATRICK, JACK F., and ANNA CRITTS KILPATRICK.   1964.   Cherokee Rituals Pertaining to Medicinal Roots. *Southern Indian Studies* 16:24–28.

KING, HAITUNG.   1975.   Selected Epidemiological Aspects of Major Diseases and Causes of Death among Chinese in the United States and Asia. In *Medicine in Chinese Cultures: Comparative Studies of Health Care in Chinese and Other Societies,* ed. Arthur Kleinman et al. Washington, D.C.: U.S. Department of Health, Education and Welfare. DHEW Publication No. (NIH) 75-653.

KLEINMAN, ARTHUR.   1973.   Some Issues for a Comparative Study of Medical Healing. *International Journal of Social Psychiatry* 19: 159–165.

———.   1975.   Explanatory Models in Health Care Relationships. In *National Council for International Health: Health of the Family.* Washington, D.C.: National Council for International Health.

———.   1978.   Clinical Relevance of Anthropological and Cross-Cultural Research: Concepts and Strategies. *American Journal of Psychiatry* 135: 427–431.

KLEINMAN, ARTHUR, LEON EISENBERG, and BYRON GOOD.   1978.   Culture, Illness and Care: Clinical Lessons from Anthropologic and Cross-Cultural Research. *Annals of Internal Medicine* 88:251–258.

KRICKUS, RICHARD.   1976.   *Pursuing the American Dream: White Ethnics and the New Populism.* Garden City, N.Y.: Anchor.

KUNSTADTER, PETER.   1978.   Ethnic Group, Category, and Identity: Karen in Northwestern Thailand. In *Ethnic Adaptation and Identity: The Karen on the Thai Frontier with Burma,* ed. Charles F. Keyes. Philadelphia: ISHI Publications.

LACOURCIÈRE, LUC.   1976.   A Survey of Folk Medicine in French Canada from Early Times to the Present. In *American Folk Medicine: A Symposium,* ed. Wayland D. Hand. Berkeley: University of California Press.

LAUER, ROGER M.   1974.   A Medium for Mental Health. In *Religious Movements in Contemporary America,* ed. Irving I. Zaretsky and Mark P. Leone. Princeton: Princeton University Press.

LAVENDER, ABRAHAM D., and JOHN M. FORSYTH. 1976. The Sociological Study of Minority Groups as Reflected by Leading Sociological Journals. *Ethnicity* 3:388–398.

LEIGHTON, ALEXANDER, and DONALD A. KENNEDY. 1959. Pilot Study of Cultural Items in Medical Diagnosis—A Field Report (July 1, 1957). Washington, D.C.: U.S. Department of Health, Education and Welfare, Division of Indian Health, Health Education Branch.

LEWIS, CHARLES E. 1976. OEO Neighborhood Health Centers: Comprehensive Health Care for Low-Income Inner-City Residents. In *A Right to Health: The Problem of Access to Primary Care*, ed. Charles E. Lewis, Rashi Fein, and David Mechanic. New York: Wiley.

LIEBERSON, STANLEY. 1963. *Ethnic Patterns in American Cities*. Glencoe, Ill.: The Free Press.

LITT, EDGAR. 1970. *Ethnic Politics in America*. Glenview, Ill.: Scott, Foresman.

LUCE, GAY. 1971. The Importance of Psychic Medicine: Training Navaho Medicine Men. In *Mental Health Program Reports—5*, ed. Julius Segal. Washington, D.C.: National Institute of Mental Health, Department of Health, Education and Welfare.

MALONEY, CLARENCE, ed. 1976. *The Evil Eye*. New York: Columbia University Press.

MCDERMOTT, WALSH, et al. 1960. Introducing Modern Medicine in a a Navajo Community. *Science* 131: 97–205, 208–287.

MCKENZIE, JOAN L. 1974. A Descriptive Study of the Traditional Folk Medical Beliefs and Practices among Selected Filipinos in Seattle. Master's thesis, School of Nursing, University of Washington.

MCKENZIE, JOAN L., and NOEL J. CHRISMAN. 1977. Healing Herbs, Gods, and Magic: Folk Health Beliefs among Filipino-Americans. *Nursing Outlook* 25:326–329.

MECHANIC, DAVID. 1968. *Medical Sociology: A Selective View*. New York: The Free Press.

———. 1969. Illness and Cure. In *Poverty and Health: A Sociological Analysis*, ed. John Kosa, Aaron Antonovsky, and Irving K. Zola. Cambridge, Mass.: Harvard University Press.

———. 1972. *Public Expectations and Health Care: Essays on the Changing Organization of Health Services*. New York: Wiley.

———. 1976. *The Growth of Bureaucratic Medicine. An Inquiry into the Dynamics of Patient Behavior and the Organization of Medical Care*. New York: Wiley.

MULLINGS, LEITH. 1978. Ethnicity and Stratification in the Urban United States. *Annals of the New York Academy of Sciences* 318:10–22.

NOVAK, MICHAEL. 1972. *The Rise of the Unmeltable Ethnics*. New York: Macmillan.

———. 1977. *Further Reflections on Ethnicity*. Middletown, Pa.: Jednota Press.

OLENDZKI, MARGARET C. 1974. Medicaid Benefits Mainly the Younger and Less Sick. *Medical Care* 12:163–172.

PADILLA, ELENA. 1958. *Up from Puerto Rico.* New York: Columbia University Press.

PARSONS, TALCOTT. 1975. Some Theoretical Considerations on the Nature and Trends of Change of Ethnicity. In *Ethnicity: Theory and Experience,* ed. Nathan Glazer and Daniel P. Moynihan. Cambridge, Mass.: Harvard University Press.

PATTERSON, ORLANDO. 1975. Context and Choice in Ethnic Allegiance: A Theoretical Framework and Caribbean Case Study. In *Ethnicity: Theory and Experience,* ed. Nathan Glazer and Daniel P. Moynihan. Cambridge, Mass.: Harvard University Press.

PATTISON, E. MANSELL. 1973. Exorcism and Psychotherapy: A Case of Collaboration. In *Religious Systems and Psychotherapy,* ed. Richard H. Cox. Springfield, Ill.: Thomas.

PELLING, HENRY. 1960. *American Labor.* Chicago: University of Chicago Press.

PERLO, VICTOR. 1975. *The Economics of Racism.* New York: International Publishers.

PLAJA, ANTONIO ORDONEZ, LUCY M. COHEN, and JULIAN SAMORA. 1968. Communication between Physicians and Patients in Outpatient Clinics: Social and Cultural Factors. *Milbank Memorial Fund Quarterly* 46 (part 1):161–213.

POLGAR, STEVEN. 1963. Health Action in Cross-Cultural Perspective. In *Handbook of Medical Sociology,* ed. Howard E. Freeman, Sol Levine, and Leo G. Reeder. Englewood Cliffs, N.J.: Prentice-Hall.

QUESADA, GUSTAVO M., and PETER L. HELLER. 1977. Sociocultural Barriers to Medical Care among Mexican Americans in Texas. *Medical Care* 15.5 (suppl.):93–101.

ROSENSTOCK, IRWIN M. 1966. Why People Use Health Services. *Milbank Memorial Fund Quarterly* 44:94–127.

ROTH, JULIUS A. 1969. The Treatment of the Sick. In *Poverty and Health: A Sociological Analysis,* ed. John Kosa, Aaron Antonovsky, and Irving Kenneth Zola. Cambridge, Mass.: Harvard University Press.

RUBEL, ARTHUR J. 1964. The Epidemiology of a Folk Illness: *Susto* in Hispanic America. *Ethnology* 3:268–283.

————. 1966. *Across the Tracks: Mexican Americans in a Texas City.* Austin: University of Texas Press.

RUIZ, PEDRO. 1976. Folk Healers as Associate Therapists. In *Current Psychiatric Therapies,* vol. 16, ed. Jules H. Masserman. New York: Grune and Stratton.

RUIZ, PEDRO, and JOHN LANGROD. 1976. The Role of Folk Healers in Community Mental Health Services. *Community Mental Health Journal* 12:392–398.

SAMORA, JULIAN, LYLE SAUNDERS, and RICHARD F. LARSON. 1961. Medical Vocabulary Knowledge among Hospital Patients. *Journal of Health and Human Behavior* 2:83–92.

SCHERMERHORN, RICHARD A. 1970. *Comparative Ethnic Relations: A Framework for Theory and Research.* Chicago: University of Chicago Press.

————. 1978. Preface to Phoenix Edition of *Comparative Ethnic Relations: A Framework for Theory and Research*.

SCOTT, CLARISSA S. 1974. Health and Healing Practices among Five Ethnic Groups in Miami, Florida. *Public Health Review* 89:524–532.

————. 1975. The Relationship between Beliefs about the Menstrual Cycle and Choices of Fertility Regulating Methods within Five Ethnic Groups. *International Journal of Gynaecology and Obstetrics* 13:105–109.

SHAW, R. DANIEL. 1958. Health Concepts and Attitudes of the Papago Indians. Tucson, Arizona: Health Program Systems Center, Division of Indian Health, Public Health Services.

SHILOH, AILON, and IDA COHEN SELAVAN, eds. 1973. *Ethnic Groups of America: Their Morbidity, Mortality, and Behavior Disorders. Vol. 1—The Jews*. Springfield, Ill.: Thomas.

————. 1974. *Ethnic Groups of America: Their Morbidity, Mortality, and Behavior Disorders. Vol. II—The Blacks*. Springfield, Ill.: Thomas.

SNOW, LOUDELL. 1974. Folk Medical Beliefs and Their Implications for Care of Patients. *Annals of Internal Medicine* 81:82–96.

————. 1977. Popular Medicine in a Black Neighborhood. In *Ethnic Medicine in the Southwest,* ed. Edward H. Spicer. Tucson: University of Arizona Press.

————. 1978. Sorcerers, Saints and Charlatans: Black Folk Healers in Urban America. *Culture, Medicine and Psychiatry* 2:69–106.

SOLON, JERRY. 1966. Patterns of Medical Care: Sociocultural Variations among a Hospital's Outpatients. *American Journal of Public Health* 56:884–893.

SPICER, EDWARD H. 1977a. Southwestern Healing Traditions in the 1970s: An Introduction. In *Ethnic Medicine in the Southwest*. Tucson: University of Arizona Press.

SPICER, EDWARD H., ed. 1977b. *Ethnic Medicine in the Southwest*. Tucson: University of Arizona Press.

STEIN, HOWARD F., and ROBERT F. HILL. 1977. *The Ethnic Imperative: Examining the New White Ethnic Movement*. University Park: Pennsylvania State University Press.

SUCHMAN, EDWARD A. 1964. Sociomedical Variations among Ethnic Groups. *American Journal of Sociology* 70:319–331.

————. 1965a. Social Patterns of Illness and Medical Care. *Journal of Health and Human Behavior* 6:2–16.

————. 1965b. Stages of Illness and Medical Care. *Journal of Health and Human Behavior* 6:114–128.

————. 1966. Health Orientations and Medical Care. *American Journal of Public Health* 56:97–105.

VAN DEN BERGHE, PIERRE L. 1974. Introduction In *Class and Ethnicity in Peru,* ed. P. L. van den Berghe. Leiden: E. J. Brill.

————. 1976. Ethnic Pluralism in Industrial Societies: A Special Case? *Ethnicity* 3:242–255.

WEAVER, THOMAS. 1970. Use of Hypothetical Situations in a Study of

Spanish American Illness Referral Systems. *Human Organization* 29:140–154.

WEIDMAN, HAZEL H. 1976. The Constructive Potential of Alienation: A Transcultural Perspective. In *Alienation in Contemporary Society,* ed. Roy S. Bryce-Laporte and Claudewell S. Thomas. New York: Praeger.

———. 1978. Miami Health Ecology Project Report: A Statement on Ethnicity and Health, vol. 1. Department of Psychiatry, University of Miami School of Medicine (mimeographed).

WILLIAMS, R. A. 1974. Black-Related Diseases: An Overview. *Journal of Black Health Perspectives* 1:35–40.

ZBOROWSKI, MARK. 1952. Cultural Components of Response to Pain. *Journal of Social Issues* 8:16–30.

———. 1969. *People in Pain.* San Francisco: Jossey-Bass.

ZOLA, IRVING K. 1964. Illness Behavior of the Working Class. In *Blue Collar World,* ed. Arthur Shostak and William Gomberg. Englewood Cliffs, N.J.: Prentice-Hall.

———. 1966. Culture and Symptoms—An Analysis of Patients' Presenting Complaints. *American Sociological Review* 31:615–630.

———. 1972a. Studying the Decision to See a Doctor: Review, Critique, Corrective. *Advances in Psychosomatic Medicine* 8:216–236.

———. 1972b. The Concept of Trouble and Sources of Medical Assistance —To Whom One Can Turn, with What and Why. *Social Science and Medicine* 6:673–679.

1
Urban Black Americans

JACQUELYNE JOHNSON JACKSON

FROM THE EARLIEST TIMES in this country, diseases and health-care patterns among blacks varied, depending on their differing statuses, extant economic and disease conditions, and the skills of medical practitioners. Prior to the Civil War, when contagious diseases were widespread and most blacks were slaves, masters were typically responsible for the health of blacks. Nonetheless, many blacks treated their own illnesses and those of other slaves as well. Usually slaves received better treatment than free blacks. However, during raging epidemics of contagious diseases (such as smallpox, cholera, and yellow fever) free blacks often received gratis vaccinations and medical care, and their neighborhoods were cleaned. (See, for example, Savitt 1975 on antebellum Virginia.)

After slavery was abolished, blacks generally became responsible for their own health care (see May 1971 on the availability of medical care to blacks in Louisiana between 1862 and 1868). It was apparently at this time that "root work" crystallized out of the traditions of classical medicine and European and African beliefs to become part of the folk medical system of not only blacks but also poor whites in the South (Webb 1971; Rocereto 1973; Wintrob 1973; Snow 1974). As Puckett has observed, when "the treatment of disease was taken out of the hands of the master and given again to the Negroes, their desire to avoid expensive medical attention focussed their attention again on the all-powerful 'root doctor' or 'hoodoo-man' as the healer of diseases" (1926.167). Obviously this "desire" on the part of blacks was largely forced upon them by the economics of industrialization and the psychological trauma of defeat for Southern whites, who had never developed a tradition of responsibility for the health care of destitute persons of their own race (May 1971:158–159).

For many years following slavery, mainstream medical care was often inaccessible to urban blacks in the United States, largely because of racism and poverty. Despite the paucity of black health professionals and hospitals, most of their white counterparts simply refused to accept black patients. Anderson, a black physician, held that both blacks and whites agreed "that the health of the Negro is largely the responsibility of the Negro medical profession" (1935:17). Some years later, Bartley declared that "the black population must look to the Negro [sic] physician for health care" (1972:264), and Sampson, agitated by increasing admissions of black patients to white hospitals, stated strongly that "black institutions are essential for health care delivery in urban communities" (1974:65). In contrast to the vested interests expressed in these professionals' views, most blacks have not regarded their health care as the province only of physicians, nor as the sole province of black physicians. In fact, the race of the physician has remained unimportant to most black patients, an issue that will be discussed at greater length later in the chapter.

Whatever the racial preferences of physicians and patients may be, it is clear that historically most of the nation's health schools deliberately barred their doors to blacks, even when they were highly qualified, thereby reducing severely the number of black physicians and other health professionals available to treat black *and* nonblack patients.[1] This form of racism also greatly retarded the dispersion of biomedical knowledge among blacks, although such factors as the legal extinction of racial segregation and expanding federal funds for health care have undoubtedly improved the accessibility of mainstream medical care to urban blacks in recent years.

This increased accessibility is fraught with new issues, one of which concerns the type and amount of knowledge about ethnicity a practitioner needs to be an effective deliverer of mainstream medical care to urban blacks, some of whom rely heavily on folk or popular medicine for the treatment of certain illnesses or make simultaneous use of folk, popular, and mainstream medical care systems. White (1977), who views blacks as culturally distinct outsiders to the mainstream medical system, believes that the lack of information about black health beliefs and practices in medical and nursing schools has caused blacks to receive inadequate care and has frustrated health-care providers in individualizing care. Moreover, Branch would only accredit nursing schools whose students, faculty, and curricula were ethnically diverse, and all accredited health service facilities would require "ethnic representation among staff and for staff to be proficient in caring for people of color" (1977:51).

Although insufficient data as well as the changing nature of urban blacks prevent any definitive statement concerning the extent to which increased knowledge about ethnicity might improve the medical care of urban blacks, this chapter provides some information and impressions about urban blacks that should prove useful to deliverers of their mainstream medical care. At the very least, it may increase awareness and dialogue about the problems involved. This undertaking is responsive to Yerby's observation that both black and white medically underserved populations will benefit, among other things, through increased "effectiveness and efficiency of the care provided" (1977:512). It should be clear at the outset that sufficient answers to most of the issues raised in this chapter are not yet available.

Identification of the Ethnic Group

Definition of Urban Blacks

Blacks are individuals who racially define themselves as such or who are so defined and treated by socially significant others. Some people dislike the term "black" and prefer designations such as "Afro-American" or "Negro." During the past century, the dominant term has shifted from "black" to "colored" to "Negro" and, once again, to "black," probably reflecting an unfulfilled hope among younger blacks that a shift in nomenclature reduces racism. Mainstream medical practitioners should, however, be cautious in labeling patients as black, particularly in face-to-face interactions. Many older blacks especially resent any identification of themselves as black, preferring instead to be called "colored" or "Negro," depending on the term to which they attached dignity during their formative years. In spite of these important variations, I shall as a convenience use only the term "black" in this chapter. "Urban blacks" will be defined as those who reside in towns, cities, or suburbs that are (generally) incorporated and contain at least 2,500 inhabitants.

Immigration and Sociocultural Contact

Unlike all other American ethnic groups, the African ancestors of urban blacks were *involuntary* immigrants, the first of whom were brought to Jamestown, Virginia, in 1619. Mostly West Africans, the bulk of the imported slaves during the next several centuries came from "the western coastal belt of Africa from the Senegal River in the north, around the Great Bend to the Guinea Coast, along the Bight of Benin and southwards beyond the Congo to the Portuguese territory of Angola," some times after preliminary conditioning in the Caribbean Islands or South America (Herskovits 1966:115–116).

The slaves were concentrated in the South, primarily on rural plantations, and the slave trade and natural increase expanded their numbers. Frequent tribal and racial miscegenation modified their gene pool and affected their predisposition for genetic diseases. Freed and free blacks also existed at the time, principally in cities such as Boston, New Orleans, New York, and Philadelphia.

More blacks migrated to urban areas after the Civil War, but the great upsurge of blacks in urban areas began about 1916, during World War I, and ended briefly by about 1935. World War II then accelerated black urban migration, especially westward. Today about three-fourths of all blacks live in metropolitan areas; and, in contrast to earlier years, most urban blacks are now urban-born.

The growth of the urban black population has been largely internal. That is, given the historical restrictions on black immigration to the United States during this century, about 98 percent of the present black population is native-born. However, most black immigrants are also urban dwellers. These immigrants are chiefly Anglo-speaking West Indians, although the influx of both legal and illegal aliens among Haitians has increased in recent years (particularly into Miami), and the number of African blacks has also grown in various metropolitan areas. This chapter is not concerned with immigrant blacks; however, a major problem frequently encountered in the literature is the failure to distinguish between foreign-born and native-born black research subjects.

Contact of urban blacks with the major American social and cultural institutions is considerable. Their native language is English, which they and other Americans speak in various ways, and they have contributed to the English vocabulary, as seen, for instance, in the now rather widespread adoption of the phrase "right on." They gave rise to jazz and the blues. Their ancestors influenced heavily the presence or preparation of many American foods, such as peanuts, yams, okra, rice, and chicken.

Most urban blacks with religious affiliations are Protestants (mainly Baptists), and many helped force American Christianity during the black civil rights movements both to reduce the gaps between its real practices and its ideal tenets that emphasized the equality of all persons and to alter its conceptions of the entitlements of "God's chosen people." In addition, a number of low-income and a few middle-income urban blacks, particularly in the large cities, are members of the American Muslim Mission (formerly the World Community of Al-Islam).

Blacks have also influenced folk and mainstream American health institutions. Webb (1971) believes that voodooism, which originated in Africa, was brought to Louisiana by blacks and spread to whites, a directionally different pattern from that postulated in North Carolina by Whitten (1962). Daniel Hale Williams, a black physician, independently performed a pericardiorrhaphy in 1893 (he was unaware of an earlier procedure performed in 1891 by Henry C. Dalton that was not reported until 1895) and "proved that the thoracic cavity was suitable territory for surgical intervention" (Beatty 1971:175–176). Charles Drew, another black physician, was the first person to develop a method for preserving blood plasma (between 1939 and 1941 at the Columbia University Medical Center, New York). He also pioneered in the establishment of blood banks. Drew was in charge of the American program for getting plasma to Great Britain during World War II, and his work was especially helpful in saving lives during the Battle of Dunkirk. Other blacks have also contributed to health developments and technologies, and many black physicians have been active in the National Medical Association (NMA) since its inception in 1895. Unlike the American Medical Association, the NMA was an early and strong advocate for national health insurance, in part because black physicians, whose median income was lower than that of their white counterparts, sought earlier the economic advantages of national health insurance.

A serious problem through the years has been the undue subjugation of urban blacks to the fluctuations of the larger American marketplace. The massive European immigration of the late nineteenth century reduced the economic opportunities of blacks, just as the cutoff of that immigration during World War I briefly increased them. Similarly, urban black unemployment rose greatly during the depression of the 1930s and declined again during World War II. Since then, employment opportunities for urban blacks in the secondary labor market have been dismal, partially because of competition from illegal aliens, principally Mexicans (Jackson 1979). Following the gains of the black civil rights movements of the 1950s and 1960s, however, employment opportunities for upwardly mobile blacks in the primary labor market have improved and have intensified black social stratification, a critical point often overlooked by those viewing blacks monolithically.

Despite gains in the desegregation of education and housing, these are still two major areas with low interracial interaction, even when blacks and whites attend the same schools or live in the same neighborhoods. (In general the meaning of neighborhood, of course, has shifted markedly toward greater impersonality.) Few additional gains in education and housing are likely to occur for the urban black masses in the foreseeable future, and the concentration of lower-class blacks in central cities will increase.

Overall, then, urban blacks have had significant contacts with and made significant contributions to major American social and cultural institutions. Yet racial segregation remains relatively widespread, particularly for lower-class blacks in central cities. Although greater contact with and participation in the major institutions of the United States are increasingly characteristic of middle-class and upper-class blacks, lower-class blacks are becoming more isolated or segregated from both other blacks and mainstream white groups. Today, many metropolitan lower-class blacks have more contact with predominantly lower-class immigrants or first-generation Americans than with other blacks or whites.

Demographic Profile

Demographic profiles help to provide useful information about different ethnic groups. However, an inherent danger of such profiles is that people who are not members of the ethnic group often perceive individual group members stereotypically, as if they fitted precisely the typical group traits. Inappropriate responses arise from medical practitioners, for example, when they treat middle-class black patients as if they were welfare patients, because they assume that most blacks are poor —an overgeneralization from the fact that a substantially larger proportion of blacks than whites are poor.

No typical urban black individual exists. This point should not be forgotten in the trend toward selective physical examinations for high-risk factors based on age, sex, race, familial history, and environmental exposure. For example, Chatman has warned against the usual assumption that endometriosis is rare in black women: "When dealing with pelvic pain, abnormal vaginal bleeding, and/or abnormal suggestive pelvic findings in the black woman, physicians are urged to maintain an acute awareness that endometriosis does occur in black women. A high index of suspicion is needed. We should strive to eliminate any residual prejudicial diagnostic posture with reference to pelvic inflammatory diseases. Routine rectovaginal examinations are important for more accurate diagnosis. Moreover, liberal use of diagnostic laparoscopy is essential" (1976: 987–988).

Since the abolition of slavery, the black population has undergone dramatic demographic changes, including phenomenal growth (though its present proportion within the total population of the country is substantially smaller than during slavery), geographic expansion throughout the nation (including a massive rural to urban shift), female excessiveness, and aging. The educational, occupational, employment, and income levels of the black population have also become more diversified.

AGE AND SEX DISTRIBUTION   The 1979 estimated midyear population for blacks, adjusted for the net census undercount, was 27.9 million, or 12.3 percent of the total United States population. Table 1.1 shows the age and sex distribution of the black population and sex ratios for various age groupings. Without the adjustment for the net census undercount

Table 1.1 Age and sex distribution of the estimated midyear U.S. black population, 1979, adjusted for net census undercount.

Age group (years)	Percentage			Sex ratio[a]
	Total	Female	Male	
Under 5	9.4	9.1	9.8	102.1
5–9	9.6	9.3	9.9	101.9
10–14	9.9	9.6	10.2	100.9
15–19	10.8	10.5	11.1	101.1
20–24	10.3	10.1	10.6	99.9
25–29	8.8	8.7	8.9	98.1
30–34	7.0	6.9	7.1	97.2
35–39	5.8	5.8	5.8	96.4
40–44	4.9	4.9	4.9	95.2
45–49	4.7	4.7	4.7	95.2
50–54	4.3	4.4	4.3	92.2
55–59	4.0	4.1	3.8	88.0
60–64	3.1	3.3	2.8	82.6
65–69	2.7	3.0	2.4	77.7
70–74	1.8	2.1	1.6	70.1
75–79	1.1	1.3	0.9	63.7
80–84	0.8	1.0	0.5	50.0
85+	0.9	1.2	0.5	40.9
Total number (thousands)	27,920	14,310	13,611	95.1

Source: U.S. Bureau of the Census (1980).
a. Number of males per 100 females.

(which still represents only an estimate), the sex ratio would have been much lower. For example, for all ages, the unadjusted sex ratio would have been 91.3 instead of the adjusted ratio of 95.1 as shown in table 1.1. Although both the black and white populations are aging, blacks as a group remain younger than whites overall. The median ages in 1979 were 25.8 years for black females, 24.2 years for black males, 32.2 years for white females, and 29.7 years for white males.

Female excessiveness, which is also higher among blacks than whites, has indirect implications for health care. For instance, male scarcity may exacerbate poverty and such health problems as alcoholism and cancer of the cervix among female household heads. Male scarcity, which also can result from different geographic distributions of the black female and male populations, may increase the probability of a greater number of partners for sexually active women. In turn, the existence of multiple sex partners is associated with increased prevalence of cancer of the cervix Another problem related to female excessiveness is that the probability of younger female household heads seeking medical care at the onset of serious medical symptoms that involve little or no discomfort is generally low. The low sex ratios among the elderly, or those over age 65, suggest that being married and living with a spouse is less common among this group than among their younger adult counterparts. In fact, many elderly blacks are widowed or live alone, and elderly persons living alone tend to use medical facilities (including emergency rooms) more frequently than their peers who do not live alone. Among blacks, female excessiveness is much greater in urban than rural areas, and, within urban areas, is greatest in the Northeast and lowest in the South.

RESIDENTIAL LOCALITIES   Whereas almost all blacks resided in the South in 1900, only 53 percent lived there in 1977. About 74 percent of blacks, as compared with 66 percent of whites, lived in metropolitan areas in 1977. Central cities claimed about 55 percent of blacks but only 24 percent of whites. In 1978, almost 77 percent of all black households were in metropolitan areas. Some geographic mobility occurs among blacks, but most movers typically remain relatively close to their regular or customary medical-care providers, assuming that they have a regular source of health care. This is so because most of these movers change residences within the same city or town. Residential instability is more characteristic of poor than non-poor urban blacks.

EDUCATION   Many medical professionals still stereotype black patients as functional illiterates, even though most blacks no longer fit that category. Among successive age cohorts of blacks, as among other ethnic groups, the median length of formal education has increased. Today about half of all blacks over 25 years of age are at least high school graduates, and increasing numbers are also college graduates.

The rising educational levels of blacks necessitate continuing modifications in the delivery of health services to them. Physicians can and should use more medical terms in discussing their disorders with them (for example, specifying diabetes mellitus instead of "sugar"). Because quantity and quality of education are not necessarily synonymous, however, physicians must also consider the comprehension level of each patient in selecting the most appropriate modality for educating the patient about specific medical problems. In some cases, audiovisual aids should supplement verbal descriptions.

EMPLOYMENT AND INCOME   Most black adults work or are seeking work. In March, 1980, among persons over 16 years of age, about 45 percent of black females and 62 percent of black males were in the United States civilian labor force, as compared to 48 percent of white females and 75 percent of white males. The larger proportion of white than black females in the civilian labor force is a recent trend, despite the fact that a larger proportion of black than white females occupy the role of family head. However, among both black and white participants in the civilian labor force, as increasing proportion are women. For example, in March, 1980, 47.5 percent of the black and 41.4 percent of the white civilian labor forces were females. Blacks constituted 9.5 percent of all black and white participants in the civilian labor force who were over 16 years of age in March, 1980.

A slight majority of whites, but less than one-third of blacks, were white-collar workers in 1980, which helps to explain racial disparities in income. Lack of data depicting true income (that is, real money and in-kind transfers, such as Medicaid, food stamps, and housing subsidies) prohibits accurate comparisons of racial gaps in individual or family total income. Nevertheless, the median incomes of black individuals and families continue to remain lower than those of comparable whites. Black females, when compared with white females and black and white males, still have the lowest median incomes.[2] For instance, in 1978, the median total money income for individuals of $3,707 for black females was somewhat less than that of $4,117 for white females, and considerably less than than of $6,861 for black males and $11,453 for white males. Further, the median total money income in 1978 for year-round, full-time workers of $9,020 for black females was again somewhat less than that of $9,732 for white females, and considerably less than that of $12,530 for black males and $16,360 for white males. Some people think that black males are more disadvantaged economically than are black females, because the disparity in median income is greater between black and white males than between black and white females. However, this is a spurious argument which belies the lowest economic standing of black females and assumes that the median income of black females should not be the same as that of white males. This assumption helps to explain why, of black and white females and males, black females are at the highest risk for poverty. In fact, a substantially large number of black females are still poor.

In recent years, however, poverty has declined greatly among blacks in the United States. Between 1959 and 1978, for blacks of all ages, the proportion in poverty declined from 55.1 percent to 30.6 percent. During the same time period, the decline among blacks who were over 65 years of age was from 62.5 percent to 33.9 percent; among blacks living in families, from 54.9 percent to 29.5 percent; and among related children under 18 years of age living in families, from 65.5 percent to 41.2 percent.

MARITAL AND FAMILIAL STATUS   The majority of blacks marry eventually, but their average age at first marriage has risen in recent years because of factors such as increased education and poor economic conditions. In 1980, more than three-fifths of blacks between 20 and 24 years of age had never married. The never-married proportion was higher among males. Among blacks over 20 years of age, a majority of the women, but only a minority of the men, were *not* living with spouses. Separations and divorces have soared among blacks during the past few decades. These trends of both increased age at first marriage and marital dissolutions are also apparent in the larger United States population, but they are more pronounced among urban blacks.

Of the 5.8 million black families in the United States in 1978, 75.1 percent resided in standard metropolitan statistical areas (SMSAs), and 98.5 percent of all black families were non-farm families. Among the non-farm families, about 56 percent were husband-wife families, and more than 39 percent were female-headed. In 1977, only 46 percent of black family heads were year-round, full-time workers (58 percent of the males, 28 percent of the females). Children under 18 years of age, living in families in which they were related to the household head, were far less likely to be poor in male headed (19.9 percent) than in female-headed (65.7 percent) households. Moreover, an unusually large number of poor black children became unwed parents during their adolescent years. Given the increasing proportion of black female-headed families (44 percent in central cities in 1978) and of minor children living only with their mothers, considerable attention needs to be focused on improving the economic conditions of black female family heads (Jackson 1971, 1973) in order to help improve the health conditions of these women and their children.

Evaluation of the Existing Data

I did not undertake an exhaustive search of the literature about the medical beliefs and practices of urban blacks, since this chapter is not intended to be a critique of the available literature. The two major resources used for bibliographic information were a computerized search of relevant literature since 1965[3] and subject-catalogue entries under *black* and *Negro* in the National Library of Medicine. Unfortunately, a number of studies that include blacks as subjects are not identified as such either in library catalogues or in indexes to various health journals.

The search produced more than a thousand items. However, most were journal articles not restricted to *urban* blacks, and most lacked an empirical or experimental base (for example, Miller and Algee's 1978 treatise on noncompliance among black, poor, and aged patients). The sparse entries strengthened my impression that relatively little is yet known about the diversified medical beliefs and practices of urban blacks. This suspicion was sustained when I examined holdings of the National Library of Medicine related to folklore and noted the considerable dependence of investigators of black folk medicine on the same few findings from extremely small and nonrepresentative samples.

Segments of the Black Population Represented in Available Studies

Studies of black medical beliefs and practices date back to colonial America (see Savitt 1975). The principal subjects then were either plantation slaves with access to contract physicians or blacks living in relatively close proximity to medical schools, or what passed as such. Some of the diagnoses recorded were racist and nonscientific, as in the case of Samuel Cartwright's identification of "two new diseases peculiar to Negroes: one, which he called 'drapetomania,' was manifested by the escape of the Negro slave from his white master; the other, which he called 'dysaesthesia Aethiopis,' was manifested by the Negro's neglecting his work or refusing to work altogether" (Szasz 1971:228–229).[4] These early studies tended to emphasize both the epidemiological aspects of black diseases and prevailing treatment patterns, including the use of conjurers. Given current medical knowledge, many of their findings were faulty, but they did emphasize ethnic differences in health patterns. Many epidemiological differences observed during the early days of slavery were undoubtedly linked to substantial racial differences in both gene pools and environmental exposure. Slaves were observed to be much less vulnerable to malaria than whites but far more vulnerable to syphilis, to which whites probably first exposed them.

Since most urban black research subjects in post-slavery times have been either users or neighbors of major northern medical centers (typically in Boston, New Haven, and New York City), most studies about medical beliefs and practices among urban blacks have in fact concentrated on native-born blacks who were migrants to Northern cities. In recent years, both the growing numbers of foreign blacks and the numerical preponderance of urban-born over migrant American blacks have produced a more diversified black population in many United States cities. As a result of this diversity, the need to control for the migratory and nativity statuses of urban black research subjects has become essential. Yet few studies that incorporate these controls can be cited.

Two examples of studies with adequate control for immigration and migration are Malzberg's study (1965) of mental illness among blacks in New York, in which his subjects were classified as native-born, migrant, or immigrant; and Kleinman and Lukoff's study (1978) of factors affecting drug use among native-born blacks, West Indian blacks, and whites residing in a New York City ghetto. Both studies found substantial differences between native-born and immigrant blacks. A third study outside the North was carried out in Maricopa County, Arizona, where Doto and her colleagues (1972) found that the frequency of positive coccidioidin reactions among school children was significantly lower among nonlifetime than lifetime black and white residents. A nonepidemiological but also useful example is Weidman's separate sampling of Southern, Haitian, and Bahamian black subjects in the Miami Health Ecology Project (1978).

Most urban black research subjects have also been lower-class, typically women and children. This bias has been due partially to greater research efforts placed on childbirth, child care, and related subjects. Most studies about mental disorders have also concentrated on lower-class blacks, frequently without comparisons between the sexes. The studies dealing with alcoholism and drug abuse, for example, have focused mainly on lower-class or military males, and those most concerned with cardiovascular or cerebrovascular disorders have also concentrated on males.

During the past two decades, the expansion of urban black samples in research studies has been substantial. The geographic area covered has also been much wider, with an increasing number of studies coming from major medical centers in the South, such as Johns Hopkins University. More community subjects who were not patients have been used. Subjects have been selected from a larger number of age, socioeconomic, and other demographic groupings. Urban blacks have also been subjects in various national probability samples undertaken by the National Center for Health Statistics, although published reports by that agency rarely provide specific data for blacks, let alone urban blacks.[5]

Interpretative and Inferential Problems

For many years, the major interpretative and inferential problems of most studies involving urban black subjects included generalizations from nonrepresentative and usually extremely small samples, such as Webb's use (1971) of 21 black patients, 2 white patients, and 10 white nurses in a study of folk medicine in Southern Louisiana; inappropriate racial comparisons that confounded social class and race; and insufficient investigations of the interactions between health institutions and health patterns. Few blacks were included in follow-up, longitudinal, or explanatory studies. Moreover, the often considerable time lag between data collection and publication frequently reduced the utility of valid and reliable results about health behaviors for subsequent cohorts of blacks. Three illustrations of these types of problems may be illuminating.

1. In a mental health workshop conducted in 1979, my co-leader informed us that pregnant black women today typically practice pica. This generalization contradicts available data indicating that most pregnant

black women (even among the poor) do *not* do so. Further questioning revealed that the black male co-leader had inappropriately generalized from a nonrepresentative sample of black women in St. Louis, many of whom were migrants from rural Arkansas and Mississippi. This is not to contend that no pregnant black women practice pica; but we do need to avoid overgeneralization in order to develop useful cues for clinicians to use in differentiating between patients who may and those who may not practice pica. Only then can health professionals avoid raising the question and thereby insulting women who are not pica-prone, yet help to reduce practices detrimental to pregnancy outcomes by raising the question among those who are prone. The diminishing phenomenon of pica among pregnant black women is now probably most prevalent among poorly educated women who rely heavily on folk traditions for their health behaviors and live in isolated rural or urban migrant enclaves.

2. Most studies using self-report data to compare black and white health statuses conclude all too often that blacks are in poorer health without making any distinctions between subjective and objective health measures, or between measures of disease and measures of illness. It is quite probable that lower-class people tend to perceive themselves as being more ill than do people of higher social class, and are, for example, more likely to report a greater number of disability days.[6] Given the typically larger proportion of black than white lower-class subjects in health interview studies, many of these studies' conclusions about the poorer health of blacks, based on self-report data, are suspect. An additional problem with such studies is the failure to control adequately for social class in racial comparisons.

3. Frankel's useful study about folk beliefs related to childbirth among poor urban black women in Philadelphia (1977) is based on data collected in 1968 and 1969. About a third of those women practiced pica, and most greatly feared and morally disapproved of abortions. These attitudes and practices have surely changed somewhat among successive cohorts of young pregnant black women in Philadelphia slums, but current information is not available. Mainstream medical professionals serving new groups of young black women cannot assume that Frankel's findings of a decade ago remain valid today, yet many mainstream medical practitioners ignore changes over time among blacks and assume that any finding about any black at any time remains applicable for all similarly situated blacks over time.

Many other illustrations of the problems identified above could be given, but the critical point is that they have diminished somewhat in recent years and, it is hoped, should be totally extinguished in the future, regardless of the researcher's race. Further, more researchers should adopt Lieberson's edict (1974) to use intergenerational controls as a standard procedure in studying Northern (to which I add Southern) black residents.

Intraethnic Diversity

A tendency to concentrate on racial comparisons in studies involving black subjects has often obscured the need for intraethnic comparisons among blacks. More consideration of intraethnic diversity may reduce the weight attached to the influence of ethnicity on given phenomena, or at least may reveal more clearly when ethnicity is or is not significant. Although relatively few studies of medical beliefs and practices of urban blacks have focused on intraethnic diversity, those that do demonstrate considerable differences. Studies on similar topics but using different samples also reveal intraethnic diversities.

Essentially, factors producing divergences in other ethnic groups—such as education, geographic location, sex, and religious affiliation—also affect urban blacks (see Fabrega and Roberts 1972). It is nevertheless important to point out that although these sources of intraethnic diversity may prevail across ethnic groups, their relative weightings may differ. In a study of depression among 97 black and 417 Mexican American women in a Southwestern inner city in 1971 and 1972, for example, Quesada, Spears, and Ramos (1978) found that socioeconomic status (the best single predictor), marital status, and age explained 18 percent of the variance in depression among black women, whereas alienation (the best single predictor) and socioeconomic status explained 16 percent of the variance among Mexican American women. Although much of the variance was left unexplained by the independent variables utilized in the study, the point remains that depression, relatively high in both groups, was reported as being influenced by different factors in each ethnic group.

Epidemiological Characteristics

Available Epidemiological Data: Cautions and Biases

Incredible as it may seem, a search for epidemiological data about major and minor diseases or the acute and chronic conditions of urban blacks is generally fruitless. Such studies simply do not exist on a national, state, or local level. Furthermore, though the number of epidemiological studies concerning the prevalence of diseases among urban blacks is growing, most are confined to relatively small geographic locations and are concerned primarily with either hypertension or cancer (see, for example, Kashgarian and Dunn 1970; Kotchen et al. 1974; Hypertension Detection and Follow-Up Program Cooperative Group 1977). Thus, a comprehensive national picture of the epidemiological status of urban blacks either now or in the past is clearly impossible.

The closest one can come to constructing a national portrait of the epidemiological characteristics of blacks is through use of various data collected by the National Center for Health Statistics (NCHS) from studies conducted at different times involving household interviews, medical examinations, and vital statistics. But even these NCHS data are quite insufficient in varying ways. Most relatively current data are not reported for blacks, who are subsumed in the "total," "female," "male," "all other," "all other female," or "all other male" categories. Clearly the "all other" category (sometimes termed "nonwhite") is misleading whenever it is treated as if it applied only to blacks. In addition, the reliability of population extrapolations from the small samples of "all others" are frequently unreliable.

The NCHS does occasionally produce publications containing specific data by various breakouts (such as age and income levels for "all others," or even for blacks), but by the time these publications appear, they are outdated and are primarily useful for comparing temporal changes in the stability of patterns. Three examples of the critical failure to provide appropriate racial breakouts, and, for blacks, further breakouts differentiated by geographic location and other relevant demographic characteristics, are *Current Estimates from the Health Interview Survey: United States—1977* (Howie and Drury 1978), *Health Characteristics by Geographic Region, Large Metropolitan Areas, and Other Places of Residence, United States 1973–74* (Gentile 1977), and *Acute Conditions, Incidence and Associated Disability, United States, July 1975–June 1976* (Choi 1978).

In addition to the insufficiency of timely data, cautions about epidemiological information also include inadequate descriptions and analyses of intra-black diversities, and gaps caused by failures to collect certain appropriate data. A further caution concerns sample size and determination. The NCHS treats ethnic groups as if they were merely members of the total population of the United States, regardless of color, and does not sample them as separate populations. The large subpopulation of whites is adequately sampled by this method, but not small subpopulations, such as blacks. I think that sampling blacks as a separate population (and not as a subpopulation) would increase the likelihood of better data with more reliable estimates. In this way, instances such as Cypress's reporting of some estimates for blacks with more than a 30 per cent relative standard error in her NCHS study of office visits for circulatory diseases (1979) could be reduced. My contention about treating blacks as a separate population is germane whenever investigations are predicated on substantial racial differences, or when the need is present to determine if racial differences exist. Furthermore, oversampling is not the answer when racial comparisons are to be made, because the size of the oversampled unit must be reduced for such comparisons, or the remaining units must be overweighted.

A further caution is that mortality data often constitute the primary index of black morbidity patterns. Mortality data, which Kadushin regards as "especially reflective of the system of medical care" rather than "the effects of forces prior to getting sick" (1967:330), are really not adequate proxies for morbidity data, but they are better than nothing. One problem in using mortality data is that the unitary manner of recording cause of death disregards multiple or contributory causes. Thus, for example, the contributing influence of hypertension on mortality is underreported. Another problem is misdiagnosis of the cause of mortality. Richter and his colleagues observed that "stroke may be misdiagnosed, particularly on death certificates when the victim has not attended a medical facility" (1977:225).

An additional problem is that the NCHS does not publish mortality data by socioeconomic status in addition to race, age, and sex. I believe that such breakouts would be extremely helpful to epidemiologists, although this opinion is controversial. Terris, for example, believes that it is

> very difficult to justify racial classification of mortality statistics on the ground of its usefulness to epidemiologists. I have a working knowledge of the epidemiology of a number of diseases which show significant differences by race, including cancer of the cervix, stomach, and esophagus, tuberculosis, sarcoidosis, cirrhosis of the liver, and prematurity; knowledge of racial differences has played little or no role in advancing the understanding of their epidemiology. Furthermore, the important epidemiological breakthroughs which have been achieved recently in the non-infectious diseases —cancer of the lung, chronic bronchitis and emphysema, dental caries, retrolental fibroplasia, radiation epidemiology, and coronary heart diseases—occurred without assistance from the white-nonwhite classification of mortality statistics. The remarkable achievements in delineating the epidemiology and methods of control of infectious, nutritional, and occupational diseases were similarly obtained without such assistance. The science of epidemiology will not be undermined by the disappearance of the white-nonwhite dichotomy in health statistics; on the contrary, it may be spared the necessity of disproving the various racist hypotheses which arise therefrom. (1973:479)

Chase, in opposition to Terris's position, has indicated strongly that data collection by "race, color, and ethnic group [is] still useful in the unfinished business of diminishing" racial and socioeconomic differentials in health patterns (1973:836), but she fails to deal sufficiently with Terris's objections to warrant acceptance of her position. Basically, I accept Terris's position that race is not a significant factor in the cause of disease; however, I think that racial breakouts should still be retained, along with measures of socioeconomic status, in order to continue to demonstrate their etiological insignificance until the time arises when such a demonstration is no longer necessary.

The major biases producing the lack of comprehensive epidemiological data about urban blacks are not, of course, entirely racial. Comprehensive epidemiological data for urban whites are also often unavailable, although good fragmentary data do exist. *There is every reason for mainstream medical practitioners to urge the NCHS and other related agencies to increase the collection, analysis, and interpretation of comprehensive epidemiological data for all segments of the United States population, including those on urban black females and urban black males of various age groupings.*

Some biases in epidemiological data can also be pointed out in areas where the NCHS now provides racial breakouts. Racial separations in data generally occur when the subject being studied is fertility patterns, particularly with respect to illegitimacy or other areas in which blacks are viewed as deficient. Biases also exist for diseases whose prevalence is typically higher among blacks than whites, such as sickle-cell anemia, hypertension, or psychoses (where labeling is a major factor affecting presumed racial differences), even though other conditions in fact occur more frequently among blacks. In short, epidemiological data about blacks are more likely to exist for conditions that are perceived as being exotic or deviant. The argument here is not to wipe out racial breakouts for these conditions, but to extend them to all conditions for which data are collected.

Finally, as is true of data not about blacks, biases include unintentional and intentional misreporting, underreporting, and nonreporting of data.

Major Causes of Death Among Blacks

As already indicated, an adequate discussion of the prevalence of major diseases among urban blacks is impossible because of the absence of sufficient data. However, a limited discussion based on mortality data and fragmented morbidity data about blacks or "nonwhites," can nevertheless be provided.

TWO-YEAR ANNUAL AVERAGES FOR DEATH RATES, 1976–1977 Table 1.2 shows death rates from all causes for black and white females and males by age groupings. In each sex group, except for those over 80 years of age, the age-specific death rates were higher for blacks. It is notable that the age of racial crossover (the point where the death rate is lower for blacks than for whites) has been increasing continuously, suggesting that it may disappear within the next few decades and thus narrow racial gaps

Table 1.2   Two-year average annual death rates per 100,000 resident population for black and white females and males, by age, United States, 1976–1977.

Age group (years)	Black females	White females	Black males	White males
All ages	733.0	788.4	1,044.2	1,004.2
Under 1	2,602.2	1,145.6	3,135.4	1,474.0
1–4	91.6	55.4	113.4	70.8
5–19	41.0	36.7	84.6	74.3
20–34	147.0	66.4	344.7	171.3
35–49	466.2	208.2	903.4	380.2
50–64	1,466.4	791.2	2,620.3	1,591.2
65–79	4,664.1	2,997.4	6,835.3	5.649.2
80+	7,976.6	11,020.0	10,904.2	15,033.1

Source: After U.S. Department of Health, Education, and Welfare (1978: 171); raw data for 1977 from the National Center for Health Statistics.

in life expectancy in the United States (Jackson 1980). Its disappearance would connote greater similarity in the health conditions of blacks and whites.

Table 1.2 also shows striking differences by race in mortality rates particularly for those under 1 year and between 20 and 49 years of age. Black rates in these categories were more than twice as high as white rates.

LEADING CAUSES OF DEATH, 1977   Table 1.3 shows the ten leading causes of death for black and white females and males of all ages. For comparative purposes, death rates are shown for each cause in each group, even if the specific cause is not a leading cause for that group. (For example, suicide was not a leading cause of death for black females, but it was for the remaining groups.) The presentation of data for all causes of death for all ages masks the fact that within each sex category rates are higher for blacks than whites for all persons below 80 years of age.

As shown in table 1.3, diseases of the heart, malignant neoplasms, cerebrovascular diseases, and accidents were the four leading causes of death for each race-sex group. The remaining causes of death differed somewhat in kind or rank order. Diabetes mellitus, infant mortality, influenza and pneumonia, cirrhosis of the liver, homicide, and arteriosclerosis (in rank order) rounded out the ten leading causes of death among black females. (Comparable causes among white females were influenza and pneumonia, arteriosclerosis, diabetes mellitus, cirrhosis of the liver, suicide, and infant mortality). For black males, the causes in rank order were homicide, infant mortality, influenza and pneumonia, cirrhosis of the liver, diabetes

Table 1.3   Death rates per 100,000 resident population for all causes of death and leading causes of death for black and white females and males, all ages, United States, 1977.

Cause of death	Black females	White females	Black males	White males
All causes	730.3	783.2	1,036.6	998.1
Diseases of the heart	268.8	338.6	326.5	429.6
Malignant neoplasms	130.9	193.0	198.1	192.7
Cerebrovascular diseases	87.1	96.5	81.4	73.2
Accidents	26.6	28.4	80.3	66.7
Diabetes mellitus	25.2	16.5	15.4	12.9
Certain causes of infant mortality	23.1	7.0	31.9	10.3
Influenza and pneumonia	17.2	22.0	30.0	25.9
Cirrhosis of the liver	13.4	9.1	26.3	18.3
Homicide	13.2	2.9	59.7	8.7
Arteriosclerosis	8.3	16.6	7.5	11.7
Nephritis and nephrosis	8.2	2.9	9.1	3.8
Congenital anomalies	7.3	5.1	8.9	6.4
Suicide	3.0	7.3	10.7	21.4
Bronchitis, emphysema, and asthma	2.9	6.1	7.9	16.5

Source: Raw data from the National Center for Health Statistics.

mellitus, and suicide. (The descending order for white males was influenza and pneumonia; suicide; cirrhosis of the liver, bronchitis, emphysema, and asthma; diabetes mellitus; and arteriosclerosis.)

Because a large proportion of deaths among both blacks and whites are now caused by diseases of the heart and malignant neoplasms, especially among older groups, tables 1.4 and 1.5 provide race-sex comparisons for specific age groups in 1950, 1960, 1970, and 1976.

DISEASES OF THE HEART, 1950–1976. Table 1.4 shows that death rates for blacks from diseases of the heart were usually much higher than white rates, a pattern that has persisted for many years. However, the general decline in black mortality rates, especially for younger groups, may be a partial function of the fact that better mainstream medical care has been increasingly available to blacks. It is also possible that greater efficiency in diagnosing and managing hypertension in recent years has been stimulated by the National High Blood Pressure Education Program (NHBPE), which was begun in 1972 with the major goal of decreasing by "50 percent every five years the number of people with diastolic blood pressures of 105 mm Hg or greater" (Ware 1977:18). Miller, however, believes that the decrease in hypertension mortality was not caused by drugs because "the decreasing mortality rate began prior to wide usage

Table 1.4 Death rates per 100,000 resident population caused by diseases of the heart for black and white females and males, by age, United States, 1950–1976.

Year and race-sex group	All ages	Age group (years)								
		Under 25	25–34	35–44	45–54	55–64	65–74	75–79	80–84	85+
1950										
Black females	289.9	11.4	52.8	190.6	542.5	1,239.8	1,783.6	3,499.3[a]	—	—
White females	290.5	4.2	13.8	43.0	144.0	472.6	1,473.6	3,237.2	5,166.9	9,085.7
Black males	348.4	9.8	53.2	202.6	641.8	1,471.6	2,232.6	4,107.9[a]	—	—
White males	434.2	4.2	21.7	114.4	429.0	1,101.4	2,396.3	4,248.7	6,186.6	9,959.6
1960										
Black females	268.5	5.4	35.7	127.6	370.4	983.0	1,742.9	2,545.0	3,743.1	5,650.0
White females	306.5	1.7	8.1	23.5	105.3	391.2	1,275.2	2,848.9	5,062.0	9,280.8
Black males	330.6	5.3	42.9	171.0	526.5	1,283.6	2,242.8	3,422.8	4,078.6	7,113.3
White males	454.6	2.1	17.2	108.8	420.4	1,076.8	2,358.8	4,099.6	6,340.5	10,135.8
1970										
Black females	261.0	4.8	25.2	94.8	295.5	722.9	1,619.6	2,625.8	3,536.8	5,003.8
White females	313.8	1.4	5.6	23.5	92.5	323.6	1,074.1	2,473.6	4,221.5	7,839.9
Black males	330.3	5.4	42.7	189.0	519.4	1,154.4	2,314.7	3,504.9	4,305.1	5,367.6
White males	438.3	2.2	12.8	93.0	370.1	997.1	2,235.1	3,939.0	5,828.7	8,818.0
1976										
Black females	237.4	4.2	15.8	60.4	220.8	572.7	1,397.2	2,869.9	2,884.4	4,344.0
White females	305.5	1.6	4.0	18.4	75.1	273.8	859.4	2,120.3	3,616.3	7,244.5
Black males	296.9	5.7	31.8	139.1	440.8	1,032.0	2,002.2	3,565.5	3,721.8	5,182.1
White males	399.4	2.5	10.4	75.2	306.6	845.8	1,927.4	3,603.3	5,219.4	8,692.9

Source: U.S. Department of Health, Education, and Welfare (1978:180–183).

a. Computed rate is for all persons 75 and over.

of . . . drugs. It has only been in recent years that effective anti-hypertensive agents have been used on a large scale. More importantly, less than half of the hypertensives have been diagnosed, and of these, less than half are taking medication which is less than 50 percent effective" (1973: 17).

Without quibbling about the effectiveness of antihypertensive drugs and NHBPE, it should be noted that NHBPE does not presently advocate racially differentiated preventive and treatment measures. Recent findings from the Bogalusa Heart Study of black and white children in a small urban area in Louisiana, however, indicate probable racial differences in metabolic backgrounds for hypertension, which would then suggest the need for racially differentiated preventive and treatment modalities (Voors et al. 1979). It is clear that more emphasis needs to be placed on research investigating probable biological differences attributable to ethnicity.

Based on data collected between 1973 and 1975 from a nationwide screening program of elevated blood pressure (diastolic pressure of 90 mm Hg or higher), Stamler and his colleagues (1976) indicated that the prevalence rate of elevated blood pressure per 1,000 was highest for black males (307.1), followed by black females (297.9), white males (269.7), white females (223.1), all other males (219.8), and finally, all other females (178.4). Although these rates were not age-specific, they are higher than the self-reported averages for the three age groups shown later in table 1.7, which suggests again that some hypertensives are unaware of their conditions. In a study of noninstitutionalized black and white welfare recipients, 65 to 74 years old, conducted in Cook County, Illinois, Ostfeld and his co-workers (1971) reported higher prevalence rates per 1,000 for hypertension (at initial examination, systolic pressure of 160 or higher and diastolic pressure of 95 mm Hg or higher) for black women (464) than for black men (376). However, as Coulehan (1979) implied in a study to be discussed in more detail later, any race-sex comparisons of hypertension should be controlled for arm circumference.

MALIGNANT NEOPLASMS, 1950–1976.   Table 1.5 shows racial variations in mortality rates for malignant neoplasms. With the exception of females under 25 or over 65 years of age, female mortality rates were consistently higher among blacks than whites between 1950 and 1976. Male mortality rates were higher among blacks between the ages of 25 and 64 in 1950 and 1970, between ages 30 and 64 in 1960, and over age 30 in 1976. In addition, mortality rates between 1950 and 1975 decreased among black females under 65 years of age but increased among black males 35 or more years of age.

Various environmental and other factors, including increased black

Table 1.5   Death rates per 100,000 caused by malignant neoplasms for black and white females and males, by age, United States, 1950–1976.

Year and race-sex group	All ages	Under 25	25–29	30–34	35–39	40–44	45–49	50–54	55–59	60–64	65+
1950											
Black females	111.8	6.5	19.7	50.6	89.2	156.6	227.3	339.5	449.9	530.1	513.0
White females	139.9	7.8	14.8	27.3	53.9	97.4	153.1	221.1	314.5	419.4	768.4
Black males	106.6	7.1	15.3	21.1	39.3	74.3	147.5	288.5	425.2	580.1	696.1
White males	147.2	9.7	15.0	20.6	32.7	57.2	110.4	194.7	327.9	506.0	986.0
1960											
Black females	113.8	6.0	18.4	43.1	75.9	132.4	210.7	308.4	384.8	518.5	591.4
White females	139.8	7.0	12.7	24.2	47.9	86.7	143.8	211.6	281.7	382.6	718.4
Black males	136.7	6.7	15.0	21.7	47.7	101.2	177.9	324.4	461.4	740.1	980.4
White males	166.1	9.7	16.4	21.1	33.8	59.7	114.5	219.9	360.1	559.3	1073.4
1970											
Black females	117.3	5.1	15.4	27.0	64.6	124.7	183.2	280.3	370.7	444.7	668.4
White females	149.4	6.0	12.4	25.1	44.3	85.0	140.4	216.5	279.0	380.8	702.0
Black males	171.6	6.8	13.9	20.3	51.1	107.5	195.3	344.6	511.9	802.8	1097.4
White males	185.1	8.5	13.7	19.1	33.6	65.3	122.9	225.4	397.4	617.0	1221.2
1976											
Black females	126.8	4.2	12.3	25.8	48.4	100.3	177.3	290.6	377.7	491.1	730.3
White females	162.0	4.7	10.3	20.3	38.6	71.0	131.3	209.5	306.3	420.7	744.9
Black males	193.5	6.0	11.4	18.4	40.0	108.8	223.2	418.2	666.6	970.4	1475.0
White males	199.2	6.8	12.1	16.4	29.8	58.7	124.7	225.1	382.7	630.5	1318.3

Source: U.S. Department of Health, Education, and Welfare (1978:192–195).

longevity and better reporting, have influenced the rising black cancer mortality rates. Henschke and his colleagues indicated that "environmental factors could well explain the marked changes in the black cancer mortality rates between 1950 and 1967" (1973:768). Factors such as earlier detection and better treatment have influenced the diminishing black cancer mortality rates, depending on the age groups examined. Some of the apparent racial variation may also be explained by different patterns of drug abuse, smoking, or sexual intercourse. But comparisons based on adequate controls of socioeconomic status (especially occupation) and other predisposing variables may well show that race does not explain black-white variations in cancer patterns, with the possible exception of skin cancers. In a comparison of cancer patients in public and private hospitals, using data from the California Tukor Registry, Linden concluded that "the factor responsible for the level of early diagnosis was social class rather than race" (1969:268).

Using the National Cancer Incidence surveys of 1947 and 1969, Seidman, Silverberg, and Holleb (1976:5) compared incidence rates for cancers of various sites among black and white females and males. For all sites, the black male rate of 248.0 per 100,000 in 1947 rose to 337.2 in 1969, a 36.0 percent change over time. This increase is undoubtedly due in part to an increase in the longevity of black males between these two time periods. Comparable data for white males were 282.0 to 300.8 (6.7 percent); for black females, 287.0 to 242.9 (−15.4 percent); and for white females, 294.0 to 255.5 (−13.1 percent). Cancer sites that showed an increased incidence among black males over time were the esophagus, colon-rectum, pancreas, lung, prostate, kidney, and bladder. (With the exception of the esophagus, similar but smaller increases occurred among white males.) The sites at which increases were observed for black females included the esophagus, colon-rectum, pancreas, lung, breast, and kidney. (The white female increases were also of lesser magnitude than those among black females.)

SUICIDE RATES, 1977   The age and sex variations in black and white mortality rates, especially for suicide, help reinforce the case for the necessity of breaking out mortality data by race-sex-age categories. Table 1.6 shows suicide rates by age for black and white females and males. The groups differ by the age of peak periods for suicide. The curvilinear relationships between age and suicide for black and white females and the linear one for white males are quite different from the very weak relationship between age and suicide for black males. Different peak periods of emotional crises during the life cycle seem to occur for each of the groups, with black females being most vulnerable during the years coinciding with the early years of marriage and child rearing.

Table 1.6   Suicide rates per 100,000 resident population for black and white females and males, by age, United States, 1977.

Age (years)	Black females	White females	Black males	White males
All ages	3.0	7.3	10.7	21.4
Under 15	0.2	0.2	0.3	0.9
15–24	3.9	5.5	14.1	23.0
25–34	6.1	9.4	15.8	26.6
35–44	4.8	11.2	14.8	24.7
45–54	4.0	13.6	11.5	27.3
55–64	3.5	6.1	12.6	31.0
65–74	1.6	9.3	10.9	38.1
75+	2.2	9.4	16.6	48.8

Source: Raw data from the National Center for Health Statistics.

How reliable are suicide data? Warshauer and Monk concluded from their study of the accuracy of New York City suicide data for the period 1968–1970 that it is "unwise to compare official suicide rates for different groups or geographic areas unless a careful study is made of the way in which deaths are assigned and classified as suicide . . . Studies are needed to determine how and to what extent the investigation, reporting, and classification of suicide deaths . . . before and after 1968, affect the differences in suicide rates between whites and blacks, or between the occupational or age groups. Until this is done, official suicide statistics . . . should be accepted with extreme caution" (1978:388).

Given the need for more reliable data, Rockwell and O'Brien's concerns (1973) about upgrading physicians' knowledge about suicide is welcome, since physicians are those who most often treat suicidally prone individuals. However, although these researchers were aware of the fact that urban black and white suicide rates were becoming somewhat more similar, they nevertheless stressed, without any racial differentiation, that persons over 60 years of age constituted the most vulnerable suicidal group. This is generally not true for urban blacks. Hendin's observations about differential age peaks and the etiology of suicide among blacks and whites are instructive here: "Among young black urban adults between the ages of 20 and 35, suicide has been considerably higher than among their white counterparts. However, this fact was ignored or obscured by the attention and concern generated by black homicide in the same age group and *because among older age groups suicide was a much greater problem among whites*" (1978:105; emphasis added).

Hendin's position is certainly more plausible and empirically more sound than the one taken by Edland and Duncan, who, in a study of suicides in Monroe County, New York between 1950 and 1972, concluded that "Negroes rarely commit suicide, and a suspected suicide in this group raises the suspicion that the death may actually be a concealed homicide" (1973:366). This conclusion is a good example of how racial bias affects research outcomes. Many physicians who harbor racial biases may also be unduly suspicious of certain conditions merely because they occur in blacks. Thus, it is important to remember that not only do some black women develop endometriosis, but some blacks also commit suicide.

Hendin posits environmental differences as the source of black-white variations in suicide patterns in the United States.

With both black homicide and black suicide, one is dealing basically with a problem of the ghetto, i.e., with the poorest socioeconomic group among the black population . . . A sense of despair, a feeling that life will never be satisfying confronts many blacks at a far younger age than it does most whites. For most discontented white people the young adult years contain the hope of a change for the better. The rise in white suicide after 45 reflects, among other things, the waning of such hope that is bound to accompany age. Those blacks in the ghetto who survive past their more dangerous years between 20 and 35 have made some accommodation with life—a compromise that has usually had to include a scaling down of their aspirations. (1978:105, 109)

Morbidity Data: Prevalence Rates and Restricted Activity

Table 1.7 contains prevalence rates for certain chronic conditions for nonwhites and whites. The data were the latest available in published form as of May, 1979. No breakouts by sex were available. Only 18 of the 39 racial comparisons (or 46.2 percent) were higher for nonwhites than for whites. It is possible that the apparently better perceptions of health conditions among Asian Americans deflected black perceptual rates. That is, the nonwhite and black rates are not necessarily synonymous. Some of the non-black nonwhites were also, no doubt, recent immigrants, but these data do not permit that determination.

TUBERCULOSIS In addition to the rates in table 1.7, other data showed that the 1976 tuberculosis case rates per 100,000 resident population were 64.2 for nonwhite males and much lower, 33.3, for nonwhite females. The larger the size of the city, the higher was the rate (U.S. Department of Health, Education, and Welfare 1978), which is in line with reported problems about low birth weights, lack of immunizations, and the like.

Table 1.7 Prevalence rates per 1,000 for selected chronic conditions reported in NCHS health interviews by nonwhites and whites, by age, United States, 1968–1976.

Condition and year data collected	Nonwhites				Whites			
	Under 17 yrs.	17–44 yrs.	45–64 yrs.	65+ yrs.	Under 17 yrs.	17–44 yrs.	45–64 yrs.	65+ yrs.
Hernia of abdominal cavity (1968)	—	—	13.3	33.9	—	—	29.9	61.0
Ulcer of stomach or duodenum (1968)	—	—	32.6	—	—	—	33.5	—
Arthritis (1969)	—	41.4	221.8	424.8	—	40.2	202.4	376.3
Asthma (1970)	38.2	25.2	44.5	42.9	29.8	26.3	31.9	35.2
Chronic bronchitis (1970)	22.7	14.2	23.5	26.0	41.8	24.5	36.6	42.5
Hearing impairments (1971)	11.1	29.7	88.7	237.5	13.3	44.2	116.8	299.4
Vision impairments (1971)	7.9	27.2	99.6	245.7	9.6	32.6	59.1	200.9
Impairment of back or spine except paralysis (1971)	—	33.0	80.7	81.9	—	51.3	66.8	65.8
Heart conditions (1972)	9.0	27.5	91.6	185.2	10.8	24.2	88.4	200.0
Hypertension without heart involvement (1972)	—	62.3	196.8	248.7	—	34.4	119.1	194.6
Diabetes (1973)	—	12.8	70.0	104.5	—	6.8	39.6	75.9
Dermatophytosis and dermatomycoses (1976)	1.5[a]	3.2	1.8[a]	—	1.9	3.6	3.0	—
Neoplasms of the skin (1976)	0.5[a]	0.4[a]	2.9[a]	3.0[a]	0.5[a]	3.1	11.9	18.3
Chronic infections of skin and subcutaneous tissue not elsewhere classified (1976)	1.5[a]	1.4[a]	1.4[a]	—	0.7	1.9	1.1	—
Eczema, dermatitis, and urticaria not elsewhere classified (1979)	28.7	28.1	27.1	10.3[a]	40.3	40.1	34.5	33.3
Psoriasis and similar disorders (1976)	1.8[a]	3.1	6.2[a]	3.4[a]	2.4	10.2	14.3	14.7

Table 1.7 (continued).

Condition and year data collected	Nonwhites				Whites			
	Under 17 yrs.	17–44 yrs.	45–64 yrs.	65+ yrs.	Under 17 yrs.	17–44 yrs.	45–64 yrs.	65+ yrs.
Other inflammatory conditions of skin and subcutaneous tissue (1976)	2.7[a]	9.9	10.0	16.7[a]	4.6	9.7	10.3	20.2
Corns and callosities (1976)	2.0[a]	32.7	90.5	102.5[a]	0.7[a]	19.2	47.2	66.1
Other hypertrophic and atropic conditions (1976)	4.1	6.0	5.1[a]	3.0[a]	4.9	8.1	9.4	13.3
Diseases of nail (1976)	1.4[a]	14.9	28.0	51.7	6.1	20.3	28.1	47.1
Diseases of sebaceous glands not elsewhere classified (1976)	8.7	19.5	9.3	0.5[a]	24.7	44.0	12.0	7.6
Other diseases of skin and subcutaneous tissue not elsewhere classified (1976)	3.7	6.5	8.0	9.4[a]	2.3	6.4	6.1	11.5
Arthritis not elsewhere classified (1976)	2.1[a]	41.7	291.8	482.8	2.3	46.1	251.6	431.9
Rheumatism, nonarticular and unspecified (1976)	—	1.0[a]	9.3	32.5	0.2[a]	2.2	6.7	14.3
Osteomyelitis and other diseases of bone (1976)	1.4[a]	2.8[a]	5.3[a]	4.9[a]	2.0	6.3	17.0	19.1
Displacement of intervertebral disc (1976)	0.4[a]	7.2	18.5	14.3[a]	0.2[a]	13.4	27.6	19.2
Bunion (1976)	0.1[a]	8.7	27.8	32.5	0.3[a]	4.0	16.1	31.9
Synovitis, bursitis, and tenosynovitis (1976)	0.9[a]	6.6	24.7	17.2	1.3	17.9	45.9	31.7
Gout (1976)	—	1.2[a]	18.7	27.1	0.0[a]	4.2	18.4	23.8

Source: U.S. Department of Health, Education, and Welfare (1976); Bonham (1978).

a. Unreliable estimates.

LIMITATION OF ACTIVITY DUE TO CHRONIC CONDITIONS   The data in table 1.8 show the percentage of blacks and others of non-Spanish origin with limitation of activity because of chronic conditions, by different levels of income and age in 1976. These data indicate that in general, income was inversely related to and age positively related to limitation of activity.

Table 1.8   Percentage of blacks and others of non-Spanish origin with limitation of activity because of chronic conditions, by family income and age, United States, 1976.

Income and age (years)	Blacks	Others, non-Spanish origin[a]
All incomes		
All ages	14.8	14.6
Under 17	3.7	3.9
17–44	10.5	8.7
45–64	32.3	23.4
65+	52.8	44.6
Less than $5,000		
All ages	24.9	31.3
Under 17	4.8	5.7
17–44	16.7	14.5
45–64	51.8	49.0
65+	59.4	52.7
$5,000–$9,999		
All ages	12.3	19.0
Under 17	4.1	4.5
17–44	10.0	10.8
45–64	29.1	31.9
65+	46.5	42.9
$10,000–$14,999		
All ages	9.7	11.8
Under 17	2.8	3.9
17–44	8.1	8.8
45–64	24.4	22.6
65+	41.2	39.0
$15,000+		
All ages	7.1	9.0
Under 17	2.8	3.4
17–44	6.1	6.6
45–64	14.3	15.8
65+	40.7	38.2

Source: Moy and Wilder (1978).
a. Includes all persons who were neither black nor of Spanish origin.

When the data were age-adjusted for specific income levels, the black percentages were slightly higher than those of all others under $5,000 (24.9 percent versus 23.0 percent), slightly lower for the categories $5,000–$9,999 (16.0 percent versus 16.6 percent) and $15,000+ (10.4 percent versus 10.8 percent), and the same for $10,000–$14,999 (13.3 percent).

The data in table 1.9 represent the number of days of bed disability per

Table 1.9 Days of bed disability per person per year for blacks and others of non-Spanish origin, by family income and age, United States, 1976.

Income and age (years)	Blacks	Others, non-Spanish origin[a]
All incomes		
All ages	9.0	6.8
Under 17	3.9	5.0
17–44	8.5	5.1
45–64	16.9	8.0
65+	18.5	14.6
Less than $5,000		
All ages	12.3	11.7
Under 17	5.0	6.7
17–44	11.7	7.5
45–64	22.3	16.9
65+	19.7	15.9
$5,000–$9,999		
All ages	7.7	8.4
Under 17	3.5	5.3
17–44	7.5	6.1
45–64	15.4	11.4
65+	19.7	14.2
$10,000–$14,999		
All ages	5.9	5.9
Under 17	3.5	4.5
17–44	6.5	5.3
45–64	10.6	7.3
65+	0.9[b]	12.3
$15,000+		
All ages	7.5	4.9
Under 17	3.8[b]	4.8
17–44	7.2	4.0
45–64	14.3	5.4
65+	14.8[b]	13.2

Source: Moy and Wilder (1978).

a. Includes all persons who were neither black nor of Spanish origin.

b. Figure does not meet standards of reliability or precision.

person per year for blacks and for others of non-Spanish origin. The unreliability of the data (due to inadequate sampling sizes) for elderly blacks in the two highest income groups and for the youngest age group in the highest income category for blacks hampers comparisons by age and income levels. Though the general pattern is similar to limitation of activity, in that age is positively related and income is negatively related to number of days of bed disability, these relationships are not as pronounced. For example, among blacks, the bed disability rate among those 45 to 64 years of age in the top income group was higher than in the income group immediately below it. When the data were age-adjusted, the bed disability rate was higher among blacks than among all others for the lowest and highest income groups, lower in the $5,000–$9,999 income group, and the same for those whose family incomes were between $10,000 and $14,999.

These rates for limitation of activity by chronic conditions and days of bed disability are important in that, contrary to popular beliefs, they show clearly that blacks are not adversely affected solely on the basis of race. Social class is highly influential in affecting chronicity and disability.

SICKLE-CELL ANEMIA AND TRAIT   It is currently estimated that roughly 1 in 500 black children born in the United States has sickle-cell anemia (see, for example, Culliton 1972). This estimate, repeated frequently in recent literature, seems to have come latest from Neel (1950, 1951). Pearson and O'Brien, who urged "routine screening of the cord blood of black and *Puerto Rican* infants for sickle-cell anemia," indicated that the estimate of 1 in 500 was "based on a prevalence rate of 8 percent of sickle cell trait in black American populations and on a one-fourth probability with each pregnancy" (1972:1201; emphasis added). Webb indicated that although most persons with sickle-cell anemia are black, "some are Caucasions of Mediterranean origin. Sickling of the blood has also been reported in American Indians, and in inhabitants of South India, the Middle East and the Caribbean countries" (1972:198). With regard to sickling-related immunity to malaria, the Vietnam war provided an opportunity to reexamine race-specific incidences of malaria (Fisher et al. 1970).

Although I was unable to locate prevalence rates for sickle-cell anemia for American Indians or other affected groups residing in the United States, it seems apparent that deliverers of mainstream medical care to ethnic groups will have to be increasingly conscious of the effects of racial amalgamation. For example, in instances of amalgamation between blacks and Indians, some offspring racially classify themselves as blacks, whereas others are categorized as Indians. Those presenting themselves in the former category would be much more likely to be viewed as subjects for sickle-cell testing, but it may also be appropriate for the latter category too.

Obstetricians remain divided in their opinions about primary sterilization of women with sickle-cell disease. Fort and his colleagues, white members of the Department of Obstetrics and Gynecology, University of Tennessee College of Medicine, believe that "the expected rate of reproductive success, when considered in conjunction with the negative attributes concerning motherhood, does not justify a young woman with sickle cell disease being exposed to the risk of pregnancy. We advocate primary sterilization, abortion if conception occurs, and sterilization for those that have completed pregnancies. Patients with sickle-cell disease should be unhesitatingly thus counseled" (1971:327). These researchers reported a maternal mortality rate of 10 percent for their sickle-cell disease patients who were pregnant. In marked contrast, Foster, the black chairman of the Department of Obstetrics and Gynecology at Meharry Medical College, Nashville, Tennessee, believed that the high maternal mortality rate reported by Fort and his colleagues reflected insufficient prenatal care. Foster, who supports options to risk pregnancies among women with sickle-cell disease, stressed that "one of our greatest concerns of management when sickle-cell disease is a complication relates to the type of advice and counsel provided to black patients regarding potential risks they incur when pregnant. Too often, the counsel provided is highly inadequate, misleading, and, on occasion, dangerous. In order to obtain the very best maternal and child health outcomes for these patients, there must be provided accurate screening, informed counseling, and exemplary clinical management. Without this sequential three-pronged approach, maternal mortality figures can be expected to approach those reported [by the University of Tennessee College of Medicine]" (1977:20).

Findings about complicating risks associated with pregnancy in women with the sickle-cell trait are also inconclusive, as evidenced, for instance, by Rimer's report (1975) of heightened incidence of premature rupture of the membranes at Charlotte (North Carolina) Memorial Hospital, and Foster's indication (1977) that the phenomenon had not been observed at Meharry.

Fertility, Infant Mortality, and Related Patterns

The total fertility rate (the sum of birth rates by age, multiplied by 5) declined from 4,541.8 in 1960 to 2,253.3 in 1976 among black females 10 to 49 years of age. Nevertheless, the black rate remained higher than that of whites, primarily because of earlier sexual activity, proportionately more low-income persons in the group, and less access to safe abortions among blacks than whites. As the abortion rate among all women in the United States has risen steadily in recent years (20.5 per 1,000 women 15 to 44 years of age in 1976), a disproportionately high proportion (about one-third) of these abortions were performed on nonwhite women. Yet, if results obtained in Georgia (Rochat, Tyler, and Schoenbucher 1971) prevail elsewhere, it is probable that there is less decline in abortion mortality among blacks than whites.

LOW BIRTH WEIGHT   Aside from accidents, the disorders most prevalent among black infants are related to low birth weights and congenital anomalies. Although the data are inconclusive, low birth weights seem to be related to prenatal care.

Taffel's findings (1978a) about prenatal care among blacks in 1969 and 1975 showed some increase in prenatal care over time. The proportion of pregnant black females beginning prenatal care in the first trimester rose from about 43 to 56 percent in the reporting 42 states and the District of Columbia. The proportion without prenatal care was almost cut in half during the same period, from 5.1 to 2.7 percent. Early prenatal care was more likely with second than first or higher order pregnancies. Women who were not at least high school graduates were far less likely than their more educated counterparts to seek prenatal care.

Among many lower-class women, a major deterrent to prenatal care has been a prevailing belief that the natural function of childbearing requires no medical intervention until the delivery stage. But even among those who may have desired care, other problems deterred them, including inadequate funds or lack of free access, difficulty in arranging medical visits, and the "forbidding settings and brusqueness" of some maternity clinics. Moreover, many unwed mothers attempted to conceal pregnancies as long as possible (Taffel 1978a:4–5).

Using data from 38 reporting states and the District of Columbia, Taffel (1978a) reported that the 1975 average of 11.1 prenatal visits of metropolitan women was higher than those of 10.3 for nonmetropolitan women, but the risk of low birth weight was higher among metropolitan black infants. Poverty is more abject in central cities, where home-grown foods are also generally absent. Within cities, then, there is clearly a need for more current and useful data for each census tract about the prevalence of various conditions, including infant mortality. Poverty and not race may be critical in certain respects, except as these factors relate to the availability and atmosphere of maternity or pediatric clinics. In addition, it would be helpful to determine the proportion of black infant mortality attributable to sickle cell in order to provide better information for reducing that mortality in metropolitan and other areas.

Gallagher's study (1978) of black and white prenatal, infant, and family care in three Kentucky counties provides a good example of racial comparisons under conditions adequately controlled for socioeconomic status. Also cognizant of the interaction of race and social class, Gallagher constructed a black-white comparison group of mothers who were residents of the same predominantly urban county, and who were matched by social class, age, and number of children. The few statistically significant racial differences that emerged were largely functions of the social system, such as the exclusion of blacks from one hospital, which led to racial differences in hospital use.

Although much remains to be learned about the etiology of low birth weight and infant mortality, the availability of black low-income pregnant women or mothers and their babies in areas with major medical centers encourages research (see, for example, Watkins 1968; Terris and Gold 1969; Bergner and Susser 1970; Erhardt and Chase 1973; Osofsky and Kendall 1973). It is quite likely that reasonable solutions facilitating the reduction of prematurity or infant mortality among poor black women will be available for effective action in the near future.

CONGENITAL ANOMALIES   Using data from 46 reporting states and the District of Columbia, Taffel (1978b) also described and analyzed black and white birth with congenital anomalies. In general, incidence rates for black females and males at birth were lower than for the total population by sex. (All congenital anomalies for the total population of females at birth were 677.6 per 100,000; for black females, 640.7; for all males, 938.2; and for black males, 800.1.) Polydactyly was the modal anomaly among blacks. The expected relationships between congenital anomalies and other variables were found; that is, they were more prevalent among males and more likely to be associated with low birth weights, older mothers, first births, plural deliveries, close spacing of pregnancies, and poorly educated mothers. Taffel indicated that "it was not possible to determine to what extent the reported racial difference in the level of anomalies was associated with socioeconomic differences" (1978b:6). Various reporting difficulties also precluded resolution of the issue of racial differences in the true incidence of congenital anomalies.

Some similarities exist between patterns of congenital anomalies and birth injuries in that the latter are also higher among males. Birth injuries are also higher among whites: the 1974 rates were 217.9 and 191.3 per 100,000 live births for whites and blacks, respectively. Injuries, as expected, were also much greater among very small and very large than among moderately-sized babies for both racial groups.

Although most blacks have lacked medical sophistication concerning the problems associated with low-birth-weight babies, for many years they have believed that these babies are unhealthy or at high risk for serious disorders or death. Conversely, they have equated "good-sized" babies with healthy babies, unless physical defects were present. They have therefore urged food on their infants and cautioned expectant mothers "to eat enough for two," initiating a pattern that predisposed some children to obesity in later life.

Risk Factors among Blacks

IMMUNIZATION AND INFECTION STATUS OF CHILDREN, 1976 Table 1.10 shows the percentages of nonwhite and white children in two age groups who had been immunized against or affected by measles, rubella, diphtheria-tetanus-pertussis, polio, and mumps within central cities. Among metropolitan blacks, immunizations were least likely among the poor in central cities. Earlier, Hinman noted that a recent upswing in measles was "affecting primarily 5–9 year-old black city dwellers" (1972: 500). The more recent data in table 1.10 probably reflect insufficient vaccinations among this group. In order to combat this trend of insufficient immunization among black children, pediatricians might emphasize the importance of completing immunizations each time injections are given and arrange to have postcards sent out or telephone calls made at appropriate times to remind mothers of the need for subsequent or new im-

Table 1.10 Immunization and infection status of nonwhite and white children, 1–9 years of age, civilian noninstitutionalized population living in central cities, Standard Metropolitan Statistical Areas, United States, 1976.

Immunization and infection status	Nonwhites		Whites	
	1–4 yrs.	5–9 yrs.	1–4 yrs.	5–9 yrs.
Measles				
% infected	5.4	14.6	6.0	12.5
% vaccinated	54.0	61.4	66.8	76.3
Rubella				
% infected	10.1	16.3	9.1	19.3
% vaccinated	51.7	64.9	63.4	70.0
Diphtheria-tetanus-pertussis				
% 3+ doses	49.4	61.2	71.5	78.4
% no doses	4.4	2.2	4.4	1.6
Polio				
% 3+ doses	38.4	52.1	61.7	73.3
% no doses	15.4	9.3	8.4	3.7
Mumps				
% vaccinated	41.0	40.7	47.9	49.3

Source: U.S. Department of Health, Education, and Welfare (1978:209).

munizations. Not all black children, of course, are under the regular care of pediatricians, so other methods must be tried as well.

Based on their experiences in the Watts Multipurpose Health Center and elsewhere, Bates, Lieberman, and Powell (1970) indicated that immunizations, preventive medicine, and annual examinations were unaffordable luxuries for the poor, including poor blacks. In an analysis of records of a random sample of registered families at the same center, Lieberman (1974) found a sizable proportion of all the family members under 17 years of age without adequate immunizations. In addition to finding that those most distant geographically from the center were least likely to obtain care there, Lieberman concluded that "after acute environmental problems are being satisfactorily solved, patients are more willing to consider the preventive aspects of care being offered" (1974: 54). Thus another challenge to pediatricians may be to help improve environmental conditions for many poor blacks. For example, politically active pediatricians may wish to help strengthen the educational curricula of public elementary and secondary schools in central cities by emphasizing publically the need for good education in a child's developmental years.

In Tulsa, Oklahoma, Stewart and Hood found that "indigenous persons (a) can effectively improve the immunization level of the population of hard-core areas, (b) can become more effective with experience, and (c) should be continuously employed in these areas" (1970:184). Further, "health representatives who 'speak the language,' have similar value systems, a desire to raise the general health level of the Negro community, and have the same racial characteristics should be better able to assist in raising immunization levels than persons who do not possess these characteristics" (1970:179). This view may challenge pediatricians to help identify and train indigenous workers.

However, in another context concerning health behaviors, Holder observed that "it is naive to believe that a person who is a member of a population group can always influence his peers to act in some specific manner or is necessarily superior to an outsider, such as a professional worker, in ability to influence" (1972:349). Wan and Gray (1978) examined the use of immunizations (poliomyelitis and diphtheria-pertussis-tetanus) among preschool children in five low-income urban areas and found that having a regular source of care was significant, that age was the best predictor of immunizations, and that children having neighborhood health centers and public health clinics as their regular sources of care had immunization rates comparable to those with private physicians as their regular source of care. It is likely that the periodic assignment of public health nurses to nursery, elementary, and secondary schools and day-care centers to provide necessary immunizations to children on site would be extremely helpful. Unfortunately, far too many school districts today simply dismiss insufficiently immunized children from school until proof of requisite immunizations is produced.

OBESITY   Table 1.11 contains self-reported and clinically determined obesity data for black females and males in 1974. The clinical diagnosis, based on triceps skinfold measurements, was defined as falling above the sex-specific 85th percentile measurements for persons 20 to 29 years of age. In general, obesity was substantially greater among females than males, a not unexpected finding. Among the males, those who were least

Table 1.11 Self-reported and clinical determinations of obesity among black females and males, by age and income levels, United States, 1974.

Determination of obesity, age, and income	Percentage	
	Black females	**Black males**
Self-reported obesity		
17–44 years		
Less than $5,000	45.3	14.2
$5,000–9,999	42.5	18.8
$10,000–14,999	46.2	19.5
$15,000+	49.9	28.7
45–64 years		
Less than $5,000	48.8	8.5
$5,000–9,999	59.9	23.7
$10,000–14,999	48.6	27.5
$15,000+	49.8	40.8
65+ years		
Less than $5,000	17.4	14.0
$5,000–9,999	39.0	14.0
$10,000–14,999	23.8	49.4
$15,000+	32.9	29.5
Clinically determined obesity		
20–44 years		
Below poverty level	27.6	11.1
Above poverty level	24.0	14.6
45–64 years		
Below poverty level	49.4	3.7
Above poverty level	40.0	12.4
65–74 years		
Below poverty level	23.2	4.6
Above poverty level	36.3	7.0

Source: U.S. Department of Health, Education, and Welfare (1978:215).

obese were also poor. Overall, income had a more pronounced effect on obesity among males. Ostfeld and his colleagues (1971) reported substantially higher prevalence rates per 1,000 among black women (548) than black men (325) in their study of obesity among noninstitutionalized welfare recipients of ages 65 to 74 in Chicago.

CIGARETTE SMOKING AND DRINKING   Table 1.12 shows the percentages for three different cigarette smoking patterns among blacks over 20 years of age, by sex, in 1965 and 1976. As expected, current smokers were proportionately greater among males; well over half of the non-elderly males smoked in 1976, as did more than a third of the women in the same age range. In a retrospective study of predominantly low-income black females in Buffalo, New York which investigated social and psychological correlates of smoking behavior among the women, Warnecke and his co-workers indicated that "black females are more likely than white females to smoke and less likely to have quit" (1978:401). They also indicated that greater smoking in urban than in rural areas was generally well documented.

Table 1.12   Cigarette smoking statuses among black females and males, 20+ years of age, United States, 1965 and 1976.

Year, sex, and age (years)	Never smoked (%)	Former smoker (%)	Current smoker (%)
1965			
Black females, 20+	59.6	6.0	34.4
Black males, 20+	27.0	12.1	60.8
1976			
Black females			
20–24	60.1	5.0	34.9
25–34	48.6	8.9	42.5
35–44	49.1	9.6	41.3
45–64	50.0	11.9	38.1
65+	77.4	13.3	9.2
Black males			
20–24	43.1	4.1	52.8
25–34	28.9	11.8	59.4
35–44	27.3	13.8	58.8
45–64	21.7	28.6	49.7
65+	40.5	33.0	26.4

Source: U.S. Department of Health, Education, and Welfare (1978:220–221).

Data about alcohol consumption among blacks 12 to 74 years of age in the period 1971–1975 showed that almost two-thirds had taken at least one drink during the year preceding the interview. About 12 percent drank every day or almost every day; about 12 percent, two or three times weekly; about 24 percent, one to four times monthly; and the remaining one-fifth drank less than one drink monthly (U.S. Department of Health, Education, and Welfare 1978). Among their white counterparts, a higher proportion (73 percent) had taken at least one drink during the preceding year, but a much smaller proportion (6 percent) drank daily or almost daily. Slightly more than 12 percent of whites reported drinking about two or three times weekly, almost 24 percent about one to four times monthly, and almost 22 percent less than one per month (U.S. Department of Health, Education, and Welfare 1978). Excessive drinking is generally regarded as being more common among blacks than whites. If so, it may be due to greater stress in this population.

In a study of black male adults born in St. Louis between 1930 and 1934, Robins, Murphy, and Breckenridge (1968) found that only 4 percent had always been non-drinkers. About two-thirds of the subjects took their first drink prior to becoming 17 years old, and about 59 percent had been heavy drinkers at some point in their lives. About 28 percent reported some medical complication associated with drinking, most often tremulousness. Their longitudinal study showed that the subjects, as boys, who were at greatest risk for becoming heavy or problem drinkers were those whose delinquency began later and who failed to complete high school. These risk factors were similar to those found among white boys who later became heavy or problem drinkers.

Concepts of Disease and Illness

Major Nosological and Etiological Taxonomies

The descriptions and analyses of folk medicine among urban blacks that I located contained limited information about theories of disease and illness and types of treatment used, and relatively little information about the prevalence of use of nonmainstream medical care or of particular problems or benefits associated with that care. Almost no empirical attention has been given to ways in which major nosological and etiological taxonomies or ideas used by urban blacks from folk, popular, and biomedical sources merge or interdigitate. In this regard, however, it is important to recall the frequent time lag between new scientific discoveries or developments and the public's awareness of them. Consider Kampmeier's notion about a medical remedy for syphilis, where his "introduction to antisyphilitic treatment was in 1921 as an apprentice to a physician who treated many syphilitic patients. Neoarsphenamine was given weekly accompanied by a unique method of mercurial inunction.

Unguenti Hydrargyri was spread thickly with a tongue blade upon the patient's bared back from nape to lumbar area, and from one posterior axillary line to the other. Then a clean *woolen* undershirt was put on and patted into the ointment, the whole to be worn a week without removal in the heat of an Iowa summer, to be repeated week after week; its efficacy was attested to by the salivation produced" (1974:1350). Many contemporary physicians have doubtless never heard of this medical prescription. The point is that much of the content of folk medicine has been derived from the mainstream medicine of another day, just as mainstream medicine has borrowed much from folk medicine.

Charles James, a black physician who has been in private practice in Charlotte, North Carolina for almost three decades, believes that most urban black physicians are aware of the various concepts of disease and illness held by their patients. Consciously or unconsciously, they must conduct at least informal research to improve their own understanding of their patients, a factor important in providing effective care. These physicians, who are frequently knowledgeable about the cultural environments of their patients, often share their findings informally with each other but rarely publish them.

ETIOLOGICAL CONCEPTS Snow (1978), whose writings about black folk medicine are based primarily on small and nonrepresentative samples in Phoenix, Arizona and Lansing, Michigan, reports no distinction between science and religion in the low-income black folk health system, where, she claims, symptoms are regarded as irrelevant in diagnosing problems. Instead, the system focuses on the etiology of the illness, which may be variously attributed to divine punishment, worry, or sorcery. But James believes that biomedical definitions typically underlie the major nosological taxonomies used by urban blacks, who often broadly classify their diseases in simplified terms: for example, ischemic or coronary heart disorders become "heart trouble." Sometimes diseases are labeled etiologically, as in the transformation of diabetes mellitus into "sugar diabetes" or just "sugar."

Etiological ideas are based on folk, popular, and biomedical sources, depending on the types of knowledge that are most prevalent among specific groups of urban blacks. Older cohorts tend to rely more heavily on folk or popular sources, as do many rural migrants. Younger cohorts, who are generally better educated, rely more heavily on biomedical sources, although many of them still retain folk and popular conceptions. This fact is important in that most persons—urban or rural, black or white—often treat themselves for illnesses they believe will respond adequately to self-treatment.

Snow (1974) believes that hexing as an etiological notion crystallized as a part of the black folk medical system following slavery. A composite of classical medicine and European and African beliefs, it was not unique to blacks, however. Hexing or "root work" was also widespread among Southern whites (see Webb 1971; Rocereto 1973; Wintrob 1973). Ignoring the admixture, however, Whitten attributes the origin of occult beliefs and practices among blacks in the Piedmont region of North Carolina solely to whites, holding that they were "part of a pattern of magical thought brought to the Piedmont by the seventeenth- and eighteenth-century colonists from Europe. From the white colonists these beliefs and practices diffused to the Negroes among whom they persist" (1962:312). (Whitten apparently felt that such beliefs and practices no longer persist among whites.)

Among urban blacks, considerable attention is also focused on the etiological role of stress in inducing physical and mental illnesses. Many blacks believe that stress (especially that induced by the effects of racism) causes hypertension. Although etiological uncertainty exists among physicians, many black (and perhaps other) physicians also cite racism as being at least a contributory cause. Ostfeld, who disputes the notion that rapid social change and accompanying stress tend to elevate blood pressures, contends that there is "no reason to believe that social pressure in itself causes changes in [blood] pressure"; rather, the elevation is more closely "related to changes in diet and physical activity than to social pressures" (1977:61).

Many blacks also believe that diabetes is induced by "worriation," and some ministers have reinforced this notion in their sermons or when they visit the sick. Interestingly, some recent research results from studies by Robert S. Sherwin and his associates, as well as David Diebert and Roy DeFronzo and their associates (all at Yale University School of Medicine), lend some support to the etiology of "worriation." Specifically, their results showed that "the activity of insulin in the human body is exquisitely sensitive to small amounts of the stress hormone adrenalin," a discovery they believe has important implications for the widespread use of early diabetes testing and perhaps for better understanding of the nature of this common and serious illness (*New York Times* 1979:C1–C2).

ILLNESS LABELS   In a study that included 120 Southern black, predominantly poor households in the catchment area of a pediatric Comprehensive Health Care program at the University of Miami School of Medicine, Miami, Florida, Weidman (1978) presented a "Southern Black Ethnic Symptom and Condition List" in which *etic* refers to the scientific understanding of terms (or the outsider's perspective) and *emic* refers to the subcultural understanding (or from within). Since then,

Weidman has deleted 12 of the 23 symptoms and conditions in the original list because her subsequent work has led her to believe that the conceptions of those symptoms and conditions were not unique to Southern blacks as represented by her sample of largely poor, inner-city black residents of Miami. It may well be that further work will reveal that the symptoms and conditions remaining in Weidman's list (table 1.13)

Table 1.13 "Southern black" ethnic symptoms and conditions

Condition or symptom	Description[a]
Tedder(s)	A scalp condition characterized by whitish, dry, scaly patches accompanied by loss of hair from the affected area; occurs primarily on children's heads, spreads into clusters, and is highly communicable.
Gas	Stomach gas in greater amounts than usual, characterized by a feeling of fullness and sometimes pressure in the chest area; also pockets of gas which cause pain in other parts of the body and shoulder. It occurs after having missed a meal and also because of certain "heavy" foods which are "slow to digest."
Falling-out	A condition characterized by a sudden collapse, during which the eyes usually remain open but "not seeing" and with hearing unimpaired. May be preceded briefly by weakness, "swinging" or "swimming in the head." The semiconscious state is usually of brief but of varying duration. It is said that "high blood" is the primary cause of falling-out; although "low-blood" may also be implicated. (For a more complete discussion, see Weidman 1979).
Ear noises	A condition characterized by a "ringing" or "buzzing" in one or both ears. Not usually discussed, because such sounds may mean "death"; sometimes interpreted as "spirits calling."
Bruised blood	Blood that is "left" in one spot, following a blow or bruise of some sort, becoming darker in color because it no longer moves.
High blood	A state in which the blood collects high in the body and tends to stay there, sometimes causing "swimming" or "swinging" in the head; also, a state in which the blood rushes to the head and causes "falling-out" spells. Less commonly, a state in which the "pressure" or blood volume is high throughout the body.

Table 1.13   (continued).

Condition or symptom	Description[a]
Low blood	A state in which there is not enough blood to allow the body to function properly; also, a condition characterized by a lack of "iron" and other nutrients required to nourish the body adequately.
Bad blood	A diseased condition of the blood which can occur from various types of contamination (natural, supernatural, hereditary); may be reflected in behavior or physical problems. Because *etic* "syphilis" connotes promiscuity and association with "low class" types of persons, "bad blood" is a preferable term for older individuals, but it is a category broader than "syphilis."
Clots	A condition in which portions of the blood stop moving, settle in a localized area, and become thick and dark in color; frequently associated with abdominal and leg cramps during menstruation. Also associated with references to "thickened blood" and "cold."
Unclean blood	A state in which impurities have collected in the blood after a period of time, i.e., during the winter months, when the blood is "thickened" and carries more "heat."
Thin blood	A state in which the blood is not thick enough to nourish and heat the body properly; said to cause a person to feel "chilly" all the time; related to "low blood" and/or insufficient "iron" in the blood.

Source: Adapted from Weidman (1978:Appendix E).

a. For more detailed descriptions, see the original source as well as Weidman 1979.

are also not uniquely defined by "Southern blacks." In fact, I suspect that they are not.

Some overlap between folk, popular, and biomedical nosology may be apparent in Weidman's classification, which is not exhaustive, but the origins of the terms among the blacks sampled were generally not given. (Might not "run-down condition" have been an *etic* term at one time?) Moreover, the extent to which the terms are common among urban low-income blacks across the United States presently remains unknown.

James noted some of the terms mentioned by Weidman in his description of equivalent meanings of folk and biomedical terms and added others, such as "dropsy," which translates roughly into edema. He stressed that some patients who appear to understand concepts actually misunderstand them, as in the case of "low blood" and "high blood," which many blacks believe are mutually exclusive. This notion of the exclusivity of "high blood" and "low blood" is also reported by Snow (1976).

LEARNING NOSOLOGICAL AND ETIOLOGICAL CONCEPTS   The social contexts in which discussions of nosology and etiology occur include both discussions involved in the socialization of children about preventive health measures and informal discussions among lay persons when a member of the group becomes ill or diseased. James remembers that when he made house calls years ago in Tennessee, all of the household members (and frequently neighbors as well) would gather around the patient and would often remain there during the physician's medical examination. After he left the patient's side or was leaving the house, one person usually confronted him and asked him to "level" about the patient. This meant that the physician should describe the patient's condition and prognosis, including "anything else to be known that should not be told to the others" —that is, the patient, family members, or neighbors (C. James, personal communication).

Many black ministers also discuss nosology and etiology with their congregants and others. Sata, Perry, and Cameron (1970) described the etiological notions of mental illness held by 25 black store-front church ministers in Baltimore as covering a wide range, from interpersonal problems to brain injury to demoniac possession. Some urban blacks also discuss their conditions with pharmacists, as well as with friends or relatives. Increasingly, many of their friends or relatives are employed in health-care or health-related settings.

Concepts of disease and illness are learned in various ways, but largely through direct experience. Many concepts that do not now appear to be biomedically oriented were nevertheless acquired from medical sources. That is, some concepts were acquired from medical sources that had various levels of medical knowledge and were not updated by new medical knowledge, in part because such new knowledge is not disseminated sufficiently to the general public; others were acquired from biomedical sources that attempted simplistic explanations for patients.

PRACTICAL IMPLICATIONS FOR CLINICIANS   Although the information available about the nosological and etiological concepts used by urban blacks is still insufficient, some changes have obviously taken place since Puckett wrote that "with the possible exception of trouble in teething . . . the great Negro ailment seems to be rheumatism . . . a very inclusive term with the Negroes, taking in almost every unfamiliar ache from a crick in the neck to tertiary syphilis" (1926:360). Snow was also probably naive in asserting that "*every* health professional who sees low-income southern patients, black or white, soon learns the necessity of taking on another vocabulary in order to communicate effectively" (1976:54). Leaving aside the considerable overlap between the popular terminologies of patients and health professionals, it is clear that some of the health professionals serving low-income black and white Southern patients were themselves raised in or exposed to environments similar to those of their patients. Snow's argument may be good fodder, however, for those who advocate the necessity of training low-income blacks as physicians so that they may better serve their own kind.

When physicians discuss concepts of nosology and etiology with their urban black patients, they should evaluate each patient to determine which concepts can be used most appropriately. For instance, if a patient believes firmly that a given condition is caused by a hex, the understanding physician might work adequately within that framework wherever possible. Tingling specifically advised that if a black patient seemed to feel "something strange" happening to him, the physician might ask, "Do you mean that someone is working roots on you?" or "Could it be roots?" (1967:489). Many of Rocereto's black subjects believed that "you should teach the nurses to ask if a patient knows how he got sick or what he thinks made him sick. You just can't ask every black person outright if root work did it, because they all don't believe in it" (1973:425). This kind of advice is in line with Harrison's edict that physicians "must deal with individuals and persons, and not with disease, disorder, and disability *per se*" (1972:349). Johnston believes that "when scientific knowledge is presented so that it appears incompatible with a patient's traditional beliefs, the traditional way will probably win, and the best health information may be rejected" (1977:78). Thus physicians clearly have an obligation to find some congruence, whenever possible, between folk and biomedical knowledge in order to enhance the well-being of the patient. Sometimes, however, the search for congruence will be detrimental to the patient and must be dealt with effectively.

Intraethnic Variation

Occupational variations produce intraethnic variations in concepts. Urban blacks who are the most knowledgeable about biomedical concepts of disease and illness are, of course, physicians and, perhaps, nurses. Other factors contributing to intraethnic variation include the usual demographic characteristics and type of religiosity, although the influence of these factors is not yet clear.

Becoming Ill

Classification and Understanding of Symptoms

Empirical data about the extent to which contemporary urban blacks use folk and biomedical traditions in interpreting and understanding symptoms are scarce, as are data about the probably considerable overlap between the two traditions. Considering both the historical exclusion of blacks from mainstream medicine and the increasing scientific developments within medicine over time, it is not unusual to expect that older blacks would utilize both folk and biomedical traditions and transmit them culturally to younger generations. Indeed, White (1977) claims that folk medicine has remained within the "black community" because of humiliation, lack of money, and lack of trust in health workers.[7]

What is generally known about urban blacks is that they regard good health as an individual responsibility for normal adults (on occasion, the good health of husbands is also the responsibility of wives), and, for others, as the responsibility of parents or guardians. The absence of good health is usually attributed broadly to two conditions: the failure to take adequate care of oneself and aging. In the case of poor health in an elderly person, failure is often attributed to earlier lack of adequate care. Adequate care includes adherence to such physical and moral norms as sufficient nutrition, rest, cleanliness (which is "next to godliness"), and the ten commandments. Beliefs are frequently quite specific about the techniques conducive to good health (for example, hair is to be shampooed with a certain frequency, menstruating women should never go swimming, no one should ever go to bed on a full stomach, and fish and buttermilk should not be ingested simultaneously).

Snow (1978) differentiated between modern scientific medicine and folk medicine among low-income blacks, as noted earlier, by indicating that proponents of the latter made no distinction between science and religion, viewed illnesses as preventable with appropriate individual care, regarded symptoms as irrelevant (the cause was the most important aspect), and regarded the distinction between somatically and mentally expressed illnesses as irrelevant. However, she failed to consider the prevalence of these attitudes among low-income blacks, nor did she identify precisely the characteristics of low-income blacks who adhered stringently to folk medicine by rejecting modern scientific medicine, as opposed to those who shifted from one pattern to the other, depending on the situation. In addition, it is quite likely that a much larger proportion of low-income blacks than Snow suspected do not regard symptoms as irrelevant in diagnosing illnesses. Moreover, as Rocereto (1973) pointed out, those who believe in spells being case also believe that spells can be avoided if one obtains adequate food, rest, and exercise, all good preventive health measures. Unfortunately, the data are insufficient to determine the validity and reliability of Snow's findings, although Weidman (1978) indicated considerable similarities between both sets of findings about folk medicine, as to some extent did Krug (1974).

Management of Symptoms

Given the absence of substantial information, I developed in collaboration with John B. Nowlin, a Duke University physician with some experience in treating urban blacks, a theoretical diagram of the possible process of symptom management among urban blacks (figure 1.1). It should, of course, be subjected to empirical investigation, using representative samples of urban blacks. (Although the diagram was developed for urban blacks, if it has any applicability, it is applicable to other ethnic groups as well. That is, there is no reason to believe empirically or experimentally that the global approach to symptom reduction as presented here would differ substantially among contemporary ethnic groups in the United States, regardless of geographic location.)

Our model begins with the perception of a symptom or symptoms, implying that one's health has deviated from normality or perceived normality. The individual then evaluates the significance of the symptom. Many important factors influence the interpretative process, such as the extent of discomfort and the determination of the symptom as life-threatening; other important variables include prior history of symptoms as well as personality patterns and life-styles. The interpretation leads to the decision to initiate further action or to take no action. If further action is deemed necessary, the two general modes of action are (1) self-treatment and (2) treatment by others. The two general categories for treatment by others are (1) nonmedical and (2) medical. Generally, when the symptom is defined as a medical problem warranting biomedical treatment, the individual will seek help most often through the mainstream medical system, turning first to the regular source of care or, if that source is not available (or if no such source exists), to an emergency room. In a study that included 125 urban, low-income blacks in California, Weaver and Inui (1975) obtained their recommendations of sources of care for five hypothetical medical problems. Mainstream medical-care sources were overwhelmingly selected: 99.2 percent for "needs shots"; 97.4 percent for venereal disease; 94.9 percent for problems with pregnancies; 93.3 percent for a badly cut leg; and 82.5 percent for conditions in which the patient is "nervous, emotionally upset."

If the treatment outcome is judged successful (that is, if abatement of symptoms occurs), then the process is terminated. But if treatment is perceived as a failure, vacillation among alternative sources of health care is likely to occur, either in some successive order or by the simultaneous use of two or more alternatives. The major goal is symptom abatement.[8] Without doubt, Mechanic's observation "that the nature of symptoms is the most powerful factor influencing the definition of illness and the seeking of care" (1969:201) applies to urban blacks, regardless of their socioeconomic or other demographic or psychological characteristics. I suspect, however, that an analysis of relevant variables—including attitudes, values, and delivery-system characteristics, in conjunction with Mechanic's ten factors related to patterns of symptomatic response

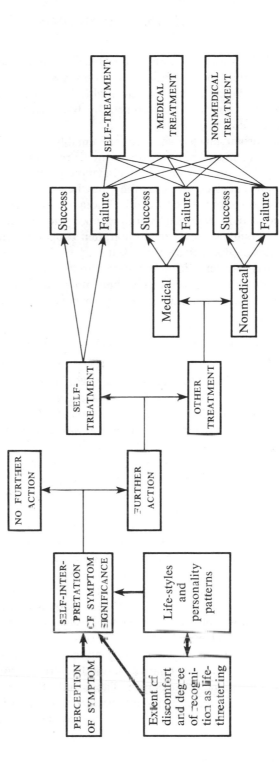

Figure 1.1 Process of symptom management.

(1969:195)—would show considerable differences between urban blacks who are eligible for Medicaid and those whose incomes are substantially higher. Middle-class blacks are probably influenced much more strongly than their lower-class counterparts by biomedical knowledge and disruption of activity.

Some urban blacks who are presumably knowledgeable about the causes of various symptoms do misinterpret them, however, frequently thinking that some serious physical symptoms are actually psychosomatically induced, given the stress they may be experiencing from familial or or work conditions. Consequently, though it is plausible to assume that more educated urban blacks are more knowledgeable about their symptoms, it should not be forgotten that their situations can cause them to err in diagnosing themselves. Indeed, it may well be the case that increased third-party payments for low-income urban blacks have caused them to seek medical help more quickly than other blacks for acute conditions. The former are certainly less likely to have full-time, year-round employment.

Initial Discussion of Symptoms

Unfortunately, the available data do not indicate the persons with whom urban blacks first discuss their symptoms for clarification or further definition. When intolerable discomfort arises in the presence of others, and particularly when it is obvious to others, it is likely that most individuals first discuss their symptoms with one or more of the persons within their midst, unless, for some reason, they wish to conceal any form of illness. The nature of the symptom and its previous history will influence discussion or lack of discussion, as well as influencing the selection of the person first approached for discussion or the significant other who initiates such a discussion.

Some limited data about help sought for acute conditions among nonwhites in 1973–1974 (Verbrugge 1979) are useful here. The average annual incidence of acute conditions among nonwhites during that time period was 30,968,000. About 56 percent of those cases were medically attended, and advice from non-physicians was sought in about 24 percent of the medically attended cases. Of the remaining cases in which no medical attention was obtained, advice was sought in about 25 percent of the cases. In cases where advice from a non-physician was sought, whether or not the case was ever medically attended, about 67 percent sought advice from a friend or relative, about 19 percent from a nurse, and 14 percent from some other person. These and other data suggest strongly that most urban blacks tend to discuss their symptoms with persons whom they consider knowledgeable, and that most seek medical care if symptoms are connected with physical origins and produce intolerable discomfort. Older persons are more likely to have ongoing relationships or appointments with physicians. Children, of course, typically discuss their symptoms first with fellow household members, or, if in school, with peers or appropriate school personnel.

Tolerance for Symptoms

One gap in the understanding of the health behaviors of urban blacks is the lack of sufficient knowledge about their tolerance for symptoms or their correlates. In a review of literature on ethnicity and health behavior related to response to symptoms, including pain, Twaddle and Hessler did not identify any studies specific to blacks but suggested that "for the present, it seems clear that different groups have different orientations that create different criteria for deciding that a health problem exists" (1977:105–106). They overlooked the few studies that have included black subjects.

In an investigation of symptoms that caused 208 black and 510 white mothers of elementary school children in a Delaware sample (79 percent urban) to keep their children home from school, a majority of the black mothers (ranging from 54.8 to 100 percent) said they would retain their children at home for fever alone or fever and one or more other ailments (sore throat, headache, stomachache, diarrhea, cough, earache, or running nose) as well as for diarrhea, "hurting all over," dizziness, chest pain, earache, sore throat, stiff neck or back, stomachache, rashes, constipation, headache, or nervousness (Slome et al. 1977). Almost half said they would keep the children home if they were fatigued. Employment of the black or white mother was a contributing factor in that housewives were significantly more likely to keep a child at home because of stomachache, fatigue, or constipation. Although the difference was not statistically significant, unskilled mothers tended to be more likely to keep their children at home for given symptoms than did mothers employed in skilled capacities.

With regard to age, sex, and racial differences in pain tolerance, Woodrow and his colleagues (1972) tested 41,119 subjects (including 3,336 black females and 2,057 black males) undergoing a Kaiser-Permanente Automated Multiphasic Screening examination and found that within each sex group, average pain tolerance was significantly higher among whites than blacks. Orientals had the lowest pain tolerance. They also found that pain tolerance decreased with increasing age for each racial group, as measured by mechanical pressure on the Achilles tendon. They suspected that tolerance to cutaneous pain increases, while tolerance to deep pain decreases, with advancing age. Socioeconomic status, as measured by educational level, did not seem to be related to pain tolerance. In comparing their findings with several other studies (Chapman and

Jones 1944; Merskey and Spear 1964; Winsberg and Greenlick 1967), Woodrow and his colleagues concluded that "the uniformity of our [racial] findings within every age group and for both sexes . . . considerably reduced the chance that our observation was an artifact" (1972: 555). Recognizing differences between experimental and clinical pain, Woodrow and his associates also indicated that "the differences in pain tolerance in our study are due to underlying differences in our subject groups. The extent to which these differences in pain tolerance are culturally determined or biologically determined is still unknown" (1972: 553).

In a review of studies about cultural factors and pain responses, Wolff and Langley (1968) indicated a number of findings contradictory to those of Woodrow and his colleagues. According to their review, if Chapman and Jones (1944) had corrected for skin temperature in their investigation of pain responses among 18 Southern Negroes and 18 Americans of northern European ancestry, the resulting racial differences would have been insignificant. Further, Chapman and Jones (1944) determined that the Russian Jewish, Italian, and Negro subjects were similar in pain threshold, but the Negroes, unlike the Russian Jews and Italians, did *not* complain. Wolff and Langley also stressed that Merskey and Spear's study (1964) of the pain reactions of 28 white and 11 Afro-Asian male medical students in England showed no significant racial differences in pain threshold, pain reaction point, and reaction interval—a point that underscores the need for controlling for socioeconomic status, or at least occupational status, when one is making racial comparisons.

Whatever its determinants, the pain felt by black patients should not be minimized by health-care providers; nor, of course, should these providers reprimand or belittle black patients if they react (or if they are believed to react) to a pain-producing procedure or symptom in a more extreme fashion than white patients are perceived to do. Moreover, physicians, nurses, and other health-care personnel should not lie to black patients by indicating that given painful procedures will not be painful. This has frequently happened in the past when small children were given painful immunizations. Although the fear of immunization has probably diminished considerably among current cohorts of young black children, James recalls that many years ago, but within his professional lifetime, black children were often informed by their parents and other adults as well that if they did not behave, the parents would have a physician administer a shot (C. James, personal communication). This meant that physicians, in treating such children, had the additional task of reeducating them to understand that illness was not a sin, but a disturbance of the body. More important than the understanding, of course, was the significant effort that had to be placed on changing the belief.

Coping with Illness outside the Mainstream Medical System

Within the family, the wife/mother is most often charged with the responsibility for protecting the health of family members. She is expected to help them maintain good health by appropriate preventive measures, such as making certain they eat properly and dress appropriately for different weather conditions. She is also expected to monitor the conditions of their health regularly, in order to identify symptoms of illness. When these symptoms are recognized, she is the one who usually determines the course of action to be followed, in consultation with the affected family member. If the person who is ill must remain at home and requires care, as in the case of a child who is not sent to school, it is usually the mother who is responsible for providing or arranging for the care. Even when both parents are employed, it is still the mother, not the father, who is likely to be absent from work. In one-parent families, however, when the mother is employed and more than one child is present, one or more of the children may be required to remain at home to provide care. Furthermore, such parents may be less stringent in defining children as ill. In intact families, where the major direct care is typically the mother's responsibility, joint parental decisions are usually made about obtaining medical care.

When family members are disabled, the mother or wife is still most often responsible for providing needed care. Other family members are expected to help, with specific assignments determined by the nature of the disability or the type of care required. Sometimes neighbors or friends are also expected to provide assistance, such as running errands and providing relief for family members.

Problems arise especially when the wife or mother becomes ill, since she is generally expected to remain well in order to care for other family members. If a husband is present, he then becomes responsible for her care, a responsibility he may, in turn, delegate to a female child or other relatives. When older couples or persons living alone are ill and require home care, a female family member (usually the oldest daughter, if there is one) is expected to provide the care.

When the chief breadwinner is ill and unable to work, problems arise in a variety of ways; the problems are most often economic, but interpersonal relationships can be adversely affected, leading to psychological problems as well. Some urban black families do, of course, have sufficient insurance or access to pensions to tide them over financially, but even they are not immune to resulting psychological and social problems.

The illnesses, diseases, or symptoms most often treated within the home involve those not perceived as being serious or requiring medical intervention; those for which no other sources of care are perceived as being available; or those that have occurred previously (in which case a decision may be made to follow previous medical advice without further medical consultation). In some instances, "leftover" medication is still on the shelves and is brought out for use, regardless of its age. Home remedies are administered on the basis of diagnoses made either by the person who is ill or by others he consults, and on the basis of beliefs about the efficacy of these remedies. Patterns of self-administration vary widely among urban blacks, as can be seen in the range of home remedies used to treat colds. Self-prescribed home medications are generally taken prior to medical consultation, but they may be continued after consultation and taken along with prescribed medications, even though the patient may not inform the physician of this fact.

Some urban blacks use ginseng roots to treat indigestion, horehound roots for diabetes, and poke salad weed (or pokeweed) as a spring tonic for "cleansing the system." Some use "burnt flour" (or flour heated in the oven) for diarrhea. Attention to the bowels is frequently a major concern of elderly blacks, some of whom use "purgatives," which are also used by some urban blacks of various ages for colds, upset stomachs, excessive drinking, and constipation. Catnip tea may be used to prevent hives and to treat infants with colic. Colds are treated in various ways, not only with purgatives but most often now by bed rest, juices, and a combination of over-the-counter drugs designed to provide congestive relief. The so-called childhood diseases, such as chicken pox, measles, and mumps, are usually treated at home. A number of poor or poorly educated urban blacks still borrow prescription drugs from each other, but the extent of this practice—and its adverse consequences—remain unknown.

When family members are perceived as being ill and incapable of carrying out their role responsibilities, they are usually relieved of those duties readily. Urban blacks tend to be sympathetic toward people who are ill. However, some urban blacks resent sick people, and ambivalent feelings may be present. In some instances, urban blacks are not aware of the proscribed behaviors accompanying given conditions, and therefore fail to relieve sick people of conflicting roles. These kinds of problems arise especially when medical conditions preclude lifting heavy objects or mopping floors.

Lay Consultation and Referral

Little information is available about patterns of consultation within the family and about the personal network used by the afflicted person in order to identify and label an illness, recommend treatment, and refer to sources of care outside the home. When the affliction occurs within the home, the mother or wife, if present, is the one most often consulted for aid. However, many family members become ill outside the home, at school or at work, where other persons are consulted. Quite often, the person within the family who is primarily responsible for the overall health care of family members is informed about decisions already made, or receives advice to be acted upon. For example, a child may be sent home from school with instructions about his illness and an indication as to whether or not medical intervention is available. Basco and her colleagues (1972) and Slome and his associates (1977) have provided some useful data about the presence of symptoms in children which cause their mothers to keep them away from school; unfortunately, these studies did not provide data about which symptoms exhibited by the first and third graders at school would cause school personnel to send them home.

Within the family, women are probably the most influential people in medical consultations (although this pattern seems to be changing somewhat as the women's movement and other societal changes modify traditional sex roles). I also suspect that in a substantial number of intact black families, both spouses participate in joint decisions about medical treatment for their offspring, and probably for each other. If the afflicted persons are elderly, the oldest daughter is usually the most influential family member. An important point that needs to be reemphasized is that although many urban blacks do not seek medical care for all of their real or imagined illnesses, most do seek medical care from mainstream practitioners when they believe they are seriously ill or are confronted with life-threatening conditions.

Delay in seeking lay or professional consultation upon recognition of symptoms depends on a wide variety of interacting variables, the most critical of which are probably perceived seriousness of the condition, extent of discomfort, a belief that treatment would produce symptom abatement, and ready access to treatment (including immediate treatment or a reasonably short waiting period). Women tend to delay consultation longer for themselves than they typically do for other family members. Both low-income and middle-income urban blacks are likely to delay medical consultation if they believe their symptoms represent dreaded diseases, such as cancer. In this respect, Jackson and Nixon, two black physicians in San Francisco, indicated that

> the black person often fears going to a medical facility because he has a great fear of diagnoses such as cancer or other dread illness. He also fears that he will be told by the physician that he cannot work. Additionally, when a diagnosis is made, he fears that the therapy will make the conditions worse or even fatal. One frequently hears in the black community such terms as "never cut into a cancer," "spinal ancsthesia will cause one to become paralyzed," etc. These confusions are often based on some degree of fact. However, little attempt has been made to separate the facts from the fiction. The result is that many members of the community dread going to

a medical facility because of the possibilities of unacceptable diagnosis or unacceptable treatment. (1970:59)

Although Jackson and Nixon did not provide empirical support for their assertions or indicate how widespread the beliefs they identified were (or what black subgroups held them), their observations raise anew concerns about the typical pat response that racial discrimination is a major cause for later presentation and diagnosis of serious illnesses among blacks than among whites. Obviously, the effects of racial discrimination are factors in these phenomena, but subcultural factors not specifically attributable to racial discrimination must also be considered.

More information about variables influencing the seeking of care would be helpful, but the process itself is very complex and depends heavily on the health attitudes and behaviors of the participants, including the importance placed on preventive health measures as well as the strategies used for prevention. Certainly, it is simplistic merely to conclude that the global concept of institutionalized racism is sufficient to explain the pattern of proportionately more blacks than whites presenting themselves for treatment at more advanced stages of diseases, as in the case of cancer.

Nonmainstream Medical Care outside the Home

When urban blacks decide they must go outside the home for medical care but do not seek mainstream medical care, they typically turn to friends or relatives. Verbrugge (1979) reported that 67 percent of nonwhites seeking advice from non-physicians for acute conditions in 1973–1974 turned to friends or relatives, while 13 percent consulted a nurse and the remaining 20 percent consulted other persons. In some instances, they were advised to see a physician. Some followed that advice; others did not. (No measures of the quality of advice were provided by Verbrugge, nor was there any analysis of characteristics that might have differentiated between those who did and those who did not follow advice to consult a physician.)

Weidman (1978) also found that the blacks in her Miami study rarely sought health advice from nonmainstream sources or a druggist. That is, during the 12 months preceding the interview, less than 6 percent of them had sought health advice or treatment from a druggist, faith healer, spiritualist, fortune teller, a woman who knew about remedies, or a root doctor, or through praying for oneself or using self-administered home remedies. More specifically, of the 583 persons in the households for whom data were available, only 14 were reported as having engaged in prayer, 13 had consulted a faith healer, 4 had visited a spiritualist, and 2 had consulted a druggist. Weidman feels that her data are suspect, believing that the subjects tended to respond by conforming to sanctioned white patterns. I, on the other hand, feel that her conclusion is suspect, given both her use of indigenous interviewers and the fact that the sanctioned patterns to which she referred were not unique to whites. Unfortunately, Weidman failed to include Southern white subjects in her study, which prohibited native black/white comparisons.

Some of the folk healers to whom some urban blacks occasionally turn have been described by Saphir and colleagues (1967), Stewart (1971), Hall and Bourne (1973), Scott (1974), Cappannari and associates (1975), Golden (1977), Snow (1978), and Weidman (1978). Unfortunately, these investigators do not generally provide sufficient descriptions and analyses of the characteristics of the urban black users of folk healers, as well as other data that would be helpful in understanding their structural and behavioral components. Moreover, the methodologies employed to investigate black folk healers have been extremely ineffective in providing much good information, in part because these folk healers apparently—and perhaps justifiably so—do not trust the researchers or are unwilling for various other reasons to be research subjects. None of the studies provides information about either the current number of black folk healers in the United States or their demographic characteristics. In all probability, the ratio of such healers to the total black population is much smaller now than in earlier years, when, for example, Puckett (1926) estimated that about a hundred elderly black women and men in Atlanta were professional voodooists. It also seems likely that in earlier times males were more prominent (and probably numerically more dominant) than now among black folk healers.

Information on the interacting attitudes and behaviors involved in the selection and use of folk healers and on the efficacy of the folk treatment is generally unavailable as well. However, Cappannari and associates (1975) and Saphir and colleagues (1967) do provide descriptions and analyses of the use of folk and mainstream medical systems by two young black adults, one a female in Nashville, the other a Southern-born male in Buffalo. All of these studies concerning folk healers indicate or intimate that among the factors influencing the selection of folk healers are beliefs that the etiology of the illness involves sorcery, which cannot be cured by mainstream practitioners. Snell (1967), however, suggested that hypnosis is an effective therapy for the hexed patient, and its use by psychiatrists does not require the therapist to accept any belief in hexing, nor to pretend to the patient that such a belief exists. He based his opinion on the treatment of 20 black patients who believed they were hexed and were treated at Grady Memorial Hospital, Atlanta.

Some urban blacks seeking nonmainstream medical care do not do so out of a belief in sorcery; rather, their religious beliefs exclude certain forms of mainstream medical care, as in the case of Jehovah's Witnesses, who eschew blood transfusions. James indicates that some of his patients who belong to the United Church of Prayer frequently wear a picture of "Sweet Daddy Grace" (the now deceased founder) under their clothing, and that they and a number of other urban blacks use mainstream medical care simultaneously or in alternation with nonmainstream care (C. James, personal communication). In such cases, the physician must be alert to the feasibility of merging the joint sources of care and must respect the patient's wishes. Difficulties arise most often when the patient is a child. In some instances physicians must seek court orders to overrule parental decisions, as in cases where medical judgment indicates that blood transfusions are necessary to maintain life.

James also indicates that many urban blacks apparently recognize that depression, anxiety, and tension are conditions that often resist superficial treatment by physicians who do not have time to treat them. Consequently, some patients defining themselves as emotionally ill will not perceive their conditions as being amenable to cure or relief by physicians (or by busy physicians); or they may initially turn to physicians, become dissatisfied with what they perceive as treatment failures, and then turn to alternative sources of care, such as root workers or faith healers. In some cases, they may rely instead on self-treatment. A key consideration here may be the increased need of many urban residents simply to find sympathetic and helpful listeners. If we assume that the consulted physician is competent in treating depression, anxiety, and tension, Norman's contention that "each ghetto resident at least should have a responsible physician whom he knows and trusts, who is unhurriedly attuned to his needs and aspirations and who understands and is concerned with his domestic and employment situations" (1969:1274) is well taken. The important issue of patient overload may be raised here, too, since it seems to be the case that a number of physicians who accept Medicaid and Medicare payments tend to have patient overloads, only in part because some patients overuse physicians services.

Though the search for symptom abatement for emotional problems, as suggested by James, may characterize many urban blacks, undoubtedly some class differences exist. When Ring and Schein (1970) sampled 388 households in a black middle-class community in Philadelphia, they found that 87.4 percent of the respondents said they would consult either a physician (48.4 percent), psychiatrist (19.2 percent), hospital (16.2 percent), or clinic (3.6 percent) for a mental or emotional problem. Of those who had experienced problems of obesity, severe headaches, allergies, dependence on medication, insomnia, excessive drinking, marked anxiety, depression, insecurity, or hostility (N = 110 households) during the previous six months, 84.5 percent had consulted a doctor, and 11 percent had gone to a hospital or clinic. These respondents were definitely oriented toward mainstream medical care rather than toward nonmainstream caretakers for emotional problems. Although these data do not permit any analysis of the effect of income on the use of professionals for mental or emotional problems, when Kulka, Veroff, and Douvan (1979) analyzed 1976 national survey data (in which a few black subjects may have been included, but in which there was no racial breakout), they concluded that when education was controlled, the relationship between income and the use of psychiatric treatment was insignificant.

I suspect that James is correct in saying that many black folk healers are actually used as psychotherapists. To that extent, they may be helpful in treating certain forms of emotional distress. The extent to which they also treat somatic problems, however, is moot. Rocereto distinguished between good and bad root doctors: the good ones recognized "when the person needed the services of a medical doctor because the illness was beyond the capabilities of the root doctor" (1973:423–424). But Stewart (1971)—whose findings were based on an extremely poor research design, a very small and nonrepresentative sample of blacks (probably confined to rural areas or small towns) in Georgia, and inexperienced interviewers- -suggested that many black users of folk healers apparently seek aid for various physical illnesses, such as dysentery, rheumatism, "high blood," headaches, bursitis, kidney problems, cancer, and hemophilia. Stewart's findings, as well as those of Snow (1974), may be geographically unique in some respects. For example, Krug, who agreed with many of Snow's findings, found some of them inapplicable to a small, rural black community in North Carolina:

> One important exception had to do with the hierarchy of healing practitioners. Writes Dr. Snow, "Because the 'medical' doctor gives medicines, he or she is in the same class as the herb doctor, the housewife, or the neighbor who happens to know a lot of home remedies." My informants saw M.D.'s as the legitimate and most trustworthy source of medical care. Many placed the M.D. higher in status than the minister (with some exceptions). Except in the case of illness resulting from a curse—in which case someone had to be found who could remove the curse—physicians were the first to be consulted at the initial sign of a significant symptom. Trust was tentative, however, and when the patient felt the doctor did not really understand the problem, non-M.D. practitioners were often consulted for the understanding car they provided. (Krug 1974:705)

James believes that the use of folk healers by some urban blacks presents both problems and benefits to mainstream medical practitioners. Some of the major problems for the mainstream physician include delayed seeking of care, use of competing and conflicting remedies, and noncompliance with the medically prescribed treatment. Physicians who are unaware or unaccepting of folk healers may be ineffective in combining the folk and biomedical systems in a way that can benefit the patient. In line with James's observation, Hillard and Rockwell (1978), in describing their successful treatment of a well-educated black rural woman in the South who experienced dysesthesia as a conversion reaction and believed herself to be a victim of witchcraft, also emphasized the need for physicians to be aware of a belief in roots. Tingling (1967) illustrated successful psychiatric treatment in Rochester, New York of a 20-year-old black male diagnosed as a catatonic schizophrenic, when the psychiatrists respected his family's belief in roots.

Often forgotten is the fact that many folk healers also encourage patients to use both systems, depending on the perceived illness and treatment procedures available to them. Some, of course, do not. Many folk healers also encourage what they perceive as preventive health measures, such as the wearing of asafetida bags to prevent illness, including diseases such as poliomyelitis.

Encounters with Mainstream Medical Practitioners

Medical-Care Settings

Though the proportion of blacks who use folk healers remains unknown, the majority of all blacks now visit a mainstream physician at least annually. Table 1.14 shows the percentage of blacks and all others (that is, non-blacks not of Spanish origin) who visited a physician in 1976, by family income and age. About three-fourths of both groups of all incomes and all ages saw a physician in that year. Although the visits were undoubtedly motivated by varying conditions, income does not appear to have any substantial effects on physician visitation. A major implication of this kind of data is that being black no longer adversely affects access to a physician. Or, to put it more bluntly, those who in the past have been discontent because blacks visited physicians less frequently than whites should now shift their concerns from the quantity of visits to the quality of care received when visitations occur, particularly in view of the fact that the 1976 age-adjusted percentage of visitations for all incomes was 74.2 percent for blacks and 76.2 percent for all others. Furthermore, the 1976 age-adjusted percentage for all incomes for short-stay hospital episodes during the previous year was the same for blacks and for all others (10.6 percent).

Most contemporary urban blacks using mainstream medical care are seen by office-based physicians, a number of whom are in solo practice. In the period 1975–1976, the number of visits by nonwhites per 1,000 population to physicians was 4,626, of which 2,768.4 were visits to a physician's office, 1,103.9 were visits to a hospital outpatient department, 293.9 were telephone consultations, 52.0 were visits to a company or industry clinic, and 33.8 were home visits by the physician (U.S. Department of Health, Education, and Welfare 1978). When asked their prefer-

Table 1.14 Percentage of blacks and others of non-Spanish origin who visited a physician at least once, by family income and age, United States, 1976.

Income and age (years)	Blacks	Others, non-Spanish origin[a]
All incomes		
All ages	73.5	76.2
Under 17	67.6	76.2
17–44	76.9	75.6
45–64	76.1	75.2
65+	78.8	80.2
Less than $5,000		
All ages	75.7	77.8
Under 17	68.2	74.7
17–44	80.6	78.7
45–64	78.2	75.6
65+	80.3	79.7
$5,000–$9,999		
All ages	70.1	75.3
Under 17	62.3	72.9
17–44	75.6	75.8
45–64	73.4	72.8
65+	79.9	80.6
$10,000–$14,999		
All ages	74.4	75.5
Under 17	68.5	76.0
17–44	79.3	75.4
45–64	73.3	73.5
65+	84.9	81.1
$15,000+		
All ages	78.5	77.4
Under 17	77.9	78.2
17–44	78.3	76.1
45–64	81.0	78.3
65+	73.3	81.5

Source: Moy and Wilder (1978).

a. Includes all persons who were neither black nor of Spanish origin.

ences of health sites, 66 percent of Gylys and Glylys's sample of low-income backs in Toledo, Ohio (1974) specified office-based private physicians, 12 percent preferred health clinics, and 22 percent had no preference between the two types of sites.

In 1977, the average number of visits per person for nonwhites to office-based physicians was 2.0 as compared to 2.8 for whites. The number of visits increased with age, from 1.3 visits per person for nonwhites under 15 years to 2.9 per person for those over age 65. (The comparable number of visits for whites was 2.2 per person for those under 15 and 4.3 for those over 65.) The average number of visits per year was higher for females than for males in 1977 (Ezzati 1980).

Using NCHS Health Interview Surveys between 1971 and 1973, Wolinsky (1978) attempted to determine what variables (predisposing, enabling, illness-morbidity) significantly predicted the sources of health care used by respondents. His health utilization measures focused specifically on hospitals, dentists, and physicians. Using a sophisticated methodology, Wolinsky found that the predisposing and enabling variables, which included race and other traditional measures of social class, were generally insignificant in explaining variations in health use. Education and income were positively related to dental use. Users of physicians were more likely to be younger, married, and in smaller-sized families. Fink and his colleagues (1969) found that race was not significantly associated with patient movement from psychiatric consultation to treatment; however, the patient's discomfort and prognostic assessment of treatment were associated. Wolinsky indicated that relatively little was yet known about the causal nexus of health-care utilization; that the variables which best explained usage were the illness-morbidity characteristics; and that his findings implied "that sociocultural characteristics are not important factors in the causal nexus of health service utilization" (1978: 394). He further suggested that unmeasured variables such as attitudes, values, and delivery-system characteristics might be relevant and should be matters for research.

James suggests a definite division, generally unrelated to socioeconomic status, between patients using private physicians and those using clinics. He suspects that a number of patients suffering from chronic disorders such as hypertension, obesity, and diabetes feel more comfortable utilizing clinics than private practices, even though compliance may be achieved better in private practice. Unfortunately, Gylys and Glylys (1974) did not identify the discriminating characteristics between their black subjects who did and did not prefer health clinics, nor do similar studies. James also suggests that a number of urban black elderly persons prefer clinics because they use the visit as a social event. They like to make relatively frequent clinic appointments so they can see and visit with friends coming to the clinics. Moreover, they gain a sense of importance by being taken to the clinic and welcomed by the physicians and nurses (C. James, personal communication).

Often, visits to the clinic provide patients with someone to listen to them. In their study of postmenopausal urban black women, Walls and Jackson(1977) found that loneliness was a significant factor distinguishing between women who did and did not use physicians for symptoms related to menopause.

I could not find any hard data about the preferences of urban blacks for "gatekeepers" (the persons who determine if the patient needs any care, if so, make case assignments or referrals) within medical settings, but I think that an increasing number prefer the physician as the gatekeeper. This preference is contrary to what occurs in the growing number of neighborhood health facilities for the medically indigent, where the gatekeepers are often paraprofessionals. This generalization needs to be modified by the presenting condition or type of services sought; for instance, it seems to be the case that an increasing number of medically indigent black women prefer family planning clinics to private physicians for obtaining contraceptive mechanisms. James thinks, however, that many family planning centers are encouraging tubal ligations among such women, who remain improperly informed about the reversibility of this procedure or problems associated with reversibility (C. James, personal communication).

Expectations in the Medical Encounter

What do urban blacks want from mainstream medical practitioners? James indicates that patients seek relief and an assurance that they have no serious disorder. In effect, they seek correct diagnoses and, if treatment is warranted, curative treatment of short duration. He believes that when medications are prescribed, most patients will take them freely if the dosage period is short and side effects are minimal or absent. However, when long-term medication or medication with undesirable side effects is prescribed, it is often difficult to convince patients that compliance is essential to their well-being. Such attitudes and behaviors reinforce his notion that patients desire rapid and effective cures. James's ideas are supported by Davis's indication (1966) that patients expect explanations, comfort, and cure. Symptom abatement is a major feature of the theoretical model of the process of symptom management presented in figure 1.1.

Increasingly, most urban black patients also seek ready access to their physicians (and not to non-physicians). They are discouraged by difficulties in obtaining appointments, long waiting intervals when they arrive for scheduled appointments, and undue delays in receiving diagnostic reports involving laboratory tests, especially when those tests may indicate serious illness. They also expect more time with the physician than they usually receive. Compliance (discussed in greater detail in the following section) is also adversely affected when these expectations are not met.

Urban blacks usually want to know the diagnosis of their condition, even if the condition is terminal. This does not mean, however, that all of them readily accept proffered diagnoses. Some will seek additional opinions from other mainstream practitioners; others who are given poor prognoses of incurable diseases may be desperate for other powers, including religious or magical ones. The determination of which patients do and do not wish to be informed realistically about their conditions is a highly individualized process, requiring great skill and insight on the part of the attending physician.

Interactional Norms

Most urban blacks assign high prestige to the status of physician, a position endowed with authority. They expect physicians to treat them with respect. Some prefer informal and others prefer formal interactional styles within the medical setting. Although some urban black patients are treated rudely or discourteously, they do not like that kind of treatment, even if they fail to complain openly (overt complaining may lead to their being labeled "bad patients" and receiving worse care). Physicians should always make certain that their support staff treats black patients respectfully.

Some urban black patients do not view themselves as active participants in the physician-patient relationship; thus they do not communicate effectively, nor do they seek clarification of directions or comments. Some physicians assume that such patients understand their biomedical presentations and that the patients accept the scientific medical system. On the other hand, when some urban black patients participate actively in the discussion of their cases, some physicians or members of their staff resent the intrusion.

James has observed another reason for the reticence of some urban blacks in the medical encounter: namely, they are sometimes testing the intelligence of the practitioner by withholding information about their symptoms or the sources of their perceived discomfort. Such patients believe that competent physicians can determine any medical problem without aid from the patient; otherwise, they would not or should not be physicians. I have heard a number of blacks, especially elderly persons (principally from rural areas or rural migrants to urban areas), express similar beliefs about physicians, and some black physicians with whom I spoke verified this phenomenon. In this regard, Krug, then a medical student at the University of North Carolina-Chapel Hill, wrote that "the frequent 'misunderstandings' of physicians were, in all fairness, contributed to by the patients [from the small, rural black community in North Carolina], who generally relied on the physician to ask the right questions rather than volunteer their real concerns. The fact remains, nevertheless, that the people I interviewed placed great value on the time a physician spent listening to the patient (the emphasis being, of course, on how the time was used). The healing effect of appropriate words from an understanding physician was recounted again and again" (1974:705–706).

Much of the literature dealing with interactional norms involving urban blacks and clinicians has concentrated on the race of the physician or the differential effects of the race of the physician on patient behavior. For example, Satcher indicated that "the traditional social relationships of blacks and whites have been carried over to the white physician–black patient relationship. In many cases, the white physician is looked upon as an authority figure whose decisions may not be understood but are not to be questioned. This is the master-servant relationship. This feeling has inhibited communication between physician and patient for many years. Black patients frequently do not admit that they do not understand the physician's instructions. Likewise, black patients often do not express their dissatisfaction with their care. Instead, their response is noncompliance with the physician's instructions" (1973:1499). Satcher further contended that "most white physicians interpreted the master-servant relationship as a good doctor-patient relationship. Their patients were 'happy.' Black patients are almost invariably called by their first names, and they are frequently exploited for teaching sessions" (1973:1499). Indicating the increased expectations and demands of blacks for first-class medical care, Satcher stressed the growing suspicion and distrust that blacks now have of "white physicians as individuals, and the predominantly white medical profession in general" (1973: 1499). Elesh and Schollaert noted that "physicians' attitudes toward black patients appear never to have been systematically studied, but few would doubt the existence of considerable prejudice" (1972:239). Perhaps some of these observations apply equally well to black physicians when their patients are poor.[9]

Though the available data are sparse and inconclusive, it still seems to be the case that some blacks prefer black physicians, others prefer white physicians, and the majority merely prefer competent physicians, regardless of color. In a sample of 250 low-income blacks in Toledo, Ohio, for example, 72 percent expressed no racial preference for a physician, while 19 percent preferred a white physician, and a smaller proportion (9 percent) preferred a black physician (Gylys and Gylys 1974).

The issue of the preference of blacks for the sex of the physician has rarely been raised. Impressions received from various sources suggest that urban blacks tend to be more comfortable with black or white male physicians, less comfortable with black female physicians, and least comfortable with white female physicians. Urban blacks tend to grant more authority to male than to female physicians, and urban black males are those least likely to wish to be treated by female physicians, especially by nonblack ones. However, given the greater antipathy that probably exists between black and white females than between black males and white females, empirical investigations may well show that, on the average, urban black females are less receptive than their male counterparts to white female physicians.

These impressions are based on patients with physical illnesses, whose preferences for treatment may distinguish them from patients with mental or emotional illnesses. Vail's study (1978) of 32 black male and 55 black female lower-class patients in a Community Mental Health Center in Philadelphia, who were randomly distributed to 10 black and white therapists of both sexes, showed that the significant correlate of early termination of individual therapy (that is, cessation of therapy in fewer than four sessions) was the interaction between sex of therapist and sex of patient: patients remained in treatment longer when the therapist was of the opposite sex. The specific professional training of the therapists was not identified in this study.

Reactions to Medical Diagnoses

The earlier discussion of nosological and etiological concepts indicated that most urban blacks tend to have a biomedical orientation toward diagnoses. As a result, physicians who provide adequate explanations of their diagnoses will find that many of their urban black patients understand them and have some awareness of the restrictions or consequences that may be involved. Sometimes patients may not be willing to accept specific diagnoses, just as they are unwilling to accept situations in which physicians indicate they cannot determine the problem, or, if the problem is recognized, its etiology. By and large, however, most urban blacks accept diagnoses given to them and are probably not as alert as they should be to the need for second opinions, particularly when elective surgery is indicated. Moreover, too few urban black patients remain consciously aware of the possibility of physician errors, which, on occasion, do occur. Even when urban black patients accept the diagnoses given, they may still search for alternative treatment modalities.

Adherence to Biomedical Treatment

Patient Compliance

Hard data about adherence to medical treatment among urban blacks are scarce. Available empirical data show various patterns of "compliance," which Davis defined attitudinally as "an orientation or willing readiness to do what the doctor prescribes or an intention to stop doing what the doctor proscribes," and behaviorally as existing "only when the patient actually carries out his doctor's orders" (1968a:115). In addition to the sparse and inconclusive data, methodological differences between the studies about compliance hamper meaningful comparisons. However, it can be said adherence to medical treatment is a problem for many urban blacks, as it is for rural blacks or urban and rural nonblacks.

Blackwell (1973) and Gillum and Barsky (1974), among others, noted generally that physicians tend to overestimate compliance. Gillum and Barsky also indicated the great difficulty experienced by physicians in identifying and dealing with noncompliers. Undoubtedly, these generalizations apply to physicians treating urban blacks, but some of these physicians may erroneously attribute their noncompliance to race and overlook the impact of the physician on compliance.

Using a large biracial sample of Social Security disability applicants in central Ohio, Collette and Ludwig (1969) found that the attitudinal component of positive or negative medical orientation had little impact on compliance with medical advice. No relationships emerged between the respondent's demographic characteristics (including race) and compliance with advice for diet modification. However, blacks were substantially less likely than whites to comply with medical advice about obtaining eyeglasses or undergoing surgery, which may have been due to their generally low socioeconomic status (and not their race). Indicating that acceptance or rejection of differing types of medical advice was affected by different variables, Collette and Ludwig concluded that "money stands as the important variable associated with compliance" (1969:411).

In a longitudinal study of the effects of prescriptions on acceptance of scheduled clinic visits by predominantly low-income, chronically ill, black adult patients in Chicago, Tagliacozzo, Ima, and Lashof (1973) found that premature termination of treatment occurred less often among those on prescribed diets or heavy medications. About 71 percent of the sample were migrants from the deep South, 44 percent had hypertension, 45 percent had diabetes, and 60 percent had two or more illnesses. Although the precise influence of the physicians on the patients' behaviors through prescriptions remained unclear, the investigators concluded that it was probably indirect, varying according to the social and psychological characteristics of the patients.

EFFECTS OF NURSING INTERVENTION   In an experiment involving the same subject pool, in which the experimental variable was intervention by nurses to increase compliance, Tagliacozzo and her co-workers (1974) found that the method of nursing intervention did not lead to substantial increases in medical compliance. The experimental and control groups were not significantly different in regularity of attendance, follow-through on referrals to other clinics, taking of medication, weight loss, improved knowledge of illness, and conception of illness severity. In the experimental group, those responding more favorably to the nurses were more knowledgeable about their illnesses, and more likely to have more than one chronic illness. Nursing intervention helped to decrease termination among patients favorably oriented toward treatment, but increased it among those who were disfavorably oriented.

Although nursing intervention was not highly successful in the Chicago studies, Stamler and Stamler (1976) stated that the special home visiting program by nurses in a Baldwin County (Georgia) hypertension program helped increase compliance to antihypertensive medication. In fact, "it was one of the earliest and most successful efforts to use non-physician personnel in the time-consuming but vital task of health education and assistance, for improved adherence to treatment. The goal of the nurses was to get patients back on medication and adhering well enough to lower diastolic pressure below 95 mm Hg . . . Before the program started, one-quarter were on treatment, with only fifteen percent of all hypertensives under good control . . . Through the nurse's efforts the percent under treatment was pushed up to an impressive 85 percent, with 80 percent under good control" (1976:28). This apparently successful pilot program was discontinued. Of related interest were Stamler and Stamler's results (1976) from a 1962 Baldwin County hypertension survey showing that financial reasons were not the major factor reducing compliance. In fact, 30 percent of the hypertensive patients discontinued medication because they felt better.

DISTANCE FACTORS AND COMPLIANCE WITH APPOINTMENTS   Lieberman's investigation (1974) of the use of pediatric care by persons under 17 years of age who were members of families registered at the Watts Health Center in Los Angeles indicated that many of the children were never brought to the center. Those who were least likely to be brought for care were those farthest removed geographically from the center, suggesting that geographic distance affects compliance. Mushlin and Collins (1975) also suggested that adherence to clinic appointments for hospital-discharged tuberculosis patients seemed better when the distance between patients and clinics was sufficiently close. Of course, geographic distance cannot be measured merely in length, but must be determined by how long it takes the patient to reach a given health facility.

GYNECOLOGICAL AND OBSTETRICAL SERVICES   Morehead's retrospective study (1975) of medically indigent married black women in New Orleans included 155 subjects who continued to use an intrauterine device (IUD) for two years, and 115 women who terminated IUD use over the same time period. The terminators, who were younger, more mobile, and more likely to change marital partners, had a more positive attitude toward pregnancy and did not feel dependent on contraceptive availability. Considerably less tolerant of side effects, they also disliked more intensely the internal IUD string check. In contrast, the continuers were much more likely to accept discomforts as a condition of freedom from pregnancy. Characterized as having more dominant personalities and familial power, they were also more independent and responsible persons.

Lowe (1973) studied the relationship between compliance with medical regimen (that is, with regard to dietary compliance, weight gain, rest, exercise, drugs, douche, tub baths, smoking, and clinic and class attendance) and pregnancy outcomes (as measured by birth weights, Apgar sources, and maternal or infant complications) among 56 black primigravidas in North Carolina, 83 percent of whom were urban. She concluded that "compliance on all variables admittedly was poor, but the outcome of pregnancy did not appear to be influenced in any way other than that increased infant birth weight seemed related to increased maternal weight gain and that decreased infant birth weight seemed to be associated with increased ingestion of meats such as pork, bologna, and hot dogs" (1973:160).

OBESITY IN PEDIATRIC PATIENTS   Using a reformulated and expanded Health Belief model, Becker and his colleagues (1977) investigated the efficacy of the model in predicting compliance of mothers (or responsible grandmothers) to prescribed diets for obese children. Almost all the subjects, drawn from an urban, largely low-income population, were black. Substantial variations in dietary compliance and appointment keeping were accounted for by health motives, threat of disease, and benefits of action. Compliance was greater among those who were more concerned generally about their children's health, who had heightened perceptions of the potential seriousness of illnesses to their children, and who felt that they could exercise some control over factors inducing weight loss. Correlations between demographic characteristics and compliance variables showed that the only significant associations included age of the child and marital status of the mother. No significant associations were found between such factors as race, mother's educational level, family income, and household size.

HYPERTENSION AND OTHER AILMENTS   In commenting on the widespread absence of treatment for asymptomatic hypertension and diabetes mellitus in their elderly Chicago sample, Ostfeld and his associates (1971) indicated that evidence that treatment would be beneficial was not compelling and that maintaining adequate long-term therapy frequently posed difficult problems for the elderly poor, many of whom did not understand the necessity for medication or adherence to a drug regimen when they did not feel sick, a finding similar to that reported by

Stamler and Stamler (1976). Freis, who also noted the difficulty of motivating asymptomatic hypertensive patients to take medication, believed that the problem was compounded among low-income blacks: "Educational disadvantages and suspicion make the problem of communication and necessary changes in attitudes even more difficult" (1973:1).

Lack of education and other presumed demographic deficiencies of low-income blacks, however, may not be substantial determinants of noncompliance with antihypertensive regimens. Finnerty, Mattie, and Finnerty (1973) interviewed 60 dropouts from hypertensive clinics at the District of Columbia General Hospital, Washington Hospital Center, Columbia Hospital, and Georgetown University Medical Center (all in the Washington, D.C. area). The major reasons for discontinuance of clinic attendance were prolonged waiting times (2.5 hours, on the average) and poor physician-patient relationships (the average time spent with the physician was 7.5 minutes). Most of the dropouts viewed hypertension as being more severe than a cold or heart disease, and 56 percent not only were aware of the need for regular checkups but also knew that maintaining appointments was the vehicle for checkups. Although 25 percent of the patients felt they could treat themselves, the majority (58.7 percent) believed that hypertension specialists were needed, and 41 percent felt that a primary need was more physician time. Finnerty, Mattie, and Finnerty concluded that dropouts were not motivated by "lack of intelligence, disregard for their health, or . . . economic reasons. To the contrary, the dropout population emerges as an intelligent, concerned group of patients whose motivation was limited by barriers on their time and who clearly viewed the system as not directed to their concerns" (1973: 74–75). Finnerty, Shaw, and Himmelsbach stated with regard to hypertensives that "once a rigid prescriptive management plan has been instituted by the physician, the patient can be followed by a well-trained paramedical person thereby conserving valuable physician's time' (1973: 78). Ware's analysis of the problems involved in fostering compliance among hypertensives supports the conclusion reached by Finnerty, Mattie, and Finnerty that money is not a major barrier: "Even in the black community only 5 percent of the patients interviewed in this random [1974 Health Interview] survey indicated cost as a primary barrier" (Ware 1977:56).

Although Miller and Algee agreed that economics and ethnicity were not the main determinants of compliance for various disorders, they nevertheless stressed that noncompliance "pose[s] special dangers for black, poor, and aged patients" (1978:733). The fact that they provided no empirical or experimental support for this generalization suggests a well-meaning but superficial approach to problems of noncompliance, a phenomenon present to a considerable extent in Snow's assertion (1974) that it simply makes little sense to indicate to blacks that high blood pressure is a lifelong condition, and in White's plea (1977) that hypertensive blacks must understand the need for lifelong medication. As previously suggested, knowledge alone is an insufficient determinant of compliance. With respect to urban blacks who use alternative medical systems, it is important to note, however, that compliance with mainstream medical regimens can be adversely affected when folk healers advise patients to suspend all other treatment (Wintrob 1973).

A number of physicians and other health professionals believe that compliance is enhanced with personalized care or continuity of care (see Finnerty, Mattie, and Finnerty 1973; Finnerty, Shaw, and Himmelsbach 1973; Wilson 1973). Coulehan noted that "adequate therapy for hypertension demands continued compliance with a drug regimen over long periods despite a lack of symptoms. However, the hospital clinics and emergency rooms that urban blacks frequently use for health care do not foster such long-term compliance because care is frequently impersonal, fractionated according to specialty service, and characterized by a high rate of broken appointments" (1979:130).[10]

Believing that neighborhood health centers should be better settings than hospital clinics for controlling hypertension because they were designed to provide accessible, continuous, and personalized care, Coulehan (1979) investigated the effectiveness of a program at the Theiss Health Center (located in a Pittsburgh public housing project) in inducing compliance among 215 hypertensive black adults. His measures of compliance or noncompliance were continuation in the clinic program, lower blood pressure, and development of complications of hypertension. (Hypertensive patients who require drug therapy to reduce the risk of strokes but who fail to take their medication are at higher risk for such complications of hypertension as strokes.) Although 67 percent of the patients studied by Coulehan remained active in care (with most of the dropouts occurring during the first year), the program had only modest success. Coulehan, who concluded that the current treatment and follow-up procedures were unsatisfactory in inducing compliance with the medical regimen, hypothesized that either obese patients were less compliant with treatment, hypertension was more resistant to drug treatment in obese patients (especially obese black women), or the initial and final blood pressures were both falsely high owing to inadequate control for large arm circumference (1979:134).

PSYCHIATRIC CARE Some studies have also focused on lack of compliance with psychiatric regimens among urban blacks. Raynes and Warren (1971) and Raynes and Patch (1971), using data from Boston City Hospital, found that a substantially large proportion of psychiatric outpatients who failed to keep appointments (following telephone referrals) were black, and that hospital discharges against medical advice were also disproportionately higher among blacks (especially females) than among whites. Using as subjects 30 black male heroin addicts being treated in a methadone maintenance clinic, Levine and his colleagues (1972) concluded that those patients who were easily molded by external pressures to perform as expected were most successful. Sue and his co-workers (1974), in a comparison of black and white clients of community mental health facilities in the greater Seattle area, found that 52.1 percent of the blacks (as compared with only 29.8 percent of the whites) terminated after the first session. Although they contended that "there was no evidence that blacks received inexpensive or less 'preferred' services since no racial differences emerged in individual psychotherapy" (Sue et al. 1974: 797), they did admit that "blacks were [significantly] more often seen at intake by paraprofessionals . . . and less often by professional specialists . . . than whites . . . A similar finding was obtained in the type of personnel performing the therapy, with blacks working more with paraprofessional than professional staff in comparison with whites" (1974:798). Further, the strongest determinant of patient assignment to a paraprofessional or a professional was race.

It may be inappropriate to provide racial comparisons of length of therapy unless adequate controls are also established for the etiology of psychiatric disorders. As Jones (1974), among others, has suggested, lower-class or black persons may have more situational problems than whites, which means that a shorter term of therapy is needed. It may also be the case that using paraprofessionals reduces compliance among urban blacks for some disorders. Chappel and Daniels suggested the feasibility of psychiatric home visiting in order to provide "an effective nonverbal way of bridging social and cultural gaps which interfere with the development of a treatment relationship between patient and therapist" (1972: 200).

SUMMARY   The hard data available about medical compliance among urban blacks show that it is dependent on many direct and indirect variables, and that the available findings are generally inconclusive. Perhaps the model used by Becker and his associates (1977) could provide an appropriate theoretical framework for further investigations of medical compliance for chronic illnesses among various urban black subgroups.

Specific Social and Psychological Factors Related to Compliance

The various types of social and psychological factors which research will show to be validly and reliably associated at statistically and meaningfully significant levels with compliance or noncompliance among patients in general will, no doubt, also be applicable to appropriate subsets of urban blacks. In an excellent review of compliance literature, Marston found no clear-cut determinants of compliance:

When demographic variables were examined separately, little or no association was found between compliance behavior and sex, age, race, marital status, socio-economic status, or education. It is unclear whether actual severity of illness is related to compliance, although severity, as perceived by the patient, probably results in increased compliance. Increased numbers of different recommendations may be associated with more serious illnesses, and noncompliance increases with the complexity of the regimen. Knowledge alone concerning illness and its treatment has not provided sufficient motivation for patients to follow their regimens. The recent use of various personality tests to predict compliance has also been disappointing. (1970: 320–321)

Marston also advised that "some of the more promising predictors of compliance have been the types of interactions which occur between patients and physicians, and the use of fear communications . . . It seems likely that compliance with medical regimens is determined by some type of interaction effect involving demographic, illness, and social-psychological variables" (1970:321). Although some of the studies cited earlier in this section, which were published after Marston's review, concluded that specific demographic variables such as race, marital status, age, and socioeconomic status substantially affected compliance, the majority did not. Haug and Lavin's study (1978) of compliance to medical advice among a prepaid and a fee-for-service sample in a Midwestern metropolis showed that only about 9 percent of the variance within the prepaid sample was explained by race, sex, and age, and only about 9 percent in the fee-for-service group by age, education, race, and a measure of general authority. Buttressed by Davis's findings (1966, 1968a, 1968b), Marston's advice about the promising predictors of compliance remains valid today.

Even though precise information is not yet available to aid physicians, patients, and significant others in maximizing compliance, the issues of recognizing potential or actual noncompliers and increasing compliance are relevant. Gillum and Barsky believe that the suspicions of physicians about likely noncompliers

should be raised by any patient who does not regard his medical problem as serious, who will admit if questioned that he has doubts about his ability to comply, and who appears hostile, demanding, aggressive, and overly self-sufficient. Likewise, patients with many other important demands on their time, attention, and finances, and those with poor social support at home, should raise the physician's index of suspicion. Any patient on a complex regimen, or one that requires much change of basic lifestyles or habits is a likely noncomplier, as is any patient with whom the physician feels his communication or relation is ambiguous, fettered, or constrained. (1974: 1565)

Satcher's concerns (1973) about the effects of white physicians (by virtue of race alone) in reducing compliance should also be considered. Raynes and Patch (1971), for example, felt that an increase in black staff in psychiatric units would increase compliance to medical advice among black patients. However, Holder (1972) conducted a field experiment of 62 black and 60 white maternity patients in Wayne County Hospital in 1968, in which his independent variables were communication source, message, and audience characteristics, and certain beliefs and behaviors were the dependent variables. He used black and white nurses and housewives as communicators. He found that "race had no observable influence on subsequent behaviors," and his results "cast doubts concerning the superior effectiveness of indigenous communicators (adults) in eliciting compliance with recommended health behaviors" (1972:348).

Whether or not the race of the physician or other health personnel substantially affects compliance among urban blacks, it is necessary for physicians to be aware of the effects of physician-patient interaction on noncompliance, and not to explain noncompliance glibly, as most of Davis's physician subjects did (1966), by the personality of the patient. The sagacious advice of Saunders should be pondered carefully:

> The patient who withdraws from a medical relationship before the termination of the relationship is medically indicated has received poor care just as much as if a preventable error in diagnosis had been made or the wrong drug administered. The physician who, because of his manner or his lack of understanding of individual or group-related differences, is unable to establish a relationship which gives satisfaction to the patient cannot give good medical care, in the fullest sense of that phrase, however skilled he may be in the other techniques of his craft. (1954:243)

It seems logical that effectively transmitted fear communications may be quite useful in motivating at least partial compliance among patients who have been assigned some responsibility for managing their illnesses. Such communications are probably more effective when the patient perceives an illness as severe and the prescribed treatment as adequate for symptom abatement. Yet Miller and Algee contend that "patient education is a positive factor which increases compliance, but fear arousal should not be used" (1978:736). In opposition to this view, James indicates that sometimes "scaring" the patient is very effective (C. James, personal communcation). Further, although Marston notes that threatening patients is considered to be in poor taste, she concludes that "research in the use of fear communications has indicated that they, when accompanied by practical instructions for reducing or eliminating the threat, are effective in motivating people to undertake diagnostic and preventive health measures" (1970:321).

Various measures have been suggested to increase compliance; they have met with varying degrees of success, most often ruling out the demographic factors that were thought to have placed people at high risk for noncompliance, as in the case of race and socioeconomic status (see, for example, Marston 1970). It must be recognized, of course, that in addition to methodological differences reducing comparisons between compliance studies, social changes (for example, the advent of Medicare and Medicaid and the desegregation of health facilities) also make it difficult to compare studies over time. That is, although it seems clear today that race and socioeconomic status are probably not significant factors directly affecting compliance, they may have been more powerful predictors in earlier years. A major challenge to both contemporary mainstream practitioners serving urban blacks and those undertaking research about their health patterns is to increase greatly their knowledge and understanding about noncompliance, as well as developing mechanisms for reducing it. Another challenging objective is to increase congruence between physician and patient expectations.

Stamler and Stamler stress the need for a widespread program to identify, evaluate, and provide long-term comprehensive care for hypertensive patients. Its implementation would require various resources, including health team personnel: "Almost everywhere physicians will need a good deal of assistance from other personnel—nutritionists, nurses, technicians, health counsellors—and more of these will have to be recruited and given special training in the care of persons with hypertension" (1976:30). Mandel, a black pharmacist, proclaims that the problem of noncompliance among hypertensives can be solved "*only* through the cooperative efforts of pharmacists and physicians" (1977:36). It is striking that any role for the patient is missing from these suggestions. Thus, another challenge to many physicians and auxiliary staff is to recognize clearly the role of the patient in managing his chronic illness.

Patterns Influencing Adherence to Dietary Restrictions

Quoting Jean Mayer (1965), Lowe indicated that "in the United States 60 percent of the diets of Negro families were obviously inadequate, with a limited intake of protein" (1973:159). Furthermore, Lowe found that Southern urban blacks "are heavy consumers of flour, baking powder, fats (fatback), rice, grits, cornmeal, sweet potatoes, and in small amounts fish, meat (preferably salt pork, bacon, and fresh pork), and poultry. Consumption of fresh vegetables is low and consumption of citrus fruits is negligible" (1973:159).

In spite of these general features, dietary patterns vary widely among urban blacks. Jerome (1969), for example, studied black urban migrants to determine transitions from traditional Southern to intermediate to new meal patterns. After about 18 months of urban residence, the heavy breakfast, midafternoon dinner, and supper consisting of dinner leftovers are replaced by a heavy breakfast with breakfast leftovers used for lunch, followed by dinner (renamed supper) much later in the afternoon, generally occurring before 6:00 P.M. The occupationally-induced transition continues with increased urban adaptation, finally resulting in a meal pattern consisting of a light breakfast, a lunch not based on leftovers, and dinner, which combines the traditional breakfast and dinner patterns. However, adults with no outside employment typically consume leftovers from the previous day's dinner for their lunch.

In addition to these acculturational sources of dietary variations among urban blacks suggested by Jerome, religious affiliations also bring about different dietary habits. For example, members of the American Muslim Mission (formerly the World Community of Al-Islam, popularly known as Black Muslims) abstain from consuming pork and alcoholic beverages.[11] Conforming Seventh Day Adventists also do not eat pork. Some blacks are vegetarians. Many also supplement their diets with vitamins or tonics. In a study of 200 mothers of different ethnic groups, Johnston (1977) found that black mothers of female children believed more strongly in the efficacy of vitamins than did comparable whites. No racial differences emerged between mothers of male children, however.

The degree to which the regular diet of blacks is unique has probably been greatly exaggerated. Without defining soul food, White, for example, stated: "Soul food has always been popular and enjoyed by the black community. Pork is widely used and food is well-seasoned. Upon admission to the hospital, the black client is fed food that is unfamiliar and tasteless. A balanced diet can be planned using soul food" (1977:31). I queried approximately 50 urban blacks who had had previous hospitalizations about the familiarity of the hospital food: none of them had been served any unfamiliar food, but most agreed that hospital food (like the food served in dormitories) is frequently bland.

As suggested earlier in Collette and Ludwig's study (1969), the influence of race or ethnicity on adherence to medically prescribed diets is probably insignificant, especially when patients perceive illnesses as serious or life-threatening. Perhaps the greatest problems arise in dealing with obesity or alcoholism, where adherence is more closely affected by psychological (and not ethnic) factors. Undoubtedly, some differences in dietary patterns attributable to social class or cultural life-style exist among urban blacks, but I could not locate any hard data on this topic.

In most instances, when physicians impose dietary restrictions on their urban black patients, they probably do not have sufficient information available to them about the normal dietary patterns of their patients. Often they do not take the time to determine these patterns and to work out necessary dietary modifications with the patients. Patients using clinics or medical schools are frequently referred to dietitians with deferred appointments. Many dietitians who are themselves not adequately knowledgeable use "canned" programs (pamphlets, brochures, and the like) for patients, and ineffective communication occurs. For example, patients may be advised to reduce fat intake without being informed simultaneously about how greens can be cooked without fatback, or how lemon may be used to season salads in lieu of salad dressing. Many dietitians are also uninformed about individual and subcultural dietary variations among urban blacks. Of course, many physicians are also not well informed about nutrition.

Additional problems arise when medically prescribed diets are based on an assumption that patients eat three suitably prepared meals daily within the home, when many, in fact, do not eat each meal at home. The patient's daily life-style must be understood, and dietary modifications made accordingly. Physicians concerned about preventive care for children must also acknowledge that many parents are in the labor force and are not able to provide breakfasts, lunches, snacks, and dinners which they prepare themselves for their growing children. Modifications in meals must be made for children, including ones which children themselves can monitor. Given the food stamp program and other nutritional programs, it is probably not now true that many urban black children suffer from malnutrition due to the scarcity of food. Today, malnutrition must more often be attributed to bad eating habits than to the lack of any food.

Recovery, Rehabilitation, and Death
Coping with Chronic and Terminal Illnesses and Death

Patterns of coping with chronic illness and death vary widely among urban blacks. The method of coping with chronic illness is heavily dependent on the severity of illness or the extent to which it disables the patient, especially in pursuing occupational or familial roles. Patients who are not severely disabled, and who can exercise some control over the extent to which they modify their expected roles, frequently continue to carry out those roles to the best of their abilities. They are often aided by significant others.

In many cases, however, particularly among low-income urban blacks, appropriate modifications are not possible because they are beyond the capacities of the patient. For instance, chronically ill blacks who can no longer engage in manual occupations requiring tasks that are medically prohibited or otherwise impossible for them to perform will find themselves out of work. Some who have considerable seniority, or who are greatly liked by their employers, may find themselves shifted to occupations that are feasible for them, but generally urban blacks with disabling chronic illnesses who were employed prior to the onset of the incapacity find themselves unemployed. One of the problems confronting them is obtaining medical certification for their disabling condition in order to be able to draw a disability pension.

Another problem is the amount of social support the chronically ill person receives, particularly from the familial/kinship network. The importance of familial support has been well documented for various aspects of the illness phenomenon. Davis (1968b), for example, indicated that familial disorganization reduces medical compliance, and Warnecke and his colleagues (1978) underscored the need for developing quasi-family groups, similar to Weight Watchers or Alcoholics Anonymous, in helping smokers to stop smoking. In this regard, a prevailing myth is that the extended family is the predominant familial form among blacks, and that it operates effectively in providing for and protecting its members from undesirable social conditions. Not only is the extended family *not* the predominant form among either rural or urban blacks, it is also not always in a position to provide sufficient instrumental and affective aid to its members.

Nevertheless, to the extent possible, services are provided by the family either out of a feeling of obligation or voluntarily. A distinction must be made between productive and unproductive services, however. For example, some older extended family members may inform or instruct pregnant women or new mothers about appropriate prenatal and infant care, and their advice will be followed; others will instruct these women inappropriately, and their advice will still be followed. This does not mean that generational transmission of health behaviors is inappropriate (or will not occur, because it invariably will), but that increased consideration must be given to the type of knowledge being transmitted and the degree to which that knowledge is being augmented or modified by other cultural institutions, such as the schools or the health system.

Another area of decreasing familial support may be connected with the increasing labor force participation of many urban black women, which means that fewer of them are constantly at home to provide regular care for family members who are ill. An interesting problem now developing among many blacks and whites is related to their concerns that governmental programs should pay a family member as a home health aide for a family member who is ill or disabled. Currently, kin are excluded as paid personnel. Here, too, physicians must become increasingly conscious of the familial situation, and not merely assume that the presence of a woman automatically ensures around-the-clock care. Perhaps more consideration should be given to ways in which the family can be helped by nonfamilial support groups or other community efforts directed at increasing compliance to medical regimens in a variety of ways. In all instances, it should not be assumed that the wife or mother must take the primary role.

Many factors, such as age and social roles of terminally ill black urban patients, influence patterns associated with terminal illness. The data in this area are also scarce. It is likely that successful coping by a terminally ill patient is much more common among elderly than among younger blacks. As mentioned earlier, many urban blacks who suspect a terminal illness may delay medical diagnosis. When the diagnosis is made, the expected stages from denial through acceptance set in. During the denial period, many may seek alternative opinions or turn to powers considered greater than themselves to fathom the reason for the disease. Many terminally ill persons may pray and ask others to pray for them. Some accept terminal illness believing that it is "God's will," and nothing more can be done. Perhaps the degree of acceptance of terminal illness is associated with conceptions of an afterlife: those who believe they will be rewarded in the afterlife may be far more accepting than those who think they may be doomed to hell, and many blacks believe in heaven and hell. Most urban blacks probably want to know if they are terminally ill; some who are not so informed probably know "deep down." Even when they know their condition, however, some patients prefer that their families not be informed.

Kalish and Reynolds (1976), who purported that black attitudes and behaviors toward death could probably not be understood with reference to violent death (an assumption I do not share), studied 109 blacks in Los Angeles County, 51 percent of whom were female. The median age of the subjects was 45.7 years, and 86 percent of them were Protestants. Finding what they considered to be an unusually high regard for living, Kalish and Reynolds reported that 60 percent of the black subjects felt that dying people in general should be informed of their prognosis, and two-thirds of the 60 percent believed that the physician should be the informant. Seventy-one percent wanted some knowledge of their own impending death, and 49 percent thought others should be given this information. Only slightly more than half felt that they were capable of sharing this information with another person. More than 80 percent indicated no fear of death (Kalish and Reynolds 1976:104).

In comparing the black subjects with Anglos, Japanese Americans, and Mexican Americans, Kalish and Reynolds reported that blacks were "least likely to encourage family members to spend time with them during their terminal stages, if it be inconvenient," "least likely to carry out the last wishes of a dying spouse," and similar to the other groups in turning to a relative "for comfort in time of grief" (1976:106–107).

Based on a study of 40 poor black mothers in Los Angeles, Wyatt suggested that the characterization of "death of a friend" as a significant social loss "might be better understood as an artifact of the black culture than as a function of the family's economic condition. While 'death of a friend' may be significant to other ethnic groups, literature describing the importance of the extended family and significant others to the stability of the black family support system suggests that the loss of a friend is viewed in the black culture in a highly significant way" (1977:17). The two supporting sources she cited for this opinion were Billingsley (1968) and Hill (1972), neither of whom studied empirically the cultural meaning of death of a friend nor made any ethnic comparisons.

Resumption of Normal Roles after Illness

Insofar as I know, urban blacks have no rituals associated with resuming normal roles following illness. Unlike some other ethnic groups, urban blacks have no standardized cultural rituals for any events, including birth, marriage, and death. Informal processes associated with recovery or rehabilitation of persons who were ill include gradual resumption of normal roles, probably with some anxiety on the part of those who are relinquishing and assuming roles.

Malingering

Given the value placed on good health by urban blacks, most who are ill wish to recover or return to good health. Although some malingering does occur, the data are not sufficient at this time to describe the characteristics of malingerers, a subject which, incidentally, was discussed years ago by Williams (1915–16), a black physician. There are at least two important and overlapping conditions inducing malingering among urban blacks: job dissatisfaction and inadequate employment opportunities. Persons who are dissatisfied with their jobs cr cannot find adequate employment (as they define it) may tend to malinger following illnesses longer than those who are eager to return to work. Some urban blacks may also malinger when they wish to avoid resumption of familial roles.[12]

Concluding Remarks

Given the underlying assumption of this volume that ethnicity has a significant impact on health attitudes and behaviors, the major purpose of this chapter was to provide some information about the health attitudes and behaviors of urban blacks that would help the mainstream medical system improve its delivery of medical services to this group. In general, the information and impressions that have been shared indicate strongly that urban blacks constitute a highly heterogeneous group. Their considerable heterogeneity raises doubts immediately about the wisdom of classifying them collectively as an ethnic group for at least two reasons pertinent here: one is that the only applicable criterion for classifying any black in the United States as a member of the ethnic group *black* is race, or, more specifically, on the basis of highly visible physical traits, such as skin color and hair texture; the second is that urban blacks display considerable variation in their health attitudes and behaviors, and, insofar as can be determined, have no common racial-geographic origin. Nevertheless, it is important to examine urban blacks as a group, primarily because so many people within the biomedical system think of them as a collectivity, or as if they were all "just alike."

In addition to the tremendous heterogeneity of urban blacks, several other important conclusions can be reached about their health attitudes and behaviors from the foregoing review of the data.

1. Although urban blacks as a group are culturally heterogeneous, a number of people, both black and white, still believe strongly that they are culturally unique and not a part of the larger American culture. An illustration of this viewpoint is seen in Mayfield's contention that "the black child, like all children, learns how to function in his own culture. His language is the legitimate form of communication in his immediate surroundings. His diet, music, religious expression, and the like are different from those of other ethnic groups" (1972:109). In effect, I have argued an opposing viewpoint, but Mayfield's viewpoint cannot be dismissed lightly because many people, including some black and white physicians, *act* as if it were true.

2. The available data about the health attitudes and behaviors of urban blacks with regard to the folk, popular, and biomedical health systems are scant, fragmented, and inconclusive. The data that are available, however, suggest strongly that a substantially large proportion of contemporary urban blacks rely heavily, and sometimes exclusively (depending on the perceived illness), on the biomedical system for symptom abatement. Since the data are inconclusive, they do not permit definitive conclusions at this time about the effects of demographic characteristics, such as sex, age, marital status, race, and education, on behaviors geared toward good health practices among urban blacks. However, it seems reasonable to conclude that, regardless of the direct effects of these variables on health attitudes and behaviors among urban blacks in the past, various social changes that have increased the access of urban blacks to health facilities have reduced the influencing weight of the variables. Much more weight must be attached to illness-morbidity variables, as suggested by Wolinsky

(1978); and in the area of compliance with medical advice, the most promising independent variables for research include physician-patient interaction and fear communications (Marston 1970).

3. The great difficulty I had in locating good data about the health conditions of urban blacks can be attributed in part to the dearth of information collected, analyzed, and published by the major federal agencies (particularly the National Center for Health Statistics) responsible for such data. This obviously means that such data ought to be collected, analyzed, and published in the future, with appropriate breakouts for all the relevant groups which physicians, epidemiologists, and other interested persons feel are needed. As a starting point, health data are clearly needed for blacks broken out by specific geographic locations (such as suburban, inner city, and farm), age, sex, socioeconomic status (perhaps specific by occupation, education, and income), and marital or familial status.

Furthermore, good research, using representative samples of urban blacks of all socioeconomic statuses, must be undertaken to determine the health attitudes and behaviors of this group. This research must include as a study variable the health institutions and their responses to urban black patients or potential patients. In the meantime, while mainstream practitioners await the results of such research, white medical practitioners could learn much by consulting with knowledgeable black medical practitioners, a group they often overlook. This does not mean, of course, that predominantly white medical schools should attempt to make instant experts out of black medical students (who, in fact, may also know very little about black health attitudes and behaviors), but they should make use of knowledgeable experts whenever practical. Of course, there are some white practitioners who are also extremely knowledgeable about black health attitudes, and they should be identified and used as well. Many black medical students and practitioners also need to enhance their knowledge about the sociocultural context of health and illness among urban blacks, particularly with regard to low-income blacks. Nowlin believes (and I agree) that it is entirely possible that current groups of low-income Southern black patients almost constitute a health culture of their own. This raises the important question of educational impact on medical compliance.

Above all, whatever data are generated by federal agencies and by other public or private sources, publication should be timely.

4. The major issues raised in this chapter include the effects of ethnicity on the health beliefs and behaviors of urban blacks and on the medical care they receive, and, more specifically, the feasible congruence between folk, popular, and biomedical systems, as well as the effects of the race of the physician on those being treated. These issues were obviously not

resolved, but mainstream medical practitioners must be aware of them, knowing that the answers of yesterday may not suffice for today, given the role of social change among urban blacks.

5. An additional issue raised questions about biologically determined racial differences. This issue was also not resolved, but it should be given more research attention. In addition to the possibility of biological differences between blacks and whites, as suggested by Voors and colleagues (1979) and others cited in this chapter, Weaver (1976–77), among others, has raised environmental concerns that may explain racial differences in infant mortality, and Owen and Yanochik-Owen (1977) have discussed the possibility of biological differences in hemoglobin level. In addition, a number of investigators have raised the issue of the probable racial differences in mental illnesses or their etiology, although others have stressed misconceptions in this area and in the general area of differences in racial intelligence (see, for example, Pasamanick 1963, 1969). The answers are not all in. But, more important, the answers can *never* be all in, in the sense that the population of blacks does not remain static for researchers; it is constantly changing in important ways. Therefore, it behooves researchers to remain aware that findings generated on given populations of urban blacks may not be applicable to subsequent cohorts of urban blacks. Such advice is even more pertinent to mainstream practitioners, who, in the final analysis, must remember that they are not treating a group, but individual patients (and, for some conditions, significant others)—each of whom, although an urban black, is in some respects like no other person.

6. It is my opinion that mainstream medical practitioners are most effective in treating urban blacks in emergency or critical situations and least effective in treating them in situations where much of the management of the illness is really the responsibility of the patient or his guardian. To this extent, mainstream medical practitioners must learn how to increase effective physician-patient interaction in order to aid in improving the overall health status of urban blacks. When it is feasible (that is, in the best interest of the patient), paraprofessionals or non-physician personnel could also be used (an area that is still in need of much research).

7. Mainstream medical practitioners also have a responsibility to help increase the solid education of urban blacks, particularly since Elesh and Schollaert have indicated that there is "growing evidence that education can explain most (though not all) of the differences attributed to the other measures of cultural predisposition . . . The sometimes forgotten point of . . . findings [about health attitudes and behaviors when education is controlled] is that formal education creates a common culture—one which places a high value on medical care" (1972:238).

Finally, mainstream medical practitioners must remember that urban blacks also have a responsibility to improve their own health status through preventive and treatment modalities, because they must recognize that in health, as in other affairs, they should captain their own ships through prosperity and adversity. This is in line with Stokes's plea that a comprehensive national health-care plan in the United States "be tied to a program that would encourage people to take more responsibility for their own health" (1979:1).

Notes

Given the embryonic stage in which this chapter remained for a long time for various reasons, I am particularly grateful to Alan Harwood for his extreme patience and occasional push, as well as for his highly constructive guidance and comments. I acknowledge the tremendous assistance in developing some portions of the manuscript which I received from Charles James, a private physician in Charlotte, North Carolina, and from John B. Nowlin, a physician at the Duke University Medical Center. I recognize the difficulty in functioning as a mother and a writer during the preparation of this chapter in the summer of 1979, and am pleased that my daughter, Viola Elizabeth, consented to abide by rather constricting rules through most of the summer so as to facilitate my work. Finally, I dedicate this chapter to M. B., who shares freely with me his considerable knowledge and wisdom about many topics and issues, not the least of which is his continuing concern about what he regards (and I agree) as my inadequate preventive health behaviors. He knows that at least I hear him.

1. Much of the recent emphasis on increasing the number of black physicians by mainstream medical schools has been directed toward increasing the number of black physicians to serve black patients. Given this emphasis, it could be presumed that most mainstream medical schools either believe that black patients are best served by black physicians, or that black physicians are not capable of effectively serving white patients. Clearly, the democratic thrust toward preparing physicians of any race to serve patients of any race represents the proper course for mainstream medical schools now and in the future.

2. The percentage increase in the median income over time in recent years, however, has been greater for black females than for black and white males or white females. For example, data for the years 1970 and 1976 from the U.S. Bureau of the Census show that the median total money income in constant 1976 dollars for year-round, full-time workers 14+ years of age in the United States was $6,651 and $7,831 respectively for black females (as compared to $8,116 and $8,376 for white females; $9,434 and $10,222 for black males; and $13,850 and $14,272 for white males). The percentage change was 11.8 percent for black females, 8.3 percent for black males, 3.2 percent for white females, and 3.0 percent for white males.

3. The assistance of Silas Jackson of the National Library of Medicine's Interactive Retrieval Service is greatly acknowledged in generating the computerized bibliographic compilation for review. In addition, Gary Thompson,

a postdoctoral fellow in the Center for the Study of Aging and Human Development, Duke University, 1978–1980, was extremely helpful in compiling a bibliography from holdings available at the Duke University Medical Center Library. Carolyn Brown also provided assistance in checking the bibliographic entries used in this chapter, as did Dr. Alan Harwood's staff.

4. A more recent manifestation of diseases contrived by racial prejudices is seen in Clifford Allen's concern about heterochromophilia, a condition he described as "the compulsion in human beings to choose a mate of different colour" (1968:243). "The condition," Allen wrote, "appears to be rather more than a fetishism since no single article of clothing, etc., is the basis of the attraction, but the whole woman. Indeed, it appears to be in the nature of imprinting in human beings . . . caused by the colour of the nurse in babyhood." Worried about its increase, he stated further that "it seems to be that apart from the implications as to its origin the condition is rare and not of great importance, but since we are getting more coloured women nursing white babies these days there is a likelihood of its becoming much more common" (1968:243).

5. For verification of this point, consult the indexes published by the National Center for Health Statistics (e.g., U.S. Department of Health, Education, and Welfare 1979) which indicate the variables, including ethnicity, contained in published reports. One major problem is that the U.S. government acts on the one hand as if ethnicity were important, but on the other hand, fails to collect relevant data about ethnicity and, in this case, about health patterns.

6. For further discussion of this issue, see especially Kadushin (1964, 1967) and Antonovsky (1967).

7. Kadushin (1964, 1967) argues forcefully that in modern societies such as the United States, the effects of social class on contracting a disease have diminished greatly, but that social class still influences heavily behaviors *after* the onset of illness. An opposing view is found in Antonovsky (1967). I believe the influence of social class has diminished, but it is still influential in terms of exposure to various diseases. An illustration is that poor elderly persons who are living in inadequate housing and are unable to maintain sufficient warmth or coolness are much more likely to be susceptible to pneumonia than are their elderly counterparts residing in adequate housing who have sufficient money to pay their rising utility bills.

8. An additional logical possibility at the point when both medical and nonmedical treatments have failed is to discontinue all treatment entirely. Though this alternative is possible, it was omitted from figure 1.1 on the assumption that people are motivated to seek relief from pain. In the case of some minor ailments, however, it is possible that no further treatment may ensue.

9. In an examination of factors influencing the spatial distribution of physicians in Chicago in 1960, Elesh and Schollaert attributed the tendency of some physicians to locate among their own ethnic groups to the fact that "in a competitive situation, they seek to take advantage of whatever preferences members of their ethnic groups have for giving their business to members of

the same group" (1972:237). However, in the case of many black physicians, they would have had no patients if they did not treat black patients. Thus, black physicians have generally not been able to avoid practicing in black areas. Elesh and Schollaert did find that some physicians, chiefly general practitioners, internists, pediatricians, and obstetricians/gynecologists, avoided practice in black areas, but they felt the avoidance could be reduced considerably if the aggregate income in the area were extremely high.

10. Sometimes urban blacks may be misled about mainstream medicine by the mass media. Compare, for example, the quote from Coulehan with the following apparent interpretation of it in *Jet* (August 9, 1979, 56:28): "The principal reason for the soaring death and disease rates is that the hospitals and clinics and emergency rooms that urban Blacks frequently use do not usually provide adequate programs to counter high blood pressure and cancer, experts say." Other misinformation contained in the same *Jet* article indicated that "Blacks have a lower average birth rate than Whites" and "the leading cause of death among Black males is murder." The need for better health education through the mass media that reach many urban blacks should be apparent.

11. Information received in a personal communication from C. Eric Lincoln, an expert on the World Community of Al-Islam, indicated that considerable modifications had occurred among the Black Muslims since the death of the founder, Elijah Mohammed. One change is less adherence by the members to regulations promoting overall health status, with the exception of proscriptions common throughout the Moslemic world, such as not eating pork or drinking alcoholic beverages.

12. I suspect that the best data on black malingering may be located in governmental records pertaining to veterans' or unemployment benefits, and I did not investigate this literature.

References

ALLEN, CLIFFORD. 1968. Heterochromophilia (correspondence). *British Journal of Psychiatry* 114:243.

ANDERSON, PEYTON F. 1935. The Negro Tuberculosis Patient and Surgical Treatment. *National Negro Health News* 3:16–17.

ANTONOVSKY, AARON. 1967. Social Class and Illness: A Reconsideration. *Sociological Inquiry* 37: 311–322.

BARTLEY, MARY ANNE. 1972. The Developing AFNA Plan: New Access Routes to Medical Careers. *Journal of the National Medical Association* 64:264–267.

BASCO, DOLORES, et al. 1972. Epidemiological Analysis in School Populations as a Basis for Change in School Nursing Practice—Report of the Second Phase of a Longitudinal Study. *American Journal of Public Health* 62:491–497.

BATES, JAMES E., HARRY H. LIEBERMAN, and RODNEY N. POWELL. 1970. Provisions for Health Care in the Ghetto: The Family Health Team. *American Journal of Public Health* 60:1222–1224.

BEATTY, WILLIAM K. 1971. Daniel Hale Williams: Innovative Surgeon, Educator, and Hospital Administrator. *Chest* 60:175–182.

BECKER, MARSHALL H., et al. 1977. The Health Belief Model and Prediction of Dietary Compliance: A Field Experiment. *Journal of Health and Social Behavior* 18:348–366.

BERGNER, LAWRENCE, and MERVYN W. SUSSER. 1970. Low Birth Weight and Prenatal Nutrition: An Interpretative Review. *Pediatrics* 46:946–966.

BILLINGSLEY, ANDREW. 1968. *Black Families in White America*. Englewood Cliffs, N.J.: Prentice-Hall.

BLACKWELL, BARRY. 1973. Medical Intelligence, Drug Therapy, Patient Compliance. *New England Journal of Medicine* 289:249–252.

BONHAM, GORDON S. 1978. *Prevalence of Chronic Skin and Musculoskeletal Conditions, United States, 1976*. DHEW Publication no. (PHS) 78–1548. Hyattsville, Md.: National Center for Health Statistics.

BRANCH, MARIE F. 1977. Catch Up or Keep Up? Ethnic Minorities in Nursing. *Urban Health* 6:49–52.

CAPPANNARI, STEPHEN C., et al. 1975. Voodoo in the General Hospital, A Case of Hexing and Regional Enteritis. *Journal of the American Medical Association* 232:938–940.

CHAPMAN, W. P., and C. M. JONES. 1944. Variations in Cutaneous and Visceral Pain Sensitivity in Normal Subjects. *Journal of Clinical Investigation* 23:81-91.

CHAPPEL, JOHN N., and ROBERT S. DANIELS. 1972. Home Visiting: An Aid to Psychiatric Treatment in Black Urban Ghettos. *Current Psychiatric Therapies* 12:194–201.

CHASE, HELEN C. 1973. Desegregating Health Statistics (letter to the editor). *American Journal of Public Health* 63:836–837.

CHATMAN, DONALD L. 1976. Endometriosis in the Black Woman. *American Journal of Obstetrics and Gynecology* 125:987–989.

CHOI, JAI W. 1978. *Acute Conditions: Incidence and Associated Disability, United States, July 1975–June 1976*. DHEW Publication no. (PHS) 78–1548. Hyattsville, Md.: National Center for Health Statistics.

COLLETTE, JOHN, and EDWARD G. LUDWIG. 1969. Patient Compliance with Medical Advice. *Journal of the National Medical Association* 61:408–411.

COULEHAN, JOHN L. 1979. Hypertension Followup in an Urban Black Population. *Public Health Reports* 94:130–135.

CULLITON, BARBARA J. 1972. Sickle Cell Anemia: The Route from Obscurity to Prominence. *Science* 178:138–142.

CYPRESS, BEULAH K. 1979. *Office Visits for Diseases of the Circulatory System, The National Ambulatory Medical Care Survey, United States, 1975–1976*. DHEW Publication no. (PHS) 79–1791. Hyattsville, Md.: National Center for Health Statistics.

DAVIS, MILTON S. 1966. Variations in Patients' Compliance with Doctors' Orders: Analysis of Congruence between Survey Responses and Results of Empirical Investigations. *Journal of Medical Education* 41:1037–1048.

———. 1968a. Physiologic, Psychological and Demographic Factors in Patient Compliance with Doctors' Orders. *Medical Care* 6:115–122.

———. 1968b. Variations in Patients' Compliance with Doctors' Advice: An Empirical Analysis of Patterns of Communication. *American Journal of Public Health* 58:274–288.

Doto, Irene L., et al. 1972. Coccidioidin, Histoplasmin, and Tuberculin Sensitivity among School Children in Maricopa County, Arizona. *American Journal of Epidemiology* 95:464–474.

Edland, J. F., and C. E. Duncan. 1973. Suicide Notes in Monroe County: a 23-Year Look (1950–1972). *Journal of Forensic Sciences* 18:364–369.

Elesh, David, and Paul T. Schollaert. 1972. Race and Urban Medicine: Factors Affecting the Distribution of Physicians in Chicago. *Journal of Health and Social Behavior* 13:236–249.

Erhardt, Carl L., and Helen C. Chase. 1973. Ethnic Group, Education of Mother, and Birth Weight, part 2. *American Journal of Public Health* 63(supplement):17–26.

Ezzati, Trena M. 1980. *The National Ambulatory Medical Care Survey: 1977 Summary, United States, January-December 1977.* DHEW Publication no. (PHS) 80–1795. Hyattsville, Md.: National Center for Health Statistics.

Fabrega, Horacio, Jr., and Robert E. Roberts. 1972. Social-Psychological Correlates of Physician Use by Economically Disadvantaged Negro Urban Residents. *Medical Care* 10:215–223.

Fink, Raymond, et al. 1969. The "Filter-Down" Process to Psychotherapy in a Group Practice Medical Care Program. *American Journal of Public Health* 59:245–260.

Finnerty, Frank A. Jr., Edward C. Mattie, and Francis A. Finnerty, III. 1973. Hypertension in the Inner City: I. Analysis of Clinic Dropouts. *Circulation* 47:73–75.

Finnerty, Frank A., Jr., Lawrence W. Shaw, and Clifton K. Himmelsbach. 1973. Hypertension in the Inner City: II. Detection and Follow-Up. *Circulation* 47:76–78.

Fisher, George U., et al. 1970. Malaria in Soldiers Returning from Vietnam: Epidemiologic, Therapeutic, and Clinical Studies. *The American Journal of Tropical Medicine and Hygiene* 19:27–39.

Fort, Arthur T., et al. 1971. Counseling the Patient with Sickle Cell Disease about Reproduction: Pregnancy Outcome Does Not Justify the Maternal Risk. *American Journal of Obstetrics and Gynecology* 111:324–327.

Foster, Henry W., Jr. 1977. Clinical Management: Sickle Cell State and Pregnancy. *Urban Health* 6:20, 52.

Frankel, Barbara. 1977. *Childbirth in the Ghetto: Folk Beliefs of Negro Women in a North Philadelphia Hospital Ward.* San Francisco: R & E Research Associates.

Freis, Edward D. 1973. Hypertension, A Challenge in Preventive Cardiology. *Circulation* 47:1–2.

Gallagher, Eugene B. 1978. *Infants, Mothers, and Doctors.* Lexington, Mass.: D. C. Heath.

Gentile, Augustine. 1977. *Health Characteristics by Geographic Region, Large Metropolitan Areas, and Other Places of Residence, United States, 1973–74.* DHEW Publication no. (PHS) 78–1540. Hyattsville, Md.: National Center for Health Statistics.

GILLUM, RICHARD F., and ARTHUR J. BARSKY. 1974. Diagnosis and Management of Patient Noncompliance. *Journal of the American Medical Association* 228:1563–1567.

GOLDEN, KENNETH W. 1977. Voodoo in Africa and the United States. *American Journal of Psychiatry* 134:1425–1427.

GYLYS, JULIUS A., and BARBARA A. GYLYS. 1974. Cultural Influences and the Medical Behavior of Low Income Groups. *Journal of the National Medical Association* 66:308–312.

HALL, ARTHUR L., and PETER G. BOURNE. 1973. Indigenous Therapists in a Southern Black Urban Community. *Archives of General Psychiatry* 28:137–142.

HARRISON, IRA E. 1972. Patients' Evaluation of Neighborhood Health Centers. *Journal of the National Medical Association* 64:348–352.

HAUG, MARIE, and BEBE LAVIN. 1978. Method of Payment for Medical Care and Public Attitudes toward Physician Authority. *Journal of Health and Social Behavior* 19:279–291.

HENDIN, HERBERT. 1978. Suicide: The Psychosocial Dimension. *Suicide and Life-Threatening Behavior* 8:99–117.

HENSCHKE, ULRICH K., et al. 1973. Alarming Increase of the Cancer Mortality in the U.S. Black Population (1950–1967). *Cancer* 31:763–768.

HERSKOVITS, FRANCES S., ed. 1966. *The New World Negro, Selected Papers in Afroamerican Studies by Melville J. Herskovits.* Bloomington: Indiana University Press.

HILL, ROBERT B. 1972. *The Strengths of Black Families: A National Urban League Research Study.* New York: Emerson Hall.

HILLARD, JAMES R., and J. KENNETH ROCKWELL. 1978. Dysesthesia, Witchcraft, and Conversion Reaction: A Case Successfully Treated with Psychotherapy. *Journal of the American Medical Association* 240:1742–1744.

HINMAN, ALAN R. 1972. Resurgence of Measles in New York. *American Journal of Public Health* 62:498–503.

HOLDER, LEE. 1972. Effects of Source, Message, Audience Characteristics on Health Behavior Compliance. *Health Services Report* 87:343–350.

HOWIE, LONNIE J., and THOMAS F. DRURY. 1978. *Current Estimates from the Health Interview Survey: United States–1977.* DHEW Publication no. (PHS) 78–1554. Hyattsville, Md.: National Center for Health Statistics.

HYPERTENSION DETECTION AND FOLLOW-UP PROGRAM COOPERATIVE GROUP. 1977. Race, Education and Prevalence of Hypertension. *American Journal of Epidemiology* 106:351–361.

JACKSON, JACQUELYNE J. 1971. But Where are the Men? *The Black Scholar* 3:30–41.

———. 1973. Black Women in a Racist Society. In *Racism and Mental Health,* ed. Charles V. Willie, Bernard M. Kramer, and Bertram S. Brown. Pittsburgh: University of Pittsburgh Press.

———. 1979. Illegal Aliens: Big Threat to Black Workers. *Ebony* 34:33–36, 38, 40.

———. 1980. *Minorities and Aging.* Belmont, Calif.: Wadsworth.

JACKSON, OSCAR J., and WALDENSE NIXON. 1970. Medicine in the Black Community. *California Medicine, The Western Journal of Medicine* 116: 57–61.

JEROME, NORGE W. 1969. Northern Urbanization and Food Consumption Patterns of Southern-Born Negroes. *The American Journal of Clinical Nutrition* 22:1667–1669.

JOHNSTON, MAXENE. 1977. Folk Beliefs and Ethnocultural Behavior in Pediatrics. *Nursing Clinics of North America* 12:77–84.

JONES, ENRICO. 1974. Social Class and Psychotherapy: A Critical Review of Research. *Psychiatry* 37:307–320.

KADUSHIN, CHARLES. 1964. Social Class and the Experience of Ill Health. *Sociological Inquiry* 24:67–80. Reprinted in *Class, Status, and Power,* ed. Reinhard Bendix and Seymour M. Lipset. New York: The Free Press, 1966.

————. 1967. Social Class and Ill Health: The Need for Further Research. A Reply to Antonovsky. *Sociological Inquiry* 37:323–332.

KALISH, RICHARD A., and DAVID K. REYNOLDS. 1976. *Death and Ethnicity.* Los Angeles: University of Southern California Press.

KAMPMEIER, R. H. 1974. Final Report on the "Tuskegee Syphilis Study." *Southern Medical Journal* 67:1349–1353.

KASHGARIAN, MARK, and JOHN E. DUNN, JR. 1970. The Duration of Intra-epithelial and Preclinical Squamous Cell Carcinoma of the Uterine Cervix. *American Journal of Epidemiology* 92:211–222.

KLEINMAN, PAULA H., and IRVING F. LUKOFF. 1978. Ethnic Differences in Factors Related to Drug Use. *Journal of Health and Social Behavior* 19:190–199.

KOTCHEN, JANE M., et al. 1974. Blood Pressure Distributions of Urban Adolescents. *American Journal of Epidemiology* 99:315–324.

KRUG, EARNEST F., III. 1974. Folk Medical Beliefs (comments). *Annals of Internal Medicine* 81:705–706.

KULKA, RICHARD A., JOSEPH VEROFF, and ELIZABETH DOUVAN. 1979. Social Class and the Use of Professional Help for Personal Problems: 1957 and 1976. *Journal of Health and Social Behavior* 20:2–17.

LEVINE, DAVID G., et al. 1972. Personality Correlates of Success in a Methadone Maintenance Program. *American Journal of Psychiatry* 129:456–460.

LIEBERMAN, HARRY M. 1974. Evaluating the Duality of Ambulatory Pediatric Care at a Neighborhood Health Center. *Clinical Pediatrics* 13:52–55.

LIEBERSON, STANLEY. 1974. Generational Differences Among Blacks in the North. *American Journal of Sociology* 79:550–565.

LINDEN, GEORGE. 1969. The Influence of Social Class in the Survival of Cancer Patients. *American Journal of Public Health* 59:267–274.

LOWE, MARIE L. 1973. Relationship between Compliance with Medical Regimen and Outcome of Pregnancy. *Nursing Research* 22:157–160.

MALZBERG, BENJAMIN. 1965. New Data on Mental Disease Among Negroes in New York State, 1960–1961. Albany, N.Y.: Research Foundation for Mental Hygiene.

MANDEL, EDWIN A. 1977. The Community Pharmacist in Hypertension Control. *Urban Health* 6:36–37.

MARSTON, MARY-'VESTA. 1970. Compliance with Medical Regimens: A Review of the Literature. *Nursing Research* 19:312–323.

MAY, JUDE T. 1971. The Medical Care of Blacks in Louisiana during Occupation and Reconstruction, 1862–1868: Its Social and Political Background. Ph.D. dissertation, Department of History, Tulane University.

MAYER, JEAN. 1965. The Nutritional Status of American Negroes. *Nutritional Review* 23:161–164.

MAYFIELD, WILLIAM G. 1972. Mental Health in the Black Community. *Social Work* 17:106–110.

MECHANIC, DAVID. 1969. Illness and Cure. In *Poverty and Health: A Sociological Analysis,* ed. John Kosa, Aaron Antonovsky, and Irving Zola. Cambridge, Mass.: Harvard University Press.

MERSKEY, H., and F. G. SPEAR. 1964. The Reliability of the Pressure Algometer. *British Journal of Social and Clinical Psychology* 3:130–136.

MILLER, GEORGE D. 1973. An Epidemiological View of Hypertension. *Urban Health* 2:16–17, 36–37.

MILLER, RUSSELL L., and JOHN ALGEE. 1978. Noncompliance and Drug Toxicity in Black, Poor, and Aged Patients. *Journal of the National Medical Association* 70:733–736.

MOREHEAD, JEAN E. 1975. Intrauterine Device Retention: A Study of Selected Social-Psychological Aspects. *American Journal of Public Health* 65:720–730.

MOY, CLAUDIA S., and CHARLES S. WILDER. 1978. *Health Characteristics of Minority Groups, United States, 1976* (Advance Data, no. 27). Hyattsville, Md.: National Center for Health Statistics.

MUSHLIN, IRVING, and JOHN G. COLLINS. 1975. The Tuberculosis Patient in the Central Harlem Health District of New York City. *American Journal of Public Health* 65:959–966.

NEEL, JAMES V. 1950. The Population Genetics of Two Inherited Blood Dyscrasias in Man. In *Origin and Evolution of Man.* Cold Spring Harbor, N.Y.: Biological Laboratory, Symposia on Quantitative Biology, vol. 15.

——. 1951. The Inheritance of the Sickling Phenomenon, with Particular Reference to Sickle Cell Disease. *Blood, The Journal of Hematology* 6:389–412.

New York Times. 1979. Stress Factor Linked to Test for Diabetes. *New York Times,* 22 May 1979, pp. C1–C2.

NORMAN, JOHN C. 1969. Medicine in the Ghetto. *New England Journal of Medicine* 281:1271–1275.

OSOFSKY, HOWARD J., and NORMAN KENDALL. 1973. Poverty as a Criterion of Risk. *Clinical Obstetrics and Gynecology* 16:103–119.

OSTFELD, ADRIAN M. 1977. Rapid Socio-Cultural Change and High Blood Pressure. *Urban Health* 6.60 61

OSTFELD, ADRIAN M., et al. 1971. Cardiovascular and Cerebrovascular Disease in an Elderly Poor Urban Population. *American Journal of Public Health* 61:19–29.

OWEN, GEORGE M., and ANITA YANOCHIK-OWEN. 1977. Should There Be a Different Definition of Anemia in Black and White Children? *American Journal of Public Health* 67:865–866.

PASAMANICK, BENJAMIN. 1963. Some Misconceptions Concerning Differences in the Racial Prevalence of Mental Disease. *American Journal of Orthopsychiatry* 33:72–86.

————. 1969. A Tract for the Times: Some Sociobiologic Aspects of Science, Race, and Racism. *American Journal of Orthopsychiatry* 39:7–15.

PEARSON, HOWARD A., and RICHARD T. O'BRIEN. 1972. Sickle Cell Testing Programs. *Journal of Pediatrics* 81:1201–1204.

PUCKETT, NEWBELL N. 1926. *Folk Beliefs of the Southern Negro.* Chapel Hill: University of North Carolina Press. (Reprinted by Dover Publications, New York, 1969.)

QUESADA, GUSTAVO M., WILLIAM SPEARS, and PETRA RAMOS. 1978. Interracial Depressive Epidemiology in the Southwest. *Journal of Health and Social Behavior* 19:77–85.

RAYNES, A. E., and V. D. PATCH. 1971. Distinguishing Features of Patients Who Discharge Themselves From Psychiatric Ward. *Comprehensive Psychiatry* 12:473–479.

RAYNES, A. E., and G. WARREN. 1971. Some Distinguishing Features of Patients Failing to Attend a Psychiatric Clinic After Referral. *American Journal of Orthopsychiatry* 41:581–588.

RICHTER, RALPH W., et al. 1977. The Harlem Regional Stroke Program: An Overview. *Archives of Physical Medicine and Rehabilitation* 58:224–229.

RIMER, BOBBY A. 1975. Sickle-Cell Trait and Pregnancy: A Review of a Community Hospital Experience. *American Journal of Obstetrics and Gynecology* 123:6–11.

RING, STEPHEN I., and LAWRENCE SCHEIN. 1970. Attitudes toward Mental Illness and the Use of Caretakers in a Black Community. *American Journal of Orthopsychiatry* 40:710–716.

ROBINS, LEE N., GEORGE E. MURPHY, and MARY B. BRECKENRIDGE. 1968. Drinking Behavior of Young Urban Negro Men. *Quarterly Journal of Studies of Alcohol* 29:657–684.

ROCERETO, LAVERNE R. 1973. Root Work and the Root Doctor. *Nursing Forum* 12:415–426.

ROCHAT, ROGER W., CARL W. TYLER, JR., and ALBERT K. SCHOENBUCHER. 1971. An Epidemiological Analysis of Abortion in Georgia. *American Journal of Public Health* 61:543–552.

ROCKWELL, DON A., and WILLIAM O'BRIEN. 1973. Physicians' Knowledge and Attitudes About Suicide. *Journal of the American Medical Association* 225:1347–1349.

SAMPSON, CALVIN C. 1974. Death of the Black Community Hospital: Fact or Fiction. *Journal of the National Medical Association* 66:165.

SAPHIR, ROBIN, et al. 1967. Voodoo Poisoning in Buffalo, N.Y. *Journal of the American Medical Association* 202:437–438.

SATA, LINDBERGH S., DAVID A. PERRY, and CAROL E. CAMERON. 1970. Store-Front Churches in the Inner City. *Mental Hygiene* 54:256–260.

SATCHER, DAVID. 1973. Does Race Interfere with the Doctor-Patient Relationship? *Journal of the American Medical Association* 223:1498–1499.

SAVITT, TODD L. 1975. Sound Minds and Sound Bodies: The Diseases and Health Care of Blacks in Ante-Bellum Virginia. Ph.D. dissertation, Department of History, University of Virginia.

SAUNDERS, LYLE. 1954. *Cultural Differences and Medical Care: The Case of the Spanish-Speaking People of the Southwest.* New York: Russell Sage Foundation.

SCOTT, CLARISSA S. 1974. Health and Healing Practices Among Five Ethnic Groups in Miami, Florida. *Public Health Reports* 89:524–532.

SEIDMAN, HERBERT, EDWIN SILVERBURG, and ARTHUR I. HOLLEB. 1976. *Cancer Statistics, 1976: A Comparison of White and Black Populations.* New York: American Cancer Society.

SLOME, CECIL, et al. 1977. Should James Go to School? Mothers' Responses to Symptoms. *The Journal of School Health* 47:106–110.

SNELL, JOHN E. 1967. Hypnosis in the Treatment of the "Hexed" Patient. *American Journal of Psychiatry* 124:311–316.

SNOW, LOUDELL F. 1974. Folk Medical Beliefs and Their Implications for Care of Patients: A Review Based on Studies Among Black Americans. *Annals of Internal Medicine* 81:82–96.

———. 1976. "High Blood" Is Not High Blood Pressure. *Urban Health* 5:54–55.

———. 1978. Sorcerers, Saints and Charlatans: Black Folk Healers in Urban America. *Culture, Medicine and Psychiatry* 2:69–106.

STAMLER, JEREMIAH, et al. 1976. Hypertension Screening of 1 Million Americans, Community Hypertension Evaluation Clinic (CHEC) Program, 1973 through 1975. *Journal of the American Medical Association* 235:2299–2306.

STAMLER, ROSE, and JEREMIAH STAMLER. 1976. The Challenge to Conquer Hypertension in the 20th Century. *Urban Health* 5:24–33.

STEWART, HORACE. 1971. Kindling of Hope in the Disadvantaged: A Study of the Afro-American Healer. *Mental Hygiene* 55:96–100.

STEWART, JAMES C., JR., and WILLIAM R. HOOD. 1970. Using Workers from "Hard-Core" Areas to Increase Immunization Levels. *Public Health Reports* 85:177–185.

STOKES, BRUCE. 1979. Self-Care: A Nation's Best Health Insurance. *Science* 205:1.

SUE, STANLEY, et al. 1974. Delivery of Community Mental Health Services to Black and White Clients. *Journal of Consulting and Clinical Psychology* 42:794–801.

SZASZ, THOMAS S. 1971. The Sane Slave: An Historical Note on the Use of Medical Diagnosis as Justificatory Rhetoric. *American Journal of Psychotherapy* 25:228–239.

TAFFEL, SELMA. 1978a. *Prenatal Care in the United States, 1969–1975.* DHEW Publication no. (PHS) 78–1911. Hyattsville, Md.: National Center for Health Statistics.

———. 1978b. *Congenital Anomalies and Birth Injuries Among Live*

Births: United States, 1973–74. DHEW Publication no. (PHS) 79–1909. Hyattsvilie, Md.: National Center for Health Statistics.

TAGLIACOZZO, DAISY M., KENJI IMA, and JOYCE C. LASHOF. 1973. Influencing the Chronically Ill: The Role of Prescriptions in Premature Terminations of Outpatient Care. *Medical Care* 11:21–29.

TAGLIACOZZO, DAISY M., et al. 1974. Nurse Intervention and Patient Behavior: An Experimental Study. *American Journal of Public Health* 64:596–603.

TERRIS, MILTON. 1973. Desegregating Health Statistics. *American Journal of Public Health* 63:477–480.

TERRIS, MILTON, and EDWIN M. GOLD. 1969. An Epidemiologic Study of Prematurity. *American Journal of Obstetrics and Gynecology* 103:371–379.

TINGLING, DAVID C. 1967. Voodoo, Root Work, and Medicine. *Psychosomatic Medicine* 29:483–491.

TWADDLE, ANDREW C., and RICHARD M. HESSLER. 1977. *A Sociology of Health.* St. Louis: Mosby.

U.S. BUREAU OF THE CENSUS. 1980. Estimates of the Population of the United States, by Age, Race, and Sex: 1976 to 1979. *Current Population Reports,* series P–25, no. 870. Washington, D.C.: U.S. Government Printing Office.

U.S. DEPARTMENT OF HEALTH, EDUCATION, and WELFARE. 1976. *Health: United States, 1975.* DHEW Publication no. (HRA) 76–1232. Washington, D.C.: U.S. Government Printing Office.

———. 1978. *Health: United States, 1978.* DHEW Publication no. (PHS) 78–1232. Hyattsville, Md.: National Center for Health Statistics and National Center for Health Services Research.

———. 1979. *Current Listing and Topical Index to the Vital and Health Statistics Series, 1962–1978.* DHEW Publication no. (PHS) 79–1301. Hyattsville, Md.: National Center for Health Statistics.

VAIL, ANTHONY. 1978. Factors Influencing Lower-Class Black Patients Remaining in Treatment. *Journal of Consulting and Clinical Psychology* 46:341.

VERBRUGGE, LOIS M. 1979. *Medical Care of Acute Conditions, United States, 1973–1974.* DHEW Publication no. (PHS) 79–1557. Hyattsville, Md.: National Center for Health Statistics.

VOORS, A. W., et al. 1979. Racial Differences in Blood Pressure Control. *Science* 204:1091–1094.

WALLS, BERTRAM E., and JACQUELYNE J. JACKSON. 1977. Factors Affecting the Use of Physicians by Menopausal Black Women. *Urban Health* 6:53–55.

WAN, THOMAS T. H., and LOIS C. GRAY. 1978. Differential Access to Preventive Services for Young Children in Low-Income Urban Areas. *Journal of Health and Social Behavior* 19:312–324.

WARE, DONALD R. 1977. NIH Priorities in High Blood Pressure Control. *Urban Health* 6:18, 56.

WARNECKE, RICHARD B., et al. 1978. Social and Psychological Correlates of Smoking Behavior Among Black Women. *Journal of Health and Social Behavior* 19:397–410.

WARSHAUER, M. ELLEN, and MARY MONK. 1978. Problems in Suicide Statistics for Whites and Blacks. *American Journal of Public Health* 69:383–388.

WATKINS, ELIZABETH L. 1968. Low-Income Negro Mothers—Their Decision to Seek Prenatal Care. *American Journal of Public Health* 58:655–667.

WEAVER, JERRY L. 1976–77. Policy Responses to Complex Issues: The Case of Black Infant Mortality. *Journal of Health, Politics, Policy and Law* 1:433–443.

WEAVER, JERRY L., and LLOYD T. INUI. 1975. Information About Health Care Providers among Urban Low-Income Minorities. *Inquiry* 7:330–343.

WEBB, JULIE Y. 1971. Louisiana Voodoo and Superstitions Related to Health. *Health Services Reports* 86:291–301.

WEBB, Z. OZELLA. 1972. Sickle Cell Anemia: A Clinical Screening Survey. *Journal of the National Medical Association* 64:197–199.

WEIDMAN, HAZEL H. 1978. Miami Health Ecology Project Report, vol. 1. Miami: Department of Psychiatry and Department of Pediatrics, University of Miami School of Medicine.

———. 1979. Falling-out: A Diagnostic and Treatment Problem Viewed from a Transcultural Perspective. *Social Science and Medicine* 13B:95–112.

WHITE, EARNESTINE H. 1977. Giving Health Care to Minority Patients. *Nursing Clinics of North America* 12:27–40.

WHITTEN, NORMAN E., JR. 1962. Contemporary Patterns of Malign Occultism Among Negroes in North Carolina. *Journal of American Folklore* 75:312–325.

WILLIAMS, DANIEL H. 1915–16. The Malingerer. *Railways Surgical Journal* 22:443–446.

WILSON, JOHN T. 1973. Compliance with Instructions in the Evaluation of Therapeutic Efficacy: A Common But Frequently Unrecognized Major Variable. *Clinical Pediatrics* 12:333–340.

WINSBERG, B., and M. GREENLICK. 1967. Pain Response in Negro and White Obstetrical Patients. *Journal of Health and Social Behavior* 8:222–227.

WINTROB, RONALD M. 1973. The Influence of Others: Witchcraft and Rootwork as Explanations of Behavior Disturbances. *Journal of Nervous and Mental Disease* 156:318–326.

WOLFF, B. BERTHOLD, and SARAH LANGLEY. 1968. Cultural Factors and the Response to Pain: A Review. *American Anthropologist* 70:494–501.

WOLINSKY, FREDERIC D. 1978. Assessing the Effects of Predisposing, Enabling, and Illness-Morbidity Characteristics on Health Service Utilization. *Journal of Health and Social Behavior* 19:384–396.

WOODROW, KENNETH M., et al. 1972. Pain Tolerance: Differences According to Age, Sex and Race. *Psychosomatic Medicine* 34:548–556.

WYATT, GAIL E. 1977. A Comparison of the Scaling of Afro-Americans' Life-Change Events. *Journal of Human Stress* 3:13–18.

YERBY, ALONZO S. 1977. Black Physicians and Black Communities. *American Journal of Public Health* 67:511–512.

2
Chinese Americans

KATHERINE GOULD-MARTIN AND CHORSWANG NGIN

Identification of the Ethnic Group

THE TERM "CHINESE AMERICAN" is used to refer to people of Chinese background in the United States and encompasses the following disparate groups: (1) the Cantonese- and Toisanese-speaking Chinese who came to this country from Toishan and nearby areas in Kwangtung Province at the end of the last century and the early part of this century; (2) their English-speaking descendants; (3) Chinese English- and Mandarin-speaking students and professionals who came from schools and cities in China, Taiwan, and elsewhere in Southeast Asia to study and work in predominantly white settings in the United States; and (4) recent urban and rural immigrants from Hong Kong, Taiwan, and overseas Chinese settlements in Asia. Though these people are genetically similar, there are linguistic, cultural, and socioeconomic differences among them.

History of Migration to the United States

Although Chinese began to enter the territory that now constitutes the United States soon after the American Revolution, it was not until the 1840s and 1850s that they began immigrating in large numbers.[1] Thus, in 1850 there were 4,000 Chinese in the West; by 1860 there were 50,000; and despite extensive concurrent outmigration, by 1882 the Chinese population of the United States had reached 132,000. In California at that time, the 110,000 Chinese residents made up 75 percent of the farmworker population. The cause of this relatively rapid influx of Chinese was twofold: the demand for labor in the United States, and chaos and over-population in China.

In 1868 the United States government negotiated the Burlingame Treaty, which secured from the Ch'ing Dynasty the right of Chinese laborers to enter the United States and change their national allegiance. At the same time, however, anti-Chinese sentiment was already developing in this country. At the end of the Civil War, discharged soldiers sought jobs in the West and were joined there later by Eastern laborers who were unemployed as a result of the 1873 Panic. After the completion of the railroad, jobs were less plentiful and, for reasons of efficiency, large employers preferred to hire Chinese. As a result, disgruntled white laborers agitated against the Chinese. Local incidents of violent, anti-Chinese hostility were accompanied by legal discrimination against Chinese immigrants in the form of special taxes and regulations. In 1882 the United States government, in the Chinese Exclusion Act, repudiated the rights set forth in the Burlingame Treaty and suspended immigration of Chinese laborers (though not of certain other classes). The act also prohibited Chinese from becoming naturalized citizens. Under an additional act, passed in 1888, Chinese laborers could not reenter this country if they left, unless they had property valued at $1,000 or a lawful wife, child, or parent resident here. As a result of these exclusionary measures, inmigration of Chinese dropped sharply and outmigration increased, and by 1920 only 61,639 Chinese remained in the United States.

In 1943, however, the Chinese Exclusion Act was repealed, and under the provisions of the National Origins Quota Act (1924), 105 Chinese were allowed to enter each year. Despite these very restrictive laws, many more Chinese immigrated between the 1920s and 1960s than one might expect. War brides, displaced persons, Hong Kong refuges, and others entered under special directives and arrangements. In addition, Chinese veterans were naturalized in 1935 and could then bring over relatives, and until 1924 Chinese in the nonlaborer classes, as well as laborers who were either American-born or naturalized before 1882, had been allowed to bring wives and children.

This small but constant trickle of immigration during the early twentieth century was enlarged in 1965, when Public Law 89236 finally abolished the National Origins Quota System. As a result, 20,000 Chinese may now enter the United States annually. Between 1960 and 1970 the Chinese population of the United States increased 84 percent, with at least two-thirds of this increase attributable to immigration. More open immigration has also equalized the sex ratio of Chinese Americans, which was 13.3 males per female at the turn of the century and had changed to 1.1 males per female by 1970.

Current Population and Geographical Distribution

After the Japanese, the Chinese are the largest Asian subgroup in the United States. According to the U.S. Census Bureau (1970a), the total Chinese-American population in 1970 was 435,000, a conservative figure because of the underenumeration of illegal immigrants and non-English speakers. Furthermore, 96 percent of this population was urban. Whereas most early immigrants landed in San Francisco and moved elsewhere from there, many now go directly to New York or other large cities away from the West Coast. In the last decade, the proportion of Chinese in the West has therefore declined, though more than half still live in that geographical region. The ten states with the highest number of Chinese are California (with 39 percent of the total Chinese-American population), New York (19 percent), Hawaii (12 percent), Illinois, Massachusetts, New Jersey, Washington, Texas, Pennsylvania, and Maryland (U.S. Bureau of the Census 1977).

The proportions of foreign- and native-born Chinese differ considerably from one American city to another (table 2.1). Hawaii, for instance,

Table 2.1 Standard Metropolitan Statistical Areas with 5,000 or more Chinese population, 1970, by place of birth.

City of residence	Chinese population	Foreign-born		Native-born	
		Number	%	Number	%
San Francisco–Oakland	88,886	41,558	47	47,328	53
New York City	78,337	50,821	65	27,516	35
Honolulu	48,616	5,506	11	43,110	89
Los Angeles–Long Beach	40,914	20,742	51	20,172	49
Boston	12,129	6,131	51	5,998	49
Chicago	11,794	6,689	57	5,105	43
Sacramento	10,398	3,638	35	6,760	65
Seattle–Everett	8,083	4,080	50	4,003	50
Washington, D.C.–Md.–Va.	7,903	4,344	55	3,559	45
San Jose, Calif.	7,781	2,919	38	4,862	62

Source: U.S. Bureau of the Census (1970c).

received a very large early influx of Chinese, but it is not a common destination for contemporary immigrants, with the result that today only 11 percent of Honolulu's Chinese population is foreign-born. In general, while second-generation Chinese Americans and those of the first generation who master English and succeed economically tend to live outside Chinatowns in suburban areas, the foreign-born (both old and new immigrants) are concentrated in Chinatowns.

General Demographic Picture

TYPES OF HOUSEHOLDS   By combining U.S. Census Bureau information (1970b) with prose accounts of Chinese-American life (Wong 1945; Chu 1961; Nee and Nee 1972; Yep 1975; Kingston 1977), we can discern four major types of Chinese-American households: the single sojourner, the old immigrant couple, the new immigrant family, and the acculturated suburban family. As we will show, this last type requires little special attention from health-care providers; a physician may simply note that the risks for certain diseases among members of this subpopulation differ from those of white Americans in similar circumstances. The three other household types, however, are similar in their poverty, their language problems, and their residence in Chinatowns.

The sojourner was born around the turn of the century in Toishan. At about age 16, he joined an older male relative in the United States and worked in restaurants or laundries in Chinatown. He may have married before leaving China or returned to marry, but his hope of bringing over his wife and children or of rejoining them for retirement has been dashed by political changes in China. If he has ever left Chinatown, it was probably to work in a Chinese restaurant in a small town. He speaks little English, has little education, and lives alone in a rooming house.

The old immigrant couple demonstrates a more successful completion of the sojourner's plan. The husband was able to bring over his wife and raise his children in this country (or he may have brought his teenage children over first and only brought his wife when his parents died and no longer needed her). Some of these families succeeded in overcoming numerous obstacles and realizing their hopes. Through hard work, frugal living, and careful child rearing, they managed to send their children to college and on to white-collar careers. In other cases, the children have been impatient and unfilial; or when the husband finally brought his wife over, he hardly knew her, and she was unable to adapt either to him or to America. According to Chinese tradition, elderly parents should live with their children. In fact, however, they often find the lives of their children too American, too busy, and too distant from Chinatown. As a result, they prefer to live by themselves amid poverty but in familiar surroundings.

The new immigrant family is the modern version of this story. The recent male immigrant who has found a steady job brings his wife over to work in the garment industry. Despite two paychecks, the family income falls significantly below that for white American families. The Chinese families are "working poor": often employed at a level of skill below that for which they were trained, they have dead-end jobs that provide no benefits, no career ladder, and no leisure to improve their language or other abilities. Despite their poverty, these families rarely rely on public assistance and are often unwilling to apply, lest it hurt their chances for naturalization or for bringing over other relatives. Unless the wife belongs to the ILGWU, they probably have no health insurance, sick leave, disability, or any other assistance for illness. These families generally have more children than other American families and may also have other relatives, especially parents, to support. Many are assisting relatives in Hong Kong and China as well. Preschool children follow their mothers to sweat shops or are left at home in the care of elderly relatives or neighbors. The parents speak Chinese at home and hope their children will learn English at school in order to succeed in America.

The fourth type of Chinese-American household, *the acculturated suburban family,* may consist of an American-born parental generation or a husband/father who is a China-born scholar, engineer, or successful businessman. Both parents may be college-educated. The father is often in a professional or managerial occupation; the mother is usually a low-status white collar worker. The preschool children attend private nursery school, giving them a head start on English, while they learn Chinese (often Mandarin) at home. The parents' combined income is well above that of the median American family, and they enjoy the many health benefits of the middle and upper-middle class: medical insurance, good medical care, and probably above-average health.

LIFE IN AMERICAN CHINATOWNS   American Chinatowns are densely populated areas of restaurants, gift shops, groceries, herb shops, small businesses, family associations, and rundown residential housing; they offer security and identity to new immigrants and remain home to old immigrants who are afraid to move out. The acculturated suburban Chinese visit Chinatowns only for dining, shopping, traditional health care, civic activities, and recreation. It is the Chinatown Chinese who constitute the bulk of the recent immigrants and more traditionally oriented older migrants, and who are therefore the major concern of this chapter.

In size, San Francisco's Chinatown is by far the largest (58,696 people according to the 1970 census), followed by New York (25,840), Los Angeles (4,691), and Boston (3,323). In each case census estimates for Chinatown populations are far smaller than those given by residents and journalists. The former estimates are affected by underenumeration, particularly of illegal immigrants; the latter are inflated by guesswork. In any case, all these areas are growing rapidly: 3,000 Chinese are estimated to enter San Francisco annually; 5,000 per year are said to enter New York City; and about 1,000 enter the core Chinatowns of Boston and Los Angeles every year. The decade from 1970 to 1980 has probably produced at least a doubling of these figures.

In many of these core Chinatowns today, rents and house prices are being driven up by Chinese investors from Hong Kong, Taiwan, and elsewhere. Dilapidated housing is being replaced by glittering banks and shopping centers on land sold for exorbitant prices. This redevelopment, as well as earlier urban renewal schemes, has resulted in increased crowding and hardship for those who remain in Chinatown and in the displacement of many people to secondary areas, such as the Sunset and Richmond areas of San Francisco and Monterey Park and San Gabriel in Los Angeles. (In April, 1980, Monterey Park had an estimated 10,000 to 15,000 Chinese residents.) As these areas become increasingly Sinicized, more foreign-born Chinese feel comfortable residing there and add to their growth.

Today's immigrants to Chinatowns often copy the pattern of those who came a century ago: they arrive alone, join older male relatives, seek jobs in the service sector, and save money to bring over their wives and parents. Though both the new and old immigrants share many problems, their somewhat different backgrounds alter their reactions to the American situation. On the one hand, early immigrants are mostly from rural areas of Kwangtung Province and have very little education. Many of them learned magical and herbal ways of dealing with disease. On the other hand, new immigrants are often urbanites and come from all parts of Asia, including Saigon and Manila. They have had at least a primary and middle-school education and were taught modern health practices and a disdain for magic. However, such modern Chinese often bring over their traditionally oriented parents, who resemble early immigrants.

The characteristics of Chinatowns most relevant to medical-care delivery are the following: crowding (not only the number of people per square mile but also the number of people per room); the preponderance of males to females; the large number of elderly persons (especially single men); the inability of many residents to speak English; low educational levels; unemployment; a high proportion of men in service occupations (especially restaurants); a high proportion of women in semiskilled operative jobs (especially in the garment industry); long working hours at low wages; a lack of medical insurance; a low proportion of eligible people receiving public assistance; inadequate day care; substandard housing; and inadequate plumbing. Though the figures from disparate sources are not always comparable, it appears that Boston's Chinatown is most affected by these problems, followed by the Chinatowns of New York, San Francisco, and Los Angeles. (For greater detail on particular Chinatowns, see Yee 1970, Carp and Kataoka 1976, on San Francisco; Wu 1971, Chan and Chang 1976, Huang and Grachow 1976, on New York City; UCLA Team 1975, on Los Angeles; and Murphey 1952, Sullivan and Hatch 1970, Murphy 1972, Gaw 1975, Chang and Tang 1977, on Boston.)

Evaluation of the Existing Data

In many ways it is fortunate that the Chinese whose medical beliefs and practices have been most studied are those for whom ethnic traditions exert an appreciable influence on health status and medical care—that is, the residents of the larger Chinatowns. The group that has been studied least, the acculturated suburban Chinese, probably appear only in the Los Angeles study (see paragraph 4 below) as people who did not live in Chinatown but visited a Chinatown herbalist.

There are several problems involved in interpreting and generalizing from the existing data base because of the marked demographic changes that have occurred in the Chinese-American population since 1965. Any study done before that date cannot take into account the huge influx of new immigrants; such studies either deal with old sojourners or point out the successful adaptations of early immigrants and their children. More recent studies, on the other hand, deal with the problems of new immigrants and are written from a new perspective: rather than stressing how Chinese Americans overcame all odds to become good citizens, they stress the obstacles that American society has put in their path.

The material available on Chinese-American beliefs and practices with regard to health and illness is of several types.

1. There are two doctoral dissertations that deal with Chinese Americans in San Francisco. Both Louie's thesis (1975) and Koo's thesis (1976) contain some ethnographic material. Koo draws not only on San Francisco Chinese for her material but also on Taiwan Chinese and classical medical texts, unfortunately without clearly distinguishing her sources at each point.

2. There are several studies of a more sociological nature that have the advantage of producing results which (unlike Louie's and Koo's) are subject to statistical analysis but which have the disadvantage of using questions that are preset by the investigator and thus are possibly of little meaning to the respondents. Peter Chen's study (1976), for instance, discusses the extent to which Chinese agree with Western ideas of mental illness, but it does not discuss Chinese ideas of mental illness. Similarly, the questionnaires used by Hessler and his colleagues (1975) and by Chan and Chang (1976) imposed severe restrictions on the answers respondents could make, and different wording might have resulted in very different answers. The respondents are nowhere allowed to speak for themselves.

3. There are also some very short discussions of health beliefs and practices in the scattered writings produced either to obtain funding for some new project or to report results after funding. The arguments of these sources are biased by their objectives: accounts of prior misery and ignorance, followed by success and enlightenment, tend to be exaggerated (Murphy 1970; CACA 1972; Lurie et al. 1976).

4. We undertook a small study in 1977–78 in which patients visiting an herbalist in Los Angeles Chinatown were interviewed informally. In

addition, Ngin, who has field experience among Malaysian Chinese, worked previously in an Asian clinic in Sacramento; Gould-Martin had field experience in Taiwan; and both are acquainted with an entirely non-random assortment of suburban Chinese Americans.

Epidemiological Characteristics

Biases and Cautions Concerning the Data

The epidemiological literature on Chinese Americans is incomplete in three important ways. First, morbidity statistics are unavailable; second, diseases with very high or very low mortality rates among Chinese Americans have not been discussed in medical journals with specific reference to this ethnic population; and third, we have no recent nation-wide study of Chinese-American mortality rates that includes post-1965 immigrants.

The most useful epidemiological studies (King and Haenszel 1973; King 1975) set white mortality rates for the period from 1959 to 1962 at 100. Comparison with Chinese mortality rates for those years is then achieved by adjusting for age and giving a standard mortality ratio (SMR) for Chinese. Thus an SMR of 200 means that the mortality observed among Chinese is twice that expected on the basis of white rates. Similarly, an SMR of 50 for a certain disease means that the Chinese are experiencing half the mortality that one might expect if their rates for the disease were the same as those of whites.

There are, in addition, small epidemiological studies that draw their samples from the nation's Chinatowns, where poverty, crowding, and overwork create conditions (and diseases, such as tuberculosis) which are not specifically Chinese but which characterize ghetto populations all over the country.

General Health

For the period from 1949 to 1952, the first period for which King found reliable figures, the SMR for all causes of death was 30 percent greater for Chinese males than for white males and 13 percent greater for Chinese females than for white females. For the period from 1959 to 1962, however, the SMR for Chinese males was almost the same as that for white males, and the SMR for Chinese females was 17 percent lower. This considerable improvement over a single decade derived primarily from reduced mortality for respiratory, digestive, nervous, and circulatory diseases, infective and parasitic diseases, and diseases of early infancy (King 1975:495). The decline in mortality from this last cause helped to produce an unusually low infant mortality rate for Chinese Americans in the 1959–1962 period: SMRs of 75 and 60 for males and females respectively (Smith 1956:669; King 1975:501).

If we compare Chinese to nonwhites, a fuller picture emerges. A national study of death certificates from 1949 to 1959 revealed that while mortality from all causes for Chinese men was higher than for both white and nonwhite men, the mortality for Chinese women fell between that for whites and nonwhites (Li 1972:537). A 1956 study of Chinese-American mortality from all causes placed the rates for Chinese Americans of both sexes between the rates for whites and those for nonwhites (Smith 1956: 668).

Second-generation Chinese have a much lower mortality rate than first-generation Chinese for all causes combined, as well as for most specific diseases (King 1975:495). In California, while white and nonwhite mortality rates declined gradually from 1950 to 1960, Chinese mortality declined sharply (Breslow and Klein 1971:770).

The Chinese living in the western United States, who constitute more than half the nation's Chinese population, seem to be in better health than their peers in the rest of the country, although this apparent advantage may result from sampling error (King 1975:495). Two studies from the 1960s on health and race in California show that on various measures the health of Chinese Americans there equals or exceeds that of whites and far exceeds that of blacks (table 2.2).

Unhappily, the health advantages enjoyed in the late 1950s and early

Table 2.2 Selected indexes of health for Chinese, Japanese, whites, and blacks, California, 1960–1967[a].

Health index	1st	2nd	3rd	4th
Infant mortality, 1967	Japanese	Chinese	White	Black
Life expectancy at birth, males and females, 1959–61	Japanese	Chinese	White	Black
SMR, all causes, 1960	Japanese	White	Chinese	Black
Life expectancy, males aged 35, 1959–61	Japanese	White	Chinese	Black
Mortality from cerebrovascular-renal disease, males aged 45–64, 1960	(Oriental)	(Oriental)	White	Black
Disability, adults, Alameda County, 1965	Japanese	Chinese	White	Black
Cancer incidence, Alameda County, 1960–64	Japanese	Chinese	Black	White

Source: Adapted from Breslow and Klein (1971:772); Hechter and Borhani (1965:122).
a. 1st = best record, 4th = poorest record.

1960s by the general population of Chinese Americans (particularly in California) have probably not characterized Chinatown residents in the 1960s and 1970s. Although we possess statistics for only New York and Boston, they are undoubtedly indicative of the declining health status of most of the nation's Chinatowns since the post-1965 immigrations. In New York City, for example, death rates for Chinese are 13.5 per 1,000 compared to 10.4 for the city as a whole, and between 1970 and 1973 infant mortality among Chinese rose from 12.2 to 15.5 deaths per 1,000 live births (Huang and Granchow 1976:298). Statistics from Boston's Chinatown indicate even more striking increases in mortality: between 1960 and 1966 infant mortality among Chinatowners rose 150 percent (from 26.6 to 66.7), and the crude death rate rose from almost twice to more than twice the rate for other Bostonians (Sullivan and Hatch 1970: 63).

Mortality from Major Diseases

Certain causes of death are far more common among Chinese Americans than among white Americans (table 2.3); there are also causes of death that are far rarer among Chinese Americans than among white Americans (table 2.4).

Table 2.3 Standard mortality ratios over 200 for Chinese Americans, 1959–1962.

Cause of death	Chinese SMR (white rate = 100)	
	Male	Female
All causes	100	83
Infective and parasitic diseases	276	—
Tuberculosis	360	—
Neoplasms		
Nasopharynx	3,120	3,103
Liver	1,134	311
Trachea, lung, bronchus	—	261
Diabetes	202	—
Hypertensive heart disease	212	—
Ulcer of stomach	294	222
Nephritis and nephrosis	201	—
Complications of pregnancy, childbirth, puerperium	a	212
All diseases of skin and cellular tissue	252	214
Suicide	—	267

Source: King (1975:498–500).
Dashes indicate SMRs under 200.
a = not applicable.

Table 2.4   Standard mortality ratios under 70 for Chinese Americans, 1959–1962.

Cause of death	Chinese SMR (white rate = 100)	
	Male	**Female**
Neoplasms		
Breast	b	50
Prostate	31	a
Arteriosclerotic heart disease, including coronary disease	68	61
Chronic endocarditis	—	42
All diseases of the digestive system	—	58
Cirrhosis of liver	—	30
Certain diseases of early infancy	—	60
Symptoms, senility, and ill-defined conditions	—	48
Motor vehicle accidents	54	59
Other accidents	61	60

Source: King (1975:498–500).
Dashes indicate SMRs over 70.
a = not applicable.
b = SMR not computed (fewer than 5 deaths).

CARDIOVASCULAR-RENAL DISEASES   Both first- and second-generation Chinese Americans experience more coronary heart disease than their counterparts in Asia. This trend is in accordance with the experience of Japanese migrants to the United States. Diet and stress are both implicated, and the effect of acculturation on these diseases is not yet clear.

TUBERCULOSIS   According to King (1975), mortality from tuberculosis among Chinese Americans has been impressively reduced from rates in their country of origin. The SMRs in the home countries of the foreign Chinese are much higher than those for American residents, whether foreign- or native-born (table 2.5). Tuberculosis among Chinese

Table 2.5   Tuberculosis mortality of selected Chinese populations expressed in SMRs (U.S. white rate = 100).

Sex	Taiwan 1959–60 1963–64	Hong Kong 1961–64	Singapore 1959–62	U.S. 1959–62
Male	1,540	1,958	1,691	360
Female	2,480	1,907	1,373	158

Source: King (1975:498–499, 504–505).

Americans is concentrated in urban Chinatowns. In 1969 the tuberculosis rate for Chinese in Boston was 192 percent greater than for the city's population as a whole. A rate of 459.4 incident (new) cases per 100,000 was reported from 1967 to 1969, compared to 110.5 for the whole city (Sullivan and Hatch 1970:64–66). In 1972, New York City's Chinatown had 329 new tuberculosis cases per 100,000 population, compared to 28.8 for the city as a whole (Huang and Grachow 1976:298).

CANCER   Cancer is the disease most researched in the Chinese-American literature, and the cause of this interest is the enormous difference in the Chinese and white rates as reflected in the SMRs for cancers of the nasopharynx, liver, prostate, and breast. There appear to be no genetically inherited diseases peculiar to the Chinese racial group. However, trophoblastic cancer, a very rare tumor in most of the world, occurs excessively in China (Fraumeni and Mason 1974; Kaplan and Tsuchitani 1978).

Nasopharyngeal cancer (NPC) is most common among the Tanka (Boat People) of Hong Kong. In neighboring Kwangtung Province, NPC occurs 10 times more frequently than in North China and 40 times more frequently than in the United States. It is interesting to note that pigs in Kwangtung Province also get NPC (Kaplan and Tsuchitani 1978:89). Cantonese and, to a lesser extent, Fukinese have carried their risk of this disease wherever they have migrated, though the risk is somewhat diminished in each succeeding generation. Both environmental and genetic etiologies are under suspicion; these include nickel exposure, association with Epstein-Barr virus, occupation as a food service worker (especially a chef), heavy cigarette smoking, use of wood as a cooking fuel, family history of NPC, and prior history of pulmonary tuberculosis, chronic sinusitis, rhinitis, or bronchitis (Kaplan and Tsuchitani 1978:67, 68, 84). A recent Los Angeles study found that Chinese NPC patients were more likely to have certain genetic (HL-A) markers (Henderson et al. 1976). Ho's suspicion (1972) of association of NPC with salt fish consumption was lent further support by an ethnographic study in Hong Kong by Anderson (1978), who suggests that a very introverted personality and a poor early childhood diet, deficient in vitamin C and containing salt fish, characterize NPC patients.

Hepatoma, primary liver cancer, is also common in Chinese and rare in white Americans. Evidence from several studies suggests that "viral hepatitis, which occurs in high frequencies in the same areas that have high incidence of liver cancer, may predispose to liver cancer by inducing posthepatic cirrhosis and creating a population of liver cells susceptible to malignant transformation by an appropriate carcinogen" (Kaplan and Tsuchitani 1978:101). This view is reaffirmed by Szmuness and his colleagues (1978) for the New York Chinatown. It is thought that the virus is transmitted during infancy (C. E. Stevens, personal communication; Dickie 1978). Mainland Chinese studies have found no association of hepatoma with alcohol, industrial chemicals, or aflatoxin exposures; however, they suspect nitrosamines in pickled vegetables. Ducks in certain high-risk areas, where alluvial soils are rich in nitrosamines, have been found to have liver cancer. Liver fluke and schistosomiasis may also be predisposing factors in this disease.

Esophageal cancer is also excessive in certain areas of North China; in Linhsien County of Honan Province the rate is 140 per 100,000—that is, 50 times the rate in the rest of the world. Chickens in these areas are found with gullet cancer, and it is thought that items in the household diet may be responsible (Kaplan and Tsuchitani 1978:65). Esophageal cancer does not appear to be very common in American Chinese, as compared to whites.

Breast cancer rates remain relatively low among Chinese Americans but are increasing. MacMahon has suggested that the main risk factor is the length of time between menarche and the first full-term pregnancy (MacMahon, Cole, and Brown 1973). This period in turn is heavily influenced by childhood diet (a richer diet supposedly bringing on an earlier menarche) as well as extended education and employment for women (resulting in a later first pregnancy). If MacMahon is correct, then breast cancer will probably continue to increase among Chinese Americans and among Chinese elsewhere. However, rates in Japan have not reached the levels one would expect on the basis of this hypothesis.

Little is known of the etiology of prostate cancer. It is virtually absent among the Chinese.

GERIATRIC PROBLEMS   With the exception of tuberculosis, the diseases with greater prominence among Chinese Americans are those of middle and old age. In addition to fatal diseases, the elderly have chronic complaints, including high blood pressure, arthritis and rheumatism, and failing teeth, eyes, hearing, and feet (Training Project 1973:34; Wu 1974:119; Wu 1975). In addition, many are reputed to suffer from malnutrition.

NARCOTICS AND ALCOHOL ABUSE   The remaining medical problems most often mentioned in connection with the Chinese are narcotic and alcohol abuse and suicide. These problems may lead directly to death and will therefore be included in this discussion of disease entities.

A 1966 study of 137 male narcotics admissions at Lexington Hospital, Kentucky, revealed that a typical Chinese heroin addict exemplified the sojourner pattern. Unlike the other addicts, who tended to be young (32.5) and either unemployed or working at illegal activities, the Chinese addicts were older (53) and were employed in laundries and restaurants. The typical addict had been taking heroin or opium (or both) for 20 years, but recently the habit had become too expensive and he had sought treatment (Ball and Lau 1966:68–72). With the aging of this unhappy sojourner class, one would expect a decrease in this kind of narcotics problem, unless the young increasingly imitate the United States pattern of youthful narcotics abuse.

The literature on alcohol use among Chinese Americans deals not with its abuse, which seems minimal, but with the task of accounting for the absence of alcoholism: are Chinese generally abstinent, or do they follow the "Jewish pattern" of moderate social drinking, coupled with strong disapproval of excessive or solitary drinking? One author concludes that abstinence is the prevalent pattern and suggests that gambling may be substituted as a release. His study draws on the same sojourner population that supplied the narcotics patients (Chu 1972:58–68).

SUICIDE   The standard mortality ratios for suicide among Chinese Americans drop sharply from first- to second-generation American residents, though they retain the characteristically Chinese pattern of higher rates for women (table 2.6).[2]

Table 2.6   Standard mortality ratios for suicide among Chinese of various nationalities (by sex, residence, and generation).

Origin of group	Chinese SMR (white rate = 100)	
	Males	Females
Chinese-American first generation, 1959–62	174	407
Chinese-American second generation, 1959–62	76	118
Taiwan, 1959–60, 1963–64	180	400
Hong Kong, 1961–64	98	201
Singapore, 1959–62	125	198

Source: King (1975:502–503, 504–505).

In 1970 suicide rates in San Francisco's Chinatown were said to be three times the national average (Yee 1970). However, San Francisco is traditionally a high-suicide city, and a study of suicide among Chinese in San Francisco from 1952 to 1968 showed that the Chinese rate had originally been higher than the city rate but had fallen to two-thirds of the city rate (Bourne 1973). The average suicide rate for Chinese over the entire period was almost identical to that for the city (27.9 versus 27.5). The national average, however, is 10 per 100,000. (We have no information about Chinese suicide rates in low-suicide cities.)

Among first-generation Chinese-American males, Bourne found that age-specific rates showed a steep rise after age 55. Most of the male suicide victims over age 50 were unemployed or retired, in chronically ill health, and living alone in a rooming house with no wife or with a wife in China. The men under age 50 who committed suicide were often those engaged in business and having financial difficulties. Women suicide victims were often engaged in interpersonal conflict, especially unhappy marriages, and many suffered from psychiatric disturbances (Bourne 1973: 749). Thus it seems that the typical suicide victim is either a sojourner or the unhappy wife of one. It is interesting to note, moreover, that suicide and attempted suicide rates in the Los Angeles Chinatown, which has many new migrants but fewer old sojourners, are reputed to be the lowest in the city (UCLA Team 1975:67).

Not only are there distinctive rates of suicide among Chinese Americans, but their methods of suicide differ from those of whites. Most elderly foreign-born Chinese lack guns and cars, with the result that drugs, jumping, and hanging are more common methods. Women prefer hanging, because this method is believed to allow the ghost to avenge herself on those who caused her misery.

Concepts of Disease and Illness
Chinese Medicine

What is called "Chinese medicine" may be divided into three distinct but related types: classical Chinese medicine, medicine in contemporary China, and Chinese folk medicine.

Classical Chinese medicine is a static doctrine based on ancient texts. The three most famous are the *Huang Ti Nei Ching* (*The Yellow Emperor's Classic of Internal Medicine*), whose author is reputed to have lived between 2698 and 2598 B.C., the *Shang Han Lun* (*Treatise on Fevers*), and the *Shen Nung Pen Ts'ao Ching* (*Shen Nung's Classic Pharmacopoeia*), the last two written around the third century B.C.

The ideas of health and disease expounded in the *Nei Ching* are based for the most part on the concept of dynamic equilibrium between opposing forces. *Yin* and *yang* are two such principles that permeate all of nature, including biological processes. Health is conceptualized in terms of harmony between the two forces; illness is viewed in terms of an imbalance or disequilibrium (see, for example, Sidel and Sidel 1973:127–128). There are additional factors, such as the five elements or five evolving phases, expressed as wood, fire, metal, water, and earth. Corresponding to the five elements are the five organs: spleen, liver, heart, lungs, and kidneys, which are further related in a complex system of analogies and interactions with the planets, colors, tastes, directions, and so on. The material found in these classical texts provided the foundation for the traditional medicine that flourished in China for centuries and that led to a wealth of empirical observations.

Chinese medicine in contemporary China draws ideas from both classical and folk traditions but is a pragmatic and progressive system. The scientific methods of phytochemistry are applied to traditionally prescribed herbs in a search for their active ingredients. Patients preparing for open-chest surgery learn ancient breathing exercises. Acupuncture anesthesia is used for cesarean section. Traditional gymnastic exercises are an adjunct treatment for high blood pressure, tubercular infection, digestive disorders, and paralysis (Sidel and Sidel 1973:139). Chinese herb treatment is often given as an alternative to, or in combination with, Western treatment, to suit the wishes of the patient and the demands of the disease. Coordinated treatment is carried out under the supervision of professionals from both Western and Chinese medicine.[3] Even the "barefoot doctor" is trained in both (Barefoot Doctor's Manual 1977). This apparently harmonious integration of Western and Chinese medicine (both misnomers in this context) is the fruit of several decades of official effort and may disintegrate under new policies. (See Croizier [1968] for an excellent study of the relationship between traditional and modern medicine in China and Taiwan.)

These developments of Chinese medicine in China have implications for American Chinese in that advances in Chinese medicine are published in medical journals and reported in the popular press. Chinese-American laymen, who merely read about these advances in the news, take pride in the confirmation of the efficacy of Chinese medicine. Moreover, some Chinese Americans communicate with friends and relatives in China, Taiwan, and Hong Kong, and medical ideas are exchanged. For example, one elderly Los Angeles Chinatown practitioner makes regular trips back to Hong Kong to learn about new developments.

Chinese folk medicine derives many of its ideas from classical sources, but expresses them more mundanely (for example, "hot" and "cold" for *yang* and *yin*). Religion and magic enter into folk medicine, as do popular and biomedical ideas. Relying not on classical texts but on handbooks, newspapers, gossip, and tradition, folk medicine is characterized by regional differences, involution of certain theories, and integration of new ideas.

Chinese medicine as it is practiced in Chinatowns in the United States is probably closer to folk medicine than to any other system. It appears to lack the heavy religious and magical bias of folk practice in Taiwan or Hong Kong (see Topley 1970; Ahern 1975; Gould-Martin 1975), yet it is neither classical in the static sense nor modern in the progressive and empirical sense. It is merely medicine in practice, administered by practitioners who differ widely in background, knowledge, and skill and who are virtually free of the constraints of official supervision.

Concepts of Popular Chinese Folk Medicine in the United States

HARMONY   The concept basic to all traditional Chinese medical thinking is that of harmony or balance. Health and disease are not opposites; rather, health is a state of homeostasis between dangerous extremes. When a person is healthy the body is in a state of equilibrium, whereas illness results from disturbances in this harmony. Balance may be affected by internal influences, such as age, sex, and temperament, and by external ones such as weather, crisis, and disease organisms. Thus health problems are attributed to excesses of one thing or deficiencies of another: too little rest, imbalanced diet in childhood, too much work, boredom, too much tension, too many parties. The illnesses that were considered by our Los Angeles informants to be caused by these imbalances were weakness, diabetes, "fright," stomach problems, colds, heart condition, watery eyes, insomnia, and asthma.

Subsidiary to the idea of balance are several additional conceptual devices: "wind," the "hot"/"cold" polarity, "poison," blood, *ch'i,* and "fright." These concepts have physical manifestations and symbolic aspects and fit together into a relatively coherent system (with many minor local variations).

"WIND"   "Wind" has an obvious physical manifestation, but a mere draft, a fan or air conditioner, an exposure, or a symptom or illness for which the Chinese name rhymes with the Chinese word for wind will elicit this classification and explanation. "Wind" is thought to be able to enter the body during a vulnerable period, such as after childbirth when "the joints are open" or during surgery when the body is cut open (Louie 1975:131). Certain foods and drinks, such as leftovers, carbonated drinks, and milk shakes, are thought to produce "wind" in the body.

"HOT"/"COLD" SYSTEM   A second explanatory device is the "hot"/ "cold" system, a major dialectic devolving from the basic *yin-yang* polarity (Gould-Martin 1978). *Yang* and *yin* are complementary: they are described symbolically by the circular picture of two intertwined fishlike creatures, one light, one dark, each with an eye of the contrasting color. "Hot" and "cold" are more prosaic versions of this cosmological distinction; they are opposites that must be balanced and regulated so that there is not an excess of either (Louie 1975:127). Foods, medicines, and diseases are often characterized as "hot" or "cold," or, in milder forms, as "warm" or "cool." Some foods are classed as "hot" or "cold" in an obvious way: deep-fried or baked foods are "hot"; raw, refrigerated, and frozen foods are "cold." "Warming" foods, which stimulate health, tend to be nutritious, red in color, or warming in effect, like ginger and pepper. "Cooling" foods are often bitter and watery. A person's predisposition and constitution may also be characterized as "hot" or "cold," and emotional states and natural physical states, like youth and old age, may be "hot" or "cold." Naturally, changes in temperature from weather, bathing, and cold or stuffy rooms fit this classification and may be blamed for causing illness.

"POISON"   A third explanatory device is "poison," a concept related to "hot" and "cold" in a way that is not entirely clear (Gould-Martin 1978). Certain conditions may be analyzed as "poison," allergic, or irritating: wounds that enlarge rather than heal, aggravated skin diseases, allergies, and infections with pus. These conditions are thought to be aggravated by certain foods classed as irritating, "poisonous," or "wet" (for example, shellfish), which are harmless for well people but to be avoided by the ill. There are other foods to remedy these illnesses and to serve as antidotes to excesses of the irritating foods (Koo 1976:231). "Poison" is a concept in traditional Chinese medicine and "allergy" a concept of modern Western medicine, but their similarities in manifestation have allowed them to be combined into one explanation by the Chinese.

BLOOD AND *Ch'i*   There are two physiological processes (one of which Western physicians consider mythical) that are very important to many Chinese: the generation and flow of blood and *ch'i*. *Ch'i* is the energy force, the breath of life; having too much or too little of it will cause problems. Blood and *ch'i* should both flow smoothly through the body, blood through the blood vessels and *ch'i* through the meridians. At special junctions there is believed to be an interchange between blood and *ch'i* (Koo 1976:43). When the flow of *ch'i* is blocked (for instance, when a bone is broken or disease occurs), then treatment at the injury site or the proper acupuncture points will allow it to flow freely again. When *ch'i* or blood is lost, energy is lost that is hard to restore.

"FRIGHT"   "Fright," a common disease of early childhood recognizable from its symptoms (listlessness, lack of appetite, mild fever, crying) and their amelioration by specific treatments, is thought in Taiwan and Hong Kong to be caused by a child's soul becoming scattered (Topley 1970; Gould-Martin 1976:177, 201–202).

The Amalgam of Chinese and Western Medical Concepts

The Western biomedical system and the Chinese classical system are both esoteric and complex collections of abstruse theory and presumed facts, employed to explain disease and justify treatment. However, ordinary Chinese Americans use severely modified and disconnected versions of these systems which they have drawn not from technical medical journals or ancient texts, but from friends and relatives, experience with professionals, advertisements, and articles in the popular press. When the Western and the Chinese medical systems are explained by simplification and analogy, especially in the Chinese press, the profound differences between the two systems become less apparent. And indeed, there are points of contact: the humoral (hot/cold) theories are used by both Chinese and Westerners in ordinary conversation. Therefore a Chinese American has at his disposal a popularized Chinese explanation, a popularized Western one, and often some way to reconcile them, as illustrated below.

Chinese tradition	Western tradition
Emphasis on balance	Moderation in drugs, alcohol, food
"Wind" causes illness	Pollen, dust (wind-borne) cause allergy
"Heat" and "poison" are treated by cooling and poison-dispersing herbs	Bacterial infections are treated by antibiotics

Specific Implications for Health Professionals

Some of the implications of Chinese theories of disease for hospital care are quite clear: a patient should be particularly consulted about windows, air conditioners, and blankets, and Chinese patients (especially women) should not be forced to bathe or wash their hair if reluctant. A wide range of foods and drinks should be offered, again with some consultation. A Chinese patient on a liquid diet may refuse cold fruit juice or soda but accept hot bouillon; he may refuse deep-fried or raw foods but may be willing to eat the same things boiled. Furthermore, during a hospital stay the patient may want herbal soups, teas, or other special dishes from home. When there is no evidence that these foods interfere with Western treatment, they should be permitted.

Becoming Ill

The evaluation of symptoms and illness occurs against a background body image: what is in the body, what it looks like, how it functions and how it is affected by the outside world. For some organs, such as the heart and bowels, the patient has sounds or sensations that help to locate the organ in his body. For others, like the gallbladder, he has no evidence of the existence of such an organ or for its functioning. As a result, body image is largely a symbolic system with a tenuous connection to anatomy (Louie 1975:146).

Symptoms and disease are most often explained by reference to "wind," "hot," and "cold" (table 2.7). Other explanations based on *ch'i*, blood,

Table 2.7 Causes of various symptoms and diseases according to popular Chinese etiologies.

"Wind"	"Hot"	"Cold"
Arthritis	Bad breath	Anemia
Bloatedness	Blurry vision	Chills
Common cold	Conjunctivitis	Colds
Dizziness	Constipation	Dull eyes
Flatulence	Diarrhea	Influenza
Influenza	Dry cough	Frequent urination
Foam in sputum	Dry mouth and throat	Leukemia
Gurgling	Ear infection	Nausea
Headache	Fever	Poor appetite
Infantile convulsions	Mouth and gum sores	Sallowness
Leprosy	Pimples	Shortness of breath
Mental illness	Sore throat	Weakness
Paralysis	Yellow tongue	Weight loss
Rubella		White tongue
Watery eyes		

Source: Koo (1976:205–206); Chang (1974:436); Cattell (1962:76); Los Angeles informants.

and "fright" are also given. A Los Angeles informant complained of *"ch'i* stagnation," a condition that made her weak and lethargic. Another had been told by her Western doctor that blood clots were responsible for her impaired vision. A diagnosis of "fright" may be used to explain why a child is listless, cries at night, refuses food, or has a slight fever. Although this is often a "magical" problem in Asia (Topley 1970; Gould-Martin 1976:107–110, 177–179, 201–202), in America fright is treated by giving the child "Protect-infant-pill," a patent medicine readily available in herb shops and Chinese grocery stores here.

Factors Influencing Tolerance of Symptoms

The patient's attitude toward his symptoms may be heavily influenced by particular familial responsibilities. One might suppose that a person with heavy responsibilities would delay treatment in order to avoid any absence from the family or work. However, Chinese Americans sometimes seek preventive care in order to avoid any disability. For example, a 65-year-old woman who regularly visited the Sacramento Asian Clinic for checkups said that she was afraid of getting sick, because if she should become incapacitated, there would be no one to look after her blind, aging husband. In another instance, an abortion was noted in the history of a 32-year-old married, childless woman. She said that her husband, an only child, was mentally unstable. Her mother-in-law was displeased with her childlessness, but her husband's mental condition and the threat of unemployment resulting from pregnancy made her decide not to have any children.

Factors about the patient himself influence tolerance of symptoms. According to Koo (1976:22 and 148), sons receive more parental concern over minor symptoms than daughters. In the Los Angeles study, there were six men between the ages of 18 and 24 with nonemergency symptoms who were taken by their parents for treatment or were given remedies their parents thought necessary. The conditions appeared to be medically benign, and the young men were not anxious, but their parents were concerned.

People who have mental and emotional problems may somatize them and go for herbal treatments when their ailments are either a natural result of old age or the direct result of their mental condition (for example, depression leading to fatigue and "ch'i stagnation"). Chinese medical theory encourages this practice by being deficient in psychological vocabulary and by analyzing and treating somatic and psychosomatic illnesses identically. There were two instances in Los Angeles where older women complained of ch'i stagnation, but their unsympathetic daughters thought that their mothers exaggerated and had brought on their own illnesses through lack of exercise.

The recommended treatment for a symptom, or even the diagnostic procedures indicated, may deter the patient from treatment and cause him to tolerate his symptom. Most Chinese are afraid of blood loss, hospitalization, and surgery. When a Western doctor recommends surgery, the patient may decide to live with the symptom or to adhere to Chinese medical explanations and treatments (Li 1972:538). For example, a woman whose "liver fire" had caused impaired vision had been recommended for surgery, a treatment she found unacceptable because of cost. She took herbal medicines, believed to be slow-acting, while her symptoms continued.

Many older people regard the hospital as a place to die, and they confirm that view by waiting till the point of death to go there. In fact, old Chinese men living in rooming houses are most often sent to the hospital by their fellow lodgers, who do not want death to take place in the rooming house (Cattell 1962:79). The association of the hospital with surgery and death, as well as the problems of cost, language, and food, all contribute to the practice of deferring hospitalization.

If a symptom is believed to indicate a severe condition, even though it is not debilitating in itself, then it is less likely to be tolerated. Impotence in males is such a condition: it indicates a severe deficiency of *yang* and *ch'i* and therefore will be treated before more severe symptoms appear. (Frigidity in women does not indicate any such deficiency, though barrenness is a matter of concern.) "Fright" in infants may also be perceived as life-threatening if not treated promptly, though the corresponding Western diagnosis of colic calls for months of parental endurance.

Consultation about Symptoms

Symptoms are discussed within the family and with people believed to have a more than average knowledge of illness. The age and sex of these local experts are not important; what matters most is their interest in the subject matter and their accessibility to the patient. The Los Angeles study found that the choice of experts both for the identification of illness and symptoms and for recommendation of treatment is usually in accord with Chinese familial relationships. Both parents decide these matters for young children, and the father, older brother, and mother-in-law appeared as home diagnosticians for young adults. In middle age, spouses consulted one another, and older people relied mainly on themselves and secondarily on their spouses and neighbors.

Coping with Illness outside the Mainstream Medical System

Home Treatment and Health Maintenance

Home preventive treatment is performed by Chinese Americans as a matter of routine: in hot weather, people drink cooling teas and eat more "cold" and cooling foods,; in cold weather they consume tonics in the form of soups and special dishes with herbs such as chicken or pork cooked with herbs, dragon eye, and red dates. Other "hot" foods include broccoli, rice wine, liver, mushrooms, ginger, black vinegar, peanuts, and any form of pepper; these are usually taken with the evening meal. People in a naturally "cold" state (that is, old people, new mothers, or people with a "cold" constitution) are more careful to avoid "cold" things and consume tonics. People may need special foods to help them through certain stages: adolescence, marriage, and pregnancy. Young, active people who are believed to have warmer bodies will be given more cooling teas, made with "cold" foods such as winter-melon, watercress, and water chestnuts. This regimen is not for treatment of a specific ailment but for cooling the body, or as one informant put it, "to lubricate the machine." Other "cold" foods include bamboo shoots, melon, soybean sprouts, white turnips, seaweed, mustard greens, bok choy, and chrysanthemum tea (Cattell 1962:76; Chang 1974: 436; Louie 1975:128).

Often when a Chinese person first notices symptoms of illness, he tries to handle the situation himself, either by ignoring the symptoms with the hope that they may go away, or by making some minor change in diet. When the symptoms become more noticeable or when he wants sympathy or suggestions, he is likely to turn to his family members. Judging from people interviewed in our Los Angeles study (table 2.8), women are more

Table 2.8 Number of people seeking care from a Los Angeles herbalist, 1978.

Age of seeker	Number seeking care for self		Number seeking care for family member	
	Female	Male	Female	Male
Old (56 and over)	3	4	5	2
Middle-aged (36–55)	1	5	5	3
Young (under 35)	1	6	4	1
Total	5	15	14	6

Source: Los Angeles study by the authors.

likely to care for a family member than are men. Nevertheless, since in immigrant families men are far more likely to be literate in Chinese or English (or both) than women, the tasks of reading medical information, deciding among prescriptions and patent medicines, and consulting home medical manuals are very likely to involve men. The bed care and running of errands, the brewing of herbs, and the cooking of soups are more likely to be women's responsibilities.

The most common ailments to be treated at home are coughs, colds, digestive problems, and skin ailments. As we have seen, these disorders are often attributed to an imbalance in "hot" or "cold" which can be remedied by administering appropriate items of the opposite temperature class. There are many patent medicines for these conditions, and the proper herbs are well known to many people, so treatment can be undertaken without professional assistance.

In the Los Angeles study, several people were found to be using home treatments for medical problems originally attended by Western doctors. Either the recommended treatment was more drastic than the patient would tolerate, or the results of the treatment were unsatisfactory. Examples of this latter circumstance included lingering coughs and bruises, a gallbladder problem for which the doctor had prescribed rest, and a child's prolonged cold, which the patients interpreted as "fright."

Chinatown herb shops carry patent medicines from Taiwan, Hong Kong, and mainland China. Patients often get two or three brands to see which is more effective. They may also buy patent medicines to duplicate their herbal prescriptions—again to test for effectiveness.

Herbs may be bought one at a time or prepackaged in combinations (that is, in accordance with some common prescription). Most commonly, people have their own prescriptions which the herbalist prepares by cutting, grinding, and weighing out the herbs they will brew at home.

Written prescriptions of Chinese herbs come from a variety of sources and are not given up to the pharmacist when he has filled them. Prescriptions are available in the medical column of the newspaper, may be passed down in a family for generations, may be borrowed and exchanged like recipes, or may be the result of a previous visit to a Chinese practitioner. In general, one person's prescription may be used by anyone else with a similar complaint, after minor dosage changes are made according to the patient's size and condition. For example, in our study, a woman in Westwood obtained herbs for "stomach chill" from her friend in Chinatown, who had obtained the prescription and herbs from a friend in Hong Kong, who in turn had obtained the prescription from a famous Chinese physician in Hong Kong. Almost one-quarter of the people buying herbs for home treatment had borrowed a prescription. It is interesting to note that while some of the prescriptions are ancient, others are currently entering the country from Taiwan, Hong Kong, and mainland China, where there is ongoing research into the medicinal properties of herbs.

Nonmainstream Care outside the Home

TRADITIONAL PRACTITIONERS   All the major Chinatowns have numerous traditional practitioners, all of them called (in Chinese) "Chinese doctor." A "Chinese doctor" can do one or more of the following: sell herbs, diagnose minor problems from the patient's appearance and history, make pulse diagnosis, perform acupuncture, and set bones. The flood of recent immigrants, not only Chinese but also Thai, Korean, and Vietnamese, has provided a demand for and a supply of traditional practitioners. A 1975 street census of New York City's Chinatown yielded the following: 20 herbalists, 5 acupuncturists, 7 bone setters, 2 herb shops without herbalists, and 19 associated businesses that also sold herbs (Chan and Chung 1976:33). According to a recent business directory for Los Angeles Chinatown (which is much smaller than New York's), there are 15 herbalists or herb shops. At least 10 of these listings seem to be practicing "Chinese doctors," and 4 of them are Doctors of Chiropractic as well.

In the United States there is no official regulation over the training, examining, licensing, or practice of traditional Chinese practitioners, with the exception of state regulations concerning acupuncture. Practitioners vary greatly in their competence, but their caution (and the basic mildness of herbs) usually protects their patients from outright harm. Local gossip also provides a guide to effective and scrupulous practitioners.

In traditional Chinese medicine, the practitioner uses eight principles for disease differentiation, ascertaining whether the illness is *yin* or *yang* in character, whether it has external or internal symptoms, whether it is of a "cold" or "warm" nature, and finally whether it is due to an increased or reduced function. Clinical data are collected by interview, observation, and pulse reading. Questioning enables the practitioner to gain information about the patient's habits, background, and any circumstances that might affect his state of health. He also inquires about appetite, urine, stool, and general health. The practitioner observes the patient's complexion, eyes, nose, mouth, tongue, and teeth. He listens to the sound of the patient's breathing, together with his manner of coughing and speaking. By feeling the pulse, the practitioner is said to be able to determine not only the condition of the heart and aortic valves, but also whether the internal organs are in good or bad order.

Traditional Chinese methods for the treatment of illness include acupuncture, moxibustion, respiratory therapy, remedial massage, exercises, treatment of fractures and injuries, and herbal medicine. Though all these methods are used in contemporary China, Taiwan, and Hong Kong, only herbal medicine and acupuncture are common in the United States. Religious and magical healing methods, so common in Hong Kong and Taiwan, are not conspicuously present in mainland China and the United States.

Typically, the practitioner writes a prescription which the patient fills at an herb shop. A common prescription, consisting of a mixture of drugs of plant, animal, and mineral origin, is boiled in a specified amount of water, and the decoction is taken internally. Sometimes a practitioner also prescribes patent medicines, particularly those manufactured in China in recent years.

Acupuncture involves the insertion of fine metal needles into strategic groups of points on the body, often distant from the target organ. According to traditional medical theory, the acupuncture points on the skin are the spots where the meridians emerge on the surface. The theory states that the ebb and flow of vital force (*ch'i*) occur along these meridians and are intricately interconnected with the internal organs. The insertion of needles into these sites is said to equalize the balance between the opposing forces and cause therapeutic changes in the affected organ. Acupuncture anesthesia—the use of acupuncture to induce analgesia during surgery—is a technique that was introduced in China in about 1958 (Sidel and Sidel 1973:144). Although it has recently received much publicity, acupuncture for this purpose appears not to be practiced in the United States.

Most practitioners in the United States use only herbal medicine in their treatment; some also use acupuncture as therapy, while a few treat exclusively with acupuncture. In addition to the methods described above, the prevention of illness is emphasized. A patient is advised on the correct balance between work, relaxation, and sleep, and on eating a moderate, "clean," and correct diet. A simple diet is usually suggested to a patient, and special dishes (usually soups made with meats and herbs) are recommended to aid convalescence. This traditional attention to diet suggests that Western physicians might advise Chinese patients on diet as a routine aspect of therapy.

THE CHOICE OF WESTERN OR CHINESE MEDICINE   When Chinese people decide they must go beyond home treatment, they are first faced with the basic decision between Western and Chinese medicine. When symptoms include acute pain, high fever, dyspnea, bleeding, and rapid onset, then Western-style help is usually sought promptly. From the findings of Chan and Chang (1976), Louie (1975), and our Los Angeles study, it appears that Western medical care is also preferred for dentistry, fever, allergy, eye problems, heart attack, stroke, surgery, diabetes, and cancer. Chinese treatment is sought for asthma, arthritis, pruritus, bruises and sprains, lumbago, stomach problems, and hypertension. With the exception of arthritis, it is unlikely that such preferences will be consistently expressed. Generally speaking, Western medicine operates quickly for symptomatic relief. Therefore, a person can use Western medicine first and then follow up with Chinese long-term treatment.

Of 22 people questioned in our Los Angeles study, 10 used Chinese medicine at the onset of the illness, 8 used Western medicine first and followed it with Chinese medicine, and 4 used both methods simultaneously. People who used Chinese medicine first did so because they thought their conditions, coughs and colds, were better treated by Chinese medicine. Those who sought Western medicine first and Chinese second had either rejected the suggested treatment of the Western physician (surgery) or had undergone treatment but had residual symptoms, or they had conditions which the Western physician did not feel needed treatment. The four instances in which patients received joint treatment were for allergy, diabetes, asthma, and high blood pressure. All had learned from their Western physicians that their conditions could not be permanently cured, although they obtained long-term symptomatic treatment; they went to Chinese practitioners in the hope of removing the root of the problem, first by correcting the imbalance of "heat," accumulated impurities, or "wind," then by strengthening the body with tonics, and finally by treating the actual ailment.

A study of Boston's Chinatown (Hessler et al. 1975) divided its 183 respondents into five types of "health-care utilizers" on the basis of their responses to eight questions about medical beliefs: pure Western (0); predominantly Western (75); half and half (27); predominantly Chinese (57); pure Chinese (27). We feel that the impression created by this study may be misleading. Though people may *believe* in Chinese medicine, it seems highly unlikely that they would go for long periods of time without using any Western care. A study of the New York Chinatown is a better guide to patterns of health-care utilization: according to this study (Chan and Chang 1976), 82.76 percent of the survey respondents had visited only Western physicians, whereas only 17.24 percent had had experience with traditional practitioners in the previous two years. No one had seen traditional practitioners more often than physicians in the previous two years. Although a significant majority of the respondents stated that going to a traditional practitioner was cheaper, required less time, and involved fewer painful procedures, they considered Western physicians more reliable and more accessible. Furthermore, Western physicians were generally recommended by family and friends. However, this same survey found Chinese medicine to be far more common as a form of home treatment. Only 6.9 percent of the sample had had no experience with Chinese drugs, whereas 93.1 percent had used Chinese drugs for self-treatment.

Similarly, the families of five acculturated, middle-aged, suburban, professional Chinese Americans who are well known to us consult Western physicians rather than herbalists but use both Western and Chinese home treatments. Western physicians have been seen for surgery, orthodox cancer treatment (chemotherapy and radiotherapy), shingles, stroke, and hypertension. Western orthodox and unorthodox medicines are used at home: prescription drugs, sleeping pills, vitamins, laetrile, and megavitamins. Chinese medicines are also used at home: patent cold medicines for children, medicated plasters for low back pain, ginseng tea, boiled centipede soup (for cancer), herbs for shingles, and eucalyptus oil for dizziness resulting from hypertension. Knowledge of remedies such as centipedes and honeysuckle for cancer comes from reading rather than from the advice of Chinese practitioners.

From the studies and the supplementary cases cited, it would appear that the most common pattern involves the purchase and consumption of Chinese herbs and patent medicines for home treatment, in combination with a preference for seeing Western physicians for diagnosis and treatment. This pattern seems to hold for Chinese Americans generally, although those with higher incomes probably receive higher quality Western care. As for those beliefs that influence choices between Western and Chinese medicine (for example, belief in the hot/cold system), they cannot be simply correlated with obvious demographic factors (Hessler et al. 1975). Medical factors (symptoms and type of disease), convenience factors (location, hours, price, language spoken, and waiting time), and the precedent set by friends and relatives all influence the treatment decision.

Problems or Benefits Associated with the Use of Chinese Medicine

It is often suggested that the use of Chinese medicine leads to the nonuse of Western medicine. The underutilization of Western health facilities by Chinatown residents may be given as evidence for this view. As we have seen, however, those who have inquired into this matter have not found this to be the case. Indeed, Cattell (1962) found that the underutilization of Western medical facilities was due to problems in social structure and medical-care organization (Cattell 1962:69, 86). This view is echoed by Chan and Chang: "If the utilization of nearby hospital facilities is low, one cannot blame Chinese medicine and traditional practitioners. Instead, the reasons may be found in the low level of income, long working hours, and language barriers; and, in the hospitals, the long waiting time for treatment, the location, high hospital costs, unavailability of interpreters, and the attitude of the hospital's staff" (1976:135).

However, Chan and Chang believe that the consumption of Chinese medicine may have dangers; they suggest (without evidence) the following possible problems: adverse results from the use of drugs obtained without professional advice, adverse side effects from the consumption of Chinese and Western drugs simultaneously, and complication of the diagnosis by the prior consumption of Chinese drugs. They worry that the lack of standardization of Chinese practitioners has led to doctor shopping, a practice detrimental to selecting Western physicians. They also note that Chinese medical theory may increase a patient's fear of surgery and blood drawing, as well as his distaste for hospital food or the diet his physician prescribes.

Clearly there are benefits, or at least potential benefits, from the use of Chinese medicine in combination with the use of Western medicine. Chinese self-treatments, since they involve foods, herbs, and teas, are almost invariably milder than those of Western medicine. Cough syrups, for instance, consist primarily of honey and herbs to soothe the throat. The dietary changes that are prescribed for certain diseases probably increase the variability of the diet and the intake of trace minerals and vitamins. Foods that "heat" the body contain protein, those to cool it are largely composed of water. In addition to being milder, home remedies are probably comforting to Chinese people since they are those that were given to the patient as a child. Since most minor illnesses are self-limiting (for example, coughs, colds, stomach upsets, rashes), the milder, cheaper treatment of the Chinese herbalist is generally beneficial. Recommending moderation in rest, exercise, diet, emotion, work, and social life is never amiss and encourages the patient to share in the responsibility for maintaining good health.

The use of these remedies and of traditional practitioners in Chinese-American communities probably takes part of the burden off the available physicians. Ideally, traditional practitioners should serve as paramedics, treating minor problems, self-limiting illnesses, and hopeless and chronic cases where Western medicine has no solution. Unfortunately, the actual situation does not always meet this ideal.

Encounters with Mainstream Medical Practitioners

Settings

By far the most common setting for mainstream medical care for Chinese Americans, whatever their financial status, is the office of a private physician (International Institute 1968:6; CACA 1972:49; Wu 1974:120; UCLA Team 1975:85).[4] Chinese Americans tend to prefer physicians who are ethnically Chinese. Because of language and transportation problems, many Chinatown residents, fearful of getting lost, will not venture outside of Chinatown and therefore prefer local Chinese-speaking general practitioners. New York, San Francisco, and Los Angeles all have Chinatown physicians; presumably other Chinatowns do as well. In many of the Chinatowns there are only a few physicians who will see drop-in patients; these general practitioners see very large numbers of people at relatively low fees. They practice a kind of medicine different from that of the specialist who serves the middle class. Knowing that their patients lack insurance and are unlikely to sue, and limited by their own training, they are far less likely to perform extensive diagnostic tests before administering the most likely treatment. These physicians are often older men who wield sufficient power in local community politics to prevent the entry of other young physicians whose practices would be competitive with theirs.

Hospitals are usually located in or near Chinatowns, simply because both are set in urban areas. But some of these hospitals (such as French Hospital in Los Angeles) are not suited to community needs: they have no emergency service or walk-in clinics; they accept patients only by referral; and they have hours that are incompatible with the employment patterns of many of their patients. Other hospitals, such as Tufts–New England Medical Center in Boston, had similar problems in the past but then improved their services in response to the needs of the surrounding community (Sullivan and Hatch 1970:64; CACA 1972:48). As in the case with physicians, many Chinese-American patients prefer hospitals with Chinese-speaking staff and may be referred to such hospitals in preference to those nearby.

According to United States Vital Statistics, the proportion of Chinese Americans hospitalized in the last five years was well below the average level of other groups (cited in UCLA Team 1975:79). This finding was substantiated by a University of California (Los Angeles) Asian-American Public Health Team, which undertook the study of health care utilization patterns of Los Angeles Asian Americans. Judging from hospital records, even the hospitals most likely to be used by Asians appeared to be severely underutilized by them (UCLA Team 1975:128–133).

Today, community clinics in many of the nation's Chinatowns (for example, the Asian Clinic in Sacramento and the On Lok Senior Day Health Center in San Francisco) provide screening, preventive and primary care, counseling, and referral services to local residents (Lurie et al. 1976). In addition, there are free clinics and Public Health Clinics. Some of these clinics are only open during the workday; however, others keep evening and weekend hours for the convenience of their patients. Again, patients prefer those clinics with bicultural staff.

Social Service Centers located in Chinatowns (such as the one in Los Angeles) usually handle legal, economic, and social matters. Though they do not offer health services, they provide language assistance, transportation, and assistance with Medicare and Medicaid applications and thus help the patient use the mainstream health-care system (Pacific Asian Project 1977). Senior Citizens Centers, set up to provide meals and "day care" for the elderly, sometimes also offer physical examinations, physiotherapy, occupational therapy, and health care as needed (Lurie et al. 1976:39–43). Many Chinatown residents receive health care either by such community projects or with their assistance.

Expectations in the Medical Encounter

Chinese-American patients want very much to understand their illnesses. The patient wants to know the cause of the illness and how that cause is linked to the symptoms; he also wants to understand the diagnostic procedures and the treatment. It is obvious that an immigrant patient may have difficulty in both understanding the physician's explanation and linking it to the body of information and theory that he generally uses to understand his health. But the patient still regards this explanation as very important. When the physician uses only technical language, the patient is offended and frustrated. Furthermore, patients think poorly of a physician who says, "There's nothing wrong" or "It's only nerves." Since physical and mental health are so closely linked in Chinese medical theory, such an explanation does not make sense.

The Chinese patient wants a physician who talks to him using language he can understand, does not appear to be in a big rush, explains the illness, does not force tests or treatments on him that he does not want, gives remedies that are clear, simple, and easy to follow, recommends a therapeutic diet, charges a low fee (a sign of virtue in a doctor), helps him to use insurance or government money to defray the costs, is interested in him, tries hard, and offers hope. (Who would not want such a physician?) However, in the final analysis, the patient wants to get well, and a physician without the foregoing qualities who nonetheless produces a rapid and complete cure will also be favored. It is the effectiveness of Western medicine that has attracted its Chinese-American clientele, not its cognitive or psychosocial appeal.

In Asia, hospital nurses provide only strictly medical care, such as injections. Nursing tasks such as feeding, bathing, and keeping the patient comfortable are performed by family members who stay with the patient in the hospital, often sleeping on the floor. Patients who have been in Asian hospitals are therefore reluctant to ask nurses for services that are normal here. American nurses must explicitly offer bedpans, blankets, and other such assistance to these patients. They should demonstrate the use of the call button, bed hoist, telephone, television, toilet, lights, and other equipment, if necessary by sign language and play acting.

Because of language difficulties, the information given by the physician and nurse must often filter through other people before it reaches the patient. A Chinese-speaking patient who is hospitalized will usually have family members or friends around much of the time to give support and assist in interpretation. Someone in this group usually speaks English and will not only talk with the physicians and nurses but also consult with close relatives about which pieces of information are to be relayed to the patient. When the patient has to be told about his condition or about further treatment, it is this interpreter who first hears of it and then discusses these matters with other members of the family. If the diagnosis involves a terminal condition, this information is usually kept from the patient to maintain hopes of recovery; for example, to most patients the diagnosis of cancer means certain death. Because of this reaction, family members are reluctant to reveal the diagnosis to the patient. The patient in turn may cooperate in this conspiracy if he suspects cancer. In such cases, however, both patient and family members welcome further palliative treatments.

Although confidentiality is built into the American medical-care system, it is a rather foreign concept to many Chinese immigrants, whose lives take place within the sight and hearing of many relatives and neighbors. Thus it is not surprising that family members are involved in the patient's medical decisions and care.

Interactional Norms in the Medical Setting

In traditional Chinese society, interactional norms were determined largely by age, sex, and social class. The ideal doctor was traditionally a Confucian scholar, a learned gentleman who may have originally undertaken the study of medicine in order to care for his parents but who benevolently consented to treat others as well.

The long schooling that physicians undergo today results in their being treated by the Chinese with the respect accorded scholars, as long as they conform to the norms of scholarly behavior: politeness, seriousness, graciousness, and benevolence. A doctor's fee is considered an ethical matter: profit making is incompatible with the moral rectitude of a humanitarian doctor (Louie 1975:224, 227).

Modesty is very important to Chinese women. Traditional Chinese doctors never approached a woman more closely than to take her pulse or scrutinize her face, while midwives handled intimate examinations and treatments. When female physicians are not available to Chinese gynecological patients, male physicians should take care to respect their patients' modesty, should explain what they are doing and why, and should forego making jokes to relieve tension. The purpose and procedure of the examination should be explained before the patient is asked to undress. When a patient is older than the physician, it is particularly important for her to be treated with obvious respect and decorum.

Difficulties of Chinese Americans in Using Mainstream Medical Services

The prime difficulty involved in Chinese Americans' using mainstream medical services is financial. Naturally, they are not alone in such a difficulty, but they may be unaware of assistance to which they are entitled. If they do not have an advocate from a Service Center, the doctor's office or hospital should try to understand their situation and assist them. In fact, Chinese people pay most of their medical bills out of savings, and they do indeed pay their bills. A person with neither credit cards nor a checking account must be allowed to pay in cash installments. Part of the Chinese New Year's celebration includes payment of all outstanding debts, and Los Angeles Chinatown physicians affirm that they are paid then, if not sooner. However, if the patient is poor and uninsured, the severe curtailment of other expenditures required to pay large medical bills may be more detrimental to health than the treatment was beneficial.

The second difficulty Chinese Americans face is lack of time for medical treatment. Many tend to work long hours—women and old people included. They are reluctant to take time from work or household duties for long waits or for procedures they regard as inessential, such as preventive care or consultation with a social worker. Regimens that call for bed rest or frequent trips to the doctor may not be feasible.

Third, Chinese Americans are often ignorant of the functioning of the American medical system. Medical personnel must work as health educators in this area. Patients need to know that some doctors are specialists, that they can ask for a second opinion, and that they can be referred to a specialist.

Fourth, Chinese-American patients are reputed by social workers to be difficult to work with. They volunteer little information and may resent probing into personal problems, even when these problems are quite severe. They expect objective technical help with such matters as forms, medications, and jobs, and they are less receptive to verbal therapy.

Finally, and probably most important, Chinese Americans have language difficulties that exacerbate all their other problems. In most cases, a patient will not go to a physician unless a bilingual relative or friend is available. Often the only available interpreters are school children who, for obvious reasons, are inadequate. Nursing services in medical centers serving Chinese patients usually have lists of bilingual employees who have volunteered to interpret. Though this service represents a step in the right direction, it is usually inadequate. The lists are often out of date, the employees may be unable to come when needed, and Chinese patients speak a variety of mutually unintelligible dialects. In medical centers where such lists are available, such as the Los Angeles County General Hospital and the Sacramento Medical Center, the patient is still expected to bring his own interpreter. If he appears without one and none is available, he is asked to return another day. Because so few Chinese-speaking patients utilize most hospitals, the hospitals are reluctant to develop their interpreting services, thus further discouraging Chinese patients from coming.

Explanations to patients can be greatly enhanced by the use of specific pictures and diagrams. On the other hand, Western analogies and systems of organization are of little use. A patient will rarely admit ignorance or ask questions, preferring to smile and nod. Thus the health practitioner needs to provide a thorough explanation to both patient and interpreter. Demonstration of how medicine should be taken—how much and when —is also necessary for the patient who may be unable to read.

During a hospital stay, a patient can be supplied with a list or a set of cards with useful phrases in Chinese and English accompanied by diagrams or pictures. These phrases express the patient's condition or needs: pain, fever, hunger, needing to use the bedpan, wanting to lower or raise the bed, and so forth. When given to the patient, the pictures should be acted out so that their meaning is perfectly clear; then when the patient has no interpreter handy, he can call a nurse and point to the appropriate phrase. One Los Angeles patient kept such a list for three years and used it for subsequent hospitalizations (C. Kushi, personal communication).

Thorough patient education has proved of long-lasting value for Chinese Americans. For example, a Los Angeles Port-a-Pap Clinic was staffed with bicultural community women who were carefully trained. The clinic has been highly successful and the initial education has spread by word of mouth to many women.

How Chinese classical concepts of nosology and etiology influence patients' reactions to Western diagnoses has not been studied. We do know, however, that except for very rare diseases not found in Chinese medical terminology, there exist Chinese equivalents for all the words in a Western diagnosis. The principal problem is not a conceptual one but a serious practical one: how to find a person competent in translating medical terminology so that the medical diagnosis can be explained to the patient in Chinese. If the interpreter is a professional, he can translate English technical language into Chinese technical language and then explain that to the patient. If he is not, then Western practitioners need first to turn the English technical language into lay language so that the interpreter can translate that. Translation and interpretation services are commonly offered by Chinese Social Service Centers found in major American cities and are listed in a National Directory (Pacific Asian Project 1977).

Assessing a Patient's Difficulties in Using Western Medical Care

The difficulties faced by a particular Chinese-American patient in his encounter with mainstream medical care can be assessed by the health professional during initial contact. For example, a medical history can include the following key facts: place of origin, length of stay in this country, education, occupation, working hours, marital situation, occupation of spouse, living situation, insurance, sick leave, and disability pay. This type of information will allow the health professional to judge the patient's English ability, his level of understanding of Western concepts of illness and treatment, his ability to follow the suggested regimen, and his ability to pay for tests and treatment. Attempts to prevent or solve specific problems involving time, finances, or other matters can begin concurrently with medical treatment.

Adherence to Biomedical Treatment

Adherence to medical treatment is a complicated matter involving many nonmedical factors. For example, Murphy (1970:1044–1046) found that Chinese-American tuberculosis patients, released from the hospital for follow-up at a chest clinic, were unreliable about keeping their appointments. The clinic was located across town and was only open in the early morning (though many Chinese-American men work late into the night). But when the clinic was moved to the vicinity where the patients lived, and the hours were changed to early afternoon, the number of broken appointments dropped sharply. Furthermore, patients were more likely to continue Western treatment when they were not discouraged from undergoing traditional Chinese treatment as well.

Adherence to treatment among Chinese Americans may be excellent in certain instances. For example, the elderly women who attended the Asian clinic in Sacramento were very conscientious about regular blood pressure checks. These women worked as seasonal fruit pickers in the Sacramento Valley. To them, keeping healthy was a social obligation. They felt that if one of them should become ill while picking fruit, the unfortunate incident would jeopardize further employment not only of the sick person but also of other fruit pickers of the same age.

Dietary Patterns

As discussed earlier, the Chinese have a complicated classification of foods and herbs used for therapy and health maintenance. Koo (1976: 233) suggests that much of the complexity of this classification has vanished among second- and third-generation Chinese Americans, leaving an etiolated version that focuses on supplementary foods and tonics for treating minor illnesses, strengthening the blood, and increasing male sexual potency. According to our experience in Los Angeles and Sacramento, "cooling" and "cleansing" foods and herbs are also commonly used.

The normal diet for a healthy Chinese American includes a wide variety of foods and drinks, selected with reference primarily to taste, texture, color, cost, and secondarily to the balancing of "hot" and "cold." If a person is not poor, this selection process usually will result in a nutritionally balanced diet. Because of the wide variety of foods normally consumed, most Chinese can adhere to a diet with certain restrictions (for example, a low-cholesterol or low-carbohydrate diet) while still selecting foods they prefer (see Campbell and Chang 1973:248).

However, many Chinatown residents are old and poor and live alone in rooming houses. These factors limit variety and result in a diet that is high in carbohydrate and salt and low in protein and vitamins. Furthermore, even though many of these elderly people have hypertension, the recommendation to reduce soy sauce intake is quite useless, since an average meal consists of rice or noodles with highly seasoned and salted preserved vegetables, meats, or fish. These foods are convenient, because they do not require refrigeration, and are also economical, because only a small quantity is consumed at each meal. Thus a change in dietary patterns cannot be achieved without considerable help, such as that provided by a feeding program for the elderly.

During recuperation from an illness or surgery and after childbirth, Chinese Americans traditionally observe food taboos and are advised to take certain supplementary foods. These dietary practices are sometimes noted by the hospital nursing staff, who find patients refusing hospital food and consuming food brought from home (Pillsbury 1977). The only nutritional study available on this subject (Ling, King, and Leung 1975:131) is concerned with the dietary practices of pregnant Chinese-American women. Its authors found the food proscriptions and prescriptions to have little or no nutritional significance. However, Ling and her coauthors did find problems with infant diet. Chinese-American babies over five months of age were found to suffer from a low intake of both iron and total calories. This finding appeared to be due to weaning children onto white rice porridge, a practice that is not only culturally approved but reinforced by low socioeconomic status and lack of education (Ling, King, and Leung 1975:131).

Attitudes toward Prescription Drugs

More important to the Chinese-American patient's recovery is his attitude toward Western prescription drugs. Western drugs are thought to work promptly and to be strong and efficacious, but to have a high risk of side effects. Consequently, patients are likely to reduce their own medication or discontinue its use entirely as soon as they experience relief from acute symptoms. When strict, continual adherence is necessary for diseases without apparent symptoms (for example, hypertension), this behavior is very likely to undermine the treatment regimen. In the case of tuberculosis, it may even be dangerous. It is therefore important that patients understand the need for long-term use of drugs in certain cases.

Chinese patients may well be more sensitive to drugs and more likely to experience side effects than other patients, possibly because of their smaller body size. It may therefore be advisable to give Chinese patients smaller doses and to forewarn them of possible side effects and how to handle them; otherwise patients are likely to discontinue medication secretly and baffle the physician with continued symptoms. Some Chinese-American patients prefer injections to oral medication. When such a choice is possible, it should be made both to please the patient and to eliminate compliance problems.

Recovery, Rehabilitation, and Death

Patterns of Coping with Chronic Illness, Terminal Illness, and Death

Patients with chronic illness will often obtain both Western and Chinese treatments: the Western treatment, for symptomatic relief; the Chinese, in the hope of curing the underlying imbalance responsible for the illness. Failure of either treatment will not necessarily cause the patient to discontinue it. He may well accept his uncured condition as the best state now possible. According to a Chinese-American social worker, Chinese-American patients tend to have a high pain tolerance and complain little. Medical practitioners might ask patients directly about pain or dispense pain-relieving drugs on schedule to prevent needless suffering.

Furthermore, Chinese-American patients tend to be stoic and fatalistic when faced with terminal illness and death. The common reaction is, "If I'm going to die, I'm going to die. There's nothing to talk about." However, the patient's family may prefer not to tell the patient directly about his diagnosis in order to maintain hope for recovery. Although impending death is not talked about explicitly, the patient generally takes the initiative in tidying up his affairs, while cooperating in his family's conspiracy of silence. In order to respect these preferences, the physician might explain the situation to family members and ask their permission to tell the patient; or if he feels it necessary to tell the patient himself, he might do so alone so that the patient can still pretend ignorance with his family.

Malingering

We have no accurate information on the extent to which Chinese Americans may, for social reasons, be reluctant to give up sick roles or, alternatively, may be reluctant to accept them. However, the employment situation of many Chinese Americans and the experience of Chinese-American social workers suggest certain characteristics of their sick-role behavior.

Chinese Americans who work at blue-collar and service jobs rarely have any sick leave or union benefits (see Yee 1970). Since they are paid by piece work or by the day, there is little temptation to malinger and a great economic pressure to work, even when a person does not feel well. Indeed, the aged and the sick generally continue to work until it becomes impossible. However, as mentioned previously, Chinese Americans tend to somatize social and psychological complaints. It seems likely that unhappily married, unacculturated older women, who lack certain types of escape forms open to men (drinking with friends, gambling, staying away from home) would be particularly prone to explain their unhappiness as illness and treat it as such. As long as the complaints are mild, they probably limit treatment to herbs for home treatment and adjustments in diet; thus they would rarely present as patients for Western practitioners.

Concluding Remarks

We have suggested many ways in which overburdened health professionals might help their Chinese-American patients struggle through poverty, language barriers, and cultural differences to obtain quality mainstream medical care. Today the children of earlier migrants from China and Japan have the highest educational levels and probably the best health of any ethnic group in the nation, but their success was achieved at considerable psychic cost (Sue and Kitano 1973) and with little outside help. It is our opinion that alert, informed, and sympathetic health professionals can reduce this cost for current migrants, many of whose children will undoubtedly become their fellow health professionals.

Notes

We would like to thank Emma Louie, Eric Chang, Robert L. Martin, Francis Hung, and Molly Joel Coye for their helpful suggestions and Henry Chang for allowing his herb shop to be our interview location.

1. This summary of the Chinese experience in the United States is based largely on Chinn, Lai, and Choy (1969).

2. The table does not compare male to female rates; rather, it compares Chinese rates to white rates for the same sex. In whites, males are more than twice as likely to commit suicide. Thus the Chinese male rate appears lower and the female rate higher than if they were based on a population with equal suicide rates for males and females.

3. In this chapter the term "Western medicine" has been used in preference to "biomedicine" because it is a translation from the Chinese and refers to that medical system which originated in the West, regardless of where it is now practiced.

4. Information for this and subsequent sections was obtained from the staff at the Los Angeles Chinatown Social Service Center and the following health and social work professionals: Eleanor Huang, Wendell Wong, Cynthia Lee Kushi, and Alice Chu.

References

AHERN, EMILY M. 1975. Sacred and Secular Medicine in a Taiwan Village: A Study of Cosmological Disorder. In *Medicine in Chinese Cultures,* ed. Arthur Kleinman et al. DHEW Publication no. (NIH) 75-653. Washington, D.C.: U.S. Government Printing Office. (Reprinted as *Culture and Healing in Asian Societies: Anthropological, Psychiatric, and Public Health Studies.* Cambridge, Mass.: Schenkman, 1978.)

ANDERSON, EUGENE N., JR. 1978. Some Observations on Nasopharyngeal Cancer in Hong Kong. Paper presented at the Annual Convention, American Anthropological Association, Los Angeles, November 1978 (mimeographed).

BALL, JOHN C., and M. P. LAU. 1966. The Chinese Narcotic Addict in the United States. *Social Forces* 45:68–72.

A Barefoot Doctor's Manual: The American Translation of the Official Chinese Paramedical Manual. 1977. Philadelphia: Running Press.

BOURNE, PETER G. 1973. Suicide among Chinese in San Francisco. *American Journal of Public Health* 63:744–750.

BRESLOW, LESTER, and BONNIE KLEIN. 1971. Health and Race in California. *American Journal of Public Health* 61:763–775.

CACA (CHINESE AMERICAN CIVIC ASSOCIATION). 1972. Report of the Conference on the Future of Boston's Chinatown. CACA, 18 Oxford Street, Boston, Mass. 02111 (mimeographed).

CAMPBELL, THERESA, and BETTY CHANG. 1973. Health Care of the Chinese in America. *Nursing Outlook* 21:245–249.

CARP, FRANCES M., and EUNICE KATAOKA. 1976. Health-Care Problems of the Elderly of San Francisco Chinatown. *Gerontologist* 16:30–38.

CATTELL, STUART H. 1962. *Health, Welfare and Social Organization in Chinatown, New York City.* New York: Community Service Society.

CHAN, CHUN-WAI, and JADE K. CHANG. 1976. The Role of Chinese Medicine in New York City's Chinatown. *American Journal of Chinese Medicine* 4:31–45, 129–146.

CHANG, BETTY. 1974. Some Dietary Beliefs in Chinese Folk Culture. *American Dietetic Association Journal* 65:436–438.

CHANG, FRANCIS H., and STEPHEN TANG. 1977. A Neighborhood Health Center: One Community's Solution. *Civil Rights Digest* 10:19–23.

CHEN, PETER WEI-TEH. 1976. Chinese-Americans View Their Mental Health. D.S.W. dissertation, School of Social Work, University of Southern California.

CHINN, THOMAS W., H. MARK LAI, and PHILIP P. CHOY. 1969. *A History of the Chinese in California: A Syllabus.* San Francisco: California Historical Society of America.

CHU, GEORGE. 1972. Drinking Patterns and Attitudes of Rooming-House Chinese in San Francisco. *Quarterly Journal of Studies on Alcohol,* suppl. no. 6:58–68.

CHU, LOUIS. 1961. *Eat a Bowl of Tea.* New York: Lyle Stuart.

CROIZIER, RALPH C. 1968. *Traditional Medicine in Modern China.* Cambridge, Mass.: Harvard University Press.

DICKIE, ELIZABETH R. 1978. Biological and Cultural Modes of Transmission of Hepatitis B Virus. Paper presented at the Annual Convention, American Anthropological Association, Los Angeles, November 1978.

FRAUMENI, JOSEPH F., JR., and THOMAS J. MASON. 1974. Cancer Mortality among Chinese Americans, 1950–69. *Journal of the National Cancer Institute* 52:659–665.

GAW, ALBERT C. 1975. An Integrated Approach in the Delivery of Health Care to a Chinese Community in America: The Boston Experience. In *Medicine in Chinese Cultures,* ed. Arthur Kleinman et al. DHEW Publication no. (NIH) 75–653. Washington, D.C.: U.S. Government Printing Office.

GOULD-MARTIN, KATHERINE. 1975. Medical Systems in a Taiwan Village: Ong-ia-kong, the Plague God as Modern Physician. In *Medicine in Chinese Cultures,* ed. Arthur Kleinman et al. DHEW Publication no. (NIH) 75–653. Washington, D.C.: U.S. Government Printing Office. (Reprinted as *Culture and Healing in Asian Societies: Anthropological, Psychiatric, and Public Health Studies.* Cambridge, Mass.: Schenkman, 1978.)

————. 1976. Women Asking Women: An Ethnography of Health Care in Rural Taiwan. Ph.D. dissertation, Anthropology Department, Rutgers University.

————. 1978. Hot Cold Clean Poison and Dirt: Chinese Folk Medical Categories. *Social Science and Medicine* 12:39–46.

HECHTER, H. H., and N. O. BORHANI. 1965. Longevity in Racial Groups Differs. *California's Health* 22:121–122.

HENDERSON, BRIAN E., EMMA LOUIE, JENNIE SOO HOO JING, PHILLIP BUELL, and MURRAY B. GARDNER. 1976. Risk Factors Associated with Nasopharyngeal Carcinoma. *New England Journal of Medicine* 295:1101–1106.

HESSLER, RICHARD M., MICHAEL F. NOLAN, BENJAMIN OGBU, and PETER KONG-MING NEW. 1975. Intraethnic Diversity: Health Care of the Chinese-Americans. *Human Organization* 34:253–262.

HO, JOHN H. C. 1972. Nasopharyngeal Cancer (NPC). *Advances in Cancer Research* 15:57–92.

HUANG, JACOB C. Y., and FREDA GRANCHOW. 1976. Health Services Dilemma: Chinatown, New York City. *New York State Journal of Medicine* 76:297–301.

INTERNATIONAL INSTITUTE OF LOS ANGELES. 1968. Oriental American Survey Project, Summer Youth Program. International Institute of Los Angeles, Summer Youth Program, 435 S. Boyle Ave., Los Angeles, Calif. 90033 (mimeographed).

KAPLAN, HENRY S., and PATRICIA JONES TSUCHITANI, eds. 1978. *Cancer in China.* New York: Liss.

KING, HAITUNG. 1975. Selected Epidemiological Aspects of Major Diseases and Causes of Death among Chinese in the United States and Asia. In *Medicine in Chinese Cultures,* ed. Arthur Kleinman et al. DHEW Publication no. (NIH) 75–653. Washington, D.C.: U.S. Government Printing Office.

KING, HAITUNG, and WILLIAM HAENSZEL. 1973. Cancer Mortality among Foreign and Native-Born Chinese in the United States. *Journal of Chronic Diseases* 26:623–646.

KINGSTON, MAXINE HONG. 1977. *The Woman Warrior: Memoirs of a Girlhood Among Ghosts.* New York: Knopf.

KOO, LINDA CHIH-LING. 1976. Nourishment of Life—The Culture of Health in Traditional China. Ph.D. dissertation, Anthropology Department, University of California, Berkeley.

LI, FREDERICK P. 1972. Health Care for the Chinese Community in Boston. *American Journal of Public Health* 62:536–539.

LING, STELLA, JANET KING, and VIRGINIA LEUNG. 1975. Diet, Growth and Cultural Food Habits in Chinese American Infants. *American Journal of Chinese Medicine* 3:125–132.

LOUIE, THERESA T'SUNG-T'ZU CHEN. 1975. The Pragmatic Context: A Chinese-American Example of Defining-Managing Illness. D.N.S. dissertation, School of Nursing, University of California, San Francisco.

LURIE, ELEANOR, RICHARD A. KALISH, RICHARD WEXLER, and MARIE LOUISE ANSAK. 1976. On Lok Senior Day Health Center: A Case Study. *Gerontologist* 16:39–47.

MACMAHON, BRIAN, PHILIP COLE, and JAMES BROWN. 1973. Etiology of Human Breast Cancer: A Review. *Journal of the National Cancer Institute* 50:21–42.

MURPHEY, RHOADS. 1952. Boston's Chinatown. *Economic Geography* 28: 244–255.

MURPHY, BETTY. 1972. Boston's Chinese: They Have Their Problems Too! In *Chinese-Americans: School and Community Problems*, ed. Integrated Education Associates. Chicago: Integrated Education Associates.

MURPHY, PATRICIA R. 1970. Tuberculosis Control in San Francisco's Chinatown. *American Journal of Nursing* 70:1044–1046.

NEE, VICTOR G., and BRETT DE BARY NEE. 1972. *Longtime Californ': A Documentary Study of an American Chinatown.* New York: Pantheon.

PACIFIC ASIAN ELDERLY RESEARCH PROJECT. 1977. National Directory of Services to the Pacific Asian Elderly. Pacific Asian Elderly Research Project, 2400 South Western Avenue, Suite 206, Los Angeles, Calif. 90018 (mimeographed).

PILLSBURY, BARBARA. 1977. Childbirth: From Chinese Social System into the Western Hospital. Paper presented at the Annual Meeting of the Society for Applied Anthropology, San Diego, April 1977 (mimeographed).

SIDEL, VICTOR W., and RUTH SIDEL. 1973. *Serve the People: Observations on Medicine in the People's Republic of China.* New York: Josiah Macy, Jr., Foundation.

SMITH, ROBERT LINCOLN. 1956. Recorded and Expected Mortality among the Chinese of Hawaii and the United States with Special Reference to Cancer. *Journal of the National Cancer Institute* 17:667–676.

SUE, STANLEY, and HARRY H. L. KITANO, eds. 1973. Asian American: A Success Story. *Journal of Social Issues* 29.2:1–218.

SULLIVAN, CHARLES, and KATHLYN HATCH. 1970. *The Chinese in Boston, 1970.* Boston: Action for Boston Community Development (ABCD), Planning and Evaluation Department (mimeographed).

SZMUNESS, WOLF, CLADD E. STEVENS, HAFEEZ IKRAM, M. ISAAC MUCH, EDWARD J. HARLEY, and BLAINE HOLLINGER. 1978. Prevalence of Hepatitis B Virus Infection and Hepatocellular Carcinoma in Chinese-Americans. *Journal of Infectious Diseases* 137:822–829.

TOPLEY, MARJORIE. 1970. Chinese Traditional Ideas and the Treatment of Disease: Two Examples from Hong Kong. *Man* 5:421–437.

TRAINING PROJECT for the ASIAN ELDERLY. 1973. On the Feasibility of Training Asians to Work with Asian Elderly: A Preliminary Assessment of Needs and Resources Available to Asian Elderly in Seattle, WA. Washington, D.C.: U.S. Government Printing Office.

UCLA ASIAN HEALTH TEAM (PORTIA CHOI, KEITH KAWAOKA, BARBARA KITASHIMA, BOB MATSUSHIMA). 1975. Asian Americans and Health Care in Los Angeles County. Los Angeles: UCLA School of Public Health (mimeographed).

U.S. BUREAU OF THE CENSUS. 1970a. *General Population Characteristics, United States Summary.* Final Report, PC(1)–B1. Washington, D.C.: U.S. Government Printing Office.

———. 1970b. A Study of Selected Socio-Economic Characteristics of Ethnic Minorities Based on the 1970 Census. Vol. II: *Asian Americans.* HEW Publication no. (OS) 75–121. Washington, D.C.: U.S. Government Printing Office.

————. 1970c. *Japanese, Chinese, and Filipinos in the United States.* Final Report, PC(2)–1G. Washington, D.C.: U.S. Government Printing Office.

————. 1977. *Statistical Abstract of the U.S.: 1977* (98th ed.). Washington, D.C.: U.S. Government Printing Office.

WONG, JADE SNOW. 1945. *Fifth Chinese Daughter.* New York: Harper.

WU, FRANCES YU-TSING. 1974. Mandarin Speaking Aged Chinese in the Los Angeles Area: Needs and Services. D.S.W. dissertation, School of Social Work, University of Southern California.

————. 1975. Mandarin Speaking Aged Chinese in the Los Angeles Area. *Gerontologist* 15:271–275.

WU, ROBIN. 1971. New York's Chinatown: An Overview. *Bridge Magazine* 1:13–15.

YEE, MIN. 1970. Chinatown in Crisis. *Newsweek,* Feb. 23.

YEP, LAURENCE. 1975. *Dragon Wings.* New York: Harper & Row.

3
Haitian
Americans

MICHEL S. LAGUERRE

Identification of the Ethnic Group

OVER THE PAST 20 YEARS enclaves of Haitians have appeared in several American cities (Laguerre 1976, 1978a, 1978b). Although the immigrants have come from various strata of Haitian society, they share many of the same cultural standards, the same languages (Creole and French), and the same mix of religions (French-influenced Catholicism, American-influenced evangelical Protestantism, and Voodoo).

Haitian communities in the United States form separate ecological niches. Most have their own community churches, stores, restaurants, social and literary clubs, newspapers, physicians, and folk healers, all of which help the immigrants to maintain their cultural traditions. Yet these communities are not isolated from one another. Through individual members, often kinsmen or in-laws, they maintain complex networks of communication, and internal migration for marriage or employment is sufficiently common to assure that links between communities are readily maintained (Laguerre 1980a).

History of Migration

Although Haitians migrated sporadically to the United States in the nineteenth century, no significant immigration occurred during that period, largely because of the institutionalized racial discriminaton that prevailed (Souffrant 1974:133–145).[1] The first significant group of Haitian migrants, about 500 upper-class urban families, came to the

United States in the 1920s. Fleeing the atrocities that accompanied the American occupation of Haiti in 1915–1934,[2] these families settled in black neighborhoods of Harlem and have since been assimilated into the mainstream of American society (Reid 1939:97).

The Haitian population that will occupy our attention in this chapter is composed of migrants who have come to the United States since 1957, when Dr. François ("Papa Doc") Duvalier was elected President of Haiti. In that year defeated presidential candidates and their close collaborators fled the country and developed a political base in New York City with the intent of organizing guerrilla troops to invade the island. They did in fact launch several invasions of the island, but all of them failed to overthrow Papa Doc's regime. By 1964, when Duvalier was elected President for Life, most expatriate politicians realized that their chances of returning to Haiti were at best slim and began sending for their relatives. Many have continued their efforts to organize revolutionary opposition to the Duvalier regime, however.

In 1971 Papa Doc died, and his son Jean Claude Duvalier became President for Life. Since then, economic deprivation has constituted the major factor behind the emigration of both urbanites and peasants from the island. Groups of these migrants, unable to gather the necessary funds to secure Haitian passports and United States visas, have been coming to this country covertly on small sailboats. Risking their lives in long journeys on high seas, some have died during the passage, and others have been jailed for illegal entry upon arrival in the United States (U.S. Congress, House Committee on the Judiciary 1976).

General Demographic Picture

The current Haitian population of the United States is estimated to be in the vicinity of 500,000 people, including the American-born children of immigrants. Because of the sizable illegal immigration, however, there is no way of knowing the exact population figures. Estimates provide the following breakdown: approximately 100,000 are either American citizens or permanent residents; about 200,000 are children of both legal and illegal immigrants who were born in the United States and are therefore American citizens; and roughly 200,000 are illegal entrants. Among this last group, 70,000 persons are estimated to be in the process of becoming permanent residents either by marrying American residents or citizens or by other means.

The Annual Reports issued by the Immigration and Naturalization Service, which deal exclusively with the legal population, permit a number of observations about the demography of this sector of Haitian Americans. From 1962 to 1975, 63,642 Haitians were admitted to the United States as legal immigrants. Although they have settled in almost every state of the union, the vast majority (72 percent of all legal immigrants in 1975) are concentrated in New York state, primarily in New York City. Minor concentrations also occur, however, in Illinois, Florida, Massachusetts, and New Jersey.

Compared to the total United States population, the age distribution of legally admitted Haitian immigrants is disproportionately weighted in the age range of 10 to 19 years. (Annually between 1970 and 1975, 19 to 36 percent of legal immigrants were teenagers.) Female immigrants slightly outnumber males (53 and 47 percent respectively). Extensive observations of the Haitian population in New York have led me to the conclusion that the sex ratio of the legal population is representative of the illegal population as well. This situation can be explained in part by the fact that the United States Consular Office in Haiti has been more lenient in providing tourist visas to Haitian females than to Haitian males. For, unlike Mexican migrants, a large proportion of Haitians who are here illegally came as tourists with an American visa and overstayed.

In terms of origin, migrants have come from nearly every city, village, hamlet, and rural district in Haiti. Nevertheless, Port-au-Prince has been the main provider of émigrés, not only because massive migration started with Port-au-Prince residents but also because every person who wishes to migrate legally is likely to have spent some time in Port-au-Prince while securing his Haitian passport and United States visa. Thus, almost all Haitian migrants have had some experience living in an urban setting prior to emigration.

Table 3.1 Occupational structure of legal Haitian immigrants in the U.S. working force (fiscal years 1965–1974).

Year	Number admitted	Number not in work force No.	Number not in work force (%)	Total number in work force	Professional and technical No.	Professional and technical (%)	Managers and administrators No.	Managers and administrators (%)	Sales No.	Sales (%)	Clerical No.	Clerical (%)	Craftsmen No.	Craftsmen (%)
1975	5,145	2,920	(56.8)	2,225	232	(10.4)	120	(5.4)	26	(1.2)	204	(9.2)	432	(19.4)
1974	3,946	2,286	(57.9)	1,660	167	(10.1)	63	(3.8)	6	(0.4)	161	(9.7)	283	(17.0)
1973	4,786	3,291	(68.8)	1,495	223	(14.9)	69	(4.6)	13	(0.9)	144	(9.6)	219	(14.6)
1972	5,809	4,066	(70.0)	1,743	394	(22.6)	73	(4.2)	13	(0.7)	162	(9.3)	216	(12.4)
1971	7,444	4,973	(66.8)	2,471	592	(24.0)	60	(2.4)	19	(0.8)	196	(7.9)	601	(24.3)
1970	6,932	2,682	(38.7)	4,250	694	(16.3)	49	(1.2)	22	(0.5)	417	(9.8)	1,418	(33.4)
1969	6,542	3,151	(48.2)	3,391	663	(19.6)	65	(1.9)	19	(0.6)	284	(8.4)	960	(28.3)
1968	6,806	3,702	(54.4)	3,104	669	(21.6)	96	(3.1)	12	(0.4)	222	(7.2)	574	(18.5)
1967	3,567	1,996	(56.0)	1,571	307	(19.5)	60	(3.8)	9	(0.6)	121	(7.7)	163	(10.4)
1966	3,801	2,118	(55.7)	1,683	353	(21.0)	106	(6.3)	23	(1.4)	221	(13.1)	250	(14.9)

Source: Immigration and Naturalization Service Annual Reports (1962–1975).

Most Haitian immigrants have come to this country to earn money, and they can be found in almost every sector of the American labor force (table 3.1). In the first years of their stay, they are usually obliged to take lower-status, "stepping-stone" jobs to make ends meet, but as soon as they learn enough English and are able to legalize their immigration status, they quite often find themselves good permanent positions. Although there are no official statistics or even rough estimates on the income distribution of Haitian immigrants, I estimate (from interviewing 60 Haitian families in New York, Chicago, Boston, and Los Angeles) that the median income of the legal population is around $13,500 per year for a nuclear family and about $8,500 for the undocumented population.

Evaluation of the Existing Data

The data for this chapter are mainly based on my research in the major center of Haitian population in the United States—that is, the boroughs of Manhattan, Brooklyn, and Queens in New York City. This population is not only geographically dispersed but also socioeconomically heterogeneous (Glick 1975). New York Haitians generally regard Manhattan as the borough where middle-class Haitian families live, Brooklyn as lower-class, and Queens as upper-middle-class. My own observations, however, do not support these perceptions, and people belonging to different strata are found in all three boroughs. Migrants from various Haitian villages and cities do tend to cluster in the same boroughs, however; for example, in Queens there is a concentration of

Operatives		Transport equipment		Laborers		Farmers		Farm labor		Service		Private Household	
No.	(%)	No.	(%)	No.	(%)	No.	(%)	No.	(%)	No.	(%)	No.	(%)
738	(33.2)	54	(2.4)	68	(3.1)	2	(0.1)	27	(1.2)	199	(8.9)	123	(5.5)
568	(34.2)	35	(2.1)	71	(4.3)	1	(0.1)	26	(1.6)	192	(11.6)	87	(5.2)
532	(35.6)	—	—	19	(1.2)	—	—	10	(0.7)	152	(10.2)	114	(7.6)
525	(30.0)	—	—	12	(0.7)	—	—	19	(1.1)	159	(9.1)	170	(9.8)
707	(28.6)	—	—	20	(0.8)	7	(0.3)	14	(0.6)	154	(6.2)	101	(4.1)
1,230	(28.9)	—	—	9	(0.2)	21	(0.5)	2	—	169	(4.0)	219	(5.2)
718	(21.2)	—	—	17	(0.5)	9	(0.3)	6	(0.2)	178	(5.2)	472	(13.9)
715	(23.0)	—	—	16	(0.5)	1	—	10	(0.3)	144	(4.6)	645	(20.8)
400	(25.5)	—	—	10	(0.6)	—	—	2	(0.1)	76	(4.8)	423	(26.9)
447	(26.6)	—	—	21	(1.2)	5	(0.3)	12	(0.7)	94	(5.6)	151	(9.0)

light-skinned migrants from Jérémie, a city located in the southern region of Haiti, and many natives of Lascahobas, a village in the central plateau of Haiti, live in Brooklyn (Laguerre 1979a). This pattern of settlement by area of origin helps immigrants to adapt to the demands of the city and assures that they have someone living nearby whom they can call upon in time of illness or other crisis.

It is nevertheless important to note that people living in any one of these enclaves maintain ongoing relationships with friends and relatives in other enclaves and in other boroughs. For example, medical problems of Brooklyn Haitians are sometimes solved by medical practitioners living in Manhattan or Queens. Indeed, the extent and intensity of ties among people residing in different enclaves make the Haitian population in New York City a single dispersed community. In times of crisis, such as the illness of a family member, friends and relatives from other boroughs show up to help diagnose and cure the patient or advise him to see a physician or folk healer.

In terms of medical beliefs and practices, the Haitian population is not at all homogeneous. Migrants from rural districts in Haiti or from outlying island territories like Ile de la Tortue, Ile à Vache, and Ile de la Gonâve, who were not taught to see a physician when sick but to get help from folk healers, have medical traditions different from those of Port-au-Prince intellectuals, who may have been educated in France and had little contact with folk medicine. Furthermore, city people in general are more receptive and more knowledgeable about scientific medicine than rural people. Thus, the social class to which a person belongs, his education, his residential background, and his skin color (black versus mulatto) are factors that help to predict his health practices.

The research on which this chapter is mainly based entailed participation in the daily life of Haitians in the three boroughs of New York. I spent time with friends whom I had known in Haiti prior to migration, and several of these friends, mainly Haitian physicians, introduced me to friends of their own. Through this friendship base, I developed in a rather short period of time a network of informants from various strata of the New York Haitian community. The bulk of the material was gathered by interviewing uneducated and lower-class migrants (50 lay persons), as well as five Haitian physicians who have been practicing in the community. Two Haitian nurses were also interviewed.

Between January and March, 1978, I interviewed lay persons from different social classes both intensively and informally. Group interviews were also conducted. The group setting had the advantage of allowing contradictory views on the same subject to be voiced and discussed. The interviews were all held in Haitian Creole, and I usually started by explaining the nature of the questions and topics in which I was interested and then letting the informants talk freely. When they felt they had exhausted the subject, I posed specific questions and asked for clarification and additional commentary. These interviews usually provided data about theories of illness and the extent to which people continued to use folk medicine.

Extended interviews were also conducted with the health professionals in the study, some of whom were in private practice and others of whom were staff physicians at various public, private, and proprietary hospitals. These interviews focused on the particular kinds of medical ailments that these health-care providers treat among Haitians in New York. Hospital staff members who act as translators for Haitian patients seeing non-Creole-speaking physicians were also helpful in this regard.[3]

In short, the data for this chapter, which were mainly gathered in New York City and supplemented later with information from Haitians in the San Francisco Bay area, derived mainly from lower-class respondents and from observations of the health behavior of mainly lower-income patients by Haitian physicians and other middle-class Haitian Americans. It must be said that although educated Haitians and the mulatto elite were quite ready to provide information on how they think impoverished or uneducated Haitians behave in terms of health practices, they were less ready to talk about their own behavior, which (like most elites) they consider to be no one's business but their own. The material in this chapter is, in short, a preliminary statement on Haitian-American health behavior.

Epidemiological Characteristics

Epidemiological studies specifically on the Haitian population in the United States have never been carried out, partly because of the recent arrival of the Haitian population and partly because of the illegal status of many of the immigrants. The Haitian Medical Association, the headquarters of which is located in New York but which has branches in various American and Canadian cities, has mainly focused on helping newly arrived Haitian physicians to secure jobs rather than studying the medical needs of the Haitian-American population. Thus, apart from several brief reports on health practices among Haitian Americans (Scott 1974, 1975, 1978; Weidman 1976, 1978), no in-depth medical research has ever been published on the state of health of the Haitian immigrant population, and most statistical studies merge Haitians with other American blacks. However, research carried out in Haiti on diet and nutrition (Dambreville 1949; Comhaire and Comhaire 1952; Boulos 1954, 1955; Sebrell et al. 1959; Jelliffe and Jelliffe 1960, 1961; King, Sebrell, and Severinghaus 1963; King et al. 1963, 1966a, 1966b, 1968a, 1968b; King 1964, 1967, 1975; Béghin et al. 1965; Béghin, Fougère, and King 1965, 1970; Dominique 1965; Sirinit et al. 1965; King and Price 1966a, 1966b;

Duvalier 1968:451–467; Rawson and Berggren 1973:288–298; Ade 1978), pellagra (Clark 1921), tropical sprue (Klipstein, Samloff, and Schenk 1966), intestinal bacteria (Klipstein and Samloff 1966), and coronary and aortic atherosclerosis (Groom et al. 1959, 1964; Groom 1961) is of some relevance to our present concern because it sheds light on some of the chronic and tropical illnesses that are also relevant to Haitian migrants in New York.[4]

Selected Disease Patterns in Haiti

DIETARY DEFICIENCIES   Since the 1950s a high prevalence of anemia and multiple nutritional deficiencies has been observed among the rural population of Haiti in particular (see, for example, Sebrell et al. 1959). A nationwide study of 1,322 lower-class preschool children, however, found that "the edema (or kwashiorkor) index was 7 percent, suggesting that, in this age group at this socioeconomic level and in the country as a whole, approximately one out of 14 children were likely to have been suffering from kwashiorkor in the summer of 1958 at the time of the survey" (Jelliffe and Jelliffe 1960:1365). Although these findings are now 20 years old, the protein-calorie deficiencies that cause kwashiorkor still exist in Haiti, and one can assume that a certain proportion of Haitian children brought to the United States suffer from this syndrome until they are able to compensate for their earlier deficiencies. A cultural factor that contributes to protein deficiency in children (and in women as well) is the unequal distribution of protein foods among family members. For, whenever meat is served for dinner, the major part goes to the husband on the assumption that he must be well fed to provide for the household. As King and his associates found in a nutritional survey of rural Haiti, "the problem is not one of net protein deficiency in the community, but rather unwise distribution of the protein among the members of the family" (1968a:118). This same pattern of distribution persists among Haitian migrants to the United States.

Recent studies on xerophthalmia and keratomalacia carried out in Haiti have found that vitamin A deficiency is one of the leading causes of binocular blindness among Haitian children (Sears 1972:187–188; Sommer et al. 1976:439–446). Sommer and his colleagues report that "the prevalence of presumed vitamin A–related corneal scars among 5,589 pre-school age Haitian children ranged from 1.2 per 1,000 in the South, to almost 1 percent in the famine-afflicted North. These scars accounted for at least 45 percent of all corneal scars, and all bilateral corneal blindness encountered. Most lesions were acquired during the first three years of life. There was no variation by sex or ecology of the sample site" (1976:446).

Although migrants to the United States do not typically come from the very poorest sectors of the Haitian population, special attention by clinicians to possible visual problems among members of this ethnic group would seem warranted, particularly in view of the high number of self-reports of chronic "serious eye trouble" among Haitians in Miami, discussed below.

Any discussion of dietary deficiencies among Haitians must also take into account the presence of various endemic diseases on the island that significantly contribute to nutritional deficits over and above dietary factors. For example, tropical sprue, which is associated with vitamin B_{12} and sometimes folate deficiencies, "is endemic in Haiti and plays a significant role in the development of the anemia and nutritional deficiencies which are frequently encountered" (Klipstein, Samloff, and Schenk 1966: 575). Parasitosis is also importantly implicated in nutritional deficiencies on the island. Both these conditions may be encountered among Haitian immigrants and should be considered in the differential diagnosis of anemic patients (Meyers, Schweitzer, and Gerson 1977).

DISEASES OF THE CIRCULATORY SYSTEM   On the basis of a comparison of a sizable postmortem population of American blacks from the South Carolina area and Haitians from around Port-au-Prince, Groom and his associates conclude: "First . . . the Negro in Haiti has about half the degree of coronary sclerosis that the American Negro has. Second, this proportion holds for both males and females and, roughly, for all age decades over 20. And third, no such disparity exists between the two populations as to the amount of aortic atherosclerosis" (1959:264). These researchers attribute the difference in the prevalence of coronary sclerosis between the two populations to differences in diet and life-style. They claim that "the Haitian consumes less of all foods of animal origin, and considerably less protein and fat [than the American black], with about three times as much of his total intake being in the form of linoleic acid" (Groom et al. 1959:284). This claim is contradicted, however, by a dietary survey conducted in 1954, which observed a marked preference for animal fat among Haitian families (Boulos 1954). If consumption patterns of animal fats among American black and Haitian populations are indeed similar, differences in life-style between the two groups may nevertheless affect the metabolism of these foods. Thus Groom and his colleagues (1959) note that Haitians both sleep and exercise more than American blacks and point to these habits as contributing to lower rates of coronary sclerosis.

The applicability of these findings to Haitian immigrants is difficult to assess. The physicians interviewed in this study were under the impression that they saw a considerable number of Haitian patients with heart and circulatory problems, although reliable statistics are, as mentioned earlier, unavailable. Thus, whether there has been an increase in circulatory diseases among Haitians in this country and whether any presumed increase might be due to postmigrational changes in diet are both moot points. It is my impression, however, that most Haitians have retained their island patterns of physical exercise, since most immigrants walk long distances to visit friends, to go to work, and to attend church. Indeed, the island pattern has been reinforced on the continent, because many Haitians perceive public transportation in American cities as being unsafe. Thus, if circulatory diseases have increased among Haitians in this country, it is unlikely that changes in activity patterns are the principal cause. Dietary change, particularly among the younger generation of migrants, may be contributory, since "junk foods" have become common in this segment of the Haitian American population.

Morbidity among Haitian Americans

Because of the absolute dearth of hard data on the mortality and morbidity rates of Haitians in the United States, we must rely for this information on the self-reports of acute and chronic conditions among a sample of Miami Haitians (Weidman 1978:325–449) and on the impressions of the Haitian physicians interviewed in New York.

In the Miami study the five chronic conditions that were most commonly reported by Haitian respondents on behalf of all members of their households during the preceding year were (in rank order): serious eye trouble, chronic skin trouble, nervous trouble and allergy (tied), and arthritis or rheumatism (Weidman 1978:361). The most commonly reported acute conditions experienced in the preceding year were, as one would expect from nationwide figures, colds, influenza, and viral infections. In addition to the conditions incorporated in standard health-status lists, reported above, Weidman and her associates developed "ethnic symptom-condition lists" which probed the prevalence of culturally defined syndromes peculiar to each ethnic group. Within this list, the most frequently cited problems were "*gaz* or 'gas' with 31 percent of the persons surveyed reporting it. *Faiblesse* (weakness/anemia) and *vers* (worms) were tied for second and third place. There was an equal response rate for *coeur brulé* (heartburn), *mauvais sang* ('restless,' 'moving,' or 'rising' blood), *hyperacidité* (hyperacidity), and *colique* (stomach cramps/abdominal pain), tying them in fourth to seventh rank at 8.6 percent" (Weidman 1978:436).

Many of the standard conditions reported, as well as the ethnic-specific symptoms, can be fully understood only within the context of certain Haitian cultural beliefs, which will be discussed in some detail in the following sections. Nevertheless, it is important to recognize that these self-reports show a correspondence with some of the diseases reported above as being common in Haiti itself (for example, the self-reports of chronic eye and skin trouble in view of the aforementioned epidemiological studies of nutritional deficiencies; also "worms" in view of parasitosis).

Haitian physicians in New York present a somewhat different picture of morbidity among Haitian Americans. The problems with this information are, of course, manifold. In addition to the fact that separate files and thus specific figures are not kept for Haitian patients, each physician's sample of cases tends to be biased by his own medical specialty, by the socioeconomic status of his clientele, and by the obvious omission of untreated cases from the sample. For what it is worth, however, the physicians report the following diseases as being most prevalent among their Haitian-American patients: diabetes, hypertension (severe and benign), stomach ulcers, and arthritis. Isolated cases of malaria are also found, and parasitosis is detected among children who have recently migrated from Haiti and among children who have eaten food that people have brought to the United States when returning from a visit to the island.

A number of other diseases are reported by the New York physicians as posing particular problems with Haitian patients because of the manner in which they present for treatment. Late presentation, for example, seems to be common for a number of conditions for a number of different reasons. On the one hand, people suffering from hydrocele (*maklouklou*) usually delay seeing a physician out of a sense of shame about the condition. On the other hand, people who have cancer (especially of the cervix) tend to present for treatment only after the disease is beyond control, because Haitians tend not to consult physicians unless they experience pain. As a result of this latter pattern of presentation, the prevalece of untreated cancer is assumed to be quite high in this ethnic group.

According to the physicians' reports, venereal diseases are also treated quite commonly among lower-class Haitian patients, as are bladder and prostate infections among the males. However, people who suspect that they have a venereal infection often secure an injection of penicillin from a friend who works in a hospital. Since these suspected cases are treated without laboratory diagnosis and with no follow-up treatment, they are rarely cured. Various local infections, as well as psychological stress brought about by hard work, busy schedules, language problems, and so forth, may also account for complaints of male impotence among Haitian Americans.

In discussing tuberculosis in the Haitian-American population, the New York physicians interviewed were unanimous in reporting that the percentage is low. Moreover, since people who may have had the disease in Haiti were necessarily cured in order to become eligible for a permanent residence visa to the United States, the reported cases all seem to have been contracted in New York. This assumed low rate of tuberculosis among Haitian Americans may be due, however, not to a low incidence of the disease but rather to patients' culturally conditioned interpretations of the symptoms of this illness, which may well lead to a failure to seek health care. Thus, rural Haitians have been reported to use the word *tuberculose* to cover a narrower range of symptoms than are covered by the word "tuberculosis." Wiese writes that "in the indigenous medical system this term [*tuberculose*] is associated only with those symptoms which modern western medicine labels 'advanced active pulmonary tuberculosis.' The other symptoms included in our general label 'tuberculosis' are spanned by three other categories in Creole, none of which is considered serious . . . The term *'tuberculose'* does not subsume those symptoms which western medicine identifies as 'primary tuberculosis.' Haitians do not believe *'tuberculose'* is found in children" (1974: 361). It is likely that with this understanding of tuberculosis symptoms, Haitian patients present for treatment only when the disease is quite advanced.[5] Fear of the disease, which almost certainly has been observed by many poor, rural Haitians to cause death with considerable frequency, also inhibits presentation for treatment.

Concepts of Disease and Illness

Concepts of Health

The most important activities reported by Haitians in Miami for maintaining health are eating well, giving attention to personal hygiene, and keeping regular hours. Prayer and good spiritual habits were reported by 8 percent of the Haitians sampled as being important to good health (Weidman 1978:311–312).

In Haitian culture fat people are considered to be both healthy and happy. In contrast, thin people are believed to be in poor health, wasted by psychological and emotional problems. Thus, Haitian dietary habits are closely related to ideas of physical and emotional well-being.

In addition to having "cold" and "hot" qualities, foods are also considered to be either "light" or "heavy." The "heavy" type, such as corn meal, boiled plantain, or potato, should be eaten during the day and is said to provide the necessary caloric requirements for daily work. The "light" types of food, such as chocolate, bread, or soup, should be eaten for dinner. The method of preparation affects the classification of the food as well; for example, boiled green bananas are "heavy," while fried yellow banana is "light."

Because of their work schedules, Haitian Americans are generally unable to continue all their nutritional customs and practices in the United States. Since they spent most weekdays outside the home at work, they eat whatever is available near their place of work. Contrary to their traditional dietary habits, many now eat their main meal at night, like most other Americans, and a "heavy" meal has consequently replaced the traditional "light" supper.

Haitians believe that not all foods are good at all times for the human body; the use of food must be in harmony with the individual life cycle. There are foods for babies, foods for adults, foods for menstruating women, foods for the sick, and foods for the elderly. Some of the same foods can be eaten by people of all ages, but they differ in the manner of preparation or the quantity consumed. Some foods are forbidden to people at different stages of the life cycle; for example, teenagers are advised to avoid drinking too much orange or lemon juice, so as not to develop acne. Pregnant women are particularly subject to food taboos or special food practices (César 1955; Wiese 1976:196). They are permitted to *manger pour deux* ("eat for two") and may therefore gain considerable weight during pregnancy. They are also cautioned to avoid spices, but red fruits and vegetables (for example, beets, pomegranate) are thought to build up the baby's blood.[6]

Degrees of Illness

Illness episodes can range on a continuum from transitory disturbances to grave situations. A Haitian American may thus characterize his illness in one of six ways:

1. *Kom pa bon* ("I do not feel well"). This means that the illness does not confine the sufferer to bed. It is a transitory disturbance, and he should soon be well.
2. *Da tan zan tan moin malad* ("I feel sick from time to time"). This is a kind of complaint about the general state of health.
3. *Moin an konvalésans* ("I am convalescing"). This means that the person was sick and is now recuperating.
4. *Moin malad* ("I am sick"). This does not indicate the kind of illness that might cause death.
5. *Moin malad anpil* ("I am very sick"). This means that the person is in critical condition.
6. *Moin pap réfè* ("I will never be well again"). This means that the illness is terminal, and the patient will die sooner or later.

Etiological Concepts

In one of the earliest papers on ethnomedicine in Haiti, Métraux observed that rural Haitians believe that illness can be of supernatural origin (supernatural illness) or of natural origin (1953:28). Natural illnesses are known as *maladi péi* (country diseases) or *maladi bon dié* (diseases of the Lord). Natural illness is believed to be of short duration. The characteristic of supernatural illness is that it appears suddenly without the patient's having previously felt any sign of discomfort. Dow

(1965:42) has confirmed some of Métraux's observations. He reports the tendency of rural Haitians to see illness as belonging to either the supernatural or the natural domain. Indeed, he writes that "in consideration of disease, for example, the common cold, which occurs so frequently, is seen as a natural occurrence, but madness is seen as exceptional and often as supernatural in origin" (Dow 1965:40). He further reports that "supernatural illness is thought by the Haitian to be caused either by the *loa* [familial spirits] or by the Dead . . . He must placate his ancestors by offering them a feast called a *manger morts* at certain intervals. If he does not, misfortune and illness are likely to befall him" (Dow 1965:41).

Within this major dichotomy of causes, "spirits" are thus the prime source of supernatural illnesses. Among illnesses of "natural" origin, six traditional conceptions of cause can be specified: (1) type (volume, quality, and color) and movement (directionality) of the blood; (2) location and movement of "gas" (*gaz*) in the human body; (3) type (quality) and movement (directionality) of milk in the female body; (4) hot/cold disequilibrium and movement of heat and cold in the body; (5) bone displacement; and (6) the movement of diseases. Though Haitians often perceive illness as caused by factors external to the body, which, if taken into the system, can cause illness (for example, "cold" or "hot" air and foods, "gas," spirits), and even though this view seems complementary to the germ theory of disease, few Haitians of lower socioeconomic status use the intrusion of germs as an explanation of illness.

"Supernatural" Causes of Illness: Spirits

Several types of illness are believed by Haitians to be of supernatural origin, caused by angry Voodoo spirits. Voodoo ethnotheology provides a theory explaining the occurrence of such illnesses (see Laguerre 1979b, 1980b). According to the basic teaching of Voodoo ethnotheology, each Voodooist family has a spirit protector whose role is to see to the well-being of his protégés by protecting them against the malevolent power of other spirits. When one is initiated into Voodoo he must sign, so to speak, a pact with his spirit protector. The spirit expects from his protégés a ceremony every year in his honor. The annual ceremony is a basic requirement for maintaining a good relationship with every spirit protector. However, each spirit may add other requirements according to his own wishes and to his structural position in the Voodoo spirit hierarchy.

Each spirit needs this kind of recognition from his protégés for various reasons. Without it, he may be the object of mockery by other spirits and may be unable to maintain his status in the Voodoo spirit hierarchy. To maintain his status, a spirit must show that he has followers, that he is able to ward off other spirits from bothering his protégés, that his protégés recognize his power and are afraid of him, that he is able to cure his protégés when they are sick, and that every year his protégés offer a ceremonial meal in his honor. If he is able to accomplish all this, he will have the respect of other spirits as well.

There is thus a relationship of dependence between spirits and protégés. The protégés are dependent on the spirits for their protection, especially for health, and the spirits are dependent on their protégés to maintain their status in the Voodoo hierarchy. However, the protégés are more embedded in a subordinate and asymmetric relationship of dependence than the spirits are.

Illness may occur whenever a person gives an opportunity to other spirits to make fun of his spirit protector; for example, this happens when a person fails to offer the annual meal. Illness thus becomes a punishment by a spirit. A spirit may "send an illness" on his protégé or may not intervene if another spirit decides to bother his protégé. Such illness can be cured with the help of the spirit protector and is considered basically to be a punishment.

The role of the Voodoo priest in diagnosing such an illness is strategic. The priest may be able to find out through spirit possession the reasons for the spirit's anger. During the possession trance, the spirit may explain the reasons why he is not happy with his protégé and tells him what he has failed to do, the nature of his illness, and what he must do before he can be well again. He also informs the patient about the medication to be taken after he has accomplished his ritual duties.

While spirit protectors are likely to inflict physical illness on their protégés, the spirits of dead relatives take a more psychological approach to make kinsmen remember them. By appearing in dreams to remind relatives of their ritual duties (see Bourguignon 1954), they usually upset the dreamer sufficiently to cause him to provide a ceremony in the dead relative's honor.

Some illnesses are primarily the domain of Voodoo healers. A type of hypertension can be cured, according to some, only by Voodoo priests. In such a case, it is believed that the spirit of a dead person sits on the neck of the patient (*mo chita dèyè noa kou moun nan*), and only a Voodoo priest may rid the sufferer of the spirit. A handicapped patient who drools is believed to be the unwilling carrier of the spirit of a dead child and is also subject to Voodoo treatment.

In short, illness of supernatural origin is fundamentally a breach in rapport between an individual and his spirit protector. It is a response from the spirit to that breach, a way of reprimanding the protégé's behavior. In such a situation, health can be recovered if the patient makes the first step of finding out the nature of the illness through the help of a Voodoo priest and then follows the advice subsequently given by the spirit itself. The study of supernatural illness is one way to come to grips with the articulation of Voodoo as both a religious and a medical system.[7]

"Natural" Causes of Illness

BLOOD IRREGULARITIES   By far the most dangerous types of illnesses are believed to be caused by irregularities in the blood system, and beliefs about the blood are extensive among Haitians. Indeed, Weidman has called blood "the central dynamic in Haitian understandings of bodily functioning and pathological processes" (1978:522; see also 529–535). To a Haitian, blood can be *cho* ("hot") or *frèt* ("cold"); *clè* ("thin"), *fèbl* ("weak"), or *épè* ("thick"); *sal* ("dirty"); *noa* ("dark"); or *jò-n* (yellow).

San cho ("hot blood") provokes high fever, while *san frèt* ("cold blood") is the result of malaria. Métraux discusses a similar classification of fevers (1953:53), although he does not discuss the symptomatology of each type. I have also found among Haitian immigrants in New York that the blood is believed to regulate the hot/cold state of the body. The blood is said to be "hot" when a person becomes nervous or is engaged in heavy intellectual activity; blood is also "hot" when one is sleeping or doing physical exercise. The body of a woman is "hot" during the weeks after childbirth. Blood is "cold," however, when one is quiet and in a resting position, although resting itself is not a guarantee of "cold" blood. For, if a person is worrying about personal problems while in a resting position, the upper part of the body will purportedly have "warm" blood, and the lower part, "cold" blood.

San clè ("thin blood") causes pallor, and *san fèbl* ("weak blood"), physical or mental weakness (Dow 1965:42). When the blood is weak, however, one is advised to eat red foods (red meat, sugar beet) and drink red beverages, like *siro pié bèf* (a syrup made of cows legs and sugar). In contrast to "thin" or "weak" blood, the blood becomes "thick" (*épè*) when one is frightened (*sézisman*) and remains this way when one is suffering from hypertension. "Thick" blood also causes *san piké* or *pikotman* (itching).

San jò-n ("yellow blood") means that bile is flowing in the blood, and *san noa* ("dark blood") is a sign that the patient is about to die of an incurable disease. *San sal* ("dirty blood") and *san gaté* ("spoiled blood"), are both associated with venereal disease and skin eruptions (Weidman 1978:377). *San gaté,* however, has also been reported to result from "fright" (*saisissement;* Métreaux 1953:58) and thus seems similar to *mové san* ("bad blood"), which is also attributed to "fright" and is associated with skin eruptions of an urticarial appearance.

Blood is also believed to be capable of turning into water, particularly from drinking too much alcohol. The occurrence of such a situation is believed likely to cause pleurisy or tuberculosis.

In addition to these various qualities of the blood itself, illness may be attributed by Haitians to irregularities in blood flow. Thus, fear and fighting are both believed to cause blood to flow to the head, which is viewed in turn as the cause of hypertension (Weidman 1978:320). *Pèdi san* refers to loss of blood through menstruation; menstrual irregularities (either profuse menstruation or menstrual periods of irregular occurrence) are referred to as *san kap boulvèsé*.

"GAS" (*Gaz*) Many Haitians believe that "gas" may provoke pain and anemia. Gas can occur in the head, where it enters through the ears; in the stomach, where it comes in through the mouth; and in the shoulder, back, legs, or appendix, where it may travel from the stomach. When gas is in the stomach, the patient is said to suffer a *kolik* (stomach pain), and gas in the head (*van nan tèt,* also called *van nan zorey*—literally "gas in one's ears") is believed to cause headaches. When gas moves from one part of the body to another (*gaz kap maché nan do-m*), pain is produced. Thus, gas traveling from the stomach to the legs produces *doulé rimatis, frédi,* or *fréchè* (rheumatism); to the back, *do fè mal* (back pain); and to the shoulder, *gaz nan zépol* (shoulder pain). A tea made of garlic, cloves, and mint, or solid foods, such as plantain or corn, are usually advised as treatment for these conditions, since they are believed to be capable of expelling gas.

To avoid entry of gas into the human body, one must be careful about eating certain foods such as "leftovers" (*mangé domi*) and especially leftover beans. After childbirth, women are particularly susceptible to the entry of gas into the body, and in order to prevent this must tighten their waist with a belt or piece of linen. Gas is also believed to become "warm," "hot," or "cold"; however, I was unable to get information on the associated health problems that such states may cause.

MOVEMENT OF MILK The milk of a lactating mother is believed to be stored in her breast, and the mother must eat very well to be able to deliver healthy milk to her child. Although the milk is nutrient for both the mother and the baby, it can also be detrimental to the health of both if it is too "thin" or too "thick." When the milk is too thick, it is said to cause impetigo (*bouton*). It can become too thin when a mother is frightened, for example; this causes the milk to move to her head, producing an acute headache or postpartum depression in the mother and diarrhea in the baby, if the child has been breast-feeding.

HOT/COLD DISEQUILIBRIUM Illness is also believed to be caused when the body is exposed to an imbalance of "cold" (*frèt*) and "hot" (*cho*) factors. These factors may be either temperatures or foods that are classified as being "hot" or "cold." Table 3.2 presents a Haitian categorization

Table 3.2   Haitian hot/cold classification of foods.

(−3) Very cold	(−2) Quite cold	(−1) Cool
Avocado	Banana	Cane syrup
Cashew nuts	Cashew	Custard apple
Marfranc cheese	Lime	Chayote fruit
Coconut meat	Grapefruit	Orange juice
Coconut juice mixed	Lime juice	Tomato
with milk	Okra	
Coconut juice	Orange	
Grenadilla flesh	Watermelon	
Grenadilla juice		
Mango		
Pineapple		
Soursop fruit		
Starapple		
Cassava bread		

(0) Neither hot nor cold: neutral		(+1) Warm
Banana juice	Kidney beans	Eggs
Beef	Lima beans	Grapefruit juice
Beets	Malanga	Pigeon meat
Biscuits (of imported	Cow's milk	
white flour)	Goat's milk	
Breadfruit	Parsley	
Cabbage	Roasted peanuts	
Mint candy	Pigeon peas	
Carrot	Plantain	(+3) Very hot
Sweet cassava	Plantain gruel	
Foreign cheese	Pork	Cinnamon
Chicken	Sweet potato	Coffee (roasted)
Coconut candy	Brown rice	Nutmeg
Conch	White rice	"Clairin" (raw rum)
Milled corn	Rice and mushrooms	Rum
Marionade (fried	Non-iced soft drinks	
dough balls)	Imported Spam	
Eggplant	White and yellow yams	
River fish	Pumpkin	
Sea fish	Sugar cane	
Grunion		
Goat meat		

Source: Wiese (1976:196). Reproduced by permission of the Society for Applied Anthropology.

of foods in this system. Although not all of these foods are available in the United States, the diet of many Haitians in this country still includes them. Though there appears to be some kind of consensus on the hot/cold qualities of most of the tropical fruits and staples used in the daily diet in Haiti (Wiese 1976:196), immigrants in New York have different views on the hot/cold states of the food available in supermarkets. This is not to say that they no longer divide food into hot/cold categories, but rather that they may label the same items differently.

Wiese found in rural Haiti that life states are also classified into the hot/cold dichotomy: "The scaling of a particular body state appears to be related to reproductive capacity. A female is always warmer than a male; a younger person always warmer than an older" (1976:198).

In this system of causation, illness is seen as being provoked by an imbalance of "hot" and "cold" factors. Thus, "cold" and "hot" experienced in rapid succession may provoke *chofrèt* (cold or pneumonia). For example, a woman who has just ironed her hair and then opens a refrigerator is likely to become a victim of *chofrèt;* or a person who becomes warm after physical exercise may become *chofrèt* if he should eat anything that is "cold." Eating "cool" tomatoes or white beans after childbirth is believed to induce hemorrhage, and "cold," acidic orange juice is avoided in cases of menstrual disturbance. Often patients decide that they have *chofrèt* when they break out in a "cold sweat" while experiencing hot fever.

To treat a person in the hot/cold system, a patent or herbal medicine of the class opposite to the disease is administered. Cough medicines, for example, are considered to be in the "hot" category, while laxatives are in the "cold" category. When a person has a cold, his body is "hot" and he needs to take a "cold" medicine. However, someone with "cold" blood may have to take a "hot" medication to regulate his body heat, and vice versa. For example, some migraines are believed to be due to an excess of heat and blood in the patient's head. To cure such an illness, one would need to take a "cold" medicine to lower the heat and bring the blood back to its normal position.

"BONE DISPLACEMENT" (*Zo Déplasé*)   There are three types of "bone displacement" (*entorse*—"sprain," *kou viré*—"twisted" or "stiff" neck, and *biskèt tonbé*—"displaced vertebra") which cause pain and discomfort and for which health care is sought. However, Haitians usually do not seek help from medical doctors for this kind of ailment, which is believed to belong to the domain of the folk healer/chiropractor. These ailments are all treated by physical manipulation of the affected part, sometimes accompanied by warm poultices or prayer as well.

MOVEMENT OF DISEASES   Diseases, whatever their primary causes, have the possibility of secondarily expanding or moving from one place to another in the body. Over time, a disease may migrate from its primal position and cause pain in the area that it has reached. The notion of "expansion" and "relocation" of disease seems to be important in Haitian conceptions of illness, both as an explanatory device and as a motivation for seeking treatment.

Selected Illness Concepts

Weidman (1978) has reviewed a large number of Haitian terms for various symptoms and conditions and has concluded that the central concept of Haitian folk understandings of illness involves a disruption in the balanced state of blood. Various kinds of internal and exteral disruptions to the system are labeled by special terms. Some of these terms (*congestion, indisposition*)[8] are similar to words used in standard biomedical terminology, and some are generally unknown to mainstream health professionals (for example, *sézisman*).

"FRIGHT"   The concept of "fright," called *sézisman* in Creole (*saisissement* in French), indicates a disruption to the system caused by a sudden shock, such as the announcement of bad news (for example, the death of a parent) or a situation where one is fearful for one's physical well-being. It may also be caused by indignation after one has been a victim of injustice (Métraux 1953:58). When *sézisman* occurs, the blood is said to move to the head and may cause partial loss of vision or headaches. Lactating women are considered particularly prone to this illness, and it is believed to affect their milk in various ways. It is also believed to cause a temporary mental disturbance (*folie passagère*). Belief in *sézisman* as well as cases of this illness are common among Haitian Americans in both Miami (Weidman 1978:517) and New York.

OPPRESSION   The term *oppression* is used by Creole speakers as a label for asthma, although the exact referent is somewhat different from the biomedical term. According to Weidman, *oppression* "include[s] more than asthma. In many instances, *oppression* for Haitians seems to describe a state of anxiety and hyperventilation instead of asthma" (1978:448). Although the French term *asthme* is generally known to Creole speakers, and rendered as *sma* (Weidman 1978:448), it is not frequently used. *Oppression* is considered to be a "cold" state, as are many respiratory conditions.

Becoming Ill

As mentioned earlier, illness is thought by Haitians to be caused by both natural and supernatural forces. These two categories of illness have their own modalities and singular features which allow for their diagnosis. "Natural" illness refers to commonly felt symptoms that afflict for a normal duration. Such illnesses, known as "diseases of the Lord" (Dow 1965; Métraux 1953), are not considered to be the result of any breach of contractual agreements with Voodoo spirits. Illnesses of supernatural origin, however, are believed to appear suddenly, and once they appear, if nothing is done, they progress slowly through the body.

The way in which Haitians perceive and evaluate "natural" symptoms depends in part on their socioeconomic status, their past illness experience, and whether or not they had access to a physician when they were in Haiti. Employed people are less likely to seek medical attention than the unemployed, for fear of losing a day's pay; thus it is likely that the former are more tolerant of symptoms. Certain symptoms that are regarded with shame (for example, hydrocele, epilepsy, or venereal disease) may also be tolerated longer before medical attention is sought. One of the reasons a sick person may have for waiting before seeing a physician is that often he is more or less convinced that the illness is a temporary state. Through proper diet, vitamins, patent medicines, and home remedies, the patient may expect to cure himself.

What seems most central in the evaluation of illness, however (and this seems to be true for both lower- and upper-class Haitians), is a person's experience with illnesses among his close relatives: one's own symptoms are evaluated in light of the symptoms previously experienced by one's close kin. The following case history is an example of such an evaluation.

Case 1. Joseph, a former teacher at a lycée in Port-au-Prince, migrated to New York in 1970. After his arrival here he worked in a gas station. For some time Joseph had not been feeling well. His complaints included poor eyesight and physical weakness, which he attributed to working hard. What bothered him most was a small sore on his leg that did not heal. Joseph spent a lot of time reviewing his relatives' illnesses with them in order to discover if his own symptoms were similar to theirs. He particularly sought the counsel of his sister and aunt, since Haitian women are generally more knowledgeable about symptoms and cures than men. After consultation with members of his extended family, Joseph decided that his illness was not grave and that it was therefore unnecessary for him to see a physician. He had also ruled out diabetes as a diagnosis, because neither his father nor his mother had had the disease. However, he was unsure about the sickness that had terminated his father's life. Joseph's own diagnosis was "gas," and he was taking a home remedy for it. After falling into a coma, however, he was taken to the hospital and diagnosed as diabetic.

In instances of self-diagnosis like the one related above, the two symptoms to which Haitians most commonly attend are *douleur* (pain) and *faiblesse* (weakness). (See Weidman 1978:495–496, who includes dizziness and stiffness as well.) One Haitian physician reported that after years of practicing medicine among Haitian Americans, he had concluded that Haitian-American medical care revolves around the treatment of "pain" and "weakness."

In clinical situations patients generally locate pain vaguely. Because of a belief among Haitians that when one is ill, the whole body suffers, the location of pain at a particular moment is not particularly important, especially since diseases may shift position, as discussed in the previous section. In addition, the causes of pain that are suggested by patients do not usually comport with biomedical ideas of causation (for example "gas").

Physical weakness (*faiblesse*) is taken as a sign of anemia or insufficient blood. A patient who fears anemia may complain to the physician, "I do not feel like eating" (*Bouch moin an mè*), or "I cannot work" (*Pa kab travay*). Since these symptoms are usually attributed to a poor diet, patients may turn to vitamins in order to recoup their strength. In general, symptoms tend to be interpreted by Haitians of low educational attainment in terms of folk medical concepts rather than biomedical concepts.

Coping with Illness outside the Mainstream Medical System

The uneducated and lower-class Haitian American has five alternatives to choose from in his efforts to secure health services: (1) home remedies that he is aware of himself or that are provided by family and friends, (2) modern medicine in either a hospital or a private clinic, (3) a non-Voodooist folk healer, (4) Voodoo medicine, or (5) a return trip to Haiti to see a family physician or Voodoo healer there. Often the first phase in seeking a cure is to try home remedies, then to see a folk healer, and finally to request help from a Voodoo healer if one is available. Because of the financial burden, a physician may be sought only as a fourth alternative; for not only does the Haitian adult have to support himself in this country, he is still expected to send money back home. When a child is sick, however, parents do not usually wait long before seeing a physician; they may delay only if they suspect that the illness is due to teething.

Home Treatment

Most first-generation Haitian Americans (those not born in the United States) try home remedies as a first resort in treating illness. Denis (1963) and Pierre-Noël (1959) have compiled lists of the most common remedies used by Haitians of lower educational and economic status. However, it was found that some educated Haitians in New York City also used these remedies in their efforts at self-treatment.

Symptoms like fever, diarrhea, and constipation are usually treated with home remedies. Parents may also administer "worm medicine" to their children either as a preventive and precautionary measure or as a cure. Weidman writes that "some Haitian mothers would diagnose 'worms' when children gave any indication of suddenly jerking during sleep, of sleep-walking, or when they cried during their sleep. In the last instance, the assumption was they cried because of 'belly pain'" (1978: 413). As mentioned previously, people may also speak about their symptoms to family members and friends, in order to learn about medications that have proved effective in treating a similar condition in the past. In such cases the illness may be diagnosed *"de tête"* (without physical examination) and the patient advised to take a prescription medicine that the consulting relative or friend has used in Haiti or is taking currently. If necessary, a person may request relatives back home to send medication for the condition; such medication can consist of leaves, roots, or French-manufactured products that have not been approved for sale in the United States by the Food and Drug Administration. A good number of migrants believe in the efficacy of French medications (such as *kafénol* for headache) that are still currently in use in Haiti.

Within the household, the mother or grandmother and sometimes the father take responsibility for diagnosing symptoms. They keep alive the therapeutic tradition of the family, some of it consisting of information that has been passed on from parents to children for generations. Today, however, there are sometimes family conflicts between first- and second-generation members when the latter would like to see a physician but are required instead to drink home remedies prepared by members of the older generation. In New York older Haitians have lost their traditional expertise in advising on nutritional matters because they lack knowledge about American foodstuffs.

When a patient has tried everything advised by his family and friends and is still not cured, he will then be advised by the same people to see a physician, folk healer, or Voodoo priest. His decision here is often influenced by his immigration status (legal or illegal), his economic circumstances, and his access to a Voodoo priest. For to be sick means to be unable to work, and being unable to work means not receiving a paycheck. If the migrant does not have any health insurance or if his status is illegal and he therefore cannot apply for Medicaid, the possibility of going to a hospital or private physician for medical care will be remote; thus home remedies, a folk healer, or a Voodoo priest will be the preferred modes of treatment. Secondarily, illegal immigrants will consult a Haitian physician before going to a hospital.

Folk Healers

Although most "natural" illnesses are referred to the folk healer or the medical doctor, there are some "natural" illnesses, such as abscess, ulcer, and *san gaté* (spoiled blood), which are thought by Haitians to require the attention of both the medical doctor and the folk healer. Other illnesses belong exclusively to the domain of the folk healer. Although such healers may also be Voodooists, these conditions require no Voodoo rituals for a cure. *Entorse* (sprain) is one such condition; another is *lalouèt tonbé* (acute respiratory distress, attributed to the obstruction of the trachea by the uvula). Treatment by a folk healer is free; the patient must give the healer a small rock in lieu of payment.

Folk healers use three techniques in diagnosing a patient. They may first take a history from the patient, which includes data such as the length of time the person has been sick and the location and characteristics of the pain. For example, a healer may want to know if the patient's pain has always been acute, if it is periodic, and if there is any relationship between the pain and the food the patient ate the previous night. A folk healer may also examine the state of the patient's blood by looking at his eyes (which might be yellow or red), his hands, and his skin color to see if there is any sign of paleness. The third technique used by folk healers is *man-yin* (touching), which consists of palpating various parts of the body to find out if there is a displaced bone or an internal organ that needs to be placed in its proper position. The medication or other therapy the healer prescribes will be based on the characteristics of the illness as perceived through this kind of medical examination.

The treatments of folk healers may involve a number of modalities. Dietary recommendations or restrictions are usually very important. I have already discussed the use of plantains or certain teas for treating for "gas," and the hot/cold system may also be employed in selecting or rejecting foods for therapeutic purposes. Folk healers also commonly employ massage with either burnt alcohol or hot oil to treat dislocations or sprains and compresses, poultices, or baths for sores or inflammations. As in the home, laxatives are often prescribed, ostensibly to clean the intestinal tract and blood of all impurities (particularly as treatment for "dirty blood" [*san sal*]). Laxatives may be followed by an enema (*lavement*) to remove whatever is left in the lower bowel.

Dow describes an array of treatment procedures and curing techniques used by folk healers: "In treating natural illness, the *hungan* uses such methods as baths, powders, and mixtures of herbs. Most *hungans* have an extensive knowledge of the native herbs and use them both externally and internally . . . Rubbing and massage are also used. Massage is always directed toward the extremities . . . These treatments are often used in ailments attributed to wind which collects in the body, to the corruption of the blood, and to eating foods which are hotter or colder than body temperature" (1965:46–47). (See also Métraux 1953:67.)

Although it is clear from the Weidman report (1978) that Haitian migrants to Miami continue to use folk medicine and to seek the services of folk healers, this is done on a limited basis. Scott explains this phenomenon by pointing out that "medicinal preparations and elements of the traditional Haitian health care system are limited in Miami, possibly because their population is not yet large enough to support more than a handful of indigenous healers" (1974:527). Thus, the size of the Haitian enclave or its accessibility to a major center of Haitian settlement affects reliance on traditional healers.

Sometimes the use of home remedies and folk healers leads to problems and complications because patients wait too long before they see a physician. At times, however, patients seek to enhance their chances of a cure by seeing two different practitioners simultaneously and thus may be under the care of a physician and a folk healer jointly.

Voodoo Healers

The Voodooist folk healer is often a Voodoo priest who has had long training in the study of the mythology of spirits and the properties of plants for home remedial purposes. In his treatment he uses both prayers and herbal remedies, which were learned from elders through the mechanisms of oral traditions. The transmission of folk medical knowledge from one generation to the next follows specific rules and is often learned during illness episodes.

Spiritual causation may be suspected and Voodoo practitioners sought out if the symptoms of an illness recur at approximately the same time every day or if a child is born with a physical deformity. Ancestor spirits are believed to cause illness if they have been neglected by a descendant who has not contributed toward the annual ceremonial meal to commemorate them. Physical deformities, however, are more likely to be attributed to an angry spirit who has been enlisted by an enemy to perform an act of witchcraft. Many psychiatric disorders are also attributed to spiritual causes (Kiev 1961, 1962; Mathewson 1975).

Although the occasions listed above are the more typical ones for consulting a Voodoo priest, any very sick person is likely to be pressured by friends to see a Voodoo healer. Sometimes the Voodoo priest himself may activate his network of contacts to enlist a sick person as a client. Furthermore, because of the possible significance of illness as indicating a dereliction in filial duty, some Haitian Americans are ashamed of being sick and believe that their friends will look down on them if they do not seek help from a Voodoo healer. Thus in desperate situations, and to gain more personalized treatment for less money, the sick are likely to turn to such healers.

The illnesses of supernatural origin that are treated by Voodooists are said to be cured only when proper rituals to appease specific spirits are performed and when the demands of the spirits, as interpreted by a Voodoo priest, are met. The spirit may make its intentions known in two ways: through ritual possession, it may explain the nature of the illness and advise on the course of action to be taken; or the spirit may manifest itself in a dream directly to the patient and may tell the patient the nature of his illness, explaining the ritual to be performed and the herbal remedies to be taken (Laguerre 1980b).

In contrast to the hospital setting, where the patient is expected, by and large, to play a passive role, in traditional Voodoo treatment he is required to play a more active role. Dow describes in great length the treatment process in the traditional Haitian setting when he states: "The *hungan* requires the patient to assume an active role in the treatment process. He has to gather funds and may be required to purchase materials used in the treatment. Often there is a great deal of preparation involved. Furthermore, he receives sympathy and assurance from his family and friends. Since his illness creates a serious economic burden, there may be considerable pressure on him to return to his regular duties" (1965:50).

Pharmacies

There are licensed pharmacies in Haitian-American neighborhoods that specialize in herbal remedies and French medication to satisfy the needs of the community. These pharmacies have Haitian personnel and sell the same kinds of products that clients are familiar with from home. Some markets and groceries in Haitian enclaves also carry herbs that Haitians use to make teas, *tisanes* (infusions of herbs), and other home remedies.

Encounters with Mainstream Medical Practitioners

Settings for Medical Care

Haitians tend to seek medical care from Haitian physicians who have developed a good reputation on the island before migrating to the United States. Some people seek out a physician they have used previously in Haiti. Haitian physicians are usually in general practice and continue to serve a Haitian clientele. However, Haitian physicians report difficulty in receiving payment for their services from Haitian patients because of the latter's expectation that, since the two are compatriots in a foreign land, the relationship between them should be a personal one, more like that between friends or relatives. This expectation has its roots in medical practices in Haiti, where physicians have different standards for charging fees depending on the patient's economic status and on any kinship ties that may exist between them. As a result of this difficulty over fees, some Haitian physicians prefer not to attract a Haitian clientele. For many illegal immigrants who avoid public facilities for fear of being caught, however, private physicians are the main sources of care (Weidman 1978:267).

A few Haitians use the services of Medicaid clinics. However, they are generally reluctant to use such facilities because services are rendered free of charge and are therefore considered to be inferior. In addition, Medicaid clinics are generally understaffed, and the likelihood of finding a Creole-speaking person working in one to act as translator is slim.

In general, Haitian Americans utilize hospitals for care because of their strong belief that hospitals are the final resource centers for solving medical problems. However, they go to the hospital only when they have become convinced that their lay diagnosis (made with the help of friends and relatives) was wrong. As one lower-class informant put it, "I have tried every single herbal remedy, and I still could not be cured. So I decided to go [to] the hospital." The particular hospital is selected on the advice of associates, who generally know which facilities have Haitian staff members.

After waiting until they are in distress to see a physician, Haitian Americans frequently go for care to the emergency room of a hospital. Sometimes the situation is considered an emergency by the medical staff, but at other times it is not. For the patient, "emergency" means that someone will take care of him upon arrival in the hospital; thus, assurance of prompt treatment in other outpatient services would undoubtedly go far in reducing use of the emergency room by Haitian patients.

The plight of the Haitian-American hospital patient is well illustrated in the following case, recounted by a Haitian nurse:

Case 2.   A Haitian woman who suffered from back pain was unable either to sit down or to walk and was confined to bed. Assuming that her illness was a temporary event, however, she did not go to a physician. Instead she made some "tea for gas" at home, which she drank in hopes of getting better. After two weeks or so, she decided to go to a hospital.

In the hospital, she passed through the regular business of registration and waiting. When she saw the physician, after a quick examination she was sent to another hospital. The time she spent waiting did not match the short time she was with the physician. She was a bit frustrated to find out that she had to start all over again at the other hospital. In the second hospital, she was placed in a wheelchair, which upset her considerably.

The woman is light-skinned and is a member of the growing middle-class Haitian population in Queens. In her first encounter with the American physician in the second hospital, she became more upset because of the kinds of questions she was asked. When asked if she had ever had syphilis, she was shocked, because this is not the kind of question she believes one should ask a person from a distinguished Catholic family. She received a second blow from the physician when she was asked to take a test for sickle-cell anemia. In her mind, she is a mulatto, not a black. Since she has never identified herself as a black, she found it degrading to take a test for an illness that she associates with blacks. On the insistence of the physician, she agreed to take the test. Later she was happy to hear that the result was negative.

During her subsequent stay in the hospital, she had to undergo surgery. She agreed to it because she did not have any other alternative. She could not read or speak English. Before the operation, she was asked to sign release papers. When the translator told her about their contents—namely, that the hospital would not be responsible should she die during the surgery —she became very frightened and emotional. She resented signing anything, because she understood the papers to say that the physician was incompetent and that she might therefore die in surgery. She could not believe that the hospital would tell her that she might die and yet expect her to go through with the operation. From her own experience in Haiti, surgeons were always very positive and helpful. Here, however, the physician, although realistic, seemed to her to be too pessimistic. In the woman's view, being pessimistic was not a good way to start an operation, because an operation is a question of life or death. A Haitian nurse came to explain to the patient that her surgery was a routine procedure and that all patients were asked to sign release papers. Furthermore, they did not mean that she was going to die. The surgery was performed without complications, and she spent a few more days in the hospital to recover.

In the days following her surgery, the woman's physician and nurses came to say hello and to compliment her on her progress in recovery. Yet this courtesy did not help her relationships with them. She appeared upset when people stopped to say hello, because she would have liked to thank them warmly for their kindness but was unable to do so because of the language barrier. Furthermore, she was never able to understand whether a visit was for social or medical purposes; in other words, she could never decipher the intentions of her medical visitors.

For this patient, as for many Haitian patients, the wheelchair is a sign of serious illness, and accepting a ride in a wheelchair is a public pronouncement of one's illness. Since illness in Haitian culture is considered an affair to be shared only among family and friends, this public display of weakness arouses considerable emotion. In Haitian culture, too, illness must be accepted heroically. A person must be strong, for being psychologically weak is a way of letting illness dominate one's body.

As this account exemplifies, surgery is greatly feared in the Haitian-American community, regardless of class, since it is viewed as a procedure that may lead to death. The patient and relatives are likely, therefore, to become quite emotional and to require considerable reassurance.

Language Problems in the Medical Encounter

In medical settings, the language problem looms large for most Haitians. When Haitians are asked if they speak French, they almost invariably say they do; yet in fact French is used only by the elite in Haiti, and the majority of Haitians in New York do not speak French, but rather Haitian Creole. Thus, if Haitian patients are assigned to a French-speaking physician, communication problems still persist.

As a result, most Haitians prefer to bring a family member or friend to help with translation, especially since they are generally reluctant to let a stranger know about their problems. Women are particularly suspicious in this regard and fear that an unknown translator may spread gossip in the community and thereby cause them embarrassment. They may even avoid consulting a Haitian physician for fear that their problems might become known among other Haitians. In spite of this desire to have a confidant act as translator, people are reluctant to ask a close associate to accompany them to a doctor if this means that the associate will miss work.

During a patient's stay in the hospital, the language problem becomes a particular source of stress. Although the patient may have the assistance of a translator in his interactions with physicians, most of the time he is left alone to communicate with the nurse and other hospital personnel as best he can. The language gap also leaves the Haitian patient isolated from other patients with whom he may share a room and with whom he would like to speak.

English-speaking Haitians may also become upset when a physician does not allow them enough time to find the proper English words for an idea they wish to convey, and they have even greater difficulty in communicating if the physician shows exasperation over their manner of speaking English. Furthermore, if the physician appears busy, the patient may be reluctant to raise questions even if he has not understood the nature of the illness after the physician has explained it.

Physician-Patient Communication

CONSEQUENCES OF PHYSICIANS' STATEMENTS   When a physician tries to send a Haitian patient to see a specialist, there is a tendency for the Haitian to go to a Haitian doctor. There are three basic reasons for this kind of behavior: (1) the language barrier, (2) the belief that the Haitian physician is in a better position to understand the patient's financial problems, and (3) a lack of familiarity on the part of uneducated Haitians with the distinction between specialists and general practitioners.

The dialogue between a physician and patient may also lead the patient to conclude that there is a need to see a Voodoo healer. Statements such as "I cannot tell what you have," "I need more tests to find out," "I don't know what you have; I am going to send you to another physician" might lead the patient to see a Voodoo healer, since the fact that the physician cannot tell what is wrong leads to the suspicion of supernatural causation.

American physicians in general do not ask their patients about the kinds of folk medication they have been taking, although they may ask patients about prescribed medication. This practice leads the patient to believe that he can continue taking home remedies because they do not conflict with any prescribed medication or dietary regimen the physician has ordered. When a physician is dealing with an ethnic patient population like Haitians, who take herbal and over-the-counter medications routinely and quite pervasively, he should make some inquiry into the nature of home remedies in order to determine if in fact any are contraindicated.

PATIENT DESCRIPTIONS OF SYMPTOMS   In his encounter with an American physician, the Haitian patient may be able to provide only a vague explanation of his illness episode, since symptoms tend to be defined in an imprecise way. For example, the ability to locate pain wherever it is felt in the body depends on one's concept of illness. For a physician, pain can be located, and this information is used in diagosis. However, Haitian patients generally perceive illness differently, so the localization of pain is not that important. The view of many Haitians is that when a person is ill, the entire body is ill. Thus, the causes of pain are not necessarily located at the site of the pain itself, and it is consequently of little importance to identify the location of pain. Furthermore, as mentioned earlier, pain is believed to shift from one location to another in the body, and its position at a particular time is thus of minor consequence.

The Haitian pattern of verbal communication tends to make considerable use of metaphoric and symbolic language, which renders cross-cultural communication even more difficult (Laguerre 1970). In medical dialogues this pattern may take the form of using euphemisms for both body parts and stigmatized diseases or symptoms. For example, the patient may use the phrase *ti pijon* (literally, "my pigeon") to refer to his penis, or the phrase *maladi tonbé* (literally, "the illness that makes you fall down") to refer to epilepsy. The patient may also be reticent for fear of making a mistake. The physician interacting with a Haitian patient may consequently experience problems in discovering exactly what the problem is, even though the patient may be trying his best to make himself understood. Thus, both patient and physician may become frustrated as the latter repeatedly requests a history of the symptoms, which the patient believes he has already made clear. Continued inability to communicate with a physician may well lead the patient to return to folk practitioners for care.

In general, Haitian patients tend to tell their physicians what illness they think they have, instead of describing or explaining their symptoms. This usually occurs because the average Haitian patient does not consult a physician to find out what kind of disease he has, but to confirm his own diagnosis. Patients seek confirmation of their self-diagnoses primarily because health is considered to be a personal responsibility, and one therefore needs to be able to diagnose oneself. Before going to a medical facility, the patient is likely to have already made a self-diagnosis; thus when describing symptoms to the health professional, the patient may tend to emphasize the ones that he thinks correspond to the disease he has in mind. Consequently, what the health professional hears is not necessarily a description of felt symptoms but the patient's interpretation of the facts to corroborate his own diagnosis.

USE OF DISEASE LABELS   In general, educated Haitian migrants use familiar biomedical disease labels. Specific terms, such as malaria, *tension* (a Creole word for both hypotension and hypertension), *poitrinaire* (tuberculosis), diabetes, and rheumatism, are sometimes used by poorly educated migrants as well, but often with meanings different from those assigned by biomedical professionals. Usually these concepts were learned in medical settings where, at the insistence of a patient or the patient's family, the physician may have provided the name of the disease that the patient was suffering from, but without explaining or describing its nature or how the disease process related to the patient's symptoms. As a result, people may use a biomedical term learned in such circumstances that does not correspond to their own symptoms. Physicians should therefore pay less attention to the biomedical concepts that patients use and concentrate instead on the task of eliciting symptoms and a history.

Expectations in the Medical Encounter

In his encounter with a physician, the Haitian patient generally wants to know quickly what he has (*rapidité de la diagnostique*—"quick diagnosis"). In addition to evaluating a physician's performance by his rapidity and effectiveness in diagnosing disease, however, Haitian patients value politeness toward the patient. The patient wants to sense that the physician is as interested in helping him as in making money.

When a Haitian consults a physician, he also wants him to use the stethoscope and perform a physical examination. If the physician does not do so, he may be considered incompetent and the patient may well try to see someone else.

Finally, when leaving a clinic or a hospital, Haitian patients want to have a prescription from the physician. Failure to secure some form of medication for the problem almost certainly undermines confidence in the clinician. Furthermore, for the lower-class Haitian, an expensive prescription is often believed to be better than an inexpensive one—an idea that may be countered by patient education about marketing practices for drugs.

Adherence to Biomedical Treatment

Adherence to biomedical treatment by Haitian Americans must be understood in terms of perception of the graveness of the illness, as well as in terms of the socioeconomic condition and legal status of the patient. An illness is considered to be grave when it has caused the death of a member of the family or a friend, or when the physician tells the patient it is. In such a case, the patient will do his best to follow whatever the physician requests of him. Certain diseases—cancer, heart disease, and diabetes—are generally regarded as grave in and of themselves. If the illness is not considered grave and the patient does not fear the outcome, he will take a more relaxed stance toward treatment. Fear of an illness does not prevent a Haitian from taking home remedies, however. Although home remedies may be classified according to folk concepts of therapy (for example, as "hot" or "cold"), prescription medicines are not.

In general, Haitian patients are most resistant to carrying through on dietary restrictions. Diabetics in particular may have problems when they come to this country, because they often do not know which of the many new foods they encounter in the United States are dietetically acceptable. Work restrictions are also particularly hard for Haitians to follow, since many have come to this country specifically to make money.

Some migrants do not adhere to biomedical treatment because of socioeconomic conditions. Although many buy life insurance policies, few buy health insurance. They also may not be aware of various forms of disability insurance available to them through their jobs. Furthermore, even when Haitian migrants have insurance they may be afraid to use it too often for fear of exceeding the amount of money they believe they are entitled to, or they may be unable to fill out the proper forms for reimbursement. As a result of these various causes of inadequate insurance coverage, a large number of Haitians return to work after a hospital stay sooner than their doctors have advised, because they must support themselves and pay their drug and other medical bills. Provision of information and advice on health insurance coverage, as well as assistance in completing necessary forms, is thus basic to the health care of many Haitians.

Undocumented Haitians face particularly critical problems in receiving adequate health care from hospitals. Their problems stem from the fact that they tend to give false identifications in order to maintain their anonymity and to change hospitals and physicians often; the physician is therefore unable to get in touch with the patient for follow-up care. Physicians are also unable to obtain medical records from other hospitals or other physicians because of the patient's desire to remain anonymous.

Recovery, Rehabilitation, and Death

When a Haitian patient is discharged from a hospital, a relative or friend will pick him up and return him to the care of his family, neighbors, and friends. People with chronic incapacitating illnesses are usually cared for at home by their families and are not placed in nursing homes.

Rituals associated with the resumption of normal roles after an illness are linked to promises the patient may have made to supernatural beings during his stay in the hospital. After a grave illness Catholic patients may pay for a mass of thanksgiving or make a pilgrimage to a shrine in the United States, Canada, or Haiti. Voodoo believers, as well, may perform a special Voodoo ceremony of thanksgiving, manifesting their appreciation to the spirits for their recovery.

Death always mobilizes the entire extended family, which includes matrilateral and patrilateral extensions and affines. Death arrangements are usually taken care of by a male kinsman of the deceased who, because of his education and fluency in English, has had experience in dealing with American bureaucracies. Such a person should preferably be the deceased's oldest son or a cousin.

Conclusions and Recommendations

The majority of Haitian Americans live in ghetto and slum districts and have the prevalent diseases and illnesses that plague ghetto residents. Poverty and membership in a low-status ethnic minority are two important factors that prevent Haitian Americans from benefiting from the American medical system (Bullough and Bullough 1972:5). Furthermore, poverty leads the majority of Haitians to use the facilities of public hospitals. These hospitals are generally overcrowded and understaffed, and the physicians who care for patients in such hospitals are likely to be in training. One cannot say that these hospitals are always equipped to help immigrants of low-status ethnic minorities adequately.

The following recommendations, however, may help physicians and other medical personnel in delivering more appropriate care to Haitian Americans.

1. Since the majority of Haitians in the United States are Creole speakers, in the urban areas where they are concentrated (for example, New York City, Chicago, Miami) they should be able to use their native language whenever they are in an encounter with medical staff. The best course of action for an area like New York, where a large number of Haitian professionals have congregated, is for hospitals to have Haitian physicians and nurses on their staff. When this is not possible, however, a physician should seek out a Creole-speaking translator. From the Haitian patient's point of view, the use of a close friend as translator is optimal; the second best option is to use Creole-speaking nurses or other hospital personnel (for example, clerical workers). It is important to recognize, however,

that some middle-class patients may be shocked to find a health worker addressing them in Creole instead of French, so that ideally a physician should discover which language the patient wishes to use: Creole, French, or English.

2. In his encounter with less educated Haitian patients, a physician should be careful to use simple vocabulary instead of technical medical terminology, which the patient may not be able to understand.

3. As mentioned previously, Haitian patients and relatives become emotional when someone is diagnosed as having a disease from which a kinsman has died. The emotionality revolving around a patient's having the same diagnosis as a deceased kinsman may be handled by the physician's probing the family history when he senses fear in the patient and his relatives, and then providing reassurance through explaining procedures carefully and indicating the probability of a cure, when the probability is relatively high.

4. Before a Haitian patient is asked to use a wheelchair, someone should explain to him that this is a routine procedure in the hospital and does not mean that he is very sick.

5. It is good practice to put Haitian patients together in the same room, especially if they do not speak English. This will make life easier for them in the hospital, in that they can support each other emotionally.

6. If a patient has a terminal illness, the physician should inform his family, who will find ways of informing the patient if they judge it necessary to do so. This same procedure should be followed in the case of surgery. An influential relative is in a better position to tell the patient what is going on.

7. Haitian patients look for friendly physicians who take a personal interest in their illness. They do not expect such physicians to blame them for their illness, even if they have been negligent. After the illness is under control, however, the physician may explain what precautions should be taken in the future.

8. Haitians do not like to try new foods. When they go to the hospital, they prefer to fast instead of eating non-Haitian food, since they are afraid that such food may make them sick. The best course of action is to provide them with rice, beans, plantains, and other foods that are part of their regular diet.

9. When taking a history, the physician is well advised to inquire if the patient has been taking medication that was prescribed for someone else. Moreover, when prescribing a potentially dangerous drug, the physician would do well to caution the patient not to pass the medication along to ailing friends without a doctor's approval.

10. Haitian patients have their own preferences for certain forms of medication. In order of preference, they are (1) injection, (2) elixirs or solutions, (3) tablets, and (4) capsules. Physicians should be aware of the preferences of their Haitian patients and, when possible, prescribe accordingly.

11. Abdominal surgery is generally feared among Haitians. Patients and their relatives become very emotional about it, and the patient may approach the operation with considerable apprehension. After surgery, it is likely that the patient will prefer to remain quietly in bed until he is com-

pletely cured, believing that any physical exercise may have a negative effect on his body system. Since such an attitude may result in postsurgical complications (pneumonia, paralytic ileus, and so on), physicians and nurses should be aware of this belief and should particularly encourage mobility to prevent such complications.

12. As a measure of preventive care, routine immunizations should be given to both children and adults.

13. Tetanus is of particular concern. Physicians should be made aware that most Haitians have never received tetanus antitoxin injections, so if they come in for emergency treatment for lacerations, they must be given the antitoxin and not tetanus toxoid, which is what is usually administered since physicians assume that the patient has already been immunized (Roger Jean-Charles, personal communication).

14. Health education and screening for hypertension through church and other Haitian organizations are strongly recommended.

15. For preventive care, diet counseling—mainly to reduce the intake of salted and fatty meats and fish, and to discuss obesity among women—is also recommended.

16. In light of the fact that Haitians have a tendency to use diagnostic terms to talk about their problems with physicians rather than describing their symptoms and what they really feel, physicians treating a Haitian clientele should become aware of the diagnostic terms used and should concentrate on getting at patients' symptoms. When taking a history, the physician should inquire: "What do your family and friends think you have?" This approach will help to introduce the subject of how the patient defines his illness and enable the physician and patient to move on to what other sources of care he may have received and what help he thought he got from these various sources. In eliciting this information, however, the physician should remain nonjudgmental about the other sources of care, unless he truly sees them as pathogenic.

Notes

This chapter is part of a book-length manuscript on *Ethnicity as Dependence: The Haitian Community in New York City*, a project financed by the Institute for Social Research and the Jesuit Community Research Board of Fordham University; The Institute for Urban and Minority Education, Teachers College, Columbia University; and The Rockefeller Foundation. I am most grateful to Charles Harrington, Lambros Comitas, Vera Rubin, Norman Whitten, and Joseph Fitzpatrick. My deepest gratitude goes to Alan Harwood for his invitation to write this chapter, his helpful suggestions, insightful comments, and editorial assistance. Finally, I acknowledge the help of Serge Francois, M.D., Pierre Paul Antoine, M.D., and Constant Pierre Louis, M.D. I also appreciate the comments of Sue Gould, R.N., Roger Jean-Charles, M.D., and Benjamin Siegel, M.D., who read the chapter in draft form.

1. During the Haitian revolution (1791–1803), many French colonists emigrated to the United States, bringing some of their slaves with them. The

émigrés settled mostly in Norfolk (Va.), Philadelphia, New Orleans, Charleston (S.C.), and New York (Moreau de Saint Méry 1947).

2. During the American occupation of Haiti peasants were forced to work without pay building public roads (Castor 1971). Several nationalist leaders, among them Charlemagne Peralte, as well as some of their supporters and followers were killed by U.S. Marines. These leaders organized various *kako* (guerrilla) groups throughout the island, whose sole reason for existence was to fight against the American occupation and to liberate the Republic.

3. This chapter has also benefited from the comments of members of various Haitian clubs in the city, who had the material read to them at a meeting and were asked to provide whatever remarks, disagreements, or suggestions they wished.

4. For a recent review of the literature on public health in Haiti, see also Noël 1975:157–172.

5. In her doctoral dissertation, Wiese (1971) has provided an extensive analysis of Haitian ways of dealing with tuberculosis and an elaboration on the meaning of tuberculosis for rural Haitians. For a recent study of tuberculosis among Haitian children, see Laven (1977).

6. For more discussion of food taboos and the way they affect the health of teenagers and pregnant, lactating, or menstruating women, see Marcelin (1954).

7. Much of the scholarship on Voodoo has focused on its religious aspect. However there is now some interest in studying Voodoo as a medical system (see Delbeau 1969; Conway 1978; Scarpa 1975; Daniel 1977).

8. For the occurrence, etiology, and treatment of "indisposition," see Philippe and Romain (1979) and Charles (1979).

References

ADE, E. 1978. Notes sur la population et l'économie d'Haiti: Importance de la malnutrition et des problèmes sanitaires en cet endroit. *Cahiers de Nutrition et de Diététique* 13:21–26.

BÉGHIN, IVAN, et al. 1965. Le Centre de Récupération pour Enfans Malnourris de Fond-Parisien (Haiti): Rapport préliminaire sur le fonctionnement du Centre et résultats de quatre premiers mois d'activité. *Annales de la Société Belge de Médecine Tropicale* 45:557–576.

BÉGHIN, IVAN, W. FOUGÈRE, and KENDALL W. KING. 1965. Enquête clinique sur l'état de nutrition des enfants prescolaires de Fond-Parisien et de Ganthier (Haiti): Juin 1964. *Annales de la Société Belge de Médecine Tropicale* 45:577–602.

———. 1970. *L'alimentation et la nutrition en Haiti.* Paris: Presses Universitaires de France.

BOULOS, CARLOS. 1954. Une enquête alimentaire en Haiti. *Bulletin de l'Association Médicale Haitienne* 6:3.

———. 1955. *Alimentation et grossesse.* Réunions Obstétricales Mensuelles de la Maternité Isaie Jeanty. Port-au-Prince: Imprimerie Théodore.

BOURGUIGNON, ERIKA. 1954. Dreams and Dream Interpretation in Haiti. *American Anthropologist* 56:262–268.

BULLOUGH, BONNIE, and VERN L. BULLOUGH. 1972. *Poverty, Ethnic Identity and Health Care.* New York: Appleton-Century-Crofts.

CASTOR, SUZY. 1971. *La ocupación norteamericana de Haiti y sus consecuencias (1915–1934).* Mexico: Siglo Veintiuno Editores SA.

CÉSAR, CARMONTEL. 1955. *La nutrition chez les femmes enceintes.* Réunions Obstétricales Mensuelles de la Maternité Isaie Jeanty. Port-au-Prince: Imprimerie Théodore.

CHARLES, C. 1979. Brief Comments on the Occurrence, Etiology and Treatment of Indisposition. *Social Science and Medicine* 13B(2):135–136.

CLARK, G. F. 1921. First Report of Pelagra in Haiti. *The U.S. Naval Medical Bulletin* 15:813–814.

COMHAIRE, SUZANNE, and JEAN COMHAIRE. 1952. La alimentación en la región de Kenscoff, Haiti. *América Indígena* 12:177–203.

CONWAY, FREDERIC JAMES. 1978. Pentecostalism in the Context of Haitian Religion and Health Practice. Ph.D. dissertation, Anthropology Department, The American University, Washington, D.C.

DAMBREVILLE, CHARLES. 1949. L'alimentation des travailleurs. *Premier Congrès National du Travail,* Port-au-Prince, Haiti.

DANIEL, CHRISTOPHE JOCELYN. 1977. La médecine traditionnelle en Haiti. Thèse de Doctorat, Lettres, Université de Bordeaux.

DELBEAU, JEAN CLAUDE. 1969. La médecine populaire en Haiti. Thèse de doctorat, Lettres, Université de Bordeaux.

DENIS, LORIMER. 1963. Médecine populaire. *Bulletin du Bureau d'Ethnologie* 4:37–39.

DOMINIQUE, GLADYS. 1965. *Table de composition d'aliments pour Haiti.* Bureau de Nutrition, Départment de la Santé Publique et de la Population, Port-au-Prince, Haiti.

DOW, J. 1965. Primitive Medicine in Haiti. *Bulletin of the History of Medicine* 39:34–52.

DUVALIER, FRANÇOIS. 1968. *Oeuvres essentielles, éléments d'une doctrine.* Port-au-Prince: Imprimerie de l'Etat.

GLICK, NINA B. 1975. *The Formation of a Haitian Ethnic Group.* Ann Arbor, Mich.: University Microfilms.

GROOM, DALE. 1961. Population Studies of Atherosclerosis. *Annals of Internal Medicine* 55:51–62.

GROOM, DALE, et al. 1959. Coronary and Aortic Atherosclerosis in the Negroes of Haiti and the United States. *Annals of Internal Medicine* 51:270–289.

———. 1964. Haitian, American Negroes Reveal Differences in Coronary Disease at Adolescence. *Journal of the American Medical Association* 188:32–33.

JELLIFFE, D. B., and E. P. PATRICIA JELLIFFE. 1960. Prevalence of Protein-Calorie Malnutrition in Haitian Preschool Children. *American Journal of Public Health* 50:1355–1366.

———. 1961. The Nutritional Status of Haitian Children. *Acta Tropica* 18:1–45.

KIEV, ARI. 1961. Folk Psychiatry in Haiti. *Journal of Nervous and Mental Diseases* 132:260–265.

———. 1962. Psychotherapy in Haitian Voodoo. *American Journal of Psychotherapy* 16:469–476.

KING, KENDALL W. 1964. Development of All-Plant Food Mixture Using Crops Indigenous to Haiti: Amino-Acid Composition and Protein Quality. *Economic Botany* 18:311–322.

———. 1967. *These Children Do Not Have to Die.* Bureau de Nutrition, Département de la Santé Publique et de la Population, Port-au-Prince, Haiti.

———. 1975. Nutrition Research in Haiti. In *The Haitian Potential: Research and Resources of Haiti,* ed. Vera Rubin and Richard P. Schaedel. New York: Teachers College Press.

KING, KENDALL W., et al. 1963. Height and Weight of Haitian Children. *American Journal of Clinical Nutrition* 13:106–109.

———. 1966a. Un mélange de protéines-végétales (AI-1000) pour les enfants haitiens. *Annales de la Société Belge de Médecine Tropicale* 46:741–754.

———. 1966b. Response of Preschool Children to High Intakes of Haitian Cereal-Bean Mixtures. *Archivos Latinoamericanos de Nutrición* 16:53–64.

———. 1968a. Food Patterns from Dietary Surveys in Rural Haiti. *Journal of the American Dietetic Association* 53:114–118.

———. 1968b. Two Year Evaluation of a Nutritional Rehabilitation (Mothercraft) Center. *Archivos Latinoamericanos de Nutrición* 18:245–261.

KING, KENDALL W., and NELSON O. PRICE. 1966a. Mineral Composition of Cereals and Legumes Indigenous to Haiti. *Archivos Latinoamericanos de Nutrición* 16:213–219.

———. 1966b. Nutritional Value of Haitian Forages. *Archivos Latinoamericanos de Nutrición* 16:221–226.

KING, KENDALL W., W. H. SEBRELL, and E. L. SEVERINGHAUS. 1963. Lysine Fortification of Wheat Bread Fed to Haitian School Children. *American Journal of Clinical Nutrition* 12:36–48.

KLIPSTEIN, FREDERICK A., and I. M. SAMLOFF. 1966. Folate Synthesis by Intestinal Bacteria. *American Journal of Clinical Nutrition* 19:237–246.

KLIPSTEIN, FREDERICK A., I. M. SAMLOFF, and ERIC A. SCHENK. 1966. Tropical Sprue in Haiti. *Annals of Internal Medicine* 64:575–594.

LAGUERRE, MICHEL S. 1970. Brassages ethniques et émergence de la culture haitienne. *Laurentian University Review* 3:48–65.

———. 1976. Migrations et vie rurale en Haiti. Port-au-Prince: Institut Interamericain des Sciences Agricoles de l'Organisation des Etats Américains.

———. 1978a. Ticouloute and His Kinfolk: The Study of a Haitian Extended Family. In *The Extended Family in Black Societies,* ed. Dimitri Shimkin, Edith M. Shimkin, and Dennis A. Frate. The Hague: Mouton.

———. 1978b. The Impact of Emigration on Haitian Family and Household Organization. In *Family and Kinship in Middle America and the*

Caribbean, ed. A. F. Marks and R. A. Romer. Assen, The Netherlands: Van Gorcum.

――――. 1979a. The Haitian Niche in New York City. *Migration Today* 7:12–18.

――――. 1979b. Etudes sur le vodou haitien. Montréal: Presses de l'Université de Montréal (Collection des Travaux du Centre de Recherches Caraibes).

――――. 1980a. Haitians. In *The Harvard Encyclopedia of American Ethnic Groups,* ed. Stephan Thernstrom, Ann Orlov, and Oscar Handlin. Cambridge, Mass.: Harvard University Press.

――――. 1980b. *Voodoo Heritage* (foreword by Vera Rubin). Sage Library of Social Research. London: Sage Publications.

LAVEN, G. T. 1977. Diagnosis of Tuberculosis in Children Using Fluorescence Microscopic Examination of Gastric Washings. *American Review of Respiratory Disease* 115(5):743–749.

MARCELIN, MILO. 1954. Cent croyances et superstitions. *Optique* 7:48–56.

MATHEWSON, MARIE A. 1975. Is Crazy Anglo Crazy Haitian? *Psychiatric Annals* 5(8):79–83.

MÉTRAUX, ALFRED. 1953. Médecine et vodou en Haiti. *Acta Tropica* 10:28–68.

MEYERS, SAMUEL, PHILIP SCHWEITZER, and CHARLES D. GERSON. 1977. Anemia and Intestinal Disfunction in Former Residents of the Caribbean. *Archives of Internal Medicine* 137:181–186.

MOREAU DE SAINT MÉRY, MEDERIC LOUIS ELIE. 1947. *American Journey,* trans. Kenneth Roberts and Anna M. Roberts. New York: Doubleday.

NOËL, PIERRE. 1975. Recent Research in Public Health in Haiti. In *The Haitian Potential: Research and Resources of Haiti,* ed. Vera Rubin and Richard P. Schaedel. New York: Teachers College Press.

PHILIPPE, J., and J. B. ROMAIN. 1979. Indisposition in Haiti. *Social Science and Medicine* 13B(2):129–133.

PIERRE-NOËL, ARSÈNE V. 1959. *Les plantes et les légumes d'Haiti qui guérissent: Mille et une recettes pratiques.* Port-au-Prince: Imprimerie de l'Etat.

RAWSON, IAN G., and GRETCHEN BERGGREN. 1973. Family Structure, Child Location and Nutritional Disease in Rural Haiti. *Journal of Tropical Pediatrics* 19:288–298.

REID, IRA DE A. 1939. *The Negro Immigrant: His Background, Characteristics and Social Adjustment, 1899–1937.* New York: Columbia University Press.

SCARPA, A. 1975. Appunti di etnoiatria haitiana [Notes on Haitian Ethnomedicine]. *Episteme* 73:298–303.

SCOTT, CLARISSA S. 1974. Health and Healing Practices among Five Ethnic Groups in Miami, Florida. *Public Health Reports* 89:524–532.

――――. 1975. The Relationship between Beliefs about the Menstrual Cycle and Choice of Fertility Regulating Methods within 5 Ethnic Groups. *International Journal of Gynaecology and Obstetrics* 13(3):105–109.

————. 1978. The Theoretical Significance of a Sense of Well-being for the Delivery of Gynecological Health Care. In *The Anthropology of Health,* ed. Eleanor E. Bauwens. Saint Louis, Mo.: Mosby.

SEARS, M. L. 1972. Keratomalacia in Haiti. In *Causes and Prevention of Blindness,* ed. I. C. Michaelson and E. R. Berman. New York: Academic Press.

SEBRELL, W. H., et al. 1959. Appraisal of Nutrition in Haiti. *American Journal of Clinical Nutrition* 7:538–584.

SIRINIT, KOSOL, et al. 1965. Nutritional Value of Haitian Cereal Legume Blends. *Journal of Nutrition* 86:415–423.

SOMMER, ALFRED, et al. 1976. Xerophthalmia and Anterior Segment Blindness. *American Journal of Ophthalmology* 82:439–446.

SOUFFRANT, CLAUDE. 1974. Les Haitiens aux Etats-Unis. *Population* 29:133–146.

U.S. CONGRESS, HOUSE COMMITTEE ON THE JUDICIARY, SUBCOMMITTEE ON IMMIGRATION, CITIZENSHIP AND INTERNATIONAL LAW. 1976. *Haitian Emigration.* 94th Congress, 2nd Session. Washington, D.C.: U.S. Government Printing Office.

U.S. DEPARTMENT OF JUSTICE, IMMIGRATION AND NATURALIZATION SERVICE. 1966–1975. *Annual Reports.* Washington, D.C.: U.S. Government Printing Office.

WEIDMAN, HAZEL HITSON. 1976. The Constructive Potential of Alienation: A Transcultural Perspective. In *Alienation in Contemporary Society,* ed. Roy Bryce-Laporte and Claudwell S. Thomas. New York: Praeger.

————. 1978. Miami Health Ecology Project Report: A Statement on Ethnicity and Health, vol. 1. Department of Psychiatry, University of Miami School of Medicine (mimeographed).

WIESE, H. JEAN C. 1971. The Interaction of Western and Indigenous Medicine in Haiti in Regard to Tuberculosis. Ph.D. dissertation, Department of Anthropology, The University of North Carolina at Chapel Hill.

————. 1974. Tuberculosis in Rural Haiti. *Social Science and Medicine* 8:359–362.

————. 1976. Maternal Nutrition and Traditional Food Behavior in Haiti. *Human Organization* 35:193–200.

4
Italian Americans

Antoinette T. Ragucci

Identification of the Ethnic Group

ITALIAN AMERICANS INCLUDE all those immigrants to the United States from mainland Italy, from Sicily and Sardinia, and from other Mediterranean islands that are part of the Italian nation, as well as those descendants of Italian immigrants who identify themselves as Italian American. Since the United States census does not inquire about national origins beyond the second generation, the present population of this ethnic group can only be estimated. The 1970 U.S. census reports 1,008,533 first-generation Italian Americans (those born in Italy) and 3,232,246 second-generation Italian Americans—a total of 4,241,000 (U.S. Department of Commerce 1977). Estimates of the number of third-generation Italian Americans vary from three to six million, depending on the degree of endogamy (marriage within the group) one assumes among the second generation (Vecoli 1978). Thus the total population of Italian Americans probably ranges somewhere between seven and ten million.

History of Migration

Between 1820 and 1976, 5,270,000 people immigrated to the United States from Italy (U.S. Immigration and Naturalization Service 1977). During that 156-year period Italians constituted 11.2 percent of all immigrants to this country, ranking second only to Germans (14.8 percent) (U.S. Department of Commerce 1977:83). Although Italian immigration began early in this nation's history, the major influx did not occur until the 1880s. Of the total Italian migration, approximately 60 percent came during the peak migration years of 1901 to 1920. Prior to these years immigrants came mainly from northern Italy; however, beginning in the last two decades of the nineteenth century and continuing to the present, the majority have come from the predominantly agrarian and impoverished regions south of Rome.[1]

Immigration from Italy declined after the passage of the Immigration Act of 1924, which established entry quotas based on the national origins of the population in 1920. By establishing annual quotas, the McCarron-Walter Act of 1952 further discriminated against immigration from Italy and other southern and central European countries. However, repeal of this act, as well as the reforms of the 1965 Immigration and Nationality Amendments, resulted in increased Italian immigration during the 1960s. During the period from 1961 to 1976, 315,642 people entered this country from Italy. This figure represents 5.2 percent of all United States immigrants during this period and makes Italy the prime source of European immigration for this recent 26-year period (U.S. Immigration and Naturalization Service 1977).

Both World War II and the vicissitudes of the quota system have produced essentially two distinct generations of Italian immigrants in this country: those who immigrated prior to World War II (mostly in the peak years before 1920), and those who immigrated after the War. For the purposes of this chapter, these two groups will be referred to respectively as the "older" or "earlier" immigrants and the "recent" immigrants. The older immigrants are relatively unschooled and had little work experience outside their natal villages or towns before coming to this country. They tend to speak regional or provincial dialects rather than standard Italian and to have known no English on arrival in the United States (Ragucci 1971:52). The recent immigrants, unlike their predecessors, are likely to have had job experience in the industrialized cities of northern Italy and Europe before coming to the United States, to communicate in standard Italian rather than a dialect, to have had more years of formal education, to have already learned an occupational skill, and to be generally familiar with urban ways and institutions (Ragucci 1971: 86–87). Furthermore, the older immigrants tend to be those who arrived alone as adult males and were joined later by their families, whereas the majority of recent migrants have been in the 10- to 29-year age range on arrival and have entered the country either as families or as the parents, wives, children, or husbands of American citizens (U.S. Immigration and Naturalization Service 1977).

Thus, although the members of both of these immigrant groups are "behavioral ethnics" in the sense that Italian cultural standards are a pervasive part of their lives, they differ from one another in representing

Italian culture at different historical periods. The specific effects of this intraethnic cultural variation on health beliefs and practices will be pointed out in pertinent sections later in the chapter.

Geographical Distribution of the Ethnic Group

One of the striking characteristics of the Italian ethnic group has been the relative stability of its residential patterns (Ragucci 1971: 87–102; Bleda 1978; Vecoli 1978) and its preference for urban living. Italian Americans of the older generation are still highly concentrated in Atlantic seaboard cities from Massachusetts to Maryland and in the "Little Italies" of a number of Midwestern cities. The recent immigrants, like their predecessors, have entered the country mainly through the ports of New York and Boston and have settled in the same metropolitan areas. Thus, recent immigrants are found mostly in the metropolitan areas of New York–New Jersey, Massachusetts, Illinois, Pennsylvania, Rhode Island, and Connecticut. However, a sizable number have settled further afield in California, Michigan, Ohio, and Florida (U.S. Immigration and Naturalization Service 1975).

In 1970, persons of Italian nativity and parentage comprised the largest proportion of the population of foreign stock in the states of Rhode Island, Connecticut, New York, New Jersey, West Virginia, Pennsylvania, Delaware, and Louisiana (U.S. Department of Commerce 1977:35). They accounted for the second largest proportion of foreign-born in Vermont, Massachusetts, Ohio, Missouri, and Maryland.

Among white ethnics, a preference for urban living remains a distinctive trait of Italian Americans (Bleda 1978; Vecoli 1978). The attachment to the inner city and the Italian neighborhood has been, in part, a matter of economic necessity. However, the dense texture of social relationships continues to hold people despite the decline in the quality of municipal services. Pride in home ownership, the strength of family and neighborhood bonds, and a filial relationship in which children feel obligated to remain close to aging parents are all cited as variables that tend to reduce mobility among Italian Americans (Campisi 1948; Ragucci 1971:87–117; Fandetti and Gelfand 1976; Vecoli 1978).

Nevertheless, movement to the suburbs is occurring, although it has not been much studied. According to Vecoli (1978), the suburbs have probably been no more effective as a melting pot for Italian Americans than the city. However, ethnicity in the suburbs tends to express itself through participation in middle-class institutions and the Catholic Church. Moreover, the suburban migration is expressive of the growing social class differentiation among Italian Americans, particularly in the second generation. While those who remain in the old inner-city neighborhoods tend

to be blue-collar workers or others of the lower middle class, the suburbanites represent the emerging upper-middle-class professionals and
business people (Vecoli 1978).

The settlement patterns and preferences of recent immigrants have also
received little attention from researchers. However, my observations in an
Italian-American enclave in Boston revealed that recent migrants either
bypass residence in the urban setting entirely or consider it a temporary
stop before moving to the suburbs. Since rent and food costs are generally
lower in Italian neighborhoods, temporary residence in an enclave provides the opportunity for a family to pool and save its resources toward
the purchase, remodeling, or building of a house in the suburbs.

In terms of potential usage of health-care facilities, the older immigrants and the less affluent, less educated second-generation Italian
Americans tend, as already stated, to be found in urban settings, whereas
both recent immigrants and the more affluent, better educated second-
generation Italian Americans tend to be found in the suburbs. Thus, both
urban and suburban health facilities are likely to be used by Italian ethnics
whose behavior is strongly influenced by the cultural standards of the
mother country.

Demographic Profile

Because the United States census restricts data on Italian Americans to the first and second generations, statistical information on the
age structure, educational level, and income distribution of this ethnic
group is far from precise. Nevertheless, some observations may be made
from these incomplete data.

AGE STRUCTURE   For the purposes of this chapter, the changing proportions of the three generations in the Italian-American population, as
well as their respective age structures, are significant. In 1970 the median
age for the more than one million foreign-born Italians was 63.2 years,
with one-third of the total represented in the 70- to 80-year age category.
Since the post-World War II migrants constitute approximately one-third
of this first-generation population, the earlier immigrants are clearly an
aging and diminishing segment of the population (Vecoli 1978:122). The
majority of the children of these early immigrants were born between
1910 and 1935, and in 1970 they had a median age of 46.6. For the third
generation, extrapolations from second-generation data yielded a median
age of 25 in 1970. Thus, apart from the recent immigrants, the greater
proportion of Italian Americans who clearly display ethnic characteristics
behaviorally are elderly or, among the second generation, approaching
middle age.

EDUCATIONAL STATUS   Only 54.1 percent of first- and second-generation Italian-American men and women are high school graduates (U.S. Department of Commerce 1977:30). This statistic reveals the relatively few years of formal education acquired by the older immigrants and their children, particularly the women. Before World War II, second-generation Italian Americans rarely continued education beyond the number of years mandated by law. However, the disparity in education between Italian Americans and the rest of the United States population is less for those in the 25- to 34-year category (Vecoli 1978).

LANGUAGE   In 1975 Italian was spoken as the primary language in 195,000 Italian-American households, or by approximately 522,000 persons over the age of four. Italian as a second language was spoken in 785,000 households (U.S. Department of Commerce 1977:34).

INCOME AND OCCUPATIONAL STRUCTURE   Though Italian Americans tend to be low in educational attainment, their incomes are comparable, if not superior, to those of other ethnic groups. A 1973 survey reported the median income of Italian families to be $12,520, the third highest for all ethnic groups surveyed (U.S. Department of Commerce 1977:30).

These data must be interpreted with an eye toward major generational differences, however. The plight of the elderly immigrant, for example, is indicated by the large percentage of families (17.5 percent) with an Italian-born head of household 65 years of age or older that were below the poverty line in 1970 (Vecoli 1978). In contrast, only 4.5 percent of all second-generation families had incomes below the poverty line.

The solid representation of second-generation families in the middle income ranges represents not only the increasing presence of Italian Americans in white-collar occupations (particularly those in the 25- to 44-year age range) but, even more, their concentration in high-paying blue-collar jobs, such as truck driving, construction work, and the skilled trades (electricians, plumbers). In addition, a higher percentage of second-generation Italian-American women (45.5 percent) were employed than second-generation females of all other ethnic groups (40 percent). These Italian-American working women are underrepresented in professional occupations, however, and overrepresented among the ranks of operatives as compared with other second-generation employed women (Vecoli 1978).

SUMMARY   From a health standpoint, we may look at the Italian-American population as falling basically into four generational groupings: (1) an elderly, early immigrant group, living primarily in Italian enclaves in East-coast and Midwestern cities; (2) a second-generation group living in both inner cities and suburbs, whose members are primarily employed in blue-collar occupations and approaching middle age, with its attendant rise in chronic diseases; (3) a younger, better-educated third-generation group, often living in the suburbs, whose members are at the stage of life when obstetrical and pediatric care are the prime health needs; and (4) a recent immigrant group comprised of families in the young to middle age range, whose residence patterns and health needs are similar to those in the second and third generations.

Evaluation of the Existing Data

Most studies of Italian Americans that provide information on their health beliefs and practices are of three types: folkloristic studies, sociological studies, and community studies. In discussing each of these sources of information, I will indicate the principal shortcomings in the data and will also discuss the major sources of intraethnic variation in health beliefs and practices in the Italian-American ethnic group.

Sources of Information and Problems of Interpretation

FOLKLORE STUDIES   An early folklore study on Italian Americans was carried out by Williams (1938) in an attempt to synthesize the health beliefs, healing practices, and other customs of Italian immigrants residing in metropolitan New Haven, Connecticut. In her capacity as a social worker during the depression years of the 1930s, Williams had "first-hand" contact with 500 families for eleven years (Williams 1938: xv). In her study, Williams used the Pitrè collection of popular Sicilian traditions (Pitrè 1871–1913) for comparative as well as baseline information and thus erred in generalizing some customs and beliefs that were unique to western Sicily to continental Italians of diverse regional origins. Furthermore, by lumping together all immigrants from Italy, Williams ignored regional and provincial variations in health beliefs and practices that were undoubtedly present.

The folklore of health and curing has been recorded for a number of impoverished towns and villages located in southern Italy. These accounts by anthropologists and others include information about traditional and contemporary practices which may be useful for understanding the folkways and customs that immigrants may have brought with them to America. Descriptions of health beliefs and practices may be found in studies of communities located in the following regions: Calabria (Douglas 1928); Basilicato (formerly Lucania) (Levi 1947; Cornelison 1969); the Abbruzzi and Molise (Moss and Cappannari 1960a, 1960b, 1962); and western Sicily (Dolci 1959; Chapman 1971).

SOCIOLOGICAL STUDIES Most sociological studies have focused on variables relating to illness and sickness behavior in order to compare the performance of Italian Americans with other American ethnic groups (usually Irish, Jewish, German, or Yankee). The variables that have been examined in these studies include reactions to pain (Zborowski 1952; Sternback and Tursky 1965), modes of expressing symptoms (Croog 1961; Zola 1966, 1973), problems of communication between patient and physician (Zola 1963), and the enactment of the sick role (Twaddle 1969). In addition, cultural differences in value orientations and the structure of role relationships have been studied in relation to their influence on mental illness and stress within the family (Barrabe and Von Mering 1953; Opler and Singer 1956; Kluckhohn 1963; Spiegel 1971).

Although these studies are notable in pioneering the investigation of interethnic differences in illness behavior, they suffer from a number of methodological deficiencies. First, the samples used are relatively small and are drawn for the most part from clinic or hospital patients in large university-affiliated institutions in the East. Thus, people who are fundamentally well or who receive care in other kinds of settings have been overlooked. Second, the studies sample mainly second-generation Italian Americans and thus often confound generational differences by failing to include the immigrant generation in the samples and by not fully analyzing variations between and within generations (a procedure admittedly made difficult by the small sample sizes). A final problem with this group of studies, closely related to the previous one, is their tendency to minimize or ignore the possible effects of social class, education, and residence (urban enclave versus suburb) on the responses of different ethnic groups.

The reader is further cautioned that the processes of differentiation and acculturation within ethnic groups in general and Italian Americans in particular are far more complicated than the conclusions of the aforementioned studies would indicate. For example, the comparative study of the persistence of old-world cultural traits of various kinds (for example, personality, sexual attitudes, political attitudes, drinking behavior) among Anglo-Saxons and second- and third-generation Italian Americans and Irish Americans led to the conclusion that not all differences among ethnic groups can be attributed to the old-world cultural heritage (Greeley and McCready 1974:100). The groups came to America at different times in their national development, settled in different parts of the country, and have had different experiences since their arrival (Greeley and McCready 1974:92, 102), and these factors may also contribute to observed differences (see Glazer and Moynihan 1963).

In sum, sociological studies yield no data on either older or recent Italian immigrants and little appreciation of intraethnic variation. Nevertheless, they constitute some of the most important sources of information on Italian-American illness and health-seeking behaviors and attitudes. Interpreted with caution, they still present useful data on crucial issues in health care.

A few sociological studies have taken a different approach to the study of the Italian-American experience by comparing behavioral variables among families in America and their counterparts in Italy. In this way more complete data on the contemporary cultural heritage of recent migrants has been accumulated. Studies of this type include Parsons' research (1960, 1961) on the social dynamics and behavior of psychotic women in Naples, and Peterson and Migliorini's comparison (1970) of parental behavior and child-rearing practices in two groups, Sicilian parents in Palermo and American parents in Champaign, Illinois. The use of alcoholic beverages by continental Italian and first- and second-generation Italian-American men was studied by Lolli and colleagues (1958), then restudied by Blane (1977), who increased the sample to include women and third-generation Italian Americans. Although these studies are limited in scope, their major contribution is to provide data on the first generation and on intergenerational variation, both notable gaps in the research described earlier.

COMMUNITY STUDIES   Most community studies of Italian-American enclaves (for example, Whyte 1943; Gans 1962; Suttles 1968) have not dealt with health and medical practices to any extent, in spite of the fact that an important feature of the community study method, participant observation, is eminently suited to observing what people actually do when someone begins to feel unwell. The study by Gans of a low-income working-class community in Boston reports some data about Italian Americans' attitudes toward health care and the nature of the physician-patient relationship (1962:136–141). However, the analysis is limited to the perceptions of second-generation men.

Thus, little has been reported using community study techniques for the investigation of the health-defining and health-seeking behaviors of Italian Americans. Therefore, my own study carried out in an Italian-American enclave contiguous to the one studied by Gans constitutes an important source of information for this chapter. This study (Ragucci 1971, 1972), carried out in 1968 and 1969, investigated the influence on health behavior of age, education, social class, generation, and region of origin in Italy (for the immigrant generation). Participant observation, focused mainly on women, was combined with structured and unstructured interviews, compilation of health histories, and attendance at formal meetings of health-care and other community service organizations. A fifteen-month residency ensured access to a number of families residing in different sectors or neighborhoods of the community. This period of time also provided an opportunity for my participation in the full round of neighborhood activities, entry into social life and ceremonials at different seasons, and acquisition of data about health behavior and illnesses over the period of a full year.

Strategies for gaining entry into the community were aimed at promoting acceptance in the roles of friend and neighbor in order to facilitate face-to-face relationships with informants and access to situations in which health beliefs and "curing" practices were more likely to be discussed. These situations included regular attendance as an observer and participant (interpreter for recent immigrant women) at the well-child clinic; observations at local pharmacies; unstructured interviews with local pharmacists, parish priests, physicians, and visiting and health-department nurses; visits to the hospitalized sick; informal visits to neighbors; and pilgrimages with older people to religious shrines in the United States and Canada that were noted for miraculous cures. This immersion in the community permitted the naturalistic observation of behavior necessary to assess the discrepancy between idealized statements and actual behavior.[2]

Sources of Intraethnic Diversity

General determinants of intraethnic diversity (class, acculturation to general American norms, regional origins in the mother country, suburban or urban residence) all apply to Italian Americans, as will be shown in subsequent sections. My study revealed, however, that first-generation and older second-generation women (50 or more years of age at the time of the study) exhibited more similarities in health beliefs and practices than either group did with younger second-generation and third-generation women. Among these women, internalization of both popular and biomedical beliefs and practices was influenced by educational attainment, age at marriage, individual and family experience with specific diseases, degree of religiosity, and the state of medical technology and science when the woman reached maturity.

Epidemiological Characteristics

Availability of Epidemiological Information on Italian Americans

Since neither Italian-born nor American-born Italian Americans are differentiated in any national morbidity and mortality statistics, one is restricted in what one can say about disease patterns in this ethnic group. The available data generally come either from urban ethnic enclaves, where government mortality and morbidity statistics can be used on the assumption that the local population is predominantly mono-ethnic, or from the occasional retrospective studies of specific disease entities which compare Italian-American rates to national statistics or to mortality or morbidity rates for other ethnic groups. Because of the expense and effort necessary to acquire data of the former kind on a scale large enough to be useful for this chapter, only data from the retrospective studies will be reported here.

Morbidity and Mortality Rates for Selected Diseases

The available epidemiological data for the peak immigration years in the early decades of this century and for the contemporary era indicate that the leading causes of death are similar in both Italy and the United States. The immigrants and their children in the peak period were more likely to be ill with and to die from diseases of bacterial origin, whereas the current leading causes of death for both countries are those in the degenerative and long-term disease categories, that is, cardiovascular diseases and cancer (Preston, Keyfitz, and Schoen 1972). Thus the older and the recent immigrants have had different experiences and have coped with different disease and illness problems both prior to and after immigration.

MALIGNANT NEOPLASMS   A survey of hospitalized cancer patients of diverse ethnicities (Polish, German, and Italian) in Buffalo, New York revealed that Italian-born patients had higher frequencies for cancers of the bladder, pharynx, and large intestine (Graham et al. 1963).

CARDIOVASCULAR DISEASES   The relationship between ethnicity and incidence of cardiovascular disease has been studied comparatively for urban Italians and other ethnic groups both in America and abroad in order to isolate some etiological factors that may have significance in the epidemiology of these diseases. Epstein, Boas, and Simpson (1957), for example, compared the frequency of coronary heart disease among Jewish and Italian male and female older persons employed as garment workers in New York City. The groups were controlled for age, sex, place of birth, time in the United States, and type and amount of fat in the diet. No ethnic differences in the age-adjusted frequency of heart disease were observed for females, but for males the frequencies were significantly different: 7.9 percent for Italians (N = 232) and 15.8 percent for Jews (N = 372).

Although manifest coronary heart disease was twice as frequent for Jewish than for Italian men, the authors were unable to explain the predisposition of Jews toward development of the disease. Though the data eliminated the variables of serum lipid levels, hypertension, obesity, and diabetes mellitus as accounting for the demonstrated ethnic difference, the findings suggest that type and amount of dietary fat might be important. The Italian diet contained less animal and more vegetable fat than the Jewish diet; 32 percent of the total fat intake of the Italian subjects came from a vegetable source, as contrasted to 20 percent for the Jewish.

Support for a dietary explanation of the relatively low rates of heart disease reported among Italians comes from a comparative study of clinically healthy men in Naples (Italy) and Minnesota (Keys et al. 1954). Cholesterol concentrations for both samples (which were matched for age and weight) were similar for ages up to the early thirties. After that, however, the Italians maintained a relatively constant cholesterol level, while the Minnesotans showed an average rise of 2 to 3 mg per 100 ml per year, so that by the age of 50 the Minnesotans averaged cholesterol levels that were 30 mg per 100 ml higher than those of the Italians. Dietary differences between the two populations seem to account for the disparity in cholesterol levels, since 40 percent of the Minnesotans' caloric intake came from fats, whereas only 20 percent of the Italians' did. Furthermore, the latter group consumed little animal fat and no butter.

In addition to differences between Italian and American dietary patterns, other cultural and social differences have been implicated in the differing rates for cardiovascular problems between the two national groups. The findings suggest that as Italians become acculturated to American values and behavior patterns, the difference in rates for these diseases declines. A study of Roseto (Bruhn, Philips, and Wolf 1972), an all-Italian community in Pennsylvania, illustrates these patterns. This community was a focus of clinical and sociological studies starting in 1962. Prior to the study, Roseto had been considered a stable ethnic community for 80 years (Bruhn, Philips, and Wolf 1972). Death rates from myocardial infarctions in Roseto were unusually low compared to those in two nearby towns, where mortality rates approached national figures for the disease. Roseto males below age 47 showed no coronary disease, and signs of ischemic heart disease were not evident, despite their presence both in relatives who lived elsewhere and in males born in Roseto who lived in other communities (Stout et al. 1964; Wolf et al. 1973). What appeared to make Roseto distinct were a number of sociocultural features: namely, closely knit and cohesive social groups and the absence of any challenge to the traditional role of the male as head of the household. By 1970, when Roseto was restudied, death rates for myocardial infarction had reached two-thirds that of the neighboring towns. Changing social and cultural practices in the second and third generations were the suggested reasons for the increase in mortality. Similar changes in mortality rates have been observed among Italian immigrants to Australia, where they have also been attributed to stresses and changes in life-style arising from acculturation (Stenhouse and McCall 1970).

The implications of these data for health professionals working with Italian Americans might be to reinforce the traditional dietary reliance on vegetable fats in order to control cholesterol levels when the situation indicates that a dietary treatment strategy is called for.

Diseases of Genetic Origin Found Among Italian Americans

FAVISM   Favism, a severe hemolytic anemia produced by ingestion of fava beans, is caused by a genetically controlled deficiency of the X-linked enzyme glucose-6-phosphate dehydrogenase (G6PD) in the erythrocytes of susceptible subjects (Bearn 1968:1208). Like thalassemia, this deficiency occurs in malarial belts, and affected persons generally possess resistance to malaria. However, the current distribution of the deficiency in the United States is not known.

Persons with this condition are particularly susceptible to hemolytic reactions following administration of the antimalarial drug primaquine and of certain other drugs, including phenacetin (Bearn 1968:1208). Since the fava bean is used extensively by Italian-American immigrants, elicitation of health histories should include questions relative to the use of this staple, as well as antimalarial and analgesic agents.

THALASSEMIA SYNDROMES   Cooley's anemia, an inherited disorder, is found in high frequencies among populations throughout the Mediterranean region, and in parts of Italy it is considered a severe health problem (Siniscalco et al. 1966). The disease is one form of thalassemia, which is classified into two types, alpha and beta. The former type, caused by retarded production of alpha chains of globin, affects the fetus, and death occurs in utero or at birth (Conley 1979:1779). Beta thalassemia, caused by the retarded production of beta chains of globin, is manifested in two forms, homozygous and heterozygous beta thalassemia. Homozygous beta thalassemia (variously known as Cooley's anemia, Mediterranean anemia, target cell anemia, or thalassemia major) is an extremely severe illness characterized by profound anemia, marked liver and spleen enlargement, icterus, prominent frontal bossing, and physical underdevelopment (Conley 1979:1779). With the use of transfusion therapy, splenectomy, and other treatment methods, patients achieve adulthood but suffer the consequences of chronic iron overload (Lassman et al. 1974).

Heterozygous beta thalassemia, or thalassemia minor, is characterized by mild anemia, usually with microcytosis, hypochromia, stippling, and target cells. Symptoms are unusual, but some persons have anemia of moderate severity associated with jaundice and splenomegaly (Conley 1979:1779–1780).

The prevalence of heterozygous beta thalassemia in Americans of Italian ancestry is not known, although two estimates of the frequency of the trait are available. The frequency of beta thalassemia trait in a sample of high school students in New Haven, Connecticut was 2.4 percent; a frequency of 4 percent has been reported for Italian Americans in Rochester, New York, although this rate was not measured directly but calculated by use of the Hardy-Weinberg formula (Pearson et al. 1974).

The psychosocial problems and the coping strategies of Italian-American families when faced with an illness with a poor prognosis, such as thalassemia major, have not been investigated. Thus, assessment of both the epidemiological magnitude and psychosocial effects of this disease among Italian Americans must await further study.

Concepts of Disease and Illness

Italian Americans of the immigrant generation, both old and recent, tend to give detailed narratives of the onset of illnesses which relate bodily sensations, the emotional impact, and the social context of the illness episode (see Zola 1966). These narrative accounts are repeated when neighbors pay obligatory visits during hospitalization and after discharge.

The following example of one such narrative indicates the selection of symptoms for evaluation, the sequence of actions taken for clarification, and the final definition of the problem and action taken. The narrative thus serves both as an introduction to this section on concepts of disease and illness by showing how biomedical concepts are transmitted within the ethnic group, and as illustrative data for the following section, which deals more specifically with the evaluation of symptoms and other aspects of illness behavior. The narrative is by a 62-year-old woman who came to the United States from Italy at age 8. The biomedical diagnosis for the case was acute cholecystitis and the treatment instituted a cholecystectomy.

Tony came home from work [employed in a produce market] Saturday night—he was late coming home even for a Saturday. He felt tired. I fixed him a nice dinner—veal chops with potatoes and eggs poached in tomato sauce, which he likes. He wanted a light dessert, so I sliced peaches he brought from the market with some marsala wine . . . Before we finished, A—— dropped in with some home-baked Boston beans and brown bread. She makes them all from scratch, the old-fashioned way with salt pork. She knows Tony likes them. I gave him a side dish.

We decided not to visit the M——s because Tony felt tired and washed out. We stayed in and watched television and went to bed after the news at 11:00. I heard him get up two times. He said he had indigestion and couldn't sleep. He thought it was the beans that caused it. He took Brioschi, and then he tried some baking soda, which helped. At 3:30 he said he had pain in his chest. I took his temperature; it was 100°. His face was flushed around the cheekbones, but it didn't turn gray like B——'s did when he had his heart attack. So I gave him some Pepto Bismol, because it was probably indigestion . . .

But by 4:30 A.M. I was worried and felt we should call Dr. X, even though it was a Sunday and nighttime. You know doctors—they don't like to be called at night. But before I did, I called A—— [a neighbor whose husband had a heart attack several months previously]. By this time it was 5:30, so I didn't feel too bad about getting her up. She counted his pulse and said it felt strong, and compared to B—— (her husband), his color looked all right. But to be on the safe side, I called Dr. X, who said to go to the emergency ward at Mass. General. The police ambulance came, and I went with Tony. A—— said she would come to the hospital as soon as she got breakfast for the family. As soon as we got to the emergency ward, they put Tony in a side room and put tubes in his nose for oxygen. (Ragucci 1971, unpublished field notes)

Each day more detail on Tony's case would be given to neighbors and friends who dropped in to inquire about the patient's progress: the results of laboratory tests and x-rays, the wife's interpretation of what the "young doctors" (interns and residents) and specialists told her, the patient's reaction to hospitalization, and the wife's perception of the quality of nursing and medical care her husband received.

An analysis of accounts like the one given above reveals not only the cognitive and decision-making processes that lead laymen to diagnose situations differentially but also the lay referral system through which the patient progresses. These aspects of the narrative will be dealt with in greater detail in the following section; however, several observations concerning the narrative are relevant here. First, the account indicates the salience of biomedical interpretations of symptoms; and second, it highlights the role of prior experience with particular disease entities (in this case the neighbor's) in directing the lay diagnosis of symptoms. This latter observation suggests the crucial role that patient education plays in illness behavior, since the physician's information is transmitted to others and used to evaluate and classify their symptoms. The beneficial effects of painstaking educational efforts are thus multiplied beyond the direct recipients of the information.

The anecdote recounted above also illustrates a behavioral norm common to Italian Americans—namely, that a person should strive for balance or the golden mean in behavior so that he will not be thought by his peers to have gone to any extreme. The narrative also shows the importance in this subculture of freeing oneself of any possible blame for the misfortune of others. The theme expressed by the speaker is that she did what was proper and appropriate, and nothing that she did or did not do should be construed as the cause of the husband's distress.[3] These dual cultural themes of behavioral propriety and exculpation may be seen in other patient behaviors described later in the chapter.

Intraethnic Variation

Notwithstanding the importance of biomedical concepts, as illustrated in the foregoing narrative, other kinds of beliefs and practices occur among Italian Americans as well. In analyzing the data from my participant-observation study, I identified the following types of beliefs: (1) the "archaic"—what was, but is no longer; (2) the "traditional"— beliefs and actions that are a combination of the ideas and practices of "little" (folk) and past "great" traditions of medicine, that is, Greco-Roman, Salernitan, and early twentieth century medicine; and (3) contemporary or "popular" medicine—beliefs and practices that have filtered down from the present great tradition of medicine (the biomedical) as reinterpreted or redefined by laymen.

An understanding of the variability in the illness categories and health-seeking strategies used by Italian Americans can best be obtained by comparing older members of this ethnic category (that is, immigrant and second-generation adults over the age of 50) with younger adults (that is, immigrants and second, third, and later generations of Americans under the age of 50). This dichotomization of intraethnic variation developed out of my observations in Boston, where, as mentioned earlier, the members of each of the two age categories showed major convergences in belief and practice within their group and differences from the other category. In general, the beliefs of older people conform to the type described above as "traditional," while those in the younger age category are most apt to hold beliefs defined as "popular."

The proponents of traditional beliefs and practices focus on concrete, sensible aspects of the materials used for the cure and prevention of illness. They also employ magical and religious modes of coping more than the people in the younger age group do. In addition, their remedies consist mainly of elements found in nature and administered according to the traditions of the earlier medical systems. Those who use the popular form, on the other hand, not only follow beliefs and practices from modern medical theory as reinterpreted by themselves, the mass media, and other laymen, they also tend to avoid espousing magical and religious causes for illness and to use remedies consisting largely of manufactured drugs and patent medicines.

Concepts about the Causes of Illness and Disease

Beliefs about illness in the Italian-American subculture focus on five factors, although followers of traditional and of popular health practices differ in the credence they lend to specific etiological ideas. These factors are the following: (1) disease-bearing winds and currents, (2) contagion or contamination, (3) genetic or hereditary disposition, (4) supernatural and human (including iatrogenic) intervention, and (5) psychosomatic interactions. (The terms in this list are mine and are not necessarily ones that Italian Americans would use themselves.) It is notable, however, that Pitrè's list of factors that were used by nineteenth-century Sicilians to explain the causes of illness includes some of the same etiological concepts employed today—for example, atmospheric and meteorological perturbations, contagion (*contagio* or *contagiosità*), and excessive acidity (*acidità*) (Pitrè 1896:167–178). (See the section on adherence to biomedical treatment later in this chapter for a discussion of acidity with regard to contemporary dietary patterns.)

Disease is not necessarily attributed to a single cause, and the biomedically recognized multicausal basis for several disease entities is understood by many Italian Americans. Tuberculosis, for example, is believed to be caused by contact with persons who have the disease, excessive smoking, and prolonged exposure to cold and dampness. It is also believed to "run" in families, testimony to the recognition of a hereditary component in the disease. Diabetes mellitus is variously conceived as being caused by uncontrolled appetite, emotional factors, inheritance, and God's will.

DISEASE-BEARING WINDS AND CURRENTS   Older Italians show a marked preoccupation with drafts or currents of air as the chief etiological basis of a number of illnesses. The basis for this belief seems to lie in Greco-Roman humoral theory as well as the concepts of *status strictus* and *laxus* (excessive closure and relaxation of the pores), which were major explanatory principles used by Greek Stoics and Methodists (Ackerknecht 1958:64).

According to the elderly, cold, moving air may chill a bodily part, causing an irritation which in turn produces an increase in secretions such as phlegm, pus, or diarrhea. Aches and pains in any part of the body may also be attributed to a "cold" contracted in this fashion from drafts. The term used in Italian for these conditions is *raffreddore,* and in reporting symptoms to a physician, Italian speakers may refer to infections of the upper respiratory tract, muscle aches and pains, or diarrheal symptoms by the translation label "cold" with the appropriate body part (for example, a "cold in my stomach" refers to symptoms of nausea or vomiting; a "cold in my shoulder" to arthritic or muscle pain in the shoulder). A "head cold," moreover, is considered to be a precursor of pneumonia.

The body is believed to be particularly vulnerable to winds and drafts when the pores are "open." A person who is perspiring is therefore in a particularly dangerous state because the pores are "more open," and exposure to atmospheric conditions at that time is deemed inadvisable. Indeed, air entering any body cavity is thought to be injurious. For instance, the elderly maintain that people undergoing cancer surgery "die quicker" because air enters the body by way of the incision.

Ideas associated with the harmful effects of air and wind may cause conflict between older and younger Italian Americans. Grandparents frequently complain that children are not sufficiently protected from drafts, and mothers and their married daughters disagree about the proper care of children with an elevated temperature. Conflict over adjustment of ventilation in homes, offices, and factories also occurs, and older Italian Americans frequently complain that drafts from fans or air conditioners have caused them to experience "gum boils" (gingivitis or other mouth infections), pain and numbness of the extremities, sore throats, and chest colds.

Although drafts are considered a cause of illness, fresh air is considered by Italians to be a prerequisite for the maintenance of health. Incapacitated women and men who are confined to their homes complain of feeling "bloated" or "being ready to burst" and attribute this feeling to prolonged deprivation of fresh air and sunshine, rather than lack of physical activity. Difficulties experienced in adjusting to the United States also may be attributed to the different qualities of the air in Italy and America. Immigrants from both coastal and mountain villages consider the air of Italy to be "light" and therefore superior to the "heavy" air of America. Several immigrants in the study population even returned to their native towns for the cure or amelioration of such ailments as "a nervous breakdown," anemia, and, in one case, symptomotology that was suggestive of chronic leukemia. Furthermore, the elderly often conceptualize their initial feeling of being in America as a sensation of being "hemmed in" or "smothered" (expressed in dialect as *mi sentiva cupata*).

CONTAGION OR CONTAMINATION AS CAUSES OF ILLNESS   A number of conditions are believed by Italian Americans to be caused by contact with objects or persons thought to be unclean. The colloquial expression *io schifo* or *mi fa schifo* ("I am disgusted," from the verb *schifare*—to be disgusted by, to shun) is used to refer to dirty or potentially contaminating circumstances. Reciprocal food exchanges and social visiting patterns in the neighborhood are influenced by the fear of contamination; thus neighbors avoid the homes of women who are considered poor housekeepers and seldom use food prepared by them. It is notable that ideas of contamination among the elderly do not ordinarily imply transmission by germs but simply by direct contact with dirt or bodily wastes (mucus, excreta). On the basis of these beliefs about contagion, territorial boundaries and limits to social interaction are instituted by residents during epidemics. During an outbreak of influenza, for example, neighbors were observed at apartment thresholds inquiring about the ill, but few entered the apartments.

Cultural and medical lag are evidenced by the stringent social and physical isolation placed on persons known to have tuberculosis and persons who are being treated by chemotherapy. For, even though prolonged hospitalization is no longer indicated for tuberculosis, kinfolk and neighbors assume responsibility for isolating the individual from the social group. Persons who are most apt to act in this manner are immigrants of the peak and recent years and second-generation women over age 50.

The extreme fear of the communicability of disease exhibited by Italian Americans may be related to past experiences with contagious diseases. The elderly remember quarantine signs tacked on doors by the Board of Health, prolonged hospitalization in sanatoriums, and the extreme seriousness of communicable diseases in the days before penicillin and immunization. Given the density of population in many urban communities where Italians have settled, however, some of their health protective behaviors may have had salutary effects.

The urban elderly also cling to notions of avoidance which may have been more meaningful in an agrarian society. For example, the "polluting" effect of a menstruating woman on animals and plants continues to be mentioned. Data about these beliefs are incomplete, however, because women in the study were reluctant to discuss menstruation out of a strong sense of modesty and shame (*vergogna*). Teenage girls and their mothers, however, claimed that taboos about mentioning this physiological function are gradually being lost. Nevertheless, there is a continuing reticence among Italian-American women to discuss or mention menstruation in the presence of men—including male physicians.

CONGENITAL CONDITIONS AND ILLNESSES OF HEREDITARY ORIGIN   Laymen's concepts about the genetic basis of physical defects and moral deviance show generational differences among Italian Americans. The elderly consistently use the idiom of "blood" when theorizing about the cause of physical or moral "defects" (for example, unruly behavior, disciplinary problems) in the children of neighbors, friends, or relatives. In general, blood is regarded by the elderly as a plastic entity that responds to fluid, food, and inherited variables. The adjectives "weak" and "strong," "good" and "bad," "high" and "low," "hot" and "cold" are used to describe the condition of this medium.[4] A few second-generation women know about chromosomes, and high school and college students of the third generation in general indicate that they know about genetic transmission by using the term "gene."

The elderly generally agree that the shape of a child's body and his features are transmitted through both maternal and paternal lines. Some state that a child inherits the features and bony structure from the father and the fleshy parts (that is, the shape of the body) from the mother. Their observations concerning specific phenotypes did not always confirm these theories, however. (It is interesting to note that American physicians in the early 1900s held similar beliefs about female and male contributions to the phenotype; see Winslow 1907:65.)

Both genetic and environmental causes of deviant behavior occur in the idea system of Italian Americans. However, a sex-linked notion of the inheritance of character is expressed more often by older than younger people, with certain moral characteristics and behavioral disorders conceived as emanating from the female line.

Genetic or environmental folk explanations must be examined within the context of the particular situation in which they are being used. Consanguineous relatives of a deviant child are more apt to project the blame for character disorders externally and to mention the environment or "bad companions" as major determinants of delinquency or deviance from cultural norms. On the other hand, non-kin and affinal relatives tend to explain the same deviance from a genealogical frame of reference. It is notable that the chances of marriage for a son or a daughter are diminished if their "blood lines" are believed to have a genetic defect or stigma attached.

Younger women are familiar with the "old superstitions" attributing congenital abnormalities to unsatisfied desires for food during pregnancy, because their grandmothers keep these notions alive in contemporary society; they tend not to believe them, however. Immigrants from all regions expressed similar beliefs about *voglie* (desires or cravings). Older women whose origins are in Sicily express additional beliefs about pregnancy: for example, if a woman is not given food that she smells, the fetus will "move inside" and a miscarriage may result; or if a pregnant woman bends or turns her body in certain ways, abnormal fetal development may result. As a result of these beliefs, neighbors offer food delicacies to pregnant women, and family members take over household tasks that involve stooping and reaching during the period of gestation.

HUMAN AND SUPERNATURAL CAUSES   Some illnesses are attributed by Italians to human or supernatural agents or forces. Humans have the power to cause illness through *malocchio* (the "evil eye," also called *iettatura*) or by *castiga* ("curse," also called *maledizione*). In America Italians make a distinction between illnesses that are caused by *iettatore* (one who has the evil eye) and those caused by a person who curses or wishes one harm. Ailments of a more or less serious nature (for example, headaches or joint pains) may be attributed to either natural causes or *malocchio,* while illnesses that have long-term or fatal consequences may at times be attributed to the more powerful curse or *castiga.*

The person who is responsible for illness attributed to the evil eye is usually unknown. His motive to cause harm may be unintended, and he may be one's kinsman, neighbor, or a stranger. The evil eye is believed to be motivated by envy or jealousy of one's good health or fortunate circumstances. Because of the pervasiveness and unpredictability of being afflicted by the evil eye, various protective and therapeutic mechanisms have been elaborated.

Empirical observations in the enclave studied reveal that belief in the evil eye today is not as pervasive as Williams (1938:xv) noted for Connecticut Italians, nor is it limited to the first generation, as Gans (1926: 140) found in a community contiguous to the one I studied. In my experience, the generational depth for the persistence of beliefs about mystical causes of illness was two generations. However, not all Italian Americans of the first and second generations believed that the evil eye precipitates illness; some informants even discounted such beliefs as nonsense (*sciocchezze*) or idle talk (*chiacchiera*). It is notable that those informants who consistently attributed misfortune and illness to the evil eye were also those who had suffered from "nerves" or a "nervous breakdown." Many were also thought of as marginal to their peer groups and the social activities of the neighborhood. For the most part they attended settlement house activities, which were generally shunned by those with a greater degree of social integration within the neighborhood. These findings suggest a need for specifying personality variables as well as the social position of those who continue to express beliefs in this phenomenon.

Castiga ("curse"), the other major supernatural force considered by some Italian Americans as a source of illness or misfortune, is believed to be sent by either God or evil people (*gente maligni*). The latter are usually known to the afflicted, unlike the case with *malocchio.* The person who has been cursed lives in dread because there is little he can do to protect himself. Fear of the curse serves as a mechanism of social control in that maintenance of amicable relationships with neighbors and kin decreases the probability that a person or his children will become the object of *castiga.*

A *castiga* from God is generally attributed to His displeasure over the transgression of moral norms and is differentiated from *disgrazia* ("disaster," "accident"), which also connotes bad luck or lack of favor or grace with God. The latter term is used in contexts in which the speaker does not wish to impute a moral lapse to the victim of an accidental injury or incapacitating handicap. In general, the attribution of illness to punishment or divine retribution is infrequent. Nevertheless, certain feared diseases—including diabetes, tuberculosis, and cancer—lend themselves more than others to this form of interpretation and therefore are not usually disclosed or discussed in the detail typical of the illness narratives discussed above. However, people of the younger generation and others who have a knowledge of biomedical ideas about the causes of diseases avoid supernatural explanations.

The externalizing or projective mechanisms underlying occult notions of disease etiology may have been transformed in the urban milieu into iatrogenic notions. For instance, in my study there were a number of incidents in which blame for disease complications or death was attributed to health professionals. People most often cited surgeons, visiting nurses, and laboratory technicians as the causative agents. Furthermore, most of the iatrogenic explanations were realistic, though simplistic. One may try to understand those explanations as verbalizations of the defense mechanisms of projection and displacement, traditionally articulated in terms of the evil eye theory of small-scale rural society and now translated into a belief system more congruent with a complex, technological society. On the other hand, the frequency of iatrogenic explanations for illness or complications may reflect a more informed and realistic attitude on the part of these consumers of modern medical and health services.

PSYCHOSOMATIC FACTORS IN THE ETIOLOGY OF ILLNESS   Italians, as a whole, recognize that suppression of emotions, as well as stress associated with fear, anxiety, grief, and sorrow, can be causative factors in a number of ailments, including heart disease, mental depression, high blood pressure, duodenal ulcers, and skin disease. The expression *sfogare o schiattare* ("give vent to emotions or burst") is used by immigrants to indicate the therapeutic effectiveness of asserting or expressing one's feelings. The implication of the expression is that if one is unable to find an emotional outlet, feelings become locked within vulnerable body organs, which may then burst.

Most folk statements reflect the dual components of psychosomatic disorders, namely, an external precipitating factor that acts upon a locus of vulnerability within the individual's psyche and body. For example, residents in the community I studied agreed that *cordoglia* ("grief," "anguish") precipitated the development of diabetes in a widow soon after her husband died. There was also a consensus that her failure to control her intake of sweets contributed to the condition. In general, however, the elderly view the heart as the seat of emotions and therefore the primary organ affected by emotional trauma.

Ideas about the etiology of the contrasted conditions "nerves" or "nervous breakdown" (*esaurimento nervoso*) and "crazy" (*pazzo*) similarly reflect a psychosomatic orientation. On the one hand, "crazy" behavior is unpredictable, socially disruptive, and uncontrollable, and the "crazy" person is stigmatized. The condition is generally attributed to somatic causes: pathology of the brain or "a sudden rush of blood to the head." On the other hand, a nervous breakdown results from worry and anxiety which in turn affect the nerves—a more clearly psychosomatic conceptualization. "Nerves" or "nervous breakdowns" are not stigmatized, and Chapman's observation in a Sicilian village (1971:227) that "nerves" is a minor affliction of which no one is ashamed applies to many Italians of diverse regional origins. The folk treatment for "nerves" consists mainly of encouraging the person to pray (*pregare*) for help and to approach situations with the right attitude (*buona volantà*). A change in environment (for example, a return to the natal town or a vacation in a sunny climate) may also be urged, especially if the "nervous" condition is marked by depression.

Jaundice (*itterizia*), which will be discussed more fully in the following section, is considered to be a disease rather than a sign or symptom of liver, gallbladder, or blood dysfunction. It is believed to result from psychological or environmental factors, or both: namely, fright, nervousness, aggravation, or drinking cold water. A vestige of the humoral theory of Greco-Roman medicine is apparent in expressions about the emotional components of jaundice. Thus, the jealous are said to be "green with envy"; the anxious or depressed are said to have "trouble with the bile." It is noteworthy, however, that people's knowledge of the multiple causes of jaundice may be extended by their own experience, their observations of others who have the symptom, and information acquired through the news media. Thus, some informants noted that jaundice could be contracted by drinking contaminated water or receiving a blood transfusion donated by a person with a history of the condition. They also related the "yellow look" that some people were observed to develop in the terminal stage of cancer to jaundice. It is also possible, however, for experience to be interpreted as confirming a traditional etiological view; for example, news reports that an entire football team had contracted hepatitis by drinking water from a contaminated source reinforced folk theorists who related this case of "yellow jaundice" to drinking cold water.

In brief, while sometimes Italian Americans' views of the role of psychological or environmental factors in disease agree with biomedical concepts, at other times they do not. The important point, however, is that for many Italian-American patients both emotional or affective and environmental predisposing factors are an important part of their conception of their illness and must accordingly be elicited and discussed with the attending health professional.

Becoming Ill

People's evaluations of symptoms and illness are predicated on their definitions of what constitutes not only an unhealthy but also a healthy state. Within the Italian community some predictable variations exist concerning definitions of these two important states.

Concepts of Health or Well-Being

Health and the maintenance of a healthy state are perceived among Italian Americans as being influenced by a person's age and his social and occupational roles. In general, health is defined as a state of well-being. However, the expectation that one's sense of well-being will decline with age is clearly reflected in the proverb, *Passata la quarantina, un dolore ogni mattina* ("After the age of 40, one can expect a [new] pain every morning").

The elderly assess their health status not only by the presence or absence of a chronic illness or disability but also according to their physical capabilities in relation to others. Older persons thus use an age-mate or a younger person as a reference point for comparison. The relative nature of health status assessments is illustrated in the statement of an elderly informant only four weeks prior to her death: "For a woman my age, I'm strong. The doctor said my health is better than for people much younger than me. Look at A. B. She's 10 years younger, but she doesn't do the things I do."

Older people also evaluate their health according to their capacity to pursue the normal activities of daily living. The continuing ability to enjoy customary eating, sleeping, and reciprocal visiting patterns in the neighborhood is the variable most frequently mentioned as an indicator of good health and well-being. In effect, physical mobility and its attendant sense of independence is perhaps the most important single factor that distinguishes the well from the ill. The statement, "As long as we can get around without having to be obligated to others, then we can say our health is good," reflects a typical sentiment.

In contrast with the elderly, younger people (that is, those under the age of 50) appraise their own and their spouses' health by the actual presence or absence of symptoms. They express concern about the significance of certain complaints which they fear may be precursors of a long-term illness that would interfere with their parental roles as homemakers or wage earners.

In comparing their health with that of people from other generations, older persons of the immigrant generation often express the view that they were healthier and stronger as youths than young people are today. These older immigrants tend to extol and idealize the premigration conditions in their rural natal towns, especially the clear and "light" air of the hills and mountains, the hard work in the fields, the availability of fresh home-grown produce, and the necessity for walking the long distances from their households to the fields.[5]

Men and women of middle age who were raised in the densely popu-lated urban areas of the peak immigration years concede that the parental generation was healthier than theirs; they also consider younger people in their generation (second), as well as their own children, to be healthier than they were in their youth. They credit the biomedical advances of penicillin, vitamins, and immunizations for alleviating the many ailments they experienced in childhood. A comment by a middle-aged, second-generation woman illustrates this point of view: "In those days [prior to antibiotics] bad infections were treated with hot towels or flaxseed poul-tices, even onions. You never see a child now with a nose dripping yellow mucus or a draining ear or abscess. Without vitamins and penicillin, no wonder we were always sick."

In sum, Italians of all ages and social classes appear to hold a concept of health that is close to one sociological definition—"a state of optimum capacity for the performance of valued tasks and roles" (Parsons 1972: 165–187). In accordance with this view, Italian Americans see their health (well-being) as related to physiological functions, but always in the context of changing role expectations as they proceed through the life cycle. In addition, many have a positive view of biomedicine, attributing an overall rise in standards of health to its technological advances.

Evaluation of Symptoms

The illness narrative that was quoted at the beginning of the previous section illustrates the social context in which symptoms are in-terpreted, as well as the sequence of actions that led in that instance to further clarification and definition of the problem. Two important points emerge from the narrative. First, medical consultation followed after a rather typical series of lay actions for severe symptoms: individual con-cern over the condition; consultation with immediate family; adminis-tration of home remedies; determination of the seriousness of the suf-ferer's condition by the only diagnostic instrument generally available in the home, the thermometer; and finally, lay consultation with an "expert," here someone who had had recent experience with one of the symptoms (chest pain). Second, although the narrative appears to be overly de-tailed and in many places irrelevant—the sort of diffuse presentation of symptoms that Zola (1966) reports as typical of Italian Americans—many of the details are indeed pertinent (for example, the lengthy pres-entation of the evening menu, the remedies taken). This observation implies that if health professionals were to listen to the "diffuse" descriptions of a problem often presented by Italian-American patients, they not only would hear the patient's or his family's view of what is wrong (the "illness") but also would glean information relevant to a biomedical diagnosis.

Beyond the general similarities in illness behavior discussed above, Italian Americans tend to differ considerably in the ways in which they evaluate the signs and symptoms associated with altered functioning of body systems. Indeed, laymen's evaluations of particular symptoms tend to vary more than their ideas about the causation of particular diseases. Three factors tend to contribute toward this variation: (1) the social position of the sufferer and the person evaluating the symptoms, (2) the nature of the symptoms themselves, and (3) the location of symptoms in the body.

VARIATION ARISING FROM SOCIODEMOGRAPHIC FACTORS   The same general sources of intraethnic variation in health beliefs and practices discussed in the section on data evaluation also apply to the evaluation of symptoms. Thus, interpretations of the severity or importance of particular symptoms vary with the age, generation, education and, in some cases, region of origin of the interpreter.

In addition, the age of the patient is an important variable in determining the interpretation and disposition of symptoms. Thus, according to my observations, professional medical care is usually sought earlier in an illness episode for a child than for an adult. Italian-American parents who delay seeking medical attention are liable to receive censure, blame, and unfavorable comments from kin and neighbors in the event of either the death of a child or serious complications. Although the decision to seek medical help may involve consultation with grandparents, other kin, or neighbors, the major responsibility for the outcome falls on the parents. They therefore act according to the maxim, "better to be safe than sorry."

SYMPTOMS THEMSELVES AS SOURCES OF VARIATION   In addition to differences among evaluators as a source of variation in the way symptoms are interpreted, the nature of the symptoms themselves also influences how they are perceived. In certain cases, some Italian Americans may equate signs and symptoms with an illness entity. For example, *itterizia* (jaundice) may be interpreted as a disease in its own right, as a sign concomitant with an enlarged spleen, or as the "yellowish tinge" that people acquire who are terminally ill with cancer.

Symptoms may also be evaluated according to severity, intensity, and duration. Symptoms that are temporary (for example, resulting from an indiscretion in eating, exercise, or drinking) will be labeled *piccola cosa* ("a small thing") or referred to as *non è niente* ("it is nothing [to worry about]"). However hemorrhage, shortness of breath, unconsciousness, severe pain of sudden onset, unexplained swelling, and discoloration of body parts all constitute symptoms that incite prompt and sometimes emergency action.

In children, listlessness, pallor, failure to gain weight, loss of appetite, and fever are symptoms and signs that initiate social and cognitive processes for determining the cause. Home remedies may be tried, and relatives and neighbors may later be asked for validation of the immediate family's lay diagnosis. Prolonged diarrhea and vomiting, when these symptoms cannot be easily explained by a "virus that is going around" and do not appear to be self-limiting, are considered more serious, however, and professional medical help is sought without much lay consultation or home treatment. Children are considered particularly incapable of withstanding prolonged fever or lack of foods and fluids because of their small body size.

LOCATION OF SYMPTOMS AND VARIATIONS IN ILLNESS EVALUATIONS
Older immigrants differ from recent migrants in the particular organic or physiological processes to which they attend in evaluating symptoms. For example, older immigrants attribute a number of symptoms to the condition of the blood. Pallor, weakness, and acidity are associated with blood that is believed to be deficient in certain properties. (See note 4 for a more detailed discussion of blood beliefs.) In contrast, new arrivals tend to focus attention on the function or malfunction of the gastrointestinal tract and liver. Indigestion, general malaise, and flatulence are symptoms frequently attributed to stomach and liver ailments. In general, first-generation Italians of all ages ascribe most abdominal complaints to the liver.

Immigrant men and women of rural origin show precision in localizing symptoms to specific body organs and possess more knowledge about the anatomy and physiology of the body than do urban-born Italians and their American-born children; this may be attributed to the participation of the former in the slaughter and dressing of farm animals. The extensive use of organ meats in the diet, such as brain, pancreas, liver, and kidneys, also aids in the application of animal knowledge to the human body.

It is important to note here that older Italian people generally employ euphemisms to refer to certain body functions or symptoms that are considered taboo (for example, diarrhea, defecation, or menstruation, which is commonly referred to as a "headache" or *quelle affari,* "those affairs"). When it is necessary to speak about such matters, they preface the discussion with a conventional apology, *parlando con rispetto* ("speaking with respect"). (The implications of this custom for practitioner-patient communication will be discussed later in the chapter.)

Coping with Illness outside the Mainstream Medical System

Treating Illness in the Home

CARETAKING RESPONSIBILITIES IN THE FAMILY   Within the nuclear family, responsibilities for the care of the ill are allocated in different ways. In general, the wife/mother is responsible for nurturing tasks
—that is, providing for the comfort, as well as the hygienic and nutritional
needs, of an ailing husband or child. Decisions about the purchase of
medicine and medical supplies (for example, a humidifier) or about calling the physician are usually made jointly by husband and wife.

In Italian-American families a daughter, rather than a son, is expected
to assume major responsibility in caring for aged and ailing parents. (This
arrangement is a reversal of the pattern that holds in rural Italy, where a
son and daughter-in-law are expected to fulfill this obligation.) Ensuring
that the caretaker role is filled is facilitated by a preference not only for
single daughters to live at home until marriage but also for married
daughters, rather than sons, to reside near their parents. The pragmatic
aspect of the mother-daughter relationship is reflected in the following
statement: "A daughter brings comfort to the mother. You can't expect a
daughter-in-law or your son to care for you when you have a headache"
(here used to refer to any indisposition of a temporary nature).

In the case of a married daughter who acts as caretaker to her parents,
the consent of her husband is essential, since the wife's involvement in her
parental home during periods of illness often requires rearrangement of
the younger family's priorities. My observations reveal that the daughter
most likely to be recruited to the role of helper is the one with the most
"easy-going" husband. Furthermore, if the wife's father is handicapped,
the tasks of bathing, dressing, and shaving him are delegated to the son-
in-law. In reciprocation for their services, the young couple may receive
an apartment in the parental home at reduced rent and help with household expenses.

If the parental illness is a long-term one, however, the main burden of
care may be assumed by one daughter, with the remaining care being
shared by mutual arrangements with other siblings and their spouses.
Sons and daughters and their spouses allocate and rotate routine tasks.
Sons who live at a distance are often recruited to transport parents to the
clinic or doctor's office. In general, it is the younger, sturdy men who are
asked to help transfer the severely disabled person from bed to chair.

The decision to admit an aging parent to a nursing home is delayed as
long as possible. The obligation to remain close to aging parents (Vecoli
1978), fear of censure by relatives and neighbors for a lack of respect
and compassion for elderly parents, and the cost of nursing homes for
long-term care are deterrents to the use of these facilities. Once the deci-

sion for nursing home placement is made, however, the preference is for either a home with Italian-speaking personnel or one sponsored by the Catholic church (Fandetti and Gelfand 1976). In general, elderly men and women with few close kin ties are more accepting of nursing home care.

Immigrant families may face unique problems in situations of serious or prolonged illness because the family support system may be truncated due to the lack of extended kin in this country. For want of a child (particularly a daughter) to fill the helping role, a person may be sought outside the immediate family, often an American-born or English-speaking woman or godchild (*figliocca*). The system of godparenthood, called *compareggio* or *comparatico,* serves to extend the kin and friendship network. At baptism a man, the *compare* ("co-father"), and a woman, the *comare* ("co-mother"), act as sponsors for the child and maintain an ongoing kin-like relationship with their godchild's parents.

HOME REMEDIES   Today most traditional remedies are regarded as exotic by both young and old Italian Americans. However, occasionally people do revert to traditional remedies when they become disillusioned or impatient with prescribed biomedical regimens. For example, one woman in the community I studied used leeches when she became dissatisfied with the prolonged physical and drug therapy prescribed by a clinic physician for a shoulder injury.

In the late 1960s the traditional herbal remedies used by Italian Americans were limited largely to the use of chamomile and mallow infusions. Mallow is used to treat head and chest colds by "bringing out the bad humors" (secretions or fluids) and, mixed with lemon juice, to liquefy mucus. Chamomile tea is used for sedation, for relief of nervousness, and for intestinal or menstrual cramps. In addition, compresses of vinegar and water, rubbing alcohol, or sliced raw potatoes are said to be effective in relieving headaches and are used on occasion. The infrequent use of onions, either as a juice or in the form of a poultice to "break up a cold," represents a last vestige of the great medical traditions of the sixteenth century (Sigerist 1960). Today, chemically manufactured remedies have for the most part replaced the natural remedies used in the past by Italian Americans.

Family medicine cabinets are likely to contain a number of over-the-counter drugs to treat symptoms and common ailments relating to several body systems—for example, headaches, colds, constipation, muscle strain, and joint aches. More than one brand of antacid or laxative may be purchased to suit the preferences of individual family members. One popular remedy for indigestion or stomach pain is Brioschi, an effervescent antacid, which was originally formulated in Italy and now has a wide market in the United States. This product, which contains 710 mg of sodium per capful (recommended dosage 1 or 2 heaping capfuls), is labeled with a warning that it be taken only under the supervision of a physician if the user is on a sodium-restricted diet. However, problems with literacy and vision often render such warnings useless. Both young and old tend to use over-the-counter medicines either without knowledge of their possible untoward effects or in spite of the warnings printed on labels.

The kitchen cabinets of recent immigrants almost invariably contain remedies imported from Italy as well. Two of the most popular are Fernet-Branca, a preparation of bitters, and Ferro-Chino. The former is used as an aperitif and digestive; the latter is a tonic containing iron. Mineral water imports from Italy have also appeared in Italian neighborhood stores in great quantities since 1965.

Both old and recent immigrants as well as the American-born use mustard greens and dandelions during the spring as a blood "tonic." These foods are analogous to the Yankee use of sulfur and molasses for springtime "renewal" of the blood.

Lay Consultation and Referral

The lay referral system is initiated within the family, where symptoms are assessed and appropriate interventions are discussed or carried out. As mentioned earlier, I observed a more rapid response to symptomatology presented by a child than by an adult. Furthermore, working men and women are most likely to delay seeking physical examinations or reporting symptoms because clinic and private physicians' hours may not be convenient, and they may not have health-care services on the job.

Consultations about an illness may go outside the nuclear family and include kin or neighbors. Young immigrant and elderly families tend to use extended networks for consultation to a greater degree than do second- and third-generation Italian Americans; the latter tend to consult a physician directly.

Medical care without intervening lay consultation may be sought by Italian-speaking people if they have a family doctor who is of Italian origin. However, because immigrants generally lack fluency in English, several categories of helping persons have emerged to assist them in health-seeking activities. Sons and daughters, even those as young as eight years of age, help interpret the health and medical needs of parents to health professionals. This reversal of role, where the child acts as teacher and guide to a mother or father, often extends into maturity.

In the community I studied, two additional types of informal caretakers were also identified: "therapeutic women" and "lay medical specialists." Therapeutic women, who belong to the immigrant or first generation, are sought by their peers for advice and traditional treatment of such ailments as persistent headaches and skin disorders. Some women who consult them show signs of anxiety, stress, and mental depression, and in many cases friends and relatives have given up attempts to support them during periods of prolonged depression. The therapeutic women are perceived as *simpatica* (pleasant, congenial, agreeable). Their kitchens provide a setting for social visits and exchange of information not only for women in distress but also for neighborhood women in general.

Lay medical specialists, who are for the most part English-speaking women of the second generation, act as intermediaries between the "American" health-care system and elderly immigrants of the peak migration years. These women interpret prescribed medical and dietary regimens and often administer such treatments as eye drops and insulin injections. Their intermediary role with medical professionals acquaints them with the signs and symptoms of a number of diseases and disabilities and enables them to make preliminary or "differential" lay diagnoses, usually with great accuracy.

Recent female immigrants, however, tend to bypass older and second-generation women in consulting others about illness and depend instead on immigrant contemporaries (friends, relatives, or ritual kin) who have been in the United States longer than they. Second-generation women, from whose ranks the lay medical specialists are recruited, are not usually asked to serve as mediators between the new arrivals and American institutions. The apparent rejection of the teaching and helping role of these women requires further inquiry, although linguistic differences may be implicated. It is also probable that a sense of modesty or shame (*vergogna*) inhibits recent immigrants from discussing ailments of certain organ systems with the older, second-generation women.

In addition to various people who are consulted about illness, home medical references constitute another source of information about the meaning and treatment of symptoms. They are used primarily by second- and third-generation men and women. Italian radio programs, newspapers, and magazines imported from Italy are also important sources of health information in urban Italian-American communities, as are the observations and informal discussions of family members' or neighbors' symptoms and responses to therapy.

In addition to these sources of information and lay referral, dominant Italian values also play a role in determining whether and when people respond to illness. Values pertinent to this process include a strong emphasis on family solidarity, the importance of regard in the community and neighborhood, thrift, and *vergogna* (a quality that refers to modesty, bashfulness, or a sense of shame, especially as it relates to women). The role of family solidarity and neighborly regard in arriving at health-seeking actions has already been discussed; because of its importance in doctor-patient interactions, *vergogna* will be treated in the following section.

With regard to thrift, members of the recent immigrant generation, faced with the expenses of settlement in a new country, generally devote a large proportion of their wages to the furnishing and eventual purchase of a house. As a result, low priority may be given to immediate health needs. Immigrants of an earlier era have evoked criticism from their children because the parents' emphasis on saving led, according to the children, to neglect of dental and other health-care needs. The immigrants counter this criticism by asserting that their frugal habits were motivated by a dread of "going on welfare" or becoming a "charity hospital case." Today, however, Medicare has helped mitigate the economic burden of sickness for the elderly to some extent, and many of the younger, employed Italian Americans have prepaid insurance plans through their jobs.

Nonmainstream Medical Care outside the Home

In the early days of settlement in urban ethnic enclaves, healers who had emigrated from the same regions or provinces provided services that were complementary or supplementary to the mainstream medical system. These healers, who included herbalists, witch doctors, and barber-surgeons, were mostly men who received a fee for services in the form of money or a food item. Women skilled in the art of divination and removal of the power of the evil eye (*malocchio*) also practiced their art in return for a small fee. These types of folk healers are generally absent today, although a number of women who have learned techniques of curing illnesses attributed to the evil eye still carry out this symbolic mode of healing. Now, however, the elaborate procedures of the past have generally been replaced by a simplified form of treatment. The appropriate incantations, which are taught to the initiate only on Christmas Eve, are simply said while tracing the sign of the cross over the affected body part.

Illness prevention measures using symbolic notions are extremely rare in contemporary society. Amulets once worn to ward off the evil eye are now referred to as "good luck charms," and charms to prevent infectious diseases have fallen into disuse. Occasionally people do revert to traditional remedies when they become disillusioned or impatient with prescribed modern therapeutic regimens. Some incantations, prayers, and signs of the cross are made which have lost their association with the evil eye but which retain meaning for the intercession of saints and divine providence. In these cases, mothers play the primary role of healer, since these measures are generally carried out for children who have minor but distressing ailments that are not thought to require medical intervention.

Parish priests and local pharmacists also act as sources of care outside the home. The parish priest is most likely to be consulted for help with disciplinary problems, especially with sons. Often, too, priests are asked for a referral to a mental health clinic or psychiatrist. In general, however, the personality of the priest and the degree to which he is perceived as approachable determine his role in mental health matters. Unfortunately, I collected few data on the use of pharmacists in the enclave. I suspect, however, that they are used for diagnosis and referral more by males than females.

Exemption from Role Responsibilities

Family members are exempted from some tasks associated with their roles if the tasks cannot be performed comfortably. Thus, a child may be relieved of responsibility for attending school or church, and this decision is made either independently by the parents or in consultation with kin or neighbors. Sick leave and disability compensations help to case the financial burden when a breadwinner must assume a sick role.

The assumption of the sick role is probably most difficult for the wife/mother, especially when there are infants or small children. Reciprocal exchange networks for child care and meal preparation are characteristic among family, kin, and neighbors within ethnic enclaves, but these supports are probably not as available to upwardly mobile families living in the suburbs. However, in these cases a parent of one of the spouses, usually the mother but occasionally a father, will assume care of the children, even if it means traveling to a distant city.

In general, once a person assumes a dependent role, he has entered, with or without competent medical help, the "sick" role. Since people's definition of a healthy state is optimal capacity to carry out valued tasks and roles, sickness is acceptance of the inability to function in these capacities (see Zola 1964:353–354; Ragucci 1971:155–160). Most Italian Americans experience distress about the dependence imposed on them when they are sick, however. They also state that sickness imposes "obligations." However, the term *soggezione,* rather than the verb *obbligare* ("to enter into an obligation," "to bind oneself"), is used to describe this situation. The various meanings of *soggezione* are "subjection," "uneasiness," or "embarrassment," thus implying an imbalance in rights and obligations associated with the sick role. This discomfort over the dependence and obligations entailed in the sick role is important in motivating the patient to relinquish the role.

Encounters with Mainstream Medical Practitioners

Medical Settings

Urban Italians generally prefer voluntary to municipal or "city" hospitals for in-hospital care. Municipal hospitals are shunned by older people because of the connotation of charity and the notion that patients are used for experimentation, whereas they feel that in proprietary or voluntary hospitals, patient care is more often under the supervision of one's own physician. For serious illnesses or major surgery, people of all generations prefer either a "specialist" who is on the staff of a large medical center or teaching hospital or a private hospital with religious affiliation. Today most working-class Italian-American families are covered by some form of hospitalization insurance and can thus exercise some choice in the selection of hospital facility and physician. Medicare benefits for the elderly and disabled and Medicaid assistance for those who qualify mitigate the financial burden imposed by sickness.

Ambulatory care needs in the urban community that I studied were met mainly in the outpatient department (41 percent of all visits by residents to medical facilities in the early 1970s). Private physicians accounted for 28 percent of all visits; a neighborhood health center, 14 percent; and emergency rooms, 14 percent. Private dental services were used by 82 percent of families, and the remaining 18 percent used dental clinics at adjacent hospitals or dental schools (Jones and Gold 1974:152).

Although the bulk of patient visits in the enclave were to outpatient clinics, private care was generally preferred. The feeling of low status engendered by the use of outpatient and ward services was in the past and is to some extent today mitigated by the use of a prestigious voluntary hospital located near the enclave. Thus both the reputation and the location of a health facility play a large part in the selection of settings for care, and the accounts of illness experiences, discussed earlier, frequently include estimates of the prestige of the facility (Ragucci 1971:143; Jones and Gold 1974).

For general medical problems the elderly, as well as recent immigrants, prefer a physician who speaks and understands Italian and whose ancestors derive, if possible, from the same town or region. In contrast, those born in America tend to disregard the ethnic affiliation or nativity of the physician (or dentist). The handicapped and elderly infirm use local health services and personnel whenever possible. Most also feel that physicians should make house calls, and the choice of a local practitioner often depends on his willingness to provide this service.

People will resort to the use of a chiropractor or osteopath when treatment by a family physician or specialist is perceived as either slow to show results or of no benefit. The frequency with which Italian Americans resort to these practitioners is not known. In general, men in the second generation appear to use their services more than do women or those in the parental generation for treatment of such conditions as low back pain and persistent headaches.

Expectations in the Medical Encounter

Recurring themes in people's expectations of medical care include a desire for safe, competent care administered in a clean, well-ordered environment by empathic health professionals (Ragucci 1971). Health professionals are often evaluated as being either *simpatico* ("warm," "pleasant," "congenial") or *superbo* ("proud," "arrogant," "unapproachable").

Italian Americans in the enclave I studied wanted information from the physician in language they could understand. This expectation, that physicians should educate and explain matters to their patients, may be carried over from medical practice in Italy. Observations during field research in an Italian village (Ragucci 1975) revealed that the villagers, in contrast to their counterparts in America, knew more both about untoward signs and symptoms associated with antihypertensive medications and abnormal laboratory values such as those associated with an elevated blood urea nitrogen level and blood sugar. In fact, they referred to the former condition by the biomedical term "azotemia." In addition to deriving such information from their physicians, people in the village were also given copies of laboratory test results to take with them to specialists when such referral was necessary. Moreover, it was customary for local pharmacists to dispense medicines in the original package, which gave detailed information about the action, dosage, untoward effects, and other contraindications of the drug. From this information villagers were able over time to associate certain signs and symptoms as well as their sense of well-being to the action and adverse effects of the prescribed medication or therapy.

Like their counterparts in Italy, Italian Americans in general want clear, explicit explanations about disease, its cause (or causes), the organ affected, the reasons for the symptoms they experience, and the expected duration of the illness or symptoms and of the convalescent period. A physician familiar with the health-care needs of Italian Americans has observed that more patient compliance, family support, and ease in dealing with Italian illness behavior result if the professional concentrates on etiological factors that do not carry any sense of blame or guilt (D. Minotti, personal communication). Patients appreciate the time taken by nurses and physicians in drawing diagrams showing the site of pathology or the specific surgical intervention. Men and women raised in rural areas easily apply their knowledge of the anatomy and physiology of domestic animals to the human body. In addition, like their compatriots in Italy, Italian Americans prefer to be informed about their blood pressure readings when being treated for hypertension. The use of numbers provides a concrete measure by which they are able to compare progress in treatment and to "explain" certain bodily feelings, which may or may not have been the result of hypertension or drug therapy.

The knowledge imparted by health professionals is reinterpreted by patients and their relatives and incorporated into the narrative accounts of illness that are transmitted to other laymen. In this way, health education by a professional has a multiplicative effect in reaching many people. Distortion or misinterpretation may occur, however, with negative consequences for the evaluation of specific professionals or hospitals; indeed, mistrust or suspicion of professional competence may result.

The following example illustrates both the mistrust of professional competence that can arise from inadequate medical explanations and the corrective and educative function that adequate explanations can have. It derives from a conversation among immigrant, second-generation, and third-generation Italian Americans who were discussing the recent death of a neighbor. The woman had died after several days' hospitalization for a "stroke," and the issue involves the failure of the attending physician to explain the difference between hypostatic pneumonia and pneumonia of bacterial or viral origin.

Mrs. A.:   Mary [sister of the deceased] said the young doctor [a medical resident] told the family that V. died from pneumonia. She didn't even have a cold, so Mary wonders how she could have gotten pneumonia.

Mrs. B.:   You know that she came all the way to _____ Hospital from the hospital on the Cape [where she had been stricken while on vacation]. Maybe she caught cold from a draft in the ambulance or from outside [air].

Mrs. A.:   Do you believe that? I've never heard of such a thing [getting pneumonia without the prodromal symptom of a cold]. I wonder why the doctor would say such a thing. Are you sure that's what he said? She's never had any trouble with her chest.

Mrs. C.:   When I had my gallbladder operation the nurses told me I had to move my legs and take some deep breaths. If I didn't my blood would slow down, and I would have trouble bringing up phlegm to clean out the air passages. They said lying still in bed without moving or getting up would cause pneumonia . . . It hurt to cough, like a sharp knife, but I did it. They were always reminding you to cough and take deep breaths . . . Maybe that's what happened to V. The day I went to see her she couldn't move or talk. She just lay there on her side . . . (Ragucci 1971, unpublished field notes)

Interactional Norms in Encounters with Health Professionals

GENERAL FACTORS   Norms for interaction that influence encounters with health professionals vary according to the age of both the recipient and the provider of care, the social class of the recipient, and the prestige, sex, and ethnicity of the caregiver. Elderly men and women tend to have more confidence in professionals in the older age categories, and mistakes in dosage or treatment are often attributed by the elderly to young interns, nursing students, or laboratory technicians.

In comparison with Irish and Anglo-Saxon ethnics of the working class, Italian Americans of the same class were reported in one study to present their symptoms in a more diffuse manner (Zola 1964:352–353; 1966). Although all patients compared in the study had the same diagnosis, Italian Americans did not localize their symptoms as much, reported more pain, presented more symptoms to the doctor, and were more vocal about the emotional and interpersonal consequences of their conditions. As a result, their symptoms were more frequently attributed by physicians to emotional causes when no organic pathology could be detected (Zola 1964:357). This openness of Italian Americans in discussing the emotional and interpersonal aspects of their symptoms is consistent with the finding that they tend to seek medical care when their symptoms have either precipitated an "interpersonal crisis" or threatened to interfere with valued social activities (Zola 1964:353–354). In other words, they simply present the totality of their problem as they see it, from the physical symptoms to the emotional or social disturbances that have tended to trigger their visit. Whether or not organic disease can be found, the health professional's responsibility with Italian-American patients who present symptoms in this manner should optimally involve responding to this total problem and therefore probing the nature of the correlated social disturbances reported by the patient and attending to the effects of the disturbances on the patient's life situation. For example, the physician might indicate that it is all right for the patient to miss a certain number of days from work because of the illness, in order to validate the patient's nonobservance of expected roles (D. Minotti, personal communication).

An additional cultural value that may in general influence interaction between health-care workers and Italian-American recipients of care is the attitude of "shame" or "modesty" (*vergogna*). The behaviors and attitudes associated with this value are expressed in diverse social and cultural contexts. With regard to medical matters, the use of euphemisms has already been mentioned. Embarrassment and reticence in discussing disorders of the female and male genitourinary system with professionals of the opposite sex is an example that is particularly relevant to patient-professional interactions. In addition, because of feelings of *vergogna* the majority of women also prefer a female physician or nurse for care of obstetrical and gynecological problems. In contrast to most urban American medical centers, in Italy midwives assume major responsibility for prenatal care, childbirth, and postnatal care. Thus, cultural discontinuity in this country increases problems inherent in client-professional relationships already characterized by social and cultural distance.

INTERACTIONS WITH PHYSICIANS   For physicians interested in treating their patients' illnesses as well as their diseases, Italian Americans tend to make very agreeable patients, since they not only generally expect to have their illnesses attended to but also are quite open in presenting their view of the problem. Indeed, data on Italian-American working-class males indicate that they, at any rate, neither like nor respond well to physicians who assume an authoritarian, impersonal, and uncommunicative manner, and they even report having difficulty describing their symptoms to such professionals (Gans 1962:138). In general, it can be said that Italian Americans of the working class share blue-collar attitudes toward American medical services in regarding them with a combination of skepticism about physicians' competence yet respect and admiration for technological advances in biomedicine (Gans 1962:141; Zola 1964).

INTERACTIONS WITH NURSES   On the whole, Italian Americans share a rather rigid role definition of the nurse's function and ignore variations in clinical specialty and educational levels within the profession. Nursing functions are perceived mainly in terms of specific tasks, such as giving baths, administering injections, and performing procedures considered aesthetically unpleasant, such as colostomy irrigations or changing dressings—that is, tasks generally performed by hospital or visiting nurses. This narrow role perception was found to exist in the Boston community studied, even when people had had direct experience with other nursing activities through contact with school and health department personnel. The independent role of the nurse in health teaching and guidance was also not acknowledged. In essence, a nurse is perceived by Italian Americans as one who carries out a physician's orders rather than as a professional who, through education and clinical practice, possesses the ability to provide information and make judgments about health care independent of the physician.

This is not to say, however, that the nurse's knowledge, derived especially through experience in hospital settings, is totally unrecognized in the Italian-American community, and nurses (particularly those who are related by kinship and neighborhood ties) form part of patients' therapy managing groups. Nurses may be sought to validate physicians' prescribed regimens as well as to explain or clarify medical information. In general, however, nursing actions and health teaching are viewed by most laymen of Italian origin as extensions of medical care rather than as health care in its own right.

A consequence of the marked discrepancy between professional and laymen's perceptions of the nursing role is that nursing actions directed toward assisting people to resume activities of daily living (that is, giving up the sick role) lack credibility and authority (Ragucci 1971:147–152). Moreover, as nurses assume more independent roles within the health-care system for health maintenance (as opposed to cure of disease, the physician's major domain), the gap between professional and lay expectations of the nurse must be addressed if their performance in roles such as clinical nurse specialist or nurse-practitioner is to be effective.

INTERACTIONS WITH SOCIAL WORKERS   The role of the social worker is also not fully understood by many Italian Americans, and the attitude toward them is essentially ambivalent. Many families have their first contact with this category of professional during particularly stressful circumstances (for example, when experiencing difficulty in meeting the financial needs of the family). People are generally uncomfortable in their interactions with social workers, and this uneasiness may reflect not only differences in social class but also cultural attitudes toward receiving help outside the social group, as well as suspicion of their investigative or interviewing techniques, which often explore sensitive areas of personal or family life.

Diagnoses That Provoke Strong Emotional Reactions

Two diseases have particularly strong emotional and social overtones for Italian Americans: tuberculosis and cancer. The special meaning of these diseases can best be seen in the elaborate preventive measures carried out for tuberculosis and in the reluctance on the part of Italian Americans to discuss or acknowledge the presence of these illnesses in themselves or their families. Health professionals who are explaining a diagnosis of one of these diseases to a patient or who even suspect such a diagnosis should be aware of the following information.

TUBERCULOSIS   Tuberculosis (*tisi* in medical terminology, more popularly called *la tisica*) is a disease familiar to Italians from their home country. In Italy the Ministry of Public Health has maintained special anti-tuberculosis services with offices in every province (the *Consorzi Provinciali Antituberculosi*) since 1927. Furthermore, more than half the population is covered by compulsory tuberculosis insurance (Carlyle 1965:791). However, since Italian Americans have shared in the general decline in the incidence of tuberculosis over the past 20 years, their continuing fear of this disease appears to be a case of cultural lag.[6] Past experience with the disease (for example, prolonged hospitalization in sanitoriums and rigid isolation to prevent spread) have served to instill a culturally transmitted fear of the disease and to perpetuate the practice of avoiding or isolating sufferers socially, contrary to contemporary biomedical practice.

CANCER   The entity cancer, unlike tuberculosis, is a relatively new concept for Italian Americans, especially for older persons of the immigrant and second generations. As a result, they have particular difficulty comprehending the nature of the disease. The word "tumor," used by most health professionals when giving people diagnostic information about the disease, is interpreted by laymen to mean a growth or increase in size of a body organ. It is therefore difficult for the elderly to reconcile this idea with the progressive "wasting away" they perceive in friends and relatives in the terminal stage of the illness.

During my field research in an Italian-American urban community, I also noted that cancer was seldom mentioned by name. When inquiring of informants in a variety of social settings about the reason for another person's hospitalization or surgery, I was frequently told that the person had "you know what." This secrecy and reluctance to admit or disclose the diagnosis of cancer may be related to its stigmatization as a terminal illness as well as to several other notions about the disease that were prevalent in the community—namely, that cancer is contagious, inherited, or of supernatural origin as a punishment for sin.

Fertility and Birth Control among Italian Americans

One may infer from the available data that Italian Americans are not averse to family planning and limitation of family size. Although the impoverished Italian immigrants of the peak migration years had exceptionally large families, second-generation daughters reversed the pattern (Femminella and Quadagno 1978). The available data for Boston and New York reveal that not only do second-generation Italian-American women have on the average fewer than half the number of children of the immigrant generation, they also have borne fewer children on the average than Americans of native parentage (Rosenwaike 1973:275). Rosenwaike has attributed this reversal in childbearing patterns to strong assimilationist pressures. However, Gambino (1974) maintains that second-generation women limited family size for the traditional reason of promoting the economic well-being of the family: "They had children in proportion to their family incomes in America, where economic realities punished families with many children. They and their husbands decided it was better for the family to limit its number of children" (1974:163–164).

The trend toward limiting family size continues for the third generation, in spite of the fact that the majority of Italians are Catholic. In a national survey Ryder and Westoff (1971) reported that of all Catholic ethnic groups, Italians were most likely to use contraceptive methods other than the rhythm method. My empirical observations in the ethnic enclave, as well as the fertility rates reported for the area by Jones and Gold (1974), support these conclusions. A variety of family planning measures are in current usage among Italian Americans, which vary according to generation. At the time of my research, the oral contraceptive and the intrauterine device were preferred by third-generation Italian-American women. Recent immigrants in the childbearing years reported that birth control measures were mainly the husband's responsibility rather than the wife's. Recent immigrants of middle age reported that they and their peers in Italy prolonged breast-feeding and deferred weaning for two or more years as the chief means of controlling family size. Although the frequency of the practice is not known, recent immigrants (especially those from the regions of Abruzzi and Molise) prefer tubal ligation after the birth of the third or fourth child. Thus, health professionals should be prepared for Italian Americans to seek family planning and birth control information.

Adherence to Biomedical Treatment

There are no studies of compliance or cooperation in treatment regimens for Italian Americans as a group. However, inferences can be made from some of the descriptive data available. As a general rule, people are more likely to cooperate with prescribed treatment if behavior changes do not conflict with cherished social activities and cultural values and if the gap between professional knowledge and layman's knowledge is closed by adequate teaching.

With regard to compliance with orders for medication, the elderly are especially wary of modern drug preparations and are critical of physicians who prescribe "too many medicines." Analgesic medications are often regarded as narcotic, and a fear of habituation results in modification of prescribed dosages. Idiosyncratic or untoward effects may lead to categorizing the prescribed medicine as "no good" or to blaming the physician for ordering the "wrong medicine." Italian Americans, like other patients, may prematurely discontinue therapy either when improvement has occurred or when the expected effect is not perceived.

An additional problem that may arise in patients' following through on a prescribed treatment regimen is the substitution of one element or preparation for the prescribed substance. Usually the two substances are perceived as having the same effects—for example, substitution of a breakfast drink advertised as high in vitamin C content for orange juice by people on diuretics. Since the potassium content of orange juice and not the vitamin C is the critical ingredient, untoward effects may result from this practice. A similar instance occurred when soybean oil and soybean milk were equated because of the common soybean base.

Dietary Patterns and Dietary Regimens

Food customs and preferences among Italians show little change from generation to generation. "Heavy" and "light," "wet" and "dry," "acid" and "non-acid" are the major categories of contrast applied in discussing food.

HEAVY/LIGHT   The contrast of "heavy" and "light" refers to the difficulty or ease with which foods are believed to be digested, and the classification depends on both the food itself and the manner of preparation. Thus, fried foods, beef, and pork are considered "heavy," and gelatin, custard, cooked fruit, rice, and soup with the fat skimmed off are all considered "light." "Light" foods are seen as providing a rest for the digestive tract and are therefore taken when people are ill. These beliefs and practices accord closely with standard medical practice concerning diet.

WET/DRY   The Greco-Roman humoral concept of wet/dry qualities is mentioned more often in connection with the maintenance of a healthy state among Italian Americans than are hot/cold attributes. The wet/dry quality of foods refers both to their mode of preparation and to the food substance itself. The typical American meal of meat with gravy, potatoes, and cooked, buttered vegetables is considered too "dry." However, the same kinds of foods would be rendered "wet" if they were prepared in a meat soup base with vegetables such as celery, escarole, cabbage, or spinach (that is, a minestrone).

Traditional Italian-American housewives serve at least one "wet" meal per week for its laxative effect (in order to "clean the system"). Such "wet" foods as escarole and other leafy vegetables are seen as particularly effective in keeping the lower digestive tract in a proper state of hydration. Since some Italian Americans believe that the body is particularly "dry" when one is sick, serving "wet" therapeutic soups is seen as one way to promote a return to health. Furthermore, because meals served in hospitals and nursing homes are generally considered too "dry," family members supplement hospital meals by taking patients homemade therapeutic soups. The ingredients of these soups contain the essentials for proper nutrition, although the families of patients on low-sodium or low-cholesterol diets should be instructed to omit salt or to use chicken in place of ham or beef in preparing these foods.

ACID BALANCE   Skin ailments are believed by Italian Americans to be caused by an excess of acid in the body. Citrus fruits, raw tomatoes, and peaches are identified as the chief culprits and eliminated from the diet.

In addition, dairy products and wines are said not to "mix" and to cause "acid" in the stomach. For this reason, adults reserve milk consumption for between-meal or bedtime snacks.

THERAPEUTIC DIETS   In following treatment regimens, Italian Americans experience the most difficulty in modifying long-standing food habits. The difficulty is strongly related to the social significance of food in this ethnic group. Thus, to be on a therapeutic diet means to the Italian American not only that he must drastically modify lifelong habits but also that the dieter must curtail valued social activities. Some people on a diabetic diet, for example, may not admit that they have *la malattia dello zucchero* because of the social consequences of being unable to participate fully in the round of neighborhood visits where coffee and pastry are customarily served. With respect to these diets, there is also a generally poor understanding of the caloric content of foods, and the word "dietetic" on labels of prepared foods is interpreted by the majority (including people who do not necessarily read the fine print) to mean that the particular food can be consumed in unlimited quantity.

Regimens for hypertension may also cause special problems for Italian Americans, largely because of certain conceptions about high blood pressure. Many Italian Americans contrast "low blood," which may refer to either anemia or low blood pressure, with "high blood," which may refer to hypertension, "too much blood," or "too rich" blood. Because these conditions are seen as being opposite in nature, foods that are considered to be therapeutic for one are contraindicated for the other. For example, beef, liver, and eggs—all good for "low blood"—are believed to be unsuitable for victims of "high blood." In the case of the aforementioned foods, the belief agrees with biomedical restrictions in low-cholesterol diets; however, other sources of protein recommended for "low blood" would be unnecessarily contraindicated for persons with "high blood" or hypertension.

The elderly in particular have difficulty in understanding diet therapy and nutrition in general. Their vocabulary does not include such words as calorie, vitamin, or carbohydrate, and their ideas about the contents of different foods are primarily based on sensory qualities such as appearance and taste. Thus, diabetics may curtail their use of sugar and sweet desserts, but they do not comprehend why fruits with a tart taste (for example, grapefruit) are also restricted. Similarly, those on low-sodium diets usually use the criterion of salty taste to decide which foods to avoid and therefore experience difficulty in comprehending why meat and certain vegetables are contraindicated or limited.

In addition to these general difficulties with therapeutic diets, idiosyncratic interpretations of food restrictions may also produce modifications or adaptations in prescribed diets. For example, one informant justified serving tuna fish canned in soybean oil to her husband, who was on a low-fat diet and had refused tuna canned in water, with the following explanation: "When my grandson was small, he was allergic to milk and the doctor ordered soybean milk. If soybean is good for little babies, then it is all right for a grown man."

Notwithstanding the aforementioned problems with therapeutic diets, Italian folklore reflects an understanding of nutrition that at times corresponds to biomedical conceptions. Thus, customary gifts of food to the sick include oranges, fresh eggs, and fruits—foods that are believed to facilitate the healing of postoperative wounds. Liver, red wine, and dark green leafy vegetables are said to be "good for the blood," and a high intake of dairy products is believed to "make the urine hard" and lead to kidney stones.

Recovery, Rehabilitation, and Death

Recovery and Resumption of Normal Roles

The ability to relinquish the sick role and resume an independent role depends on a person's capacity to undertake the activities of daily living. People who are employed in jobs that require exposure to inclement weather, especially the cold, may (because of the aforementioned concerns about drafts and wind) delay return to gainful employment. Resumption of work activities may also be delayed if the patient stands to gain secondary benefits from it. Sick leave and disability benefits, which ensure the maintenance of a certain economic level, might in some cases delay return to the ranks of the well until benefits are used up. In addition, the blue-collar jobs in which many first- and second-generation men and women are employed often entitle people to larger compensation payments than their wages. Thus once a person is on the disability rolls, there may be disincentives for getting off. Resumption of the work role means losing Medicare coverage, even though expenses for continuing medical care are still being incurred. Many workers believe that once they are off the disability roll, it may be difficult to get back on; thus the sick role may be extended beyond the time of recovery.

Today in the more secular urban environment, recovery from a critical illness is not usually marked by special rites or celebrations. However, for immigrants of the first generation (both of the peak and the recent migration—especially those who were raised in an agrarian region), masses of thanksgiving "for a favor received" may still be requested by churchgoers. Older Italian Americans generally place more emphasis on divine intervention as the cause of recovery from illness than do younger people. Most older and recent immigrants from rural villages and towns believe in miraculous cures, and saints are seen as mediators between

God and man. Two categories of saint-healers are recognized: the "specialists" and the "generalists." The former receive petitions for intercession and help in healing specific disorders. For example, St. Rocco is the patron saint for surgical wounds and skin ulcerations, St. Blais for throat ailments, and St. Lucy for eye disorders. "Generalist" saints (for example, St. Anthony and St. Joseph) provide intervention when spiritual help is needed for a variety of health problems. In general, Italians view the roles of saints and physicians as complementary, however. Recovery from a serious illness is almost always attributed to a miracle brought about by the timely intervention of both saint and doctor.

Chronic Disease and Death

With regard to terminal illness, the attitude of fatalism ascribed by some social scientists to Italian Americans (Kluckhohn 1963; Spiegel 1972) is better viewed as the end stage of a process of unsuccessful action against adversity than as an all-pervasive resignation to incapacitation or death (see also Gans 1962:140). This statement of a 72-year-old widow mourning the death of her husband from cancer is typical:[7] "We have done all that we could to make him better . . . He had the best doctors . . . He was in the best hospital . . . He had all the medicines . . . We could do no more . . . It was his destiny to die this way" (Ragucci 1971:199).

It is difficult to make generalizations about deciding whether or not to disclose information about a poor prognosis, choosing the appropriate time, and determining the content of such a disclosure. I have observed that the manner in which disclosure is made is often more important than either the "if" or the "when" issue. People have voiced resentment toward physicians who give information in what is perceived as a cold, abrupt, or impersonal way. Others, both the patient and family members, mention with surprise and pleasure that the physician "took the time to sit down" with them to talk about the situation. Families and patients also appreciate receiving information about medical, nursing, and self-care measures that can be taken to reduce the pain and discomfort of the dying person in the home setting.

In immigrant families the oldest adult son is the person who usually assumes the responsibility of communicating with the physician about a parent's condition. Young immigrant families who lack English skills rely on relatives, ritual kin (that is, godparents, *compari*), or friends for translation and support. Disclosure of information about impending death or a poor prognosis, however, is probably best accomplished by assembling the entire family and informing them. At that time family feelings and attitudes about the manner of disclosing the prognosis to the dying person can be elicited and then acted upon.

Meeting with all family members also provides the physician and other health professionals the opportunity of assisting the family in dealing with feelings of blame or accusations of irresponsible behavior toward one another (D. Minotti, personal communication). In these situations the health-care professional's biomedical explanation of the etiology of the disease, accompanied by remarks on the inevitability of death (for example, mentioning "God's will"), frequently helps to quell accusations that arise from feelings of guilt. Reassurance that family members have fulfilled their obligations to the sick and dying and have "done the right things" is an approach that would be helpful to Italian Americans of all generational categories and social classes.

Religious and social ceremonies facilitate people's coming to terms with the ultimate reality of the death of a loved one. The mourning process and associated grief work for Italian Americans often involve participation in masses for the dead, beginning with the funeral mass and often followed by annual masses on the anniversary of the death. Health professionals may participate in the rituals and customs associated with mourning by sending a sympathy card or attending the wake, the funeral mass, or one of the masses which relatives or friends customarily request at the parish church. A telephone call to a widowed spouse or bereaved parents two or three weeks after the funeral is also important in helping people deal with feelings of guilt or remorse which may be part of the grieving process.

The custom of *lo consolo,* the meal prepared and served to the bereaved family by friends or relatives on the day of burial, is still carried out in some form by Italian Americans of all generational groups. Essentially the custom functions to express group solidarity and to reintegrate social ties among the living.

Suggestions for Professional Interventions

The goals of health professionals include two major tasks: first, to ascertain the nature and extent of the discrepancy or disparity that may exist between the viewpoints and goals of the layman and the professional, the "little" tradition and the "great" tradition of medicine; and second, to evaluate the consequences of a cultural group's basic premises about health maintenance and restoration on the actions (self-directed or professionally prescribed) taken for care and cure. In light of this information, professional interventions may then be directed toward reinforcing positive health-seeking behaviors and eliminating those with undesirable consequences.

The reader is advised that in spite of the guides to professional interventions that are implied in this account of health beliefs and actions, there are no convenient formulas or generalizations about Italian Americans that can relieve health professionals of their responsibility for a careful assessment of the health care needs of each patient or client. The heterogeneity of Italian Americans—a function of many variables including time of immigration, generation in America, region of origin, rural or urban derivation, residence in suburbia or an urban ethnic enclave, social class (income, education, and occupation), specific illness experiences, and the state of medical technology and science at different stages of people's life cycle—precludes easy generalizations and stereotyping. Given this diversity, health-care providers might do well to consider whether particular behaviors and beliefs they observe may be culturally derived and thus common for the group, or whether they are socially determined (for example, due to social class influences rather than ethnic determinants) or idiosyncratic (that is, unique and applicable only to the individual). In spite of these important caveats on overgeneralizing from the data provided, a number of strategies may be employed for working with the real cultural differences that exist.

Problems in Communication of Health-Care Needs and Symptoms

Barriers to effective health care have been identified especially for the Italian-speaking immigrant generation and the blue-collar workers who comprise a large part of the second generation.

LANGUAGE PROBLEMS AND USE OF INTERPRETERS   The lack of fluency in English may lead health professionals to underestimate immigrant Italians' ability to understand the nature of their problems and the rationale of prescribed therapy. Interpreters are usually recruited from the patient's neighborhood or kin group to act as chief informants and intermediaries; they are depended on by Italian speakers to present to the physician or nurse as complete information as possible about the "chief" complaint. My observations reveal the existence of an informal process by which people judge the interpreter's skills as reliable and trustworthy. Indeed, judgments about accurate reporting may be more problematic for health professionals than for patients. Rephrasing questions and allowing time for review, clarification, and validation of symptoms before termination of the office or clinic visit may ensure more accurate interpretation of information.

Furthermore, because of a sense of *vergogna,* modesty, and privacy, a patient may find it difficult to share her symptoms with an interpreter employed by the health agency. Translation by close family members or a trusted neighbor may alleviate this problem.

PROBLEMS RELATED TO ALLOCATION OF TIME   Second-generation Italian Americans, particularly those in blue-collar occupations, tend to report symptoms in ways that differ from middle-class norms. As described earlier, they tend to report more symptoms (Croog 1961) than do other ethnics with whom they have been compared and to phrase or describe complaints in terms of interference with social and interpersonal relationships. As a consequence, physicians tend to diagnose emotional problems more often for Italian Americans than for those of different ethnicity (Zola 1973).

Both translation issues among immigrants and the patterned manner of reporting symptoms among second-generation Italian Americans indicate that health professionals must be prepared to spend a substantial amount of time with patients and their families. The constraints placed on private practice and clinic appointment schedules may be formidable. However, professionals can help the patient focus on the salient features of illness episodes that have triggered the decision to see the physician or consult the nurse practitioner.

Moreover, structuring people's expectations about threatening events, such as surgery or intrusive medical procedures, can be done by presenting the procedure in a systematic manner, devoid of technical jargon. Explicit descriptions about the normal or usual sensations or reactions either to specific medical or surgical therapies or to a diagnostic category may also help to allay people's concerns and decrease telephone inquiries by anxious relatives to physicians and hospital units.

Culturally Relevant Health-Care Instruction for Long-Term Care

The teaching of nursing techniques for patients with long-term or terminal illness is best done with the family as a whole, rather than with one individual. In this way, the burden of daily care, especially of an aging parent, can be shared among siblings and their spouses. Admission to a nursing home can be avoided or delayed if health-care professionals consider the family's preference for home care and teach family members such measures as hygienic care of the skin and mouth, prevention of pressure sores, transfer techniques, provision for nutritional and fluid needs, and both active and passive exercises.

The services of the Visiting Nurse Association, as well as those incorporated under the hospice concept, would be acceptable to Italian Americans, particularly in coping with problems of persons in terminal stages of cancer.

Cooperation in Carrying Out Medical and Nursing Prescriptions

The experiences of Italian Americans with illness reveal that in general they are motivated to seek explanations and to understand the cause and effect relationships that underlie illness episodes. Analysis of people's "stories" or narratives reveal that they engage in a perceptual-interpretive process by which they incorporate information from a number of sources. The acceptance, modification, or rejection of a prescribed mode of therapy or health instruction depends on the meaning or relevancy it has for them.

No research has been carried out that differentiates Italian Americans from others in regard to compliance or cooperation with medical prescriptions. The high frequency with which I noted peoples' modification of dietary and other prescriptions in the community studied may be in part explained by inadequate or irrelevant teaching by health professionals. The following interventions are suggested:

1. Graphic illustrations and models should be used for teaching anatomy, physiology, and pathophysiology of specific organ systems.
2. Food portions should be concretely illustrated (for example, one cup of various types of pasta placed on a dinner plate) as part of dietary instruction.
3. In discussing the diabetic exchange list and low-sodium diets in particular, one should specifically discuss culturally relevant and valued foods.
4. Brochures and other literature prepared by pharmaceutical companies should be distributed by the physician, pharmacist, or nurse in order that patients may have additional sources of information about prescription medications—their actions, intended and untoward effects, and so on.

In conclusion, the most general advice one can give a health professional treating an Italian-American (or indeed any other ethnic) patient is to recognize and reinforce cultural health-caring behaviors that have positive consequences for health maintenance and cure.

Notes

The study of the Italian-American enclave reported in this chapter was supported by a grant from the National Institutes of Health, U.S. Department of Health, Education and Welfare. The comparative material from Southern Italy was gathered under a grant from the American Philosophical Society. I wish to acknowledge the helpful comments of Charles A. Dinarello, M.D., and Dominick A. Minotti, M.D., who read the chapter in draft form.

1. The South of Italy includes the regions of Lazio, south of the province of Rome, Abruzzi and Molise, Campania, Puglia, Basilicato, Calabria, the islands of Sicily and Sardinia, and several smaller islands.

2. Since so many of the data presented in this chapter derive from an Italian-American enclave in Boston, it would be useful if we could compare it to other "Little Italies" in the United States to see how representative this particular one is, at least in terms of standard demographic indexes. Unfortunately, however, I could find no comparable data for the same time period with which to compare the Boston data. In lieu of comparative information from other Italian-American urban enclaves, I will therefore present some basic demographic data on the study area which the reader may use in comparing my findings to any other similar enclave.

The enclave studied is commonly known as the North End. With a total population of 11,271 people (Jones and Gold 1974:155), it is predominantly a working-class community. The median family income for the area was $8,395 in 1970, slightly below the Boston average of $9,133. In spite of this relatively low median family income, however, only 9 percent of the families in the area were on public assistance (as compared to 13.8 percent for Boston as a whole). The median number of school years completed by persons 25 and over was 7.5. The neighborhood ranked twentieth out of twenty-one in percentage of adults completing high school—30 percent compared to 54 percent for Boston as a whole. The average number of children per family was 0.8, and the percentage of people 65 years of age and older was 14.3, compared with a Boston average of 12.8. The residential stability of the area is attested by the fact that 59 percent of the population over 5 years of age lived in the same house in 1965 and 1970. On the whole, the statistics reflect an area oriented to older age groups which, although fairly stable and family-oriented, is losing the younger generation, who are choosing to live elsewhere.

3. I am indebted to Dominick Minotti, M.D., for his insight and interpretation of the cultural themes in these data concerning exculpation and its association and expression through norms of "proper" behavior. He has also provided a number of other valuable suggestions that have been incorporated into the text.

4 Although I did not study blood beliefs in great detail, some data on concepts about these various dichotomous states of the blood were obtained, mainly from older immigrant and second-generation people. "Strong" blood is associated with youth and physical vigor, and "weak" blood with old age, when the blood is said to become more watery. Since the characteristics of offspring are thought to be determined by the blood, elderly parents are said to produce puny offspring because of their "weak" blood. Mixing of similar blood (for example, through marriage between cousins) is said to produce blood in the child that is "too strong," in which the additive quality of the two bloods produces physical deformities or mental retardation. Little information was obtained on "hot" or "cold" blood, although Gans, working in an enclave adjacent to mine, reports that both peptic ulcer and high blood pressure were attributed to "hot" blood (1962:139). "Good" blood generally refers to favorable heritable qualities or a hard-working, stable family. "Bad" blood, on the other hand, may refer both to potential breeding capacity and to disease states, in which the blood is believed to have been infected and must be either drawn or flushed out of the body. Finally, "high" blood may refer either to high blood pressure or to blood that is too "rich"; "low" blood refers to both low blood pressure and anemia. The high/low combination, which is common in various ethnic groups, may lead to compliance problems or a credibility gap between patient and physician if both high blood pressure and anemia should be diagnosed, since in the popular view "high" and "low" blood are mutually exclusive conditions.

5. In areas where malaria was endemic, Italian peasants were unable to live on or near the lowlands they cultivated. Although this land was the most fertile, it was also the most malarial. In response to the threat of malaria, grouping of houses on hilltops became a feature of agrarian towns. People

walked to and from the fields during daylight hours and spent the period from dusk to dawn in the comparative safety of their towns (Foerster 1919:61).

6. Health status data for the enclave that I studied indicated the incidence of tuberculosis was far below city-wide norms in 1973. Only 9 cases per 100,000 were reported that year as compared to 41 per 100,000 for the city as a whole (Jones and Gold 1974: 151–152, 156).

7. The cultural dynamic of exculpation ("it is not my fault and please don't blame me") may also be read in the widow's statement. An additional expression of the inevitability of death, in which fatalism is coupled this time with an empirical assessment of the probable consequences of treatment, comes from a 61-year-old second-generation woman in the terminal stages of cancer. The woman had refused chemotherapy on the ground that she had known people who had had "chemo": "I saw how they suffered, sores in their mouths, bleeding, hair falling out, sick and vomiting. I don't want that for me . . . I want to control my own body, not the drugs and the doctors. My husband and children tell me I should do everything I can to help myself and to do what the doctor says [i.e., start the prescribed course of chemotherapy]. But life is such that everyone has to die. I'm ready to go now: I've been annointed; the children are settled; they are good [and] will look after their father so he isn't lonely. I've had the last rites. I'm not afraid."

References

ACKERKNECHT, ERWIN. 1958. *A Short History of Medicine.* New York: Ronald Press.

BARRABE, PAUL, and OTTO VON MERING. 1953. Ethnic Variations in Mental Stress in Families with Psychotic Children. *Social Problems* 1:49–53.

BEARN, A. G. 1968. Genetic Principles. In *Cecil-Loeb Textbook of Medicine,* vol. 2, ed. Paul B. Beeson and Walsh McDermott. Philadelphia: Saunders.

BLANE, HOWARD T. 1977. Acculturation and Drinking in an Italian-American Community. *Journal of Studies on Alcohol* 38:1324–1346.

BLEDA, SHARON E. 1978. Intergenerational Differences in Patterns and Bases of Ethnic Residential Dissimilarity. *Ethnicity* 5:91–107.

BRUHN, JOHN G., BILLY U. PHILIPS, and STEWART WOLF. 1972. Social Readjustment and Illness Patterns: Comparisons between First, Second and Third Generation Italian-Americans Living in the Same Community. *Journal of Psychosomatic Research* 16:387–394.

CAMPISI, PAUL J. 1948. Ethnic Family Patterns: The Italian Family in the United States. *American Journal of Sociology* 53:443–449.

CARLYLE, MARGARET M. 1965. Italy: Administration and Economic Conditions. *Encyclopaedia Britannica,* vol. 12, pp. 787–792. Chicago: Encyclopaedia Britannica.

CHAPMAN, CHARLOTTE G. 1971. *Milocca: A Sicilian Village.* Cambridge, Mass.: Schenkman.

CONLEY, C. LOCKARD. 1979. The Thalassemia Syndromes. In *Cecil Textbook of Medicine,* ed. Paul B. Beeson, Walsh McDermott, and J. B. Wyngaarden. Philadelphia: Saunders.

CORNELISON, ANN. 1969. *Torregreca.* Boston: Atlantic Monthly Press.

CROOG, SYDNEY H. 1961. Ethnic Origins and Responses to Health Questionnaires. *Human Organization* 20:61–69.

DOLCI, DANILO. 1959. *Report from Palermo,* trans. P. D. Cummins. New York: Orion Press.

DOUGLAS, NORMAN. 1928. *In Old Calabria.* New York: Modern Library.

EPSTEIN, FREDERICK H., E. P. BOAS, and RITA SIMPSON. 1957. The Epidemiology of Atherosclerosis among a Random Sample of Clothing Workers of Different Ethnic Origin in New York City. *Journal of Chronic Diseases* 5:300–328.

FANDETTI, DONALD V., and DONALD E. GELFAND. 1976. Care of the Aged: Attitudes of White Ethnic Families. *Gerontologist* 16:544–549.

FEMMINELLA, FRANCIS X., and JILL S. QUADAGNO. 1978. The Italian American Family. In *Ethnic Families in America: Patterns and Variations,* ed. Charles H. Mindel and Robert Habenstein. New York: Elsevier.

FOERSTER, ROBERT E. 1919. *The Italian Immigration of Our Times.* Cambridge, Mass.: Harvard University Press.

GAMBINO, RICHARD. 1974. *Blood of My Blood.* New York: Doubleday.

GANS, HERBERT. 1962. *The Urban Villagers.* New York: The Free Press.

GLAZER, NATHAN, and DANIEL MOYNIHAN. 1963. *Beyond the Melting Pot.* Cambridge, Mass.: MIT Press.

GRAHAM, SAXON, et al. 1963. Ethnic Derivation as Related to Cancer at Various Sites. *Cancer* 16:13–27.

GREELEY, ANDREW M., and WILLIAM C. MCCREADY. 1974. Does Ethnicity Matter? *Ethnicity* 1:91–108.

JONES, DEBORAH, and MARSHAL GOLD. 1974. Ambulatory Health Care in the City of Boston: Needs, Resources, and Priorities. Report prepared for Regional Director, H.E.W. Region 1, by Abt Associates, Cambridge, Mass.

KEYS, ANCEL, et al. 1954. Studies on Serum Cholesterol and Other Characteristics of Clinically Healthy Men in Naples. *Archives of Internal Medicine* 93:328–336.

KLUCKHOHN, FLORENCE R. 1963. Some Reflections on the Nature of Cultural Integration and Change. In *Sociological Theory, Values and Sociocultural Change,* ed. Edward Tiryakian. New York: The Free Press.

LASSMAN, M. N., et al. 1974. Endocrine Evaluation in Thalassemia Major. *Annals of the New York Academy of Science* 232:226–237.

LEVI, CARLO. 1947. *Christ Stopped at Eboli.* New York: Farrar, Strauss.

LOLLI, GEORGIO, et al. 1958. *Alcohol in Italian Culture.* Glencoe, Ill.: The Free Press.

MOSS, LEONARD, and STEPHEN CAPPANNARI. 1960a. Folklore and Medicine in an Italian Village. *Journal of American Folklore* 63:95–102.

———. 1960b. Patterns of Kinship, Compareggio and Community in a South Italian Town. *Anthropological Quarterly* 23:24–32.

———, 1962. Estate and Class in a Southern Italian Hill Town, *American Anthropologist* 64:287–300.

OPLER, MARVIN, and JEROME SINGER. 1956. Behavior and Psychopathology: Italian and Irish. *International Journal of Social Psychology* 2:11–22.

PARSONS, ANNE. 1960. Family Dynamics in South Italian Schizophrenics. *Archives of General Psychiatry* 3:507–518.

————. 1961. A Schizophrenic Episode in a Neapolitan Slum. *Psychiatry* 24:109–121.

PARSONS, TALCOTT. 1972. Definitions of Health and Illness in the Light of American Values and Social Structure. In *Patients, Physicians and Illness,* ed. E. Gartley Jaco. New York: The Free Press.

PEARSON, HOWARD A., et al. 1974. Comprehensive Testing for Thalassemia Trait. *Annals of the New York Academy of Science* 232:135–144.

PETERSON, D. R., and G. MIGLIORINI. 1970. Pancultural Factors of Parental Behavior in Sicily and the United States. In *Readings in Child Socialization,* ed. Kurt Danziger. New York: Pergamon Press.

PITRÈ, GIUSEPPE. 1871–1913. *Biblioteca delle Tradizioni Popolare Siciliane* (25 vols.). Palermo: L. Pedone-Lauriel di Carlo Clausen.

————. 1896. *Medicina Popolare Siciliana.* Torino-Palermo: Carlo Clausen.

PRESTON, SAMUEL H., NATHAN KEYFITZ, and ROBERT SCHOEN. 1972. *Causes of Death: Life Tables for National Populations.* New York: Seminar Press.

RAGUCCI, ANTOINETTE T. 1971. Generational Continuity and Change in Concepts of Health, Curing Practices, and Ritual Expressions of the Women of an Italian-American Enclave. Ph.D. dissertation, Department of Anthropology, Boston University.

————. 1972. The Ethnographic Approach and Nursing Research. *Nursing Research* 21:485–490.

————. 1975. Comparative Study of Folk Beliefs and Practices in Southern Italy. In *Yearbook, 1974,* The American Philosophical Society, Philadelphia.

ROSENWAIKE, IRA. 1973. Two Generations of Italians in America: Their Fertility Experience. *International Migration Review* 7:271–280.

RYDER, NORMAN B., and CHARLES F. WESTOFF. 1971. *Reproduction in the United States, 1965.* Princeton, N.J.: Princeton University Press.

SIGERIST, HENRY E. 1960. *On the History of Medicine.* New York: MD Publishing.

SINISCALCO, M., et al. 1966. Population Genetics of Haemoglobin Variants, Thalassemia and Glucose-6-Phosphate Dehydrogenase Deficiency with Particular Reference to Malaria Hypothesis. *Bulletin of World Health Organization* 34:379–393.

SPIEGEL, JOHN. 1971. Cultural Strain, Family Role Patterns, and Intrapsychic Conflict. In *Theory and Practice of Family Psychiatry,* ed. John G. Howells. New York: Brunner-Mazel.

————. 1972. *Transactions: The Interplay between Individual, Family, and Society.* New York: Science House.

STENHOUSE, N., and M. McCALL. 1970. Differential Mortality from Cardiovascular Disease in Migrants from England and Wales, Scotland and Italy and Native-born Australians. *Journal of Chronic Diseases* 23:423–431.

STERNBACK, RICHARD, and BERNARD TURSKY. 1965. Ethnic Differences among Housewives in Psychophysical and Skin Potential Responses to Electric Shock. *Psychotherapy* 1:241–246.

STOUT, CLARK, et al. 1964. Study of an Italian-American Community in Pennsylvania: Unusually Low Incidence of Deaths from Myocardial Infarction. *Journal of the American Medical Association* 188:845–849.

SUTTLES, GERALD D. 1968. *The Social Order of the Slum: Ethnicity and Territory in the Inner City.* Chicago: University of Chicago Press.

TWADDLE, ANDREW C. 1969. Health Decisions and Sick Role Variations: An Exploration. *Journal of Health and Social Behavior* 10:105–115.

U.S. DEPARTMENT OF COMMERCE, BUREAU OF THE CENSUS. 1977. *Statistical Abstracts of the United States,* 98th annual edition. Washington, D.C.: U.S. Government Printing Office.

U.S. IMMIGRATION AND NATURALIZATION SERVICE. 1975. *Annual Report.* Washington, D.C.: U.S. Government Printing Office.

———. 1977. *Annual Report.* Washington, D.C.: U.S. Government Printing Office.

VECOLI, RUDOLPH J. 1978. The Coming of Age of the Italian Americans: 1945–1974. *Ethnicity* 5:119–147.

WHYTE, WILLIAM F. 1943. *Street Corner Society: The Social Structure of an Italian Slum.* Chicago: University of Chicago Press.

WILLIAMS, PHYLLIS H. 1938. *South Italian Folkways in Europe and America.* New Haven: Yale University Press.

WINSLOW, KENELM. 1907. *Home Medical Library,* vol. 3. New York: The Review of Reviews.

WOLF, STEWART, et al. 1973. Roseto Revisited: Further Data on the Incidence of Myocardial Infarction in Roseto and Neighboring Pennsylvania Communities. *Transactions of American Clinical Climatological Association* 85:100–108.

ZBOROWSKI, MARK. 1952. Cultural Components in Response to Pain. *Journal of Social Issues* 8:16–30.

ZOLA, IRVING K. 1963. Problems of Communication, Diagnosis, and Patient Care. *Journal of Medical Education* 38:829–838.

———. 1964. Illness Behavior of the Working Class. In *Blue Collar World,* ed. Arthur Shostak and William Gomberg. Englewood Cliffs, N.J.: Prentice-Hall.

———. 1966. Culture and Symptoms—An Analysis of Patients' Presenting Complaints. *American Sociological Review* 31:615–630.

———. 1973. Pathways to the Doctor—From Person to Patient. *Social Science and Medicine* 7:677–684.

5

Mexican Americans

JANET M. SCHREIBER AND JOHN P. HOMIAK

IN THE LAST TWO DECADES Mexican Americans have grown in numbers and have become more visible, overwhelmingly urbanized, and politically more sophisticated. They have made the larger public aware of a variety of inequities in their condition, conspicuous among which is their poor health status. During this time it has become progressively clearer that solutions to the health-care problems of this ethnic collectivity would profit from a more effective use of existing social science knowledge. The national Health Planning and Resources Act of 1974 (Public Law 93–641) recognizes this need and mandates cultural awareness in the planning of health-care programs for cultural minorities. Accordingly, this chapter will examine the social science and medical literature in order to assess its relevance to the practical concerns of health-care professionals providing services to Mexican Americans.

Identification of the Ethnic Group

Definition of the Group

In spite of the increasing numbers and visibility of Mexican Americans, any discussion of their condition is complicated by the problem of defining this population. Seemingly straightforward issues, such as: "How many Mexican Americans are there?" "What are their demographic characteristics?" "What is the extent of internal variation within this group?" or "How do contemporary statistics compare with past data?" do not yield unequivocal answers (Hernández, Estrada, and Alvírez 1973: 671).

Currently, three ways of defining Mexican-American status are used in federal census data. The oldest of these, first used in the 1850 census, classifies all persons born in Mexico or of Mexican parentage as Mexican American. Obviously, this definition leads to serious underenumeration of the population because it excludes persons whose grandparents, great-grandparents, or even more remote ancestors came to the United States from Mexico. To overcome the underenumeration entailed by this method of classification, two other approaches have been used: the first identifies Mexican Americans by Spanish language and surname (both items used for a 15 percent sample), and the second asks the respondent to identify himself by "origin" (a method used on a 5 percent sample).

Although the use of these two forms of data collection obviates some of the difficulties encountered with the previous census classification, these methods contain their own particular problems and, in addition, weaken the comparability of censuses through time and by geographic region (table 5.1). Thus, use of the Spanish language to define Mexican Americans presents problems in many areas of the United States where immigrants and descendants of other Spanish-speaking groups (such as Puerto Ricans, Cubans, Dominicans, Central and South Americans, and even some Filipinos) are included in this category. Moreover, because the unit of data collection for these questions is the household, statistics include persons who may not in fact have a Spanish heritage, such as Anglo spouses. Using the criterion of Spanish surname poses the additional problems of eliminating from enumeration all people of Mexican origin who marry and relinquish their Hispanic last names, while including certain Hispanic populations of New Mexico and Colorado who colonized those areas when Mexico was still New Spain and who do not identify with the Mexican-American community.

Another central issue is the problem of finding an adequate term of reference. Historically, some persons of Mexican descent, in order to avoid the negative associations of ethnic membership, called themselves "Latin Americans" or "Spaniards." Today the use of the term "Chicano," with its connotations of cultural pride and social reform, has become increasingly popular but is unacceptable to large segments of the ethnic group who do not subscribe to the rhetoric of the Chicano movement. In a survey of 666 Mexican Americans in California, half of whom were born in Mexico and half in the United States, 54 percent of respondents identified themselves as Mexican, 27 percent as Mexican American, 7 percent as American of Mexican descent, and 6 percent as Chicano (Acosta 1974:218). "Mexican American" is perhaps the most neutral term. However, some persons of Mexican descent who have resided in the United States for as long as four generations resent the implication that they are somehow still foreigners and must remind people that they are Americans; others feel that this term implies an assimilationist per-

Table 5.1 Preliminary population totals according to various measures of ethnic status for the United States, the Southwest, and selected states, 1970.[a]

	Mexican foreign stock[b]			Spanish language or Spanish surname				Persons of Puerto Rican birth or parentage	Persons self-identified as of Spanish origin
	Born in Mexico	Native of foreign parentage	Spanish surname	Spanish mother tongue	Spanish language	Others of Spanish surname	Total, language or surname		
United States	759.7	1,579.4	—	7,823.6	10,042.3	—	—	1,379.0	9,070.1
The Southwest	625.3	1,347.0	4,668.0	4,727.6	5,662.7	525.7	6,188.4	58.3	5,008.5
Arizona	31.3	82.5	246.4	259.1	306.6	26.7	333.3	1.9	264.8
California	411.0	701.0	2,222.2	2,150.6	2,738.5	363.1	3,101.6	46.1	2,369.3
Colorado	5.4	19.3	211.6	194.7	256.0	30.5	286.5	1.8	225.5
New Mexico	11.0	26.8	324.2	329.7	379.7	27.6	407.3	0.4	308.3
Texas	193.6	517.4	1,663.6	1,793.5	1,981.9	77.8	2,059.7	8.1	1,840.6
New Jersey	1.1	2.2	—	258.1	310.5	—	—	138.7	288.5
New York	4.8	7.4	—	1,266.7	1,455.9	—	—	872.5	1,352.0
Pennsylvania	1.5	3.2	—	74.8	106.6	—	—	44.5	108.9
Connecticut	0.4	0.8	—	58.4	73.4	—	—	38.1	65.5
Florida	3.0	8.0	—	381.2	451.4	—	—	29.0	405.0
Indiana	5.1	13.3	—	49.4	67.2	—	—	9.4	112.5
Illinois	50.1	67.2	—	295.1	364.4	—	—	87.5	393.2
Louisiana	1.4	3.5	—	42.6	69.7	—	—	2.7	70.5
Massachusetts	7.6	1.4	—	48.2	64.9	—	—	24.4	66.2
Michigan	7.6	23.5	—	83.5	120.7	—	—	6.8	151.1
Nevada	1.8	3.9	—	16.8	27.1	—	—	0.7	20.5
Ohio	2.6	10.7	—	66.4	95.1	—	—	20.9	130.0
Utah	1.3	6.4	—	29.6	43.6	—	—	0.7	33.9
Washington	4.4	13.5	—	47.1	70.7	—	—	1.8	57.4
Wyoming	0.6	2.0	—	13.1	18.6	—	—	0.1	13.9

Source: Hernández, Estrada, and Alvírez (1973:684–685).

a. Figures are in thousands, rounded to the nearest hundred. Data were provided to Hernández, Estrada, and Alvírez by the Ethnic Statistics Branch, Population Division, U.S. Bureau of the Census. The states selected were those having a Spanish language population of 60,000 persons or more, or in which the Spanish language population constituted at least 4 percent of the state's total population.

b. Each set of columns is an *independent* measure of ethnic status.

spective that is ultimately a "sell-out" to the Establishment. This lack of terminological consensus reflects the varying historical, social, and political experience of this population as a whole, and, as such, represents problems inherent in any generalized approach to Mexican Americans as a collectivity.

Since no satisfactory solution to the problem of terminology appears to exist at present, we will adopt the term "Mexican American" as a general designation for the population of Mexican ancestry, regardless of time or place of arrival in the United States.

History of Migration and Contact with the United States

As a group appellation, "Mexican American" includes persons whose ancestors settled in the Southwest in the sixteenth century as well as those who have been in the United States only a few weeks. Yet, compared to the European mass migrations to America, the major influx of Mexicans began rather late. The Mexican revolution, beginning in 1909, spurred the first substantial wave of permanent migrants. This migration peaked in the 1920s but stopped during the years of the depression, when large numbers of migrants were repatriated by United States agencies.

The next large influx of migrants arrived in the post–World War II period. The need for agricultural labor, as well as for unskilled workers to keep pace with the industrial expansion of the postwar years, made Mexican immigration economically attractive to segments of the larger American society at the time. Business was the only real point of contact between the two cultures, however, and American society in general was not concerned with the housing conditions, lack of schooling, or availability of health services for Mexican immigrants (Galarza, Gallegos, and Samora 1969:65).

This neglect, coupled with outright prejudice and discrimination, encouraged Mexican Americans to maintain a distance from the public institutions and governmental authorities that might deport them in the early months after arrival (Padilla and Ruiz 1973:119–134). Particularly for illegal migrants, this distancing from Anglo institutions has been reported to carry over to health-care facilities (Casillas 1978:79; Scrimshaw and Burleigh 1978:34).

Three characteristics have made Mexican-American migration patterns unique:

1. Compared to Europeans and some Asians, most Mexicans have arrived in this country relatively recently (though no more recently than other Hispanics).
2. Because of geographical proximity and low travel costs, Mexicans have followed an unusually wide variety of migration patterns to the United States. In addition to those who come as permanent legal immigrants, there

are those who come either legally or illegally for various periods of temporary employment—from the daily commuters of the border states of Mexico to the seasonal agricultural workers and long-term target laborers.
3. Immigration to the United States has been more intense from Mexico than from any other country in recent years. Indeed, Mexico has been the primary source of both legal and (purportedly) illegal immigration into this country since the 1960s (Grebler, Moore, and Guzman 1970:62–69).

Some of these migration patterns have obvious implications for the delivery of health services to Mexican Americans. For example, referrals and follow-up are difficult when families move widely and frequently. Moreover, migrant families often do not know how to obtain and are unable to afford health services. In recent years, the Migrant Health Program of the Public Health Service has been established to help cope with problems resulting from these irregular patterns of population movement.

Current Population and Geographical Distribution

Given these problems of the conceptual definition of the group and its substantial illegal immigration, it is not surprising that current estimates of the number of Mexican Americans vary. It is generally acknowledged, however, that the Mexican-American community is much larger now than most figures indicate, primarily because of three factors: (1) census undercount, (2) a high birth rate, and (3) continued immigration. The 1975 population survey estimated a population of 6.7 million persons of Mexican origin in the United States (U.S. Department of Commerce 1976). If one uses the growth rate of 3.7 percent per annum established in the 1960–1970 decade to project a current population for 1980, the estimate would be 8,034,680.

Contrary to stereotypes, the vast majority of Mexican Americans live in urban areas, predominantly in the states of California, Texas, and Illinois. However, there are also significant numbers in Arizona, Colorado, and New Mexico, as well as in the northwest and midwest states. The 1970 census reported 86 percent of Mexican Americans as living in urban areas, but this figure has probably increased to more than 90 percent in the intervening years.

Many Mexican Americans live in ethnic neighborhoods (*barrios*) with specific geographical boundaries. Housing in these areas is frequently overcrowded and only marginally provided with services. For example, in some parts of Texas a large percentage of Mexican-American homes lack running water and sewage facilities. A recent survey of 65 unincorporated Mexican-American communities, known as *colonias* (a group of *barrios*), in two counties with a population of about 34,000 persons found that 54 percent of the houses lacked treated drinking water, and none had sewers (Warner 1978:36).

Also contrary to popular stereotypes, foreign-born persons constitute the smallest proportion of the Mexican-American population in the United States (only 12 percent were born in Mexico). In the 1970 census, the overwhelming majority (58 percent) of Mexican Americans in the five southwestern states were native-born or of native parentage. The remainder (less than one-third) were native-born, but of Mexican parentage. This figure, of course, does not reflect the substantial illegal immigration.

Demographic Profile

AGE AND FERTILITY   Compared to Anglos, Mexican Americans are a young population, with proportionately more people in each age group up to 40 and proportionately fewer in the groups over 40 (table 5.2). The median age of persons of Mexican origin was 19.8 as compared to 28.6 for the total population. Because of the large number of children in the Mexican-American population, there are 80 persons in the dependent age ranges (those under 16 and over 64) for every 100 persons of working age; this compares to 65 dependent per 100 working-age persons among other whites. The fact that there are comparatively few elderly Mexican Americans makes this an even more startling statistic. Poor families with young children have enormous obstacles to fulfilling

Table 5.2 Age distribution of Mexican-origin population of the United States (March 1975).

Age (years)	Total population (%)	Mexican origin (%)
Under 5	7.7	13.7
5–9	8.3	12.5
10–17	15.7	19.5
18–20	5.7	6.6
21–24	6.9	7.8
25–34	14.4	13.8
35–44	10.8	10.7
45–54	11.3	8.1
55–64	9.3	3.8
65+	10.1	3.3
Total percent, 18 and over	68.3	54.3
Total percent, 21 and over	62.6	47.7
Total number of persons (thousands)	209,572	6,690
Median age (years)	28.6	19.8

Source: U.S. Department of Commerce (1976:5).

children's needs. There are slightly more males than females of working age, probably as a result of the disproportionate immigration of males and, to a small extent, maternal mortality.

No other ethnic group distinguished by the United States census has as high a fertility level as Mexican Americans (Uhlenberg 1973:30). In the 1970 census Mexican Americans had the highest number of children born for any urban group. Furthermore, most fertility took place within marriage, and 94 percent of young children were living with their own mothers and fathers. However, Johnson (1976) found that higher income, education, and labor force participation reduce fertility levels considerably; and for those women of Mexican ancestry who reported English as the language of the home, fertility did not differ from Anglo rates. Thus, acculturation changes the traditional pattern of high fertility.

However, the overall high rate of fertility among Mexican-American women under age 20, combined with the large family size, suggests a high risk for both maternal and infant health in this ethnic group. Indeed, both the youthfulness and the high fertility of the Mexican-American population make maternal and child health a primary concern for this group and suggest a need for greater emphasis on pediatric and obstetrical services.

SOCIOECONOMIC STATUS   Of the three component variables of socioeconomic status (income, education, and occupation), the median number of years of schooling most clearly differentiates Mexican Americans from Anglos. For Anglos in 1970, the median was one year of college; for Mexican Americans, the median was ninth grade (table 5.3). Furthermore, a full 9.3 percent of Mexican Americans had three years or less of formal education, although younger persons have in recent years achieved higher levels of education than their elders.

The income levels reported for 1970 are best understood by pointing out that 13.8 percent of Mexican Americans had incomes of less than $3,000, while only 5.7 percent of Anglos reported such low incomes. The median household income for families identifying themselves as "of Mexican origin" in the 1975 population survey was $9,559, compared to $12,836 for all American families (U.S. Department of Commerce 1976:7). This figure must be considered in light of the fact that Mexican-American families are larger than Anglo families. For an indication of income distribution among families of Mexican origin in 1974, see table 5.4.

The occupations of Mexican Americans are slowly becoming more diversified but are still most frequently of low prestige (Penalosa 1967: 410–411). The 1975 population study conducted by the U.S. Bureau of the Census found that more than 60 percent of the occupations held by

Table 5.3 Percentage of the total U.S. population and of persons of Mexican origin that completed less than 5 years of school and percentage that completed 4 years of high school or more (March 1975).

Years of school completed and age (years)	Total population (%)	Persons of Mexican origin (%)
Persons who completed less than 5 years of school		
25–29	1.0	9.8
30–34	1.0	11.8
35–44	1.9	22.1
45–54	2.5	30.2
55–64	3.5	35.7
65+	11.0	63.8
Total 25+	3.3	24.6
Persons who completed 4 years of high school or more		
25–29	83.2	46.1
30–34	78.6	42.3
35–44	71.5	32.2
45–54	63.8	24.6
55–64	51.9	15.4
65+	35.2	3.6
Total 25+	62.6	31.0

Source: U.S. Department of Commerce (1976:6).

Table 5.4 Income in 1974 of all U.S. families and of families with head of Mexican origin (March 1975).

Family income	Total families (%)	Mexican origin (%)
Less than $4,000	9.0	15.0
$4,000–$6,999	13.0	19.2
$7,000–$9,999	13.9	18.8
$10,000–$14,999	24.4	26.6
$15,000+	39.7	20.4
Total number of families (thousands)	55,712	1,429
Median income	$12,836	$9,498

Source: U.S. Department of Commerce (1976:7).

men of Mexican origin 16 years of age and older were blue-collar jobs. In comparison, however, only about 45 percent of all employed men in the United States 16 years and older were classified as blue-collar workers. There were half as many white-collar workers among employed males of Mexican origin than among the rest of the American male population. Overall, males of Mexican origin are employed in less prestigious occupations when their occupations are compared to jobs held by all men in the United States in 1975 (U.S. Department of Commerce 1976:7).

Summary

The general demographic features of low income, poor living conditions, little schooling, and ethnic segregation can affect the health of Mexican Americans in the following ways: (1) by increasing exposure to infectious diseases through crowded housing and lack of treated drinking water or sewerage; (2) by decreasing awareness of preventive measures in disease control (for example, as a result of not being able to read a health bulletin or to understand germ theory); (3) by restricting access to health care because of an inability to pay for physicians' fees, medicine, and special treatment; (4) by barring a person from health-care services through ethnic discrimination; and (5) by increasing the chances of inappropriately using the less costly types of health care (for example, lay curers or midwives).

Evaluation of the Existing Data

Studies of Mexican-American medical beliefs and behavior, which span a quarter of a century, encompass geographically dispersed groups with varying sociodemographic characteristics and represent different objectives and concerns. In this section we will survey the existing data base on Mexican-American health-care behavior by (1) canvassing its geographical distribution, (2) evaluating its coverage in terms of intraethnic diversity, and (3) assessing problems of interpretation and generalization that result from the age of particular studies and the diverse methodological orientations represented in the literature.

Nature of the Populations Studied

An effective overview of the existing literature can be gained from the listing in table 5.5, which specifies the research locale, the sociodemographic characteristics of the population studied, and the methodology of those studies that deal more or less explicitly with Mexican-American health beliefs and practices. It should be noted that the table is not an exhaustive list of research on Mexican-American health care and specifically omits epidemiological studies and programmatic statements, many of which are, however, discussed in the text.

An examination of table 5.5 reveals that most research on Mexican Americans has been done with lower-class populations (55 percent) or with mixed populations of predominantly lower- and middle-class origin

Table 5.5 Studies of Mexican-American health beliefs and practices (including epidemiology).

Study	Year	Research locale	Population	Method
Saunders, L.	1954	New Mexico	Rural/lower-class	Ethnographic
Murry, M.	1954	San Antonio, Tex.	Urban/lower-class	Survey/ethnographic
Clark, M.	1959	San Jose, Calif.	Urban/lower-class	Ethnographic
Schulman, S.	1960	Colorado/New Mexico	Rural/lower-class	Ethnographic
Jaco, G.	1960	Texas	Rural-urban/mixed class	Epidemiological
Holland, W.	1963	Tucson, Ariz.	Urban/lower- and middle-class	Survey
Schulman, S., and A. Smith	1963	Colorado/New Mexico	Rural/lower-class	Ethnographic
McLemore, S. D.	1963	Texas	Urban/lower-class	Survey
Madsen, W.	1964	Hidalgo Co., Tex.	Rural/lower- and middle-class	Ethnographic
Rubel, A.	1966	Hidalgo Co.	Rural/lower- and middle-class	Ethnographic
Sheldon, P.	1966	Los Angeles	Urban/middle-class	Survey
Karno, M.	1966	Los Angeles	Urban/lower-class	Clinical
Martínez, C., and H. Martin	1966	San Antonio	Urban/lower-class	Survey
Nall, F., and J. Speilberg	1967	McAllen, Tex.	Rural/lower-class	Survey
Kiev, A.	1968	San Antonio	Urban/lower-class	Clinical/ethnographic
Moustafa, A., and G. Weiss	1968	California	Urban/indeterminate	Survey
Weaver, J.	1969	Orange Co., Calif.	Urban/lower- and middle-class	Survey
Karno, M., and R. Edgerton	1969	Los Angeles	Urban/indeterminate	Survey
Creson, D., C. McKinley, and R. Evans	1969	Texas	Urban/lower-class	Survey
Torrey, E. F.	1969	Santa Clara Co., Calif.	Rural-urban/mixed class	Clinical
Edgerton, R., M. Karno, and I. Fernández	1970	Los Angeles	Urban/indeterminate	Survey
Weaver, T.	1970	New Mexico	Rural-urban/mixed class	Ethnographic/survey
Lurie, H., and G. Lawrence	1971	Yakima Valley, Wash.	Rural/lower-class	Clinical
Welch, S., J. Comer, and M. Steinman	1973	Nebraska	Rural/lower-class	Survey

Table 5.5   continued.

Study	Year	Research locale	Population	Method
Hoppe, S., and P. Heller	1975	San Antonio	Urban/lower-class	Survey
Weclew, R. V.	1975	Chicago	Urban/indeterminate	Survey
Kay, M.	1977	Tucson	Urban/lower-class	Ethnographic
Cheney, C., and G. Adams	1978	Houston	Urban/lower-class	Survey
Aguirre, L.	1978	El Paso	Urban/lower-class	Ethnographic
Schreiber, J., and L. Philpott	1978	Texas border counties	Rural-urban/mixed class	Survey/ethno-graphic
Farge, E.	1978	Houston	Urban/mixed class	Survey
Sandler, A., and L. Chan	1978	Los Angeles	Urban/lower-class	Survey
Keefe, S., A. Padilla, and M. Carlos	1979	Santa Barbara, Calif.	Urban/lower- and middle-class	Extended survey
Roberts, R., and E. S. Lee	1979a,b	Alameda Co., Calif.	Urban/mixed class	Survey

(30 percent). Geographically, research has centered on the states of Texas and California (43 percent and 29 percent of the studies, respectively) and on urban (60 percent) rather than rural populations. Since only a small proportion of Mexican Americans live in rural areas today, rural dwellers are quite clearly overrepresented among existing studies, although the lack of mainstream medical services and educational opportunities among this sector of the Mexican-American population tends to make their health behaviors more at variance from the general population than those of their urban counterparts and thus worthy of special study.

Much of the extant health-care literature on Mexican Americans has been subject to a critical review by Weaver (1973) which identifies three phases or "generations" of research. These phases involve relatively distinct data bases and methodological premises.

For the most part, the first and second generations of studies, carried out during the 1950s and 1960s, are characterized by the use of ethnographic methods and relatively small, homogeneous samples (Saunders 1954, 1958; Murry 1954; Clark 1959; Schulman 1960; Schulman and Smith 1963; Madsen 1964a; Rubel 1966). They also tend to treat cultural patterns as the sole explanation for observed behavior. Though these studies have yielded important and detailed information about traditional medical beliefs and practices, they have nevertheless tended to give insufficient attention to intraethnic variation and its sources.

During this earlier period of intensive ethnographic effort on primarily rural, working-class Mexican Americans, an important large-scale study of the incidence of severe mental illness among the three major ethnic groups in Texas (white, black, and Mexican American) was undertaken by Jaco (1959, 1960). This study, based on Texas mental hospital records, indicated—without direct observation or knowledge of the subculture—that Mexican Americans experienced the lowest incidence of mental illness of the three groups. Although these widely reported findings have been partially confirmed by two later studies using admission rates to mental hospitals in New Mexico and Colorado (Weaver 1973:90), they have been the subject of considerable dispute with regard to both their substance and the interpretations made of the data (see Kiev 1968: 175–189; Madsen 1969:238–242; Karno and Edgerton 1969; Edgerton, Karno, and Fernández 1970:125–126; Keefe, Padilla, and Carlos 1979: 151).

Whereas the earlier studies of Mexican-American health behavior have tended toward generalization and methodological uniformity, more recent research of the late 1960s and 1970s tends to be more methodologically diverse, using surveys of varying size as well as ethnographic data. In addition to studying folk beliefs and practices, this research has generally focused on more narrowly defined substantive areas (for example, mental health knowledge, referral patterns, utilization of medical services) and has concentrated on more varied segments of the Mexican-American population. Although these recent studies have still leaned heavily toward working-class populations in the rural Southwest, urban areas have received increasingly greater attention, and samples have occasionally included middle- and upper-income respondents. The recent research has also been more "problem-oriented" than earlier studies and has examined relationships among specific variables in order to develop causal statements about specific aspects of Mexican-American health behaviors or beliefs. In short, this "third generation" of research studies, in keeping with both the growing diversification of the Mexican-American population and funding practices of the 1970s, has sampled more widely and tended to narrow investigation to issues of immediate concern to planners of mainstream health services.

Problems of Interpretation and Generalization

Given the regional, acculturational, and socioeconomic variation existing within the Mexican-American population, it is obviously hazardous to formulate conclusions about the entire ethnic group from samples as distinct as rural villagers in New Mexico and Colorado (Saunders 1954; Weaver 1970), agricultural laborers in Texas (Madsen 1964a; Rubel 1966), indigent *barrio* residents in Arizona (Kay 1977), or middle-class urbanites in metropolitan southern California (Keefe, Padilla, and Carlos 1979). Not only do the extant studies represent different populations in terms of geographic provenience and socioeconomic status, they frequently use different definitions of "Mexican American" (see Broom and Skevsky 1952; Murry 1954:3–4; Quesada 1973) and employ divergent methodological perspectives. Moreover, no studies incorporate a significant cross section of the overall Mexican-American population or encompass the sizable Mexican-American groups living in Illinois, Ohio, or Michigan (Weaver 1973:101).

Though it may be overly critical to contend that existing research provides almost no comparable data on Mexican-American health-care behavior, it is certainly true that general conclusions with regard to the medical beliefs and practices of this ethnic group must be circumscribed and formulated with extreme caution. In this regard, careful consideration must be given to the relative age of particular studies; many are more than two decades old and are therefore insensitive to the changing demographic characteristics of the Mexican-American population. Of course, this is not necessarily a problem in instances where studies show extensive coverage of a geographic region and continuity over time, since the existence of adequate data from different points in time obviates the risk of generalizing from one "ethnographic present" to another (Kay 1977: 166). It seems clear that the data base on Mexican-American health-care behavior is most extensive and generalizable for populations in Texas, Arizona, and New Mexico, is possibly less so for California Mexican Americans, and is of questionable applicability to less studied groups throughout the remainder of the United States.

A few comments are also warranted concerning the relative strengths and weaknesses of the methods utilized in this literature. Ethnographic studies, because they focus on relatively small, homogeneous samples, have always been subject to criticism with regard to equivalence, representativeness, or sensitivity to cultural variation. On the other hand, however limited these studies may be in terms of sample size, the validity of ethnographic data is less frequently open to question, given a competent style of cultural analysis that gives proper attention to native concepts and categories and the multiple contexts that inform their meaning. By comparison, survey research, with its tendency to postulate relevant categories or variables a priori, appears weak with regard to validity. Moreover, the questionable measures by which some studies operationalize attributes such as "familism," "alienation," or "community integration" suggest that their findings should be approached with caution (see, for example, Nall and Speilberg 1967; Hoppe and Heller 1975). More apparent, perhaps, is the inadequate sample size of various survey studies and the possible sampling biases introduced by their exclusive reliance on clinic populations (McLemore 1963; Creson, McKinley, and Evans 1969). Finally, the reliability of much survey research may depend on the relative sociocultural attributes of investigator and respondent. For example, a good deal of ethnographic research attests to the fact that matters concerning traditional medical beliefs and practices constitute a sensitive area for investigation. Because folk practices are frequently unacknowledged, many respondents—to avoid either social censure or legal punishment—do not readily disclose information to unknown investigators from the dominant culture. Consequently, data reported by survey instruments or interview techniques should be accepted only with reservation (Torrey 1969; Aguirre 1978:61; Kay 1978:89).

Sources of Intraethnic Diversity

The studies discussed above suggest a number of important determinants of intraethnic variation in health-care beliefs and behavior, including socioeconomic status, level of acculturation, nativity and generational status, sex, family size, and ethnic community size and integration. It should be noted, however, that these variables are not discrete and cannot productively be considered in isolation.

Although the majority of research on Mexican-American health behavior focuses on lower-class segments of this population, a number of sources—relying on ethnographic and survey methods—report socioeconomic status as a major determinant of medical beliefs and practices (Holland 1963; Madsen 1964a:91–95; Sheldon 1966; Farge 1978; Kay 1978:91). Despite this fact, insufficient attention has been given to this source of variation, particularly with regard to the relative impact of its constituent elements (income, education, and occupation) on specific health activities and to its interaction with related sources of variation (for example, acculturation).

Level of acculturation, particularly since it is broadly correlated with social class, has also long been cited as an important index of variation in medical behavior (Saunders 1954, 1958; Clark 1959; Holland 1963; Madsen 1964b; Kay 1977). However, the concept of acculturation, although descriptively clear, lacks analytic precision because it subsumes other sources of variation known to affect health behavior, such as language use and familism (Edgerton and Karno 1971; Karno and Edgerton 1974:292). Consequently, the criteria by which acculturation is measured are often impressionistic or unevenly applied (see Murry 1954:119; Holland 1963, Madsen 1964b; Kiev 1968:14–21; Creson, McKinley, and Evans 1969:265; Kay 1977:156). It is also rarely acknowledged by researchers that acculturation, though seen as a causal factor in the context of health-care studies, is itself an effect of other cultural and noncultural variables that are poorly understood.

The factors of nativity and generational status have also been linked, either implicitly or explicitly, with intraethnic variations. However, since present-day Mexican immigrants are apparently coming from a much more urbanized and industrialized homeland than that of two or three decades ago (Penalosa 1967:407; Welch, Comer, and Steinman 1973: 210), nativity and generational status may be diminishing in importance as factors in understanding Mexican-American health practices. Nevertheless, fragmentary data suggest that these factors may still retain significance for those Mexican Americans embedded in sizable, ethnically segregated communities of largely monolingual Spanish speakers. Such persons, by virtue of their encapsulation in viable subcultural groups and their relative isolation from Anglo society, may reinforce or perpetuate more traditional behavioral patterns of health activity (Clark 1959; Kay 1977).

Although all the sources of variation mentioned above contribute to diversity in the medical beliefs and practices of Mexican Americans, it is far from clear precisely what the relative impact of specific variables is on various forms of medical behavior. In particular, evidence is equivocal as to the effect of cultural versus noncultural (for example, economic) factors on health activity (Nall and Speilberg 1967; Welch, Comer, and Steinman 1973; Weaver 1973; Farge 1975). For clinical purposes, however, the factors of lower socioeconomic class (as identified by income and educational attainment) and involvement in an ethnic community may be used as general indicators of adherence to more traditional health behaviors.

Epidemiological Characteristics

The surprisingly small number of epidemiological studies of Mexican Americans indicate a consistent pattern. According to the available data, Mexican Americans are generally in poorer health than Anglo Americans but in better health than black Americans. In addition, Mexican Americans have higher age-standardized death rates than do Anglo Americans. The same pattern is true for life expectancy, infant and maternal mortality, and nutritional deficiencies (Aranda 1971; Quesada and Heller 1977).

Cautions Concerning the Available Data

Good epidemiology requires the development of reliable sources for both numerator and denominator data, as well as investigations into risk factors and their distribution in a population. Besides the difficulty of establishing an accurate total population estimate to calculate a denominator, the absence of morbidity and mortality reports that identify the number of cases even for Spanish-surnamed persons make it difficult to calculate numerator data. Moreover, the interplay among cultural, acculturational, and economic factors that dispose Mexican Americans to low utilization of health services also affects the reporting of disease and therefore the quality of numerator data (Aranda 1971; Hoppe and Heller 1975; Menck et al. 1975:531; Quesada and Heller 1977; Rubel and O'Nell 1978).

Given these difficulties, the best information on the prevalence and incidence of disease among Mexican Americans currently comes from specially designed research projects. Yet even this research tends to focus on unrepresentative populations; for example, most epidemiological research has been directed toward child health, with a heavy emphasis on nutrition and on samples from California, Texas, and Colorado. Furthermore, none of these studies reports behavioral information on illness, utilization of health services, or treatment in conjunction with epidemiological data. This paucity of multidimensional data handicaps health planners by depriving them not only of an accurate measure of the amount and distribution of disease in Mexican-American communities, but also of the behavioral data needed to design appropriate disease control programs. It is hoped that these gaps in our knowledge can be filled in the near future.

Mortality Data

PRINCIPAL CAUSES OF DEATH   Although Mexican Americans, like the general United States population, die most commonly from heart disease or cancer, their death rates for these causes do not appear to be quite as high as those of the Anglo population (see table 5.6). However, Mexican Americans die more frequently than Anglos from cirrhosis of the liver (Johnson and Matre 1978), tuberculosis, diabetes,[1] infectious and parasitic diseases, circulatory diseases, and accidents (Aranda 1971: 104; Quesada and Heller 1977:94). Mortality rates for many of these conditions are quite clearly related to low income and poor housing conditions (Scrimshaw and Burleigh 1978:34). In addition, higher mortality rates from tuberculosis and diabetes may reflect the stoic attitudes toward nondebilitating symptoms that have generally been documented for lower socioeconomic groups (Clark 1959:195; Richardson 1972:232–233).

In spite of these general observations, Roberts and Askew's conclusion (1972:267) that virtually no comparative mortality data are available for Chicanos still appears to be basically correct. One exception, however, is an analysis of Texas death certificates from 1969 to 1971 (Fonner 1975; see table 5.6). This study not only documents a high mortality rate from accidents for Mexican-American males but also shows a startlingly high mortality from diabetes for Mexican-American females. The study also reveals high death rates from certain causes of perinatal mortality and from bacterial and parasitic disease for both males and females. In Colorado, Mexican Americans are said to die younger than their Anglo counterparts—56.7 years as compared to 67.5 years (Moustafa and Weiss

Table 5.6 Cause-specific death rates per 100,000 for Mexican Americans, standardized to those for Anglos, Texas, 1969–1971.

Cause of death	Anglos, crude death rate		Mexican-Americans, standardized death rate	
	Males	Females	Males	Females
All causes	991.86	728.36	995.01	862.80
Infective and parasitic diseases	8.59	6.28	26.87	18.70
Neoplasms, total	174.41	132.97	143.72	147.73
Trachea, bronchus, lungs	58.44	13.00	33.83	14.12
Large intestine, rectum	17.12	18.62	10.39	9.58
Other digestive sites	17.17	13.24	24.52	26.02
Lymphatic and hematopoietic	18.97	14.48	13.71	10.27
Prostate	15.86	—	11.38	—
Breast	—	24.47	—	19.53
Ovary	—	9.40	—	9.18
Cervix uteri	—	5.38	—	12.59
Diabetes mellitus	11.84	16.24	27.96	52.95
All circulatory diseases	501.80	395.77	472.70	407.62
Hypertension	7.58	9.08	8.37	13.31
Ischemic heart disease	332.19	217.23	256.78	224.99
Diseases of the arteries	27.25	26.73	24.41	27.51
Cerebrovascular disease	88.69	107.68	88.97	99.87
Other heart diseases	34.98	24.42	38.42	31.00
Other circulatory diseases	11.11	10.69	9.75	10.94
Influenza and pneumonia	29.90	25.63	36.87	36.85
Other respiratory diseases	39.67	13.12	22.75	14.08
Digestive diseases, total	35.89	27.51	53.03	41.52
Congenital anomalies	8.74	7.47	10.76	8.02
Perinatal mortality	22.25	14.07	27.81	18.21
Accidents	108.59	47.64	143.26	37.63

Source: Fonner (1975:47–54). Reprinted with permission.

1968), and in San Antonio, Texas, Mexican Americans have a higher death rate at each age level except for those over 76.

Calculations using data from standard mortality ratios in 1960 show that the mortality rates of Mexican-American females are twice as high as those of Anglo females. Moreover, they are higher than mortality rates for Anglo, black, and Mexican-American males and lower only than the rates for black females (American Public Health Association 1974:32). Findings by Roberts and Askew (1972:215) are relatively consistent with this pattern: Mexican-American mortality rates are reported as being intermediate between those of Anglos and blacks; however, in their study

Mexican-American females evidence a higher mortality rate than either Anglo or black females.

Quesada and Heller (1977:95) further elaborate these variations and question why the comparative advantage of Anglo-American females over males does not similarly obtain for Mexican Americans. In part, this difference may be attributed to relatively higher levels of female fertility, earlier inception of childbearing, higher maternal mortality, and poorer nutrition among Mexican-American women (Gilbert and O'Rourke 1968; Bradfield and Brun 1970; Bradshaw and Bean 1973; Menck et al. 1975; Cardenas, Gibbs, and Young 1976). At the same time, the increasing involvement of Mexican-American women in the labor force has eroded traditional patterns of sex-role segregation, possibly exposing females to the same occupational and environmental health hazards as males (Kiev 1968:18; Johnson 1976).

INFANT MORTALITY Although data on infant mortality are not reported by Spanish surname, Teller and Clyburn (1974) have analyzed Texas birth records for the period 1964–1972. They found that infant mortality among Mexican Americans has been higher than that among whites and lower than that among blacks, but they also noted that infant mortality rates are decreasing for this ethnic group. However, the authors acknowledge that extreme caution must be exercised in drawing implications from their data and speculate that the reported frequencies may be overly conservative as a result of unreported infant deaths among families migrating back across the border (Teller and Clyburn 1974).

A study by Campos (1978), using an indirect estimate technique, similarly suggests the conservatism of available infant mortality data. Relying on child survivorship data (that is, the number of living children compared to number of previous births) for the period 1969–1971, this study disclosed that published infant mortality rates underestimate the actual occurrence for the 11 Texas border counties. In spite of this underestimation, actual Spanish-surname infant mortality rates were found to range between 37.75 and 43.08, as compared to Anglo rates of 18.36 and 23.78 for the same area (Campos 1978:30). (See Moustafa and Weiss (1968) for similar findings in Colorado and a smaller differential between Mexican and Anglo rates in San Antonio, Texas.)

Morbidity among Mexican Americans

Since neither the Center for Disease Control nor state departments of health collect morbidity data specifically for this ethnic group, no comparative national statistics are available, and all data thus derive from specific studies. Findings from a large survey in California, however, suggest that Mexican Americans there have a morbidity experience that is somewhat more favorable than that of the general population; they reported less disability, fewer chronic conditions, and fewer symptoms or ailments than the population at large (Roberts and Lee 1980a:24).

POVERTY-RELATED DISEASES Many diseases found among Mexican Americans are associated with poverty. Bacterial and parasitic diseases and tuberculosis, for example, are related to overcrowding, inadequate housing, lack of pure water, and poor nutrition. The tuberculosis case rate for Mexican Americans in Los Angeles County (California) has been reported to be double that of the overall county rate (Aranda 1971:104). In the border areas of south Texas communicable disease rates are substantially higher than for other areas of the state (Warner 1978), and a similar picture prevails for most reportable diseases in Los Angeles County, where the rates for Mexican Americans are two or three times higher than for whites (Aranda 1971:104).

Many diarrheal diseases may be underreported for Mexican Americans, since this ailment may be accepted as a fact of life among the poor segment of the population (Clark 1959). Severe ailments like typhus and typhoid, however, are probably reported for Mexican Americans as often as they are found in all income groups.

CANCER Data on cancer incidence among Mexican Americans in Los Angeles reveal that both adult male immigrants and American-born, Spanish-surnamed persons experience lower rates for all types of cancer combined than other residents of the city (Menck et al. 1975). In keeping with the trend in most immigrant groups, however, the rates among the American-born are closer to those of other indigenous Americans.

Both immigrant and American-born Spanish-surnamed persons in Los Angeles have been found to have higher incidences than whites of malignancies of the stomach and gallbladder. Less compelling evidence also suggests higher risks for cancers of the liver, nasopharynx, nose and sinuses, male genitalia (other than testes), and connective tissue. In contrast, malignant melanomas, lymphomas, and cancers of the bladder, buccal cavity, larynx, and lung were found to be relatively uncommon in Spanish-surnamed men and women (Stern et al. 1975).

Cancer of the cervix has been observed to be frequent among Mexican-American women, particularly those born in Mexico. It has been suggested that this pattern may relate to the early age and longer duration of fertility among Mexican-born women (Menck et al. 1975:533–535; Kay 1977:156–157). In contrast with cervical cancer, consistently low rates of breast cancer have been observed for Mexican-American women in every urban area of Texas surveyed (MacDonald and Heinze 1975).

CARDIOVASCULAR DISEASES   Factors that put Mexican Americans at similar risk with other Americans for cardiovascular diseases are reported from a northern California study (Stern et al. 1975). This research discovered similar plasma cholesterol concentrations and blood pressures in both Anglo-American and Mexican-American groups. Although fewer Mexican Americans than whites were found to be heavy cigarette smokers, the advantage gained by this tendency was more or less counterbalanced by the greater prevalence of obesity and high triglyceride levels among the former group. Mexican Americans are like other lower socioeconomic groups in evidencing a higher prevalence of obesity compared to those in higher socioeconomic groups, and this trend may be reinforced by a cultural preference for a "well-fleshed" body (Schulman and Smith 1963).

Selected Health Issues

NUTRITIONAL STATUS   In general, the nutritional level of Mexican Americans is similar to that of other predominantly low income groups. Low income, large family size, low educational level, and poor sanitary conditions tend to result in poor nutritional status. Among Mexican Americans it is the quantity rather than the quality of diet that appears to be responsible for low nutritional status. Moreover, specific subpopulations are more susceptible to malnutrition: pregnant and lactating women, children under age 6, and older persons (Bradfield and Brun 1970). High rates of lactose intolerance have been observed among Mexican Americans (Woteki, Weser, and Young 1977); this should be an important consideration in dietary counseling for pregnant and lactating women particularly.

Repeating a predictable pattern, a ten-state nutrition survey conducted during the period 1968–1970 found that Mexican Americans had a deficient nutritional intake less frequently than blacks but more often than Anglos (U.S. Department of Health, Education, and Welfare 1972). In particular, this study highlighted deficiencies in vitamin A, vitamin C, calcium, and iron. Similar nutritional deficits have been reported by Bradfield and Brun (1970). Avitaminosis has been documented particularly among Mexican-American children in urban California and Colorado, as well as in rural Texas (Quesada and Heller 1977:95). In addition, Chase and his colleagues (1971:322) reported Vitamin A deficiency to be a major medical problem in the children of migrant families. Studies by Acosta (1974) and Larson (1974) cite a combination of these factors as responsible for the "undergrown" size of children in California and Texas migrant families. Somewhat conflicting data are presented in a study by Yanochik-Owen and White (1977:154), however, which found 10 percent of Arizona Mexican-American children sampled to be overweight.

Unfortunately, the dietary patterns of Mexican Americans have not been adequately described or quantified (Bradfield and Brun 1970). Using a "24-hour recall," the ten-state nutrition study found that almost one-third of low-income Mexican Americans reported no meat consumption and the highest cereal and grain consumption of all groups studied (U.S. Department of Health, Education, and Welfare 1972:307–308). Most studies using this method of data collection conclude, however, that the diet of this group is well balanced but contains less meat, vegetables, sugar, and milk and more eggs and beans than the typical Anglo diet (Lantz and Wood 1958; U.S. Department of Health, Education, and Welfare 1972)—a finding that is in striking contrast with the previously reported clinical observations of rather widespread vitamin deficiency.

An association between poor nutrition and low educational attainment is suggested in a study by Cardenas, Gibbs, and Young (1976) on primigravid Mexican-American patients in a large Texas city. This research found that more than 85 percent of the respondents could not name different types of nutrients (for example, carbohydrate, protein), and 58 percent failed to make a correct association between specific food items and their nutrient category. Only one-half named meat as an important food during pregnancy.

In sum, the available data on diet and nutrition suggest that Mexican Americans—particularly those in low-income families—may be somewhat undernourished with respect to caloric intake, vitamin A, vitamin C, iron, and possibly calcium. Because of the higher prevalence of lactose intolerance in this population, milk should not ordinarily be recommended as a dietary supplement.

MENTAL HEALTH   Culturally oriented studies of illness have always had an affinity with psychiatric research, and non-Western categories of disease have often been analyzed with the assumption that social and psychological factors constitute their primary etiological factors (see Rubel 1960, 1964). A formidable amount of research—much of it contradictory and equivocal in its findings—has been devoted to elucidating the mental health characteristics of Mexican Americans. This fact prompts at least some attention to issues of mental health in this survey.

Most researchers have hypothesized that Mexican Americans would have a greater need for mental health services than the general population because of the additional stress they presumably experience from acculturational pressures, intergenerational conflict, poverty, language barriers, limited education, and discrimination. On the contrary, however, considerable research has documented not only substantial underrepresentation of Mexican-American clients in mental health facilities (Jaco 1959; Karno 1966; Karno and Edgerton 1969; Torrey 1969; Edgerton,

Karno, and Fernández 1970; Padilla and Ruiz 1973; Keefe, Padilla, and Carlos 1979:150) but also generally low rates of psychosis among members of this group. Moreover, differences have been found in the types and severity of psychopathology experienced by Mexican Americans as compared with Anglos (Meadows and Stoker 1965; Fabrega, Swartz, and Wallace 1968). In general, Mexican Americans tend to display a more affective symptomatology with regard to severe disorders, whereas Anglo-Americans manifest a more paranoid symptomatology (Meadows and Stoker 1965:275).

This discrepancy between apparently high risk factors, on the one hand, and both low prevalence of psychoses and low utilization of psychiatric facilities, on the other, has been labeled an "epidemiological paradox" (Karno and Edgerton 1969) and has been the source of continuing controversy and debate (Madsen 1969; Flores 1978; Keefe, Padilla, and Carlos 1979:150–151). Several explanations have been advanced for this "paradox."

First, Mexican Americans may rely on different cognitive criteria than Anglo groups for perceiving and evaluating psychological difficulties. Attempts to test this hypothesis, however, have been inconclusive. Karno and Edgerton (1969) interviewed groups of Mexican Americans and Anglo Americans of similar socioeconomic status and concluded that the two groups did not differ significantly in their perceptions and definitions of mental illness. These findings are suspect, however, since the respondents were presented mainly with vignettes that described severe psychotic conditions, such as schizophrenia. Emotional and psychological problems that do not manifest themselves in thought disorder (for example, anxiety neurosis, interpersonal conflict, or personality disorder) remained outside the scope of the study and may yet be found subject to differential perception by Mexican and Anglo groups. (Karno and Edgerton's findings may also be questioned on the grounds of using an inappropriate data-gathering technique—survey questionnaires—to probe a sensitive area of inquiry.)

A study by Phillipus (1971), on the other hand, supports the hypothesis of differential interpretation of symptoms by Mexican Americans and Anglo Americans. Only 16 percent of Mexican-American teenagers interpreted hearing "heavenly voices" as evidence of hallucinations or insanity, whereas 90 percent of the Anglo teenagers in the study did so; the former group tended to view such an occurrence as a religious experience. Obviously, further research is needed to evaluate Mexican-American definitions, attitudes, and perceptions toward predominantly nonpsychotic problems such as situational and depressive reactions, anxiety problems, sexual dysfunctions, and various adjustment reactions (Newton 1978).

A second explanation prominent in the debate about the "epidemiological paradox" is that the social and familial structure of Mexican-American life buffers individuals from conflicts with the larger society and is generally protective of their mental health (Jaco 1959; Madsen 1969; Hoppe and Heller 1975:306). Although little empirical research has actually been undertaken on this buffering phenomenon, it is thought to be operative especially among more conservative lower-class families. Madsen, for example, contends that the Mexican American rarely faces crises alone and that the close-knit extended family serves as "an anxiety-sharing and anxiety-reducing mechanism in stressful situations" (1969: 239–240). More recent empirical research by Keefe, Padilla, and Carlos (1979) is somewhat ambiguous on this point. While noting that the extended family is a primary, if not *the* primary, source of emotional support for more upwardly mobile Mexican Americans, these researchers indicate that members of this group are also willing to utilize formal helping services outside the family. The authors consequently discount the presence of the extended family as the reason for an alleged lower incidence of mental illness among Mexican Americans (Keefe, Padilla, and Carlos 1979:150–151).

A third factor sometimes cited as contributory to the low rates of reported psychopathology among members of this ethnic group is the psychological and behavioral attributes of folk illnesses. These illnesses are typically regarded as "diseases of adaptation" (Klein 1978) which afford people an opportunity to satisfy repressed drives or to avoid stress from role conflict or role failure (Madsen 1964b, 1964c, 1969:232–233). In most instances, the stress-alleviating and preventive functions of these disorders are seen to dovetail with the dynamics of Mexican-American folk psychiatry, or *curanderismo* (Kiev 1968).

Other researchers contend that there is a striking discrepancy between the reported low incidence and a much higher true incidence of psychopathology among Mexican Americans (Edgerton, Karno, and Fernandez 1970:126; Torrey 1972:138). Many would argue that present studies simply lack the methodological sophistication to discern such disorders. A recent study of depression among Mexican Americans (Quesada, Spears, and Ramos 1978) suggests that although the family functions as a strong protective agent and tends to lower the actual reporting of depression, it does not insulate its members from feelings of powerlessness and the actual experience of depression. This study further argues that Mexican Americans have experienced an increase in the incidence of depression concomitant with their increasingly urbanized status but that they adopt a second identity or "mask of survival" beyond the boundaries of the family and *barrio*, which obscures the degree of underlying emotional disturbance (Quesada, Spears, and Ramos 1978:84). It should be noted, however, that earlier research on Anglo-American and Mexican-American clinical patients (Meadows and Stoker 1965) reported depressive reactions to be common among Mexican-American females but particularly rare among Mexican-American males.

Explanation of the "epidemiological paradox" has also been approached from the standpoint of utilization of health facilities. A number of studies contend either that a higher real incidence of mental illness is obscured by primary reliance on folk curers (*curanderos*) or that reliance on these folk practitioners is itself preventive of more severe psychiatric disorder (Kiev 1968; Madsen 1969; Torrey 1969, 1972:138–140; Kearney and Richman 1977; Kearney 1978; Macklin 1978). On the other hand, some researchers claim that Mexican Americans turn to private physicians, rather than either *curanderos* or psychiatrists, for help with psychological problems and that this fact accounts for their low utilization of mental health facilities (Karno, Ross, and Caper 1969; Padilla, Ruiz, and Alvarez 1975).

Again, however, the evidence concerning these various points is contradictory. Two Los Angeles studies (Edgerton, Karno, and Fernandez 1970; Padilla, Ruiz, and Alvarez 1975) would seem to indicate that *curanderismo* is on the wane. Few respondents in these studies would recommend a *curandero* to someone with an emotional problem, and about half the sample in the second study could name a mental health clinic, felt positive about it, and would be willing to use it (although few actually did so). In contrast, relatively widespread use of *curanderos* has been reported for Mexican Americans living in San Antonio, Houston, and Chicago (Martínez and Martin 1966; Creson, McKinley, and Evans 1969; Weclew 1975; Quesada and Heller 1977). Moreover, recent data fail to support the claim that Mexican Americans, more often than Anglos, take their emotional problems to private physicians for treatment (Keefe, Padilla, and Carlos 1979:151).

Finally, low utilization of mental health facilities by Mexican Americans has been related to lack of availability and inappropriate organization of services (Karno 1966; Karno and Morales 1971; Abad, Ramos, and Boyce 1974). In most instances, differences between providers and clients in terms of social class, culture, and language have been felt to make mental health services uncongenial to Mexican Americans and to deter utilization. Studies by Flores (1978) and Trevino, Bruhn, and Bunce (1979), however, indicate that when these barriers to utilization are reduced or eliminated, expected utilization tends to be achieved.

An additional mental health issue that has received some research attention among Mexican Americans is alcohol abuse. The previously cited mortality rates for cirrhosis of the liver imply that alcoholism may be a significant problem among particular segments of this population. This observation is supported by reports that *curanderos* frequently treat problems of alcohol abuse and have developed a treatment model for it within the folk medical system (Trotter and Chavira 1978).

Although there are no incidence rates or estimates of prevalence of alcohol abuse, several cultural aspects of alcohol consumption among Mexican Americans have been described. Female Mexican Americans drink less frequently and have fewer abuse problems than males. Consumption patterns, particularly for lower-class males, have been linked with the maintenance of self-identity as a *macho*. Although it has been hypothesized that pressures associated with acculturation contribute to alcohol abuse among Mexican-American males (Madsen 1964c:358–359), feelings of anomie have not been observed to predict alcohol consumption among Mexican Americans, as they do among other whites. Unfortunately, the relative lack of substance-abuse research among members of this ethnic group makes it impossible to determine the extent of particular problems in Mexican-American communities. It is hoped that adequate data will be forthcoming in the near future.

Summary

The epidemiological evidence suggests that the health status of Mexican Americans is strongly related to both poverty and other access barriers that contribute to underutilization of existing health services. This finding suggests that comprehensive health programs for this ethnic group must include provisions for social and economic changes that work toward eliminating these important contributory causes of mortality and morbidity.

With regard to mental health, the overall epidemiological data appear inconclusive. The controversy over apparent versus real incidence rates for psychopathology remains unresolved and awaits the development of more innovative methodological strategies for identification and measurement of mental disorders. Despite evidence to the contrary, it does appear that certain elements of the Mexican-American population (particularly lower-class rural and border residents) continue to have their mental health needs met by folk practitioners (Kiev 1968; Cheney and Adams 1978; Macklin 1978; Kearney 1978). At the same time, a number of efforts are being made to implement collaborative programs between modern and folk psychiatry that utilize the relevant and culturally compatible aspects of the latter (Kay 1978:91; Scrimshaw and Burleigh 1978). In addition, increasing energy is being spent to develop facilities within the mainstream mental health system that encourage utilization by Mexican Americans.

Concepts of Disease and Illness

In varying degrees, Mexican Americans subscribe to concepts from folk, popular, and scientific medicine. The folk concepts, because they lie outside the nosological system of modern medicine, prove most unfamiliar to physicians. Knowledge of folk ideas, however, is of considerable practical importance to practitioners working among Mexican-American populations. Since these concepts signal fundamentally different assumptions about the cause and treatment of disease, physicians must often demonstrate sensitivity to traditional categories of illness if they are to provide effective health care. However well intended, attempts simply to dismiss these concepts and to educate patients to present complaints in ways familiar to the practitioner are often ill-advised. Such an approach generally confirms a suspicion among Mexican-American patients that doctors lack the competence to treat a whole class of widely recognized folk disorders, thus ultimately discouraging the presentation of potentially disabling or fatal symptoms (Rubel 1960:805; Holland 1963:93; Madsen 1964a:105, Rubel and O'Nell 1978:147).

Folk Concepts of Illness and Disease

FOLK CONCEPTS OF ETIOLOGY   A comprehensive anthropological literature documents the historical derivation and present-day distribution of Mexican-American folk medicine. Foster (1953) traces its origins to the confluence of sixteenth century Spanish medical knowledge and native American beliefs during the contact period. In addition to the indigenous *materia medica,* the latter element in this syncretism involved widespread ideas about the magical and emotional causation of illness. In particular, native ideas concerning soul loss occasioned by fright, spirit intrusion, object intrusion, and breach of taboo have continued to play a significant role in illness theory, where they are attributed ultimately to emotional causes: shame, fear, disillusion, anger, or envy (Foster 1953: 203; Holland 1963:93).

The Spanish element in this belief complex is a simplified version of Hippocratic humoral pathology. Although some importance is still placed on the balance of bodily humors, the hot/cold theory remains the most prominent aspect of this tradition in contemporary illness theory (Madsen 1955; Clark 1959; 164–170; Currier 1966; Ingham 1970). According to this doctrine, the healthy body is in a state of equilibrium in terms of the contrasting qualities of "hot" and "cold." Illness is conceived as resulting from disequilibrium after exposure, either internally or externally, to excessive amounts of "heat" or "cold." Traditionally, it should be noted, "hot" and "cold" are not determined simply by temperature but by qualities believed to be inherent in individuals and in particular substances, such as medicines, foods, or objects (Madsen 1955:123; Baca 1973:75). Water, "cold" foods, air, and a cold floor are sources of extreme "cold," which must be neutralized or drawn off by eating "hot" foods, using *emplastos calientes* ("hot poultices"), or drinking herbal teas. Correspondingly, strong emotional experiences, fright, exposure to the sun, and "hot" foods are sources of excessive heat, which require treatment by rubbing the body with a raw egg ("cold"), eating "cold" foods or herbal remedies, or applying *emplastos fríos* ("cold poultices"). The classification of "hot" and "cold" substances refers, in short, to their effects on the human body (Madsen 1964a:71).

Although analyses of Mexican-American folk medicine invariably place considerable emphasis on the hot/cold contrast, there is good evidence to suggest that it is of declining significance in its traditional form (Foster 1948:51; Saunders 1954:147; Lewis 1960:12; Currier 1966: 253). Clark, for example, notes that "although there is a good deal of reliance placed on diet modification for illness, there are relatively few people who know which foods are 'hot' and which are 'cold' " (1959: 165). Although the traditional system may persist among curing specialists, there is an increasing tendency to think less in terms of the "qualities" of hot and cold and more in terms of the actual temperatures associated with foods or bodily conditions (Kay 1977:162; Sandler and Chan 1978:780–781). Accordingly, " 'hot' and 'cold' disorders are coming to be treated more frequently with herbal remedies or with topical applications which either warm or cool the affected area" (Clark 1959:165). Patent and over-the-counter medicines may be used in this fashion as well (Clark 1959:169).

Although classical humoral doctrine appears to be disappearing, the concept of homeostasis is of continuing importance to illness theory among Mexican Americans. Ill health may thus be attributed to internal or external imbalance. The structural parts of the body, for example, are conceived as having a specific place and function, and any change in their position is presumed to cause illness (Rubel 1960:808; Madsen 1964a: 71; Scrimshaw and Burleigh 1978:37). Thus, loss of blood in any amount (even the small quantities required for laboratory tests) is thought to weaken a person and precipitate illness. Blood loss is particularly feared in males, since it is thought to impair sexual vigor (Clark 1959:181; Scrimshaw and Burleigh 1978:36).

Health is also viewed as entailing harmonious relations within both the social and spiritual realms. Disruptions in social relations or transgressions of cultural injunctions are believed to have a deleterious effect on a person's emotional and physical well-being (Schulman and Smith 1963: 232; Madsen 1964a:68). Given this complex interaction of social, psychological, and material factors, folk concepts of etiology do not distinguish between psychic and somatic disorders; rather, both forms of illness are implicated in a theory of causation that combines naturalistic elements with magical and religious elements.

FOLK CLASSIFICATION OF ILLNESS   A number of ethnographers have explored the traditional folk illness taxonomies of Mexican Americans (Saunders 1954; Clark 1959:164–179; Rubel 1960, 1966:157–170; Holland 1963; Madsen 1964a; Baca 1973). Although these studies employ various analytic criteria for classification (for example, diseases of hot/cold imbalance, magical origin, emotional origin, and dislocation of internal organs), none of them discuss the semantic and organizational principles that Mexican Americans themselves use to structure their illness concepts. Rubel (1966:156–157) simply notes that traditional folk concepts are collected under the categories of *males naturales* ("natural illnesses") and *mal puesto* ("witchcraft"). The former category includes four prominent folk syndromes—*caída de la mollera* (or *mollera caída*), *empacho, mal ojo,* and *susto*—in addition to a number of less salient disorders: *bilis, latido, tripa ida, mal aire, chipil,* and *pasmo* (to be defined below). *Mal puesto,* the second major category of disorders, is a somewhat residual group, which may also be termed *brujería, hechicería,* or *enfermedad endañada.*

There is fragmentary evidence suggesting that some Mexican Americans have retained some of these traditional illness labels while discarding the folk concepts and treatments associated with them (Kay 1977: 163–164; 1979:88–92). The terms thus do not mean the same for all users. For example, some Mexican Americans apparently use the term *bilis* to describe "pain in the gallbladder" (Kay 1977:133, 164), *aire* to signify "gas" (Kay 1979:89), *(mal) ojo* to refer to conjunctivitis or nystagmus (Martínez and Martin 1966:162), or *empacho* to mean constipation, devoid of its psychosocial implications (Madsen 1964a:75). These usages thus refer to organic ailments, which are unrelated or only tangentially related to the folk illnesses of the same name. Because of the variance in usage of many illness terms, clinicians treating Mexican Americans must be alert to discover what an individual patient means if he should use one of the following terms in a history or presentation of symptoms; for only by knowing this can the clinician treat the illness along with the disease.

1. *Caída de la mollera* ("fallen fontanelle") is a condition restricted to the very young. This disorder occurs when the *mollera* (the fontanelle of the parietal or frontal bone of the cranium) falls and leaves a "soft spot" which sometimes vibrates during breathing. As reported in the literature, this phenomenon is either mechanically caused by a fall from some height or occurs during breast-feeding when the nipple is suddenly

withdrawn from the infant's mouth. The fallen fontanelle, according to folk theory, results in a downward projection of the palate, which inhibits the infant's ability to ingest food. Since presumably regular feeding cannot resume until the fontanelle is raised to its normal position, the child is usually spoon-fed during this illness.

Symptoms of *caída* include an inability to suck the breast or bottle, diarrhea, vomiting, and inordinate crying and restlessness. The disorder is also generally accompanied by a high temperature and clinically resembles dehydration (Rubel 1960:197–198; Holland 1963:92; Kiev 1968: 105). Noteworthy in this regard is a general confusion between cause and effect; that is, the concept of *caída* seems to be based on the observed loss of subcutaneous fluid over the fontanelle—a result of dehydration caused by infant diarrhea. However, in folk belief the depressed fontanelle and the exaggeration of palatal rugae resulting from fluid loss are assumed to be the primary causative factors (Clark 1959:171). People who are more exposed to mainstream care have apparently come to note the correspondence of these symptoms with dehydration and accordingly equate *caída* with *deshidratación* ("dehydration") or *carencia de agua* ("lack of water") (Kay 1977:135).

Although *caída* is ostensibly linked with a straightforward mechanical etiology, it is an emotionally loaded syndrome for Mexican-American parents, who traditionally display a central concern for children. Guilt over implied improper care or neglect often amplifies general anxiety over this condition (Kiev 1968:106). Although this disorder is not generally fatal, *caída* can result in the infant's death if it is not properly and correctly treated, since the enlargement of palatal rugae sometimes prevents the ingestion of food and liquids, causing gradual desiccation (Rubel 1960:798).

2. *Empacho* ("surfeit" or "indigestion infection") is an infirmity afflicting both children and adults and is attributed to a complex interaction between physiological and social factors. Unlike some other folk disorders, *empacho* can be confused with illnesses and pathogenic conditions recognized by scientific medicine (Quesada and Heller 1977:99). Organically, the condition is caused by a dysfunction of the digestive system, namely, a failure to pass a bolus of poorly digested or uncooked food through the intestinal tract. Consumption of certain foods—cheese, eggs, bananas, or too much white bread—is often thought by Mexican Americans to result in this condition (Clark 1959:179). The intestinal blockage results in sharp pains, "gas on the stomach," or indigestion. In some cases it is reported to cause a fever in the stomach which cannot be observed but which is indicated by great thirst. Abdominal swelling generally results from excessive drinking to quench this thirst (Martínez and Martin 1966:148). Symptoms may include lack of appetite, stomachache, diar-

rhea, and vomiting as well as fever, crying, and restlessness in children. It should be noted that the importance of this disease category in the Mexican-American folk system is no doubt reinforced by the existence of frequent enteric disease, which has fostered a pervasive concern with gastrointestinal disorders (Scrimshaw and Burleigh 1978:36–37).

When a Mexican American suffers from an *empachado* condition, it is generally believed that the illness has resulted from causing the person to eat against his will (for example, forcing a child to eat food he does not want; accepting food offered as hospitality when one is not hungry). In short, this condition results from an individual's allowing another person to override his personal autonomy and thus moving out of balance with his social milieu (Rubel 1960:799–800, 1966:166). If neglected, *empacho* is said to cause severe constipation and, in some instances, death (Kay 1977:135).

3. *Mal ojo* ("evil eye") also embodies the belief that social relations contain inherent dangers to the equilibrium of the individual. Thus a "strong" person with *vista fuerte* ("strong vision") can exert an undue influence over a "weaker" person and bring about the disorder. Children and women, as "weaker" beings, are therefore thought to be particularly susceptible to *mal ojo*. Strong glances, covetous expressions, or inordinate attention causes the entrance of a "stronger power" into the body of weaker individuals and robs them of the ability to act on their own accord. It is sometimes thought that the glance of a pregnant woman may cause an infant to become ill with fever because the "heat" of pregnancy overpowers the child's spirit (Holland 1963:93).

This syndrome appears abruptly and is manifested by rather vague symptoms, including severe headache, nervousness, inconsolable weeping, unusual fretfulness, rashes, or feverishness. In children the illness may be signaled by insomnia, trembling, and excessive crying in addition to fever. In general, *mal ojo* is not considered fatal. However, faulty treatment, sometimes attributed to physicians, allows the infirmity to advance to a grave stage, known as *ojo pasado*. This stage is often fatal because of the severe coughing and vomiting, sometimes of "green bile," that are symptomatic of its critical period (Rubel 1960:801–802, 1966:158).

It should be of considerable importance to physicians to note that *mal ojo* is often invoked only after other diagnoses and their remedies have failed. Accordingly, its symptoms are frequently persistent and may obscure underlying organic pathology, such as colic or influenza (Madsen 1964a:95; Uzzel 1974:374–375).

4. *Susto* ("fright") is by far one of the most frequently studied of all the so-called culture-bound reactive syndromes and is widely known throughout Latin America (Gillin 1948; Rubel 1964; Adams and Rubel 1967; O'Nell and Selby 1968; Klein 1978; Rubel and O'Nell 1978). Al-

though the labels *susto* and *espanto* ("soul loss") are sometimes used to refer to the same illness, older people may distinguish them as two separate disorders caused by different forms of fright. In most instances, however, they are used interchangeably, although the former term is preferred.

The disease is sometimes, though not always, linked to the Hispanic-American belief that the individual is composed of a corporeal being and one or more immaterial souls (*espíritus* or *almas*) which may become detached from the individual as a consequence of an unsettling experience. A number of untoward events, both social and nonsocial, can engender *susto*. Some may be completely physical (for example, falling into a lake or encountering a dangerous animal), others may involve social incidents, such as being attacked or deserted by one's spouse, experiences of embarrassment or humiliation, or the injury or death of a relative or close friend. The trauma of such an experience is thought to immobilize the afflicted person and result in helplessness and the inability to act or remove the cause of fear.

This syndrome affects persons of both sexes and of all age categories. In particular, it is found in children, who are believed to be susceptible even in utero (Clark 1959:177; Uzzel 1974:370; Klein 1978:24; Scrimshaw and Burleigh 1978:35). Early stages of the disorder (*susto nuevo* or *susto liviano*) are accompanied by stomachache, diarrhea, high temperature, vomiting, and other symptoms (Holland 1963:98). Persons who are *asustado* generally experience continuous periods of languor, loss of appetite and strength, weight loss, restlessness, inability to urinate, general listlessness, and lack of motivation to discharge everyday tasks and social responsibilities. Additional symptoms may sometimes be added to this basic syndrome—for example, fever, muscular pains, alteration in complexion, nausea, stomach or intestinal upsets, and vertigo (Klein 1978:23). Advanced cases (*susto pasado*) are frequently fatal and are characterized by the slow wasting away of the organism. The wasting effects of this advanced stage give the condition its other names, *mal de delgadito* and *tis* (Rubel 1960:805). Some people reportedly believe that untreated cases of *susto* can lead to tuberculosis (Martínez and Martin 1966:149).

The epidemiology of *susto* indicates a variable and complex interaction between physiological states, the experience of intracultural stress, and individual personality dispositions. On the one hand, it appears to be a culturally meaningful type of anxiety hysteria linked to role conflicts and self-perceived social inadequacies (Rubel 1964:278–282; O'Nell and Selby 1968; Kiev 1968:170; Klein 1978). This view suggests that *susto* is preeminently a social and flexible disease that serves both as an explanation and an excuse for a passive sick role. Rubel, for example, notes that in instances of adult *susto* "people . . . not only choose to assume the sick role but also elect the kinds of symptoms by which to make manifest to others an absence of well-being" (1964:280). Similarly, Uzzel emphasizes the voluntary aspects of the disorder, noting that *susto* is a role "that may be assumed by an individual primarily in order to impose his or her definition upon situations and thereby control . . . interactions" (1974:374). Inasmuch as a person afflicted with this syndrome can temporarily escape from psychological stresses engendered within a cultural framework, it is to be expected that people who experience greater role stress and who have fewer available, culturally legitimate ways to express that stress are most likely to be at risk for the disease. There is some evidence to indicate that women suffer *susto* significantly more often than men for these reasons.

At the same time, *susto* is often more than simply a culturally constituted defense mechanism. Its advanced manifestations (*susto pasado*) and the fact that children, who are too young to participate in a diagnosis, frequently experience the illness both imply a strong organic component. In this regard, a recent study has demonstrated that *asustado* persons are significantly more organically diseased *and* less adequate at discharging standard social roles than persons suffering from other illnesses (Rubel and O'Nell 1978).

These findings are of considerable practical importance to health-care providers because they indicate the necessity of diagnosing and treating both the physical and the psychological manifestations of this illness. They also imply that in dealing with conditions like *susto* and *mal ojo*, which combine symptoms of multiple origins according to biomedical concepts of etiology and nosology, the clinician is best advised to attend to the particular signs and symptoms the patient presents, rather than the labels he may attach to them (Rubel and O'Nell 1978:150). However, when the clinician is explaining the diagnosis or negotiating a treatment regimen, the patient's concepts and labels then assume critical importance.

5. The term *bilis* ("bile"), while not always used to indicate a disease, often implies that a person is in a nervous or "upset" condition. A belief borrowed from classical humoral theory maintains that bile must remain in balance for a person to enjoy good health. Any highly emotional experience (anger, fear, sorrow) that causes a person to become upset may cause bile to flow into the bloodstream, giving rise to a variety of ills. This disorder produces symptoms of acute nervous tension, chronic fatigue, and malaise (Clark 1959:175; Holland 1963:92).

6. *Latido* ("palpitation," "cachexia") is an infirmity diagnosed by severe weakness, accompanied by a "pulsating of the stomach." It is thought to be caused by going without food for long periods of time, which then results in severe pains in the diaphragmatic area that make it difficult to eat again. Advanced forms of *latido* are characterized by severe emaciation, loss of abdominal fat, and an empty stomach and intestines.

This condition makes it possible to feel the normal pulsation of the abdominal aorta on deep palpation (Clark 1959:178; Kay 1977:135).

7. *Tripa ida* is a physical condition often associated with the onset of *susto*. Despite the fact that folk nosologies characteristically treat each set of symptoms as an etiologically discrete illness (Fabrega 1974; Young 1976:8), there is some uncertainty as to whether *tripa ida* and *susto* are considered separate disorders or simply progressive stages of symptom formation in a single syndrome. *Tripa ida* is not often reported in the literature, and there is some discrepancy about its symptomatology. Kay (1977:135) contends that it may accompany "fright" or trauma and involves a "locking" of the intestines. That this "locking" produces constipation may be inferred from the fact that the condition is treated with suppositories (Kay 1977:152). Holland (1963:93), on the other hand, reports stomachache, diarrhea, high temperature, and vomiting as symptoms of *tripa ida*.

8. *Mal aire* ("bad air") is generally linked to the hot/cold theory of disease. It is thought that air, especially night air, may enter the body through its various cavities and result in illness. People in a weakened state from overheating or extreme emotion are thought to be particularly susceptible to this phenomenon. Symptoms produced by this infirmity vary but are principally associated with phenomena in which sensory and motor functions of the body are impaired. Most commonly, *mal aire* produces facial twisting or paralysis. General preventive measures include avoidance of drafts, particularly for infants, children, and pregnant women. Some concern is expressed about cutting the umbilical cord too short, thus allowing air to enter through the abdomen and umbilicus (Clark 1959:173; Currier 1966: 254; Baca 1973:73; Scrimshaw and Burleigh 1978:35).

9. *Chipil* is another ailment restricted to infants, although it is becoming increasingly rare as bottle feeding becomes more popular. It involves a belief, found widely throughout the world, that an infant may suffer from an emotional disturbance and upset stomach if the mother becomes pregnant before he is weaned (Madsen 1964a:75). Symptoms include a loss of sucking ability and excessive crying.

10. *Pasmo* ("infection") is most often described as a postpartum illness that results from the transgression of prohibitions associated with *la dieta* or *la cuarentena* (the 40-day period of convalescence following delivery). During this time women are enjoined to avoid bathing, eating foods that are "too acid," and, in particular, engaging in sexual intercourse. Violation of these injunctions is believed to result in symptoms similar to those of tetanus, kidney disease, and septicemia. Swelling around the eyes and ankles is often a primary diagnostic feature in newly delivered mothers (Kay 1977:155). In other individuals, however, *pasmo*

manifests as a rash or blisters that are associated with a rapid chilling of the body (Kay 1977:135–136). This disorder is rarely reported in the literature and may be specific only to certain areas.

11. For two reasons, *mal puesto* ("bewitchment") is a residual disease category for Mexican Americans. First, there is a declining belief in *brujería* or *hechicería* (witchcraft) among this group; and second, the label *mal puesto* is used only after several other diagnoses have been tried and their treatment proven unsuccessful. Bewitching is most commonly believed to follow from serious disruptions in social relations—for example, quarrels between lovers, unrequited love, or conflict between families or individuals (Madsen 1964a:84; Rubel 1966:168). Following a disruption of these kinds, a *bruja* or *brujo* (sorcerer) is charged with placing a hex on the offending person.

Mal puesto is assumed to be a common cause of barrenness and insanity and is usually invoked to explain schizophrenic reactions and other psychotic disorders. A person who is suspicious, moody, or begins to act strangely may be identified as *embrujada* ("bewitched"). This syndrome is also often associated with a wide range of physical symptoms that persist despite various forms of treatment and cannot otherwise be explained. As a general rule, the longer the duration of any type of illness, the more probable it is that it will eventually be diagnosed as *mal puesto* (Clark 1959:174–175; Madsen 1964a:84–85; Rubel 1966:167–168; Kiev 1968:98, Ingham 1970:82; Kay 1977:139).

Folk and Scientific Concepts of Illness

In recent years, medical anthropologists have focused much effort on understanding the interaction between traditional and modern medical systems. Almost universally, they have documented the persistence of indigenous disease concepts, despite the inroads of scientific medicine. A substantial number of cases indicate a simultaneous recognition of both folk and scientific concepts, with varying recourse to their respective etiological theories. In many respects, the orientation of Mexican Americans to scientific medicine reflects this pattern.

Members of this ethnic population recognize a number of scientific disease categories, although they do not necessarily so label them. For example, within the category of *males naturales* ("natural illnesses"), a clear distinction is made between those disorders that are unique to the folk nosology and those recognized by biomedicine. The latter include, among others, *sarampión* (measles), *la chanza* (mumps), *pulmonía* (bronchitis or pneumonia), *presión* (high blood pressure), *ataque de corazón* (heart disease), *cálculos* (stones), *ulceras* (ulcers), *reuma* (rheumatism), *mal de riñón* (kidney disease), *asma* (asthma), *tos ferina* (whooping cough), *resfriado* (cold), and *cólico* (colic) (Clark 1959:180;

Madsen 1964a:72; Rubel 1966:167; Kay 1977:126–127). Recognition of these biomedical categories, however, does not necessarily imply a corresponding acceptance of scientific etiologies. In some instances, scientific syndromes may be attributed to a derangement or imbalance in social relations. (Among older, more conservative Mexican Americans, for example, it is not uncommon to relate illness to the pathogenic impact of changing cultural conditions.) In other instances, folk theories of causation, often derived from local modifications of the hot/cold paradigm, may be used to explain standard biomedical diseases (Clark 1959: 167–168; Madsen 1964a:72–73; Kay 1977: 160–164).

At least in part, the relationship between modern and folk etiological theories may reflect Mexican-American patients' uneven exposure to the practice and theory of modern medicine. Elements of modern medical practice are readily observable to lay persons and are incorporated where they appear compatible. In contrast, scientific medical theory is typically not revealed to health-care utilizers by physicians, who often fail to disseminate diagnostic and etiological knowledge to their clients (McClain 1977:341; see also Madsen 1964a:71). This failing may have implications of varying severity for the treatment of specific ailments, since conservative Mexican Americans tend to classify and treat disease according to its cause rather than its symptoms (Madsen 1964a:71). Accordingly, a variety of Western disease entities (for example, colds, rashes, diarrheas, ulcers, and constipation) may continue to be treated according to the tenets of folk theory. Thus, informants interviewed by Kay in Tucson expressed the belief "that colds should be allowed to run; that rashes should erupt; that diarrheas should not be checked; [and] that ulcers should continually drain" (1977:163). Since some of these practices not only run counter to current medical theory but also may be harmful, clinicians would be well advised to inform patients of practices that are likely to cause further problems (for example, the consequences of allowing diarrhea to go unchecked without compensating for fluid loss—a concept that is completely compatible with homeostatic folk theories of illness).

Intraethnic Variation in Disease Theory and Knowledge

Mexican-American illness concepts and theory vary widely both among subgroups and among individuals of this ethnic collectivity. As previously noted, variations in the knowledge of and adherence to folk or scientific medical concepts are largely determined by the interaction of factors such as socioeconomic class and degree of acculturation (Holland 1963; Madsen 1964a:95; Farge 1975:410, 1978; Kay 1978:91; Scrimshaw and Burleigh 1978), rural or urban status (Kay 1977:159, 1978: 91; Farge 1978:281; Casillas 1978:79; Scrimshaw and Burleigh 1978: 37–39; Collado 1978) place of birth and generational status (Clark 1959;

Madsen 1964a; Rubel 1966), family and community integration (Clark 1959; Weaver 1970; Kay 1977:159; Cheney and Adams 1978:82–83), and sex. This last factor is related to the woman's role as "home medical specialist" (Weaver 1970:143). As a consequence of this role allocation, most medical knowledge is transmitted between mothers and daughters (Rubel 1966:180).

It is very important to recognize, however, that it is misleading to dichotomize Mexican Americans according to "traditional" or "scientific" medical orientations. In reality, the distinction is a continuous rather than a discrete one. Most Mexican Americans are, in fact, heterogeneous utilizers of medical care (Holland 1963; Weaver 1970). Although there may exist a small minority of Mexican Americans who subscribe exclusively to folk illness concepts and theory, most research indicates that even lower-class members of this group share some knowledge and acceptance of biomedical concepts but tend to maintain separate cognitive categories for "folk" and "scientific" disorders. In some instances, it appears that these categories are relatively insulated from each other, in which case people logically conclude that each class of illness can only be effectively treated by practitioners of that respective class (Holland 1963:100; Martínez and Martin 1966:150; Creson, McKinley, and Evans 1969:265). More often, however, it appears that the salience of a folk or a scientific concept depends on a variety of factors such as the nature of an illness episode, the sequencing of referral and treatment, and the ability of folk or scientific methods to effect a satisfactory outcome (Holland 1963:101; Madsen 1964a:95; Weaver 1970:143; Kay 1977:151). In short, folk or scientific beliefs may be "situationally selected" in light of any or all of these factors.

It is also important to point out that folk illness concepts tend to have broad cultural significance for many Mexican Americans. Anthropologists have long realized that illness beliefs and their associated practices are intimately woven into the pattern of a specific sociocultural existence. Illness episodes, by virtue of the manner in which they are ordered and given meaning, perform an important ontological role, namely, communicating and confirming significant ideas about the nature of social reality (Young 1976). Thus for many Mexican Americans, the diagnosis and successful management of these disorders essentially confirm traditional ideas about the nature of the individual and his proper relationship with his fellows. Madsen, for example, notes that insofar as "Anglos are believed to be immune from [folk illnesses], merely being afflicted by one is a means of cultural identification with La Raza" (1964c:433). Consequently, it is not difficult to understand how these traditional concepts of illness may serve culturally unifying functions—particularly under disruptive and stressful conditions of social change. Occurrences of folk illness have thus acquired a symbolic significance for many Mexican Americans that far transcends their importance as pathological conditions (Clark 1959:201–203; Rubel 1960:813–814; Scrimshaw and Burleigh 1978:37).

In view of the symbolic significance that some patients may attach to interpreting a particular ailment in folk terms, it is important for clinicians to discover how the patient conceives of his problem when it entails symptoms that may well receive a folk label. In those instances in which a folk illness is suspected, Kay suggests that the clinician may say to the patient: "There are different facts about bilis (pasmo, mollera, arteritis, etc.). Tell me your thoughts about this condition. In your case, what caused it? What do you think would be the best treatment?" (1979:91). If the patient's explanation differs from the clinician's, the latter may simply note that there are many illnesses with similar symptoms and that his examination indicates a particular diagnosis and treatment, which should then be explained carefully and clearly.

Becoming Ill

In all cultural settings, the transition from health to illness is as much a psychosocial as it is a biophysical process. The perception and evaluation of symptoms is significantly mediated by situational and social factors. Given that Mexican Americans (1) experience somewhat poorer health than the majority of Americans and (2) have recourse to competing interpretations of illness, it may be of some concern to health providers to understand the criteria by which members of this group perceive illness, assess symptoms, and decide whether a person is sufficiently impaired to warrant treatment.

The Concept of Health

For Mexican Americans, a healthy person is defined primarily by three factors: adequate functioning, a robust or "well-fleshed" body, and the absence of pain (Schulman and Smith 1963). As with all cultural groups, "adequate functioning" is an integral part of the image of health. For Mexican Americans, this concept implies a high level of energy output and physical activity which ensures that adult men and women successfully perform the routine tasks of everyday life. As is generally the case for most people, "health" may include the presence of signs or symptoms that indicate pathology, as long as they do not interfere with normal activity (Schulman and Smith 1963:229; S. Fisch, personal communication). Accordingly, members of this group may frequently assign little or no negative value to symptoms such as sore throat, diarrhea, or cough. In addition, they may frequently accept as "normal" the presence of a contagious person in their midst (Murry 1954:130–131; Schulman and Smith 1963:228).

Most Mexican Americans feel that life is full of traumas and difficulties that should be borne with dignity and courage. Consequently, neither men nor women easily succumb to the initial signs of illness. Moreover, since illness and health are considered more or less a matter of chance, the sick person is rarely held responsible for becoming ill, nor does he think of blaming himself for developing an infirmity (Clark 1959: 197–198). Thus, an attitude of blame on the part of the clinician is totally at variance with Mexican-American cultural expectations and should be avoided.

The Social Context of Diagnosis

In contrast to Anglo-American notions of individual responsibility for one's health, Mexican Americans involve others, particularly kinsmen, in matters concerning individual well-being. Even though a person may be convinced that he is sick enough to warrant special attention, it is customary for a Mexican American "to present his symptoms to his relatives and friends for their appraisal before he takes steps to obtain medical treatment" (Clark 1959:203). Conversely, a recalcitrant person who refuses to seek treatment despite a debilitating condition often becomes the focus of group persuasion to accept some form of care (Clark 1959: 191–192). This pattern of group consultation is particularly notable for major decisions like surgery, hospitalization, or referral to a distant specialist (Clark 1959:189–204; S. Fisch, personal communication). The practical implications of this behavior will be discussed in the sections on mainstream medical care and adherence to treatment.

The order in which family members may be consulted for particular conditions seems to be quite predictable. Almost invariably the wife/mother makes the initial assessment of a symptom. Although different patterns are reported (Holland 1963:101; Kay 1977:151), a person's inability to diagnose a disorder or to effect a quick cure generally results in consultation with kinsmen who are perceived to be particularly knowledgeable (for example, experienced older women) and then with compadres, neighbors, and finally friends (Rubel 1960:798; Weaver 1970: 142–143; Kay 1977:125). Particularly resistant or severe problems may subsequently be referred to a folk curing specialist and ultimately to a physician if alleviation of the condition has not been achieved (Holland 1963:101–102; Kiev 1968:32; Weaver 1970).

An increasingly important variant of this general pattern relates to concurrent or "dual usage" of folk and biomedical practitioners. There is fragmentary evidence to suggest that with increasing exposure to biomedical practices, many Mexican Americans have become aware of the

vagueness and indeterminacy associated with folk diagnostic procedures. By simultaneous reliance on folk and biomedical interpretations,
they are in a sense "hedging their bets" on a successful outcome (Martínez
and Martin 1966:150; Creson, McKinley, and Evans 1969:266; S. Fisch,
personal communication). In general, one might logically expect that
more severe, persistent, or recalcitrant symptoms will be handled in this
manner.

Perception and Evaluation of Symptoms

A number of studies, though fragmentary, provide data on the
evaluative components of Mexican-American illness behavior. In addition
to knowing the symptoms for a variety of minor ailments (colds, sore
throats, and so on), most female heads of household appear to recognize
the symptoms associated with folk disorders as well as certain symptoms
and signs of more serious physical illnesses. Using formal elicitation techniques with 60 lower-class Mexican-American women in Tucson, Kay
reports the recognition and use of the following signs and symptoms in
evaluating illness: *calentura* ("general fever"), *calentura local* ("local
fever"), *dolor* ("pain"), *basca* ("nausea or vomiting"), *pujo* ("grip-
ing"), *moco* ("mucus"), *tos* ("cough"), *cambio de color* ("change in
color"), and *erupción* ("rash"). Signs and symptoms used to diagnose
enfermedad emocional ("emotional illness") include *mortificación*
("worry") or *miedo* ("fear"), *desequilibrio* ("lack of equilibrium"),
tristeza ("sadness" or "depression"), *coraje* ("rage" or "hostility"),
desvarío ("delirium"), *desmayo* ("fainting"), and *ataques* ("convulsions") (Kay 1977:125–128).

Though it is reasonable to assume that some of these symptoms may be
used systematically to identify a limited range of illnesses, the identification of syndromes by particular symptoms is, in practice, generally
achieved or validated by laymen only "after the fact" (Young 1976:11).
Rubel illustrates this point with a description elicited from a young informant:

> You would have a pain in your head and would touch your hand to your
> head and say, "Mamá, Mamá," and maybe you would cry a little. Then
> mother would get some aspirins and she would put you in bed to keep
> you warm and comfortable. If you didn't hurt anywhere in your body, then
> there was nothing the matter with you. Then during the middle of the night
> mother would get up and go over to the bed and see how you were doing.
> In the morning if you didn't get out of bed, she would give you more
> aspirins, and if you were still sick, she would start on the herbs. She would
> go through all the teas that she knew, and then she would ask the neigh-
> bors. If none of these things worked, and you had tried all the teas and
> medicines that people knew of, then they figured that you suffered from

ojo. Ojo, also, is very dangerous. The people would start praying for you, and they would start rubbing your body and making a big cross on your chest with an egg. After that you might be swept with branches of a *pirul* tree. Then if this didn't help the sickness, and if you're not dead yet, they would . . . start curing you for *empacho.* All this time you were kept in bed. This is because you were to be warm and kept comfortable. You couldn't walk around because you would have your little strength drained out of you. After all this treatment and after you were well again, mother would give us a purge to clear the stomach of all the herbs; this was to allow the stomach to start new again. (Rubel 1966:156)

Thus, lay diagnosis is essentially contingent and pragmatic; according to Rubel, "as in more orthodox nosological systems, a diagnosis is, in the final analysis, validated by the favorable response a patient makes to the regimen of healing that the diagnosis demands" (1966:155–156). In addition to depicting the pragmatic nature of folk diagnosis, the passage quoted above implies that any listing of symptoms is relatively meaningless unless it stipulates the conditions under which particular symptoms are translated into illness. Even though some symptoms clearly command greater attention than do others, the relative importance given to any sign or symptom depends significantly on a variety of social and situational factors.

CLINICAL IMPLICATIONS OF LAY EVALUATION OF SYMPTOMS   Clearly, a folk orientation requires the presence of symptoms to diagnose illness, whereas this is not necessarily the case for biomedicine. A person who manifests no debilitating symptoms is generally regarded by Mexican Americans as healthy, despite the fact that the diagnostic tests of biomedicine may disclose serious pathology (for example, carcinoma, tuberculosis, or heart disease). It should be noted, however, that the concept of a "preclinical" stage of illness is not unfamiliar to folk belief. For example, it is recognized that a person may not develop the symptoms of *susto* for some time following a traumatic experience, and moreover, if prophylactic measures are initiated during this time the illness may be averted (Clark 1959:228). Given this kind of appreciation, it is not completely clear why the preclinical stages of biomedical syndromes are not more widely recognized by members of this group. This orientation does suggest, however, that clinicians treating asymptomatic patients should thoroughly explain the prodromal stages of disorders such as tuberculosis or cancer.

Because folk illness categories are typically based on vague and quite general symptomatologies, they have the capacity of being applied to rather global symptom complexes which in fact signal serious organic disorder (Rubel 1960:808, 1966:161–165; Rubel and O'Nell 1978).

A number of these disorders, such as heart disease (*mal de corazón*), cancer (*cancer*), and liver disease (*mal de higado*), are characterized by rather generalized symptoms (fatigue, weakness, malaise) which may allow them to be interpreted as *susto*. Indeed, this interpretation appears to be made quite frequently with symptoms of tuberculosis and diabetes (Madsen 1964a:105; Rubel and O'Nell 1978). It is therefore important to recognize that this tendency may prevent or delay a variety of disorders from coming to the attention of a physician. This situation emphasizes the value of careful screening when persons suspected of maintaining a strong folk orientation visit a health facility for any reason.

Variations in Response to Symptoms

In addition to the relative importance of folk or modern medical orientations, prominent determinants of different responses to and evaluations of symptoms include the social and physical characteristics of the afflicted person; the duration, location, and severity of symptoms; and the degree of interference of symptoms with social activities or familial responsibilities.

Although Mexican Americans tend to assume a stoic attitude toward illness, considerable variation exists in light of the factors mentioned above. Initially, of course, it is to be expected that considerations of class, education, and acculturation, which promote ideological commitment to anglicized and middle-class perceptions and attitudes, will be of fundamental importance. In general, men and older boys are most reluctant to submit to illness. For the latter, there is a strong urge to express their masculinity, and giving in to illness with the first appearance of symptoms is considered an admission of weakness and lack of stamina. Adult males, moreover, are generally constrained by the necessity of successfully discharging their role as wage earners. Women, on the other hand, can more easily be relieved of their social duties during illness by relatives and *comadres* ("ritual kin"), who are generally close at hand (Clark 1959: 195; Kay 1977:112).

In the case of children, particularly infants and young children, symptoms are less frequently ignored. Indeed, according to Madsen, Mexican-American parents are "particularly conscientious about taking sick children to the doctor when there is the slightest cause for alarm, even though the cost of medical treatment may impose a severe financial strain on the family" (1964a:95). Similar caution extends to pregnant women, who are at liberty to restrict their activities in order to ensure the safe delivery of a healthy child (Clark 1959:196).

Another factor in conditioning tolerance to symptoms is that of visible physical attitudes. People of both sexes who are *robusto* ("big") and have a "well-filled frame" may be expected, and may themselves expect, to demonstrate more resistance to symptoms than people who are less well endowed. It has been observed, for example, that people who are *robusto* may refuse to accept treatment for early diagnosis of tuberculosis, a disease that is typically associated with the "small and emaciated" (Schulman and Smith 1963:231–232).

Conversely, symptoms such as noticeable weight loss are often considered serious enough in themselves to warrant attention. In many cases, a person who is sufficiently thin (for whatever reason) may warrant a diagnosis of *latido* ("chachexia") (Clark 1959:178–179, 228). Similarly, a *niño galgo* ("hungry child") may be the object of much parental concern and will be considered ill if he is unable to gain weight (Schulman and Smith 1963:232).

Just as individuals with different social and physical attributes are assessed differently against the context of illness, so do particular symptoms evoke different levels of concern. A number of chronic and acute disorders may be permitted to run their course, provided they prove to be neither incapacitating nor terribly painful. A variety of intermittent symptoms may also be ignored, as is often the case with upper respiratory infections, asthma, or the early stages of tuberculosis (Clark 1959:191–196; Schulman and Smith 1963:228–232). Likewise, a number of less serious afflictions such as sore throats, diarrhea, and the like may be tolerated by Mexican Americans as long as they do not develop into more severe conditions.

In contrast, there is considerable cultural preoccupation and worry over symptoms relating to the gastrointestinal tract—for example, vomiting, bloating and belching, indigestion, gas on the stomach, or constipation. The concern over these conditions is reflected in a common practice of "cleaning the stomach" with purges two or three times a year (Clark 1959:180; Scrimshaw and Burleigh 1978:36). Similar anxiety attaches to symptoms such as fever and nervous tension or "being high-strung" (*corajudo*). The presence of ganglion masses or varicosities in the tissue of the arms and legs is regarded as evidence of a disabling nervous condition; these irregularities are taken to indicate *bolitas* ("lumps" or "little balls"), a condition in which the "nerves are out of place" (Clark 1959: 172; Klev 1968:132). It should be noted that the physical signs described above constitute the primary symptom complexes for a number of folk disorders (for example, *empacho, susto nuevo, tripa ida, bilis, ojo*).

Clinicians frequently do not view such conditions with great concern. For many Mexican Americans, however, these disorders are particularly worrisome and disabling in themselves (Kiev 1968:188; S. Fisch, personal communication) and, on this ground, should be paid special attention by medical personnel. Careful explanation of the causes of these symptoms will undoubtedly contribute toward reducing patients' anxiety concerning them.

Conclusions

Among many Mexican Americans, the extent to which rather generalized and common symptoms are interpreted in terms of a folk as opposed to a biomedical concept depends largely on their exposure to modern medicine. Moreover, the nature of this exposure is often crucial, since a person's ultimate welfare may depend on his acting in terms of a biomedical perspective. It is worth reiterating the point that physicians should play a more active educational role vis-à-vis many of their Mexican-American patients. Despite the fact that medical providers are by training often encouraged to view their role as largely technical, if they are to serve the best interests of this patient population they must assume greater responsibility for providing people with the skill to evaluate symptoms in a manner that will enable them to seek out the most effective sources of treatment.

Coping with Illness outside the Mainstream Medical System

A consideration of how people solve illness problems outside the mainstream medical system is particularly important among members of low-income populations, who may be less able to afford the high costs of medical care. It is an even more important concern among Mexican Americans, given cultural and communication barriers and often limited access to medical services. It is not surprising, therefore, that many Mexican Americans avail themselves of other sources of treatment before, during, or after seeking mainstream health services.

Treating Illness in the Home and Family

The traditional Mexican-American family is characterized by a large, close-knit kin group, including both lineal and collateral relatives (Clark 1959:156; Madsen 1964a, 1969; Rubel 1966; Kay 1977:107–109). Ties beyond the nuclear family are strong and extensive, linking grandparents, aunts, uncles, and cousins in relationships characterized by frequent material and emotional supportive exchanges. This kin network is frequently extended further by the institution of *compadrazgo* ("ritual coparenthood") in which *compadres* and *comadres* assume the rights and obligations of relatives and are assimilated into the extended family (Clark 1959:157–161). Often this kinship structure serves as a protective support system from which a person can expect cooperation and assistance in times of stress (Madsen 1964c:425). In this role the family is preeminent in the initial diagnosis and treatment of illness and significantly mediates all subsequent outside efforts at therapy and re-habilitation.

Actual treatment of folk disorders and of a variety of minor illnesses commonly occurs within the home. Folk therapies include oral adminis-tration of various herbal teas and purgatives for digestive disorders; topi-cal application of liniments, oils, and herbal mixtures as well as *sobadas* ("massage") and *ventosas* ("cupping") for muscle aches; dietary regula-tion; magical-religious cures; and the use of patent medicines, tonics, salves, and laxatives (Clark 1959:163–182; Kay 1977).

LAY TREATMENT OF FOLK DISORDERS   Although few lay therapies ap-pear to be harmful, the treatments for *mollera caída* and *empacho* present particular problems or opportunities for clinicians treating more tradition-ally oriented Mexican Americans.

Treatment of *mollera caída* involves a number of alternative proce-dures that are known and used by many Mexican-American women. Most common is the mechanical method of placing the thumb inside an afflicted infant's mouth and applying upward pressure on the distended palate. In this manner, the *bolita* (that is, the swollen palatal rugae) is supposedly restored to its proper position. At the same time, an external "pull" may also be applied to the depression in the fontanelle by exerting sucking pressure with the mouth. The child is then held upside down and the body is brusquely shaken toward the head. Finally, treatment is con-cluded by applying a poultice of either salt, fresh soap shavings, or herbs to the depression on the head, which is left in place for a few days (Clark 1959:170–171; Rubel 1960:798; Holland 1963:92; Martínez and Martin 1966:148).

From a biomedical standpoint, the health impact of the physical ma-nipulations associated with this treatment may be questionable. However, the therapy is of significance to clinicians because it is the only set of treatments that leaves visible evidence of ministering to a folk syndrome. Since the family will often seek the aid of a physician if the infant's con-dition does not quickly respond to treatment for *caída* (Rubel 1960:798), the telltale signs of treatment afford the clinician an opportunity to in-form the family in a noncondemnatory manner of the biomedical corre-lates and consequences of dehydration (Kay 1977:151, 165).

Lay therapy for *ojo* and *susto* involves substantively magical treat-ments (namely, "sweeping" or passing an egg over the contours of the body); however, the treatment for *empacho* involves empirical therapies, including massage and manipulation of the abdomen and back along the lower spinal column in order to dislodge the undigested bolus of food. In addition, an oral dosage of lead protoxide (sold as *la greta* in phar-macies) or *azogue* ("quicksilver") is administered to penetrate and soften the offending ball of food. To counteract the toxicity and "coldness" of these therapeutic agents, "hot" Epsom salts may later be taken to neutralize them. Again, depending on the individual understanding of the condition and local knowledge, this treatment may be followed by ingestion of other "hot" and "cold" agents, in a process of balance and counterbalance (for example, castor oil, herbal preparations, juices) (Rubel 1960:799). Also reportedly used as purgatives are herbal teas made from *estafiate* (larkspur or wormwood), *hojas de sen* (senna leaves), *manzanilla* (chamomile), *pamita* (tansy mustard), *yerba buena* (mint), *epazote* (saltwort or wormseed), or ashes from the food believed to have caused the *empachado* condition (Clark 1959:179; Martínez and Martin 1966: 148; Kay 1977:142–144).

In light of the various therapeutic agents and counteragents that a person may ingest during treatment, and the often unknown pharmacological properties of various herbal remedies (or the quantities in which known remedies are safe), physicians should explore with patients the nature of the treatment they have already undergone in the case of an illness of the digestive system. This is particularly important because patients infrequently volunteer such information, and lay remedies combined with medicines prescribed by a physician may potentiate one another, so the possibility of an overdose may be a genuine concern (Kay 1978:94). Accordingly, it is advisable for health-care professionals to become familiar with the properties of the locally used pharmacopoeia, both to advise against the use of certain dangerous herbs (such as *epazote*) and to guard against the inadvertent but harmful synergistic effects of herbal and prescription medicines.

Lay Consultation and Referral outside the Home

Information concerning the hierarchy of curative resources among Mexican Americans is uneven and largely impressionistic. A study by Weaver (1970:142), however, identifies two basic types of referral networks, the "extended" and the "truncated," which are more or less consistent with a number of ethnographic accounts (Clark 1959; Holland 1963; Madsen 1964a; Rubel 1966; Cheney and Adams 1978).

For the most part, the extended network, with its reliance on lay, folk, and nonmainstream medical referrals, has already been described in the section on concepts of disease and illness. In contrast, the truncated network moves the patient directly to a physician after the ministrations of the extended family and kin group have produced no noticeable improvement (Weaver 1970; Kay 1977:151). Predictably, these patterns are strongly influenced by socioeconomic class, acculturation, and situational considerations. The sequence described in the extended system is generally characteristic of lower-class and working-class Mexican-American families, both rural and urban (Clark 1959:206–208; Madsen 1964a:95; Rubel 1966:175–177), whereas the truncated style of referral tends to predominate among more anglicized and middle-class families (Weaver 1970:142–146).

This generalization, however, is not fully sustained by the evidence. For example, studies of both middle-class Mexican Americans (Holland 1963:101; Madsen 1964a:95) and lower-class Mexican Americans (Kay 1977:151; Cheney and Adams 1978:83) indicate a common pattern of consulting folk specialists after mainstream medical practitioners have been unable to alleviate a problem. In addition, conjoint consultation of folk and biomedical practitioners has been increasingly reported among lower-class Mexican Americans (Kay 1978; Casillas 1978:78; Cheney and Adams 1978:83). Indeed, the actual consultation and referral network that is utilized in any particular instance seems to be more closely related to a variety of situational factors than to social class. These factors include past experience with medical specialists (Clark 1959:206), the severity of the illness, the nature of the symptoms, and the level of anxiety of the major decision makers. What these different patterns of recourse to care imply for mainstream practitioners is that it is difficult to know, without actually asking, whether a patient may be receiving care simultaneously from a folk healer. In circumstances in which it seems advisable to establish this fact, the clinician must therefore ask directly, though in a manner that does not imply censure of the practice.

Nonmainstream Medical Care outside the Home

A wide variety of folk practitioners administer to the Mexican-American community, including *herbolarios* or *yerberos* ("herbalists"), *sobadoras* ("masseuses" or "folk chiropractors"), *señoras* ("wise women"), *espiritualistas* ("spiritualists"), *parteras* ("lay midwives"), and *curanderos* ("curers"). All these practitioners treat in accordance with the illness concepts and etiological theory outlined in the section on concepts of disease and illness.

Most instances of actual referral to these folk specialists apparently take place through a family member, relative, or friend who has had previous occasion to engage the practitioner's services or is aware of the practitioner by reputation (Madsen 1964a:90). Research conducted in Houston by Cheney and Adams (1978:82–83) documents the existence of intensive information exchange networks among *barrio* families concerning nonmainstream curative resources. This practice results in an extensive lay referral system that crosses city-wide *barrio* boundaries to identify traditional curers with varying levels and types of expertise. Evidence of similar referral practices has also been suggested by Kiev (1968), Clark (1959:206–207), and Weclew (1975:150–151).

It is not clear if there is any predictable sequence in which these various folk practitioners are consulted. Given the reported tendency of Mexican Americans to seek quick relief from symptoms, it is likely that the services of different practitioners are utilized pragmatically rather than in a definite sequence (Rubel 1966:175–177; S. Fisch, personal communication; but compare Kiev 1968:32, who reports *herbolarios* as a source of care used prior to *curanderos*).

YERBEROS *Yerberos* ("herbalists") are especially knowledgeable about home remedies and have long been an important health resource in Mexican-American neighborhoods and communities. They validate their healing abilities through "knowledge of nature"—recognizing hundreds of wild and domestic medicinal plants. The herbalist's role in the curative process is less that of a diagnostician and more that of an adjunct to home diagnosis. His medical performance, consequently, centers on providing instructions for the preparation and proper dosage of orally and topically applied remedies, which most often involve decoctions for the treatment of *empacho,* various digestive ailments, and any number of other common indispositions. Although specific data do not exist concerning the prevalence with which Mexican Americans rely on herbalists, the widespread popularity and use of herbal remedies reported in all ethnographic accounts indicate that they are a ubiquitous feature of health-care behavior.

CURANDEROS *Curanderos* or folk curers comprise the preeminent specialty among indigenous healers. It should be noted, however, that these curers do not constitute a homogeneous group; they may be distinguished not only according to their expertise with particular disorders, but also according to the types of healing powers they claim (Romano 1965). Most *curanderos,* for example, rely on empirical remedies (herbs, poultices, massage) and magical-religious treatment rather than on supernatural abilities. Other *curanderos,* however, are recognized as charismatic healers who attribute their curing abilities to divinely bestowed powers (Madsen 1964a:87; Rubel 1966:185–189; Kiev 1968:86).

The *curandero's* armamentarium includes a wide range of herbal remedies and ritual treatments, such as stylized manipulation of raw eggs and palm leaves ("sweeping") and various incantations. Moreover, in addition to the various treatments used by other folk specialists (for example, massage and poultices), *curanderos* may use inhalation and sweating therapy for viral upper respiratory infections (Kiev 1968:130–132; Kay 1977:150). There is some indication that a number of contemporary *curanderos* have also taken on a few accoutrements of modern medicine: they may maintain consulting rooms equipped with medical instruments, use stethoscopes, and give hypodermic injections of antibiotics and vitamins (Madsen 1964a:90; Casillas 1978:78).

Although the literature indicates that some variability exists, it appears that *curanderos* are most often consulted for the treatment of folk syndromes (*caída, ojo, empacho,* and *susto*), febrile illnesses in children, chronic nonremitting illnesses and symptoms, and a variety of psychologically and socially disruptive complaints (for example, depression, impotence, alcoholism) (Madsen 1964a:104–105, 1964c; Kiev 1968:32; Quesada and Heller 1977:99). Evidence concerning the willingness of *curanderos* to treat more severe organic disorders is somewhat conflicting. It is certainly true that these healers unwittingly treat chronic organic conditions that are misdiagnosed as folk syndromes (for example, tuberculosis and diabetes as *susto pasado*). Trotter and Chavira (1978) report that *curanderos* handle a number of serious ailments, including terminal cancer, tuberculosis, and the like. In contrast, however, Madsen (1964a: 90) contends that these practitioners rarely accept cases that they perceive as terminal, since the death of a patient threatens the healer's reputation, exposes him to accusations of witchcraft, and may lead to legal investigation.

There is increasing, though fragmentary, evidence to suggest that folk curers do not see themselves in competition with modern medical providers. Cheney and Adams (1978:83–84) report that all the *curanderos* contacted in their study acknowledged the use of biomedical services for themselves and their families. Likewise, Kay (1978:90) indicates that curers will avail themselves of scientific care for serious illness. In addition, both studies document the willingness of healers to refer clients to biomedical practitioners for serious ailments. Indeed, in some instances they may encourage treatment for folk syndromes by both traditional and biomedical means. *Curanderos* studied by Kay (1978:94), for example, believe that the condition labeled *caída* by folk medicine and "dehydration" by biomedicine requires therapy from both systems—that is, healers administer treatments to lift the fontanelle but also refer their patients to physicians for treatment of dehydration and diarrhea. In this way, many curers may serve to integrate patients into the mainstream medical system rather than promoting their encapsulation within the folk system.

A number of studies indicate that *curanderos* are good intuitive psychologists who display considerable insight into both intracultural and acculturational pressures and stresses (Madsen 1964c; Torrey 1969; Kline 1969). Kiev's extensive ethnopsychiatric analysis of *curanderismo* (1968:185–187) suggests that folk healers are capable of making effective use of various stock psychotherapeutic maneuvers. Indeed, there is a growing recognition of the expertise of *curanderos* in dealing with neurotic and personality disorders as well as the less severe psychoses (Madsen 1964a:114–115; Kiev 1968:185–187; Torrey 1969; Kline 1969; Macklin 1978).

Curanderos may be the preferred sources of medical care for a number of reasons. First, they typically expect a donation rather than fixed remuneration for their services, and they prescribe inexpensive herbs or balms rather than costly medications (Rubel 1966:194). In addition to sharing traditional concepts of illness, they satisfy the interactional norms expected between healer and patient. Not only do they establish a warm and intimate relationship with their clients (they may in fact be well-known members of the community), they also give importance to the social significance of illness among Mexican Americans. The patient is often treated in the presence of his family, and the *curandero* may allow the family head to decide whether and when treatment should commence and permit family members to take an active role in the treatment (Madsen 1964a:91; Kiev 1968). Since the *curandero's* interpersonal style is of considerable importance in gaining the trust and confidence of patients, it is one of the elements of folk medicine that warrants careful consideration by biomedical practitioners.

The *curandero*-patient relationship may frequently capitalize on a pattern of "paternalistic dependence" that is often said to characterize the interpersonal relations of many conservative Mexican Americans (see Quesada and Heller 1977:98). Although it is unwarranted to overgeneralize this point, Mexican Americans have frequently been reported to attempt to establish a patron-client relationship with authority figures, and curers, by virtue of their cultural role, are generally regarded as such (Romano 1965; Kiev 1968). In any event, the folk healer, rather than asking a series of objective, clinical questions, more often satisfies the patient's expectations by providing reassuring answers. (In fact, the *curandero,* because he is usually part of a stable and well-integrated community, often has intimate knowledge of the social conflicts surrounding a potential patient before he is even consulted.) In short, folk healers may take on a kind of omniscience that is seen to be lacking in the objectivity of the medical professional.

As suggested earlier, the frequency with which folk healers are used by Mexican Americans is nearly impossible to determine. Most research that attempts to measure utilization of this health resource is either highly impressionistic or relies on questionable survey and sampling methods (see Martínez and Martin 1966; Creson, McKinley, and Evans 1969; Edgerton, Karno, and Fernández 1970; Torrey 1972:136–142; Weclew 1975). Existing data suggest that there may, in fact, be regional variations in the importance of *curanderos* in the health-care system. More specifically, *curanderismo* appears to be declining outside the border states of the Southwest but to be flourishing among populations located within that region (Quesada and Heller 1977; Velimirovic 1978).

ESPIRITUALISTAS   *Espiritualistas* ("spiritualists") may treat basic folk disorders and use herbal medicine, massage, and special diets. However, these healing modalities are secondary to the treatment of both serious and minor ailments through trance and spirit mediumship. This category of healers represents a syncretism between *curanderismo* and *espiritualismo*. Their primary effectiveness appears to be limited to psychosomatic and emotional disorders. These healers are seemingly much less used than other folk specialists, although their popularity is reportedly growing among certain populations (Madsen 1964a:89; Macklin 1974, 1978; Kearney 1978).

PARTERAS   *Parteras* (lay midwives who may be both folk practitioners and marginal members of the mainstream medical system) have long been an important component of the health-care delivery system available to Mexican Americans. They deliver a significant proportion of babies in the Rio Grande Valley of Texas and other parts of the borderland states. Unlike certified nurse midwives, these folk specialists are not products of a formal educational program, although they may be subject to licensing requirements in some states (for example, Arizona).

In addition to handling pregnancies, *parteras* may also serve as an important component of the illness referral system for their clients, both during a pregnancy and during sickness events unrelated to birth. Clients may be referred to herbalists or to clinics for prenatal blood and urine tests. In some instances the midwife may refer her patient to an Anglo physician if complications are predicted (Schreiber and Philpott 1978).

The popularity of these specialists is related to both economic and cultural factors. They are not only easily accessible, particularly in rural areas, but they are often favored by low-income women because of their low cost (generally around $60 to $75 for prenatal care, delivery, and postnatal care). Although the lowering of economic barriers often encourages the use of clinics by lower-class women, many continue to prefer *parteras* who, because they are mothers themselves, are felt to understand the fears and pains attached to childbirth better than physicians, the majority of whom are males. In addition, a strong cultural element of modesty makes physical exposure to a male physician extremely embarrassing for many Mexican-American women. Finally, *parteras* are considered to be more patient and to show more interest in their clients than physicians. They may stay at home with the mother from the time labor begins in order to administer massage and provide hot teas for her comfort (Clark 1959:124–125; Rubel 1966:182; Schreiber and Philpott 1978).

SOBADORAS   *Sobadoras* ("masseuses") are specialists who treat physical ailments, relying on massage to relieve sprains, muscular pains, and joint dislocation. According to Kay (1977:150), this role in the healing hierarchy is generally occupied by a woman who learned the skill from her mother or grandmother. *Sobadoras* are believed to be particularly effective in the treatments of *empacho* and *caída,* which both involve forms of physical manipulation that may be combined with prayers and *barridas* (spiritual cleansing and "sweeping") in order to restore bodily equilibrium. The popularity of these specialists no doubt derives from a class of common ailments that are thought to involve the displacement of internal organs (Clark 1959:170–171; Holland 1963:92).

SEÑORAS *Señoras* ("wise women") are middle-aged and elderly women who are looked upon as specialists because they have absorbed more popular medical knowledge than their contemporaries. *Señoras* may demonstrate skill in the treatment of particular folk disorders (particularly those affecting infants) and may also function as midwives. Most often these healers minister to the needs of the extended family and people within the immediate community (Rubel 1966:181–182; Cheney and Adams 1978:82).

Encounters with Mainstream Medical Practitioners

It is obvious that Mexican Americans have not been full participants in the mainstream health-care system. As a predominantly low-income population, they experience a number of socioeconomic impediments to health care, and these barriers are exacerbated by sociocultural factors.

Access Barriers to Health Care

The marginal economic position of many Mexican Americans cannot be overstated. The fee-for-service structure of modern medicine frequently represents too high a percentage of family income, and despite increasing movement of Mexican Americans into the urban-industrial sector, many still lack health insurance plans or adequate medical coverage (Roberts and Lee 1980b). Time and money are limited for people with low incomes and large families, and these are often the critical factors that determine whether a patient will go to a doctor or will simply rely on home remedies or folk healers. Furthermore, both rural and urban Mexican Americans still experience problems of access because of inadequate education and social and geographic isolation (Scrimshaw and Burleigh 1978:39). In other instances, members of this group are underserved in particular areas of health care (Quesada and Heller 1977:95; Roberts and Lee 1980b).

Among Mexican Americans none are more subject to these access barriers than migrants. Moreover, even when the economic burden of health care is mitigated for them, procurement of health services still remains a problem. Thus, in a special experiment in which migrants in the area of Laredo, Texas were supplied with Blue Cross cards to cover their health-care costs while in the migrant stream, utilization rates were still lower than expected (Walker 1979). The extreme poverty, large families, and geographical mobility that Coles (1970) and others have described among migrants all go a long way toward explaining the special health problems of this subsector of the population.

The Chicano health movement has adopted broad-ranging policies to alleviate some of the major problems that Mexican Americans face in using the mainstream medical system. Consumer interest groups, migrant health centers, and regional health organizations have been developed in many states and cities to deliver medical services, disseminate health information, develop trained Chicano health personnel, and organize support for issues affecting the health of Mexican Americans. These organizations generally operate under the assumption that improvement in health care for minorities can only occur in the wake of broader social change.

Problems of Language and Communication

The ability to communicate is undoubtedly one of the most essential tools of the health-care provider. That language acts as a barrier to the full use of health services has been well documented in the case of Mexican Americans (Clark 1959:218–221; Lurie and Lawrence 1971; Cervantes 1972; Quesada 1976; Quesada and Heller 1977; Gonzálcs 1978). Although most Mexican Americans are bilingual, a minority speak little or no English. Even for many of those who are nominally bilingual, the inability of health providers to converse in Spanish is looked upon as a form of ethnocentrism that discourages interaction. In the areas of both mental and physical health care, language difficulties act as a deterrent to referral, impede the delivery of medical care, and reduce its quality (Karno 1966; Cervantes 1972; Quesada 1976; Flores 1978; Trevino, Bruhn, and Bunce 1979).

These factors may have a number of consequences for the actual clinical encounter. Given that Mexican Americans (sometimes more than members of other ethnic groups) are frightened by illness, problems of communication make it impossible for physicians to attend properly to the emotional aspects of care (Clark 1959; Lurie and Lawrence 1971: 780). Moreover, Mexican Americans, in attempting to maintain their *dignidad* ("dignity"), are often reluctant to admit their poor comprehension of English and consequent failure to understand medical instructions and explanations (Lurie and Lawrence 1971:778). Only when a medical fiasco occurs does the nature and extent of the language barrier become apparent.

Language problems are further reflected in a frequent overestimation of the speaking and technical vocabularies of patients. Even Spanish-language health materials often use terminology that has no meaning for many Mexican Americans (Clark 1959:221). In addition, attention must be directed to assuring that such materials are culturally relevant for this population, rather than for other Spanish-speaking groups such as Puerto Ricans (Kay 1977:164).

Cultural Factors in the Use of Mainstream Medical Services

In addition to linguistic impediments, certain aspects of Mexican-American culture have been suggested as factors that may discourage the use of mainstream care. Commonly cited in this regard is familism—that is, encapsulation in a close-knit kinship network. The data on this point, however, have been conflicting (compare Nall and Speilberg 1967; Hoppe and Heller 1975; Keefe, Padilla, and Carlos 1979). Though it cannot be concluded from these studies that familism actually prevents the use of mainstream medical care, it does appear to affect both the pathway to mainstream care and the speed with which members of close-knit families consult a professional health facility (Quesada and Heller 1977:95).

Interactional Norms in the Medical Encounter

ROLE OF THE FAMILY   Although there exists some question about the impact of familism on access to mainstream care, it is clear that it plays an important role in the actual medical encounter. Any diagnosis or treatment suggested by a biomedical professional (or folk practitioner) will be discussed, evaluated, and either accepted or rejected by consensus of the patient's family (Scrimshaw and Burleigh 1978:38). As might be expected, family participation is particularly significant in major decisions regarding surgery, hospitalization, or referral to a distant specialist (S. Fisch, personal communication; Clark 1959:189–204).

Obviously, this pattern of intense family involvement is of considerable importance in relations with medical professionals, who tend to deal with patients as though they were autonomous decision makers. When a Mexican American is asked to make an on-the-spot medical decision on his own initiative, he is placed in an embarrassing and impossible situation. Clinicians frequently report that trying to force such an immediate decision without allowing the patient an opportunity to consult with his family not only causes increased patient anxiety but also may result in a refusal to undergo treatment (Scrimshaw and Burleigh 1978:38). In other instances the patient, possibly in an effort to appear courteous and gracious, may seemingly agree to whatever plan the physician presents; then, however, if the family subsequently disagrees with the "approved" arrangements for a procedure, appointments may be broken without warning, much to the confusion and exasperation of medical practitioners (Clark 1959:205; Baca 1973:76).

Decisions concerning the health care of infants and children—given their central importance in Mexican-American society—may be particularly sensitive (Clark 1959:204). A clinician might logically expect that consultation with the mother is sufficient to elicit a decision concerning a child's needs for hospitalization or special treatment. However, not allowing the woman time to go home and talk matters over with the entire family (husband, relatives, and *compadres*) generally results in an unwillingness to consider the proposed action (S. Fisch, personal communication).

The implications of this familistic orientation to health-care decisions are obvious. Given that the Mexican-American family often supersedes the authority of both the individual patient and health-care personnel, the latter are well advised to exercise patience and tact and to afford the patient every opportunity to arrive at a conclusive decision within the context of his family. In fact, the physician may go a long way toward gaining the trust and confidence of patients by demonstrating his understanding of the family's importance in medical matters—for example, by suggesting such consultation or soliciting the opinions of other family members (Clark 1959:214).

EXPECTATIONS ABOUT THE PATIENT-HEALER RELATIONSHIP   Mexican Americans often regard mainstream medical encounters as unsatisfying experiences because of cultural expectations about the patient-healer relationship that are not shared or recognized by modern practitioners. Biomedical practitioners are typically educated to remain objective and affectively neutral in dealing with patients. Although Mexican Americans clearly vary in their expectations, many perceive the "professionalism" of mainstream health-care practitioners as cold, impersonal, and indicative of a lack of concern. An overly clinical attitude may, in fact, be interpreted as a sign of hostility (Clark 1959:215; Scrimshaw and Burleigh 1978:38). Members of this group expect that the physician will take a personal interest in their problems and will convey sympathy, warmth, and reassurance. The fact that these amenities are frequently not forthcoming may reinforce already-present fears of Anglo discrimination (Scrimshaw and Burleigh 1978:38).

From the physician's perspective, these expectations often conflict with notions of "efficiency." Physicians with many cases to handle work against time, and this generally involves avoiding long conversation with a patient and coming directly to the point. Such a procedure is often viewed as rude and indecorous by Mexican Americans, who expect the physician to demonstrate his good will by exchanging social amenities and inquiring into the patient's own opinion of his condition. For many members of this group, illness is such a sobering and frightening event that they do not want to be rushed. Moreover, since the anxiety level of patients may already be rather high by the time they reach the mainstream medical practitioner, such "efficiency" does nothing to allay their fears or encourage confidence in the provider.

Although practitioners have real demands on their time and abilities, they need not compromise their professional integrity or their objectivity by striking a friendly manner toward patients. The efficacy of treatment in the long run may depend more on the manner in which the health-care provider interacts with patients than on his technical abilities. Touching —in the form of a handshake, a pat on the head, or a clasp of the arm—is taken as a sign of concern and good will. The importance of attentive listening, however briefly, should also not be underestimated. Whether the physician is Anglo or Chicano, Spanish-speaking or not, if he does not listen attentively to the patient he is not considered to be a good doctor (Scrimshaw and Burleigh 1978:38).

The same expectations on the part of Mexican Americans that tend to jeopardize the dyadic patient-practitioner relationship often apply to the hospital setting as well. Lurie and Lawrence observe that many Mexican Americans "have unrealistic expectations about the role of the doctor in the hospital setting" (1971:780), largely because they do not understand the nature of hospital routines and the constraints they impose on physicians. Families assume that the doctor will take time to be friendly and supportive, since he presumably understands the fears that accompany hospitalization, and they may interpret the absence of special attention as either a lack of concern or Anglo prejudice.

This situation not only underscores the apprehension of Mexican Americans concerning hospitalization (McLemore 1963; Schulman and Smith 1963:956; Madsen 1964a:93) and the corresponding need for greater reassurance from providers during such periods, it also reemphasizes the importance of communication between practitioners and patients. For, to the extent that Mexican Americans are marginal participants in the modern medical system, they are less well informed about its "realities," poorly acquainted with its institutional procedures, and may experience greater than normal anxiety over certain facets of care (for example, surgical interventions). Thus they are dependent on health-care personnel to provide them with a set of expectations for coping with what may be a strange and ominous experience.

Another important dimension of patient-practitioner interaction involves the social distance between the parties concerned and the perceived nature of the physician's authority. Traditionally, respect for authority has an important place in Mexican-American culture. However, this concept has somewhat different connotations for conservative Mexican Americans than it does for middle-class professionals. Physicians often believe that by virtue of the prestige of their training they will be recognized as the final authority in medical matters and can therefore assume a good deal of control over the patient's behavior—in short, that they can issue directives. Such an approach is viewed as heavy-handed by many Mexican Americans and is seen as violating the notions of *dignidad* ("dignity") and *respeto* ("respect") embodied in traditional asymmetrical relationships (Quesada (1976:324).

With regard to all these interactional considerations, health-care professionals can learn a valuable lesson from the style of folk practitioners— namely, the willingness of *curanderos* to take a personal interest in their clients, to include the family in all phases of care, and to suggest rather than order their clients. To the extent that medical professionals can adopt some of these behaviors, the therapeutic relationship with Mexican Americans will be enhanced.

INTERACTION BETWEEN THE SEXES   The impact of varying role expectations is also evident in other aspects of the patient-practitioner relationship. In particular, difficulties can result from differing attitudes concerning modesty and sex roles. Reportedly, Mexican Americans of both sexes frequently experience medical treatment as embarrassing. As a result of culturally conditioned feelings of feminine modesty, Mexican-American women may be particularly sensitive about obstetrical and gynecological examinations with male physicians or nurses (Clark 1959:229–230; Rubel 1966:182). A Mexican-American husband may be reluctant to leave the examining room during such an examination of his spouse, since he feels it is necessary, as a good husband, to protect his wife's modesty (Lurie and Lawrence 1971:780). Mexican-American men are reported to experience similar discomfort in medical encounters with female practitioners when they are asked to undress or to give a urine specimen; such requests are seen as threatening to the masculinity and self-esteem of males and may be refused.

What physicians and nurses may perceive as ignorance or lack of cooperation in these instances is, however, viewed by the patient as a reasonable attempt to preserve self-dignity (Lurie and Lawrence 1971:780). This difference in viewpoint suggests that medical professionals might avoid embarrassing Mexican-American patients unnecessarily by limiting the amount of bodily exposure required during physical examinations. Moreover, requests for this exposure can be more tactfully managed by same-sex members of a clinical staff, and sexual topics may be more comfortably explored if they are not discussed in mixed groups (Clark 1959:

229–230; Madsen 1964a:92; Lurie and Lawrence 1971:779–780). Variations in attitudes undoubtedly exist in these areas; however, reported behaviors do suggest that they are best approached with caution and tact by medical personnel.

Reactions to Medical Diagnosis

Not only do Mexican Americans come to the medical consultation with a culturally determined set of interactional norms, many have their own culturally derived concepts and interpretations about particular health problems. It has already been noted that many members of this group have a fatalistic outlook toward illness. Although this attitude is no doubt changing with the wider awareness of the communicability of disease, hygiene, and preventive medicine, the view persists in some sectors of Mexican-American society. Consequently, the implication by a medical provider that the patient is somehow at fault and responsible for his condition is often received with hostility and indignation. To the afflicted person and his family, such a view is unjust or even malicious (Clark 1959:230).

It has also been observed that Mexican Americans infrequently volunteer their perceptions regarding folk medicine to health professionals. However, in those instances where patients do disclose a self-diagnosis (for example, a folk disorder), they may be insulted when it is summarily dismissed or denounced as a superstition (Madsen 1964a:92). Many Mexican Americans know that such disorders exist, because they have seen them diagnosed and successfully treated. This fact makes it much more productive for mainstream health-care personnel to play down differences in etiological concepts by making it clear that different illnesses may have similar symptoms. Indeed, a carefully explained and tactfully presented "alternative" diagnosis that culminates in successful treatment may serve an important role in shaping medical knowledge and future attitudes (Clark 1959:226, Madsen 1964a:95). Furthermore, denial by mainstream practitioners that folk disorders exist only reinforces the belief that these illnesses lie outside the physician's sphere of competence; for how can a doctor treat something he does not realize exists? Thus, skepticism or ridicule of a self-diagnosis for such disorders only encourages patients to continue other forms of treatment.

Even in instances where folk diagnoses are not revealed to the health-care provider, patients may have already defined and treated their disorder within the traditional medical framework. A thoroughly elaborated biomedical diagnosis and prognosis may similarly serve an important educational function in these cases. This presentation should be preceded, however, by a nonjudgmental elicitation of the patient's view of the illness so that appropriate likenesses and differences can be discussed.

Not only are there frequent discrepancies between the nosological and etiological concepts of patients and those of practitioners, but their emotional investment in particular symptoms is also frequently discordant. It has already been noted that Mexican-American patients may not attach particular significance to symptoms that physicians consider serious, and vice versa. Again, this phenomenon is a straightforward reflection of this group's marginal involvement in mainstream medical care, since the different meanings attached to diagnostic categories by physicians and patients are, at least in part, a function of familiarity. To the extent that the views of each remain discrepant and unexplored, however, they tend to undermine the quality of medical care in terms of both patient satisfaction and therapeutic effectiveness.

The impact on patient satisfaction, for example, may be seen when health professionals dismiss or treat lightly those symptoms that Mexican Americans regard as particularly threatening. The failure of clinicians to clarify and dispense reassurance over such conditions often leaves patients unsettled and feeling as if further action is required. Indeed, from the patient's perspective, reassurance that his symptoms are not pathological may be as important as the diagnosis and treatment of "real" disease (Clark 1959:229; S. Fisch, personal communication). In both instances, however, the importance of the physician as a source of information and counsel comes into focus. If the cooperation, trust, and confidence of patients are desired, medical professionals must be more conscious of providing accurate and understandable explanations in terms of symptoms, prognosis, and treatments.

Adherence to Biomedical Treatment
Structural and Interactional Factors

It is certainly not surprising to find that adherence to biomedical treatment is affected by many of the same structural, attitudinal, and cognitive factors that deter entry into the health-care system. Problems of economics and transportation clearly have a deterrent effect on follow-up care, and in many cases, if inexpensive generic drugs are not specified in pharmaceutical prescriptions, members of large families may well find it impossible to comply with a treatment regimen because of competing primary necessities (Quesada 1976).

It is also apparent that the interactional and communicational aspects of the provider-patient relationship have no small impact on compliance. Clinicians may themselves contribute to patient attrition because they relate to patients in an authoritarian or impersonal manner. On the other hand, nonadherence to treatment may simply be a consequence of inadequate explanation on the part of a health-care provider or the inability of a patient to understand instructions—a communicative gap that may be masked by a silent or overly agreeable facade (Quesada 1976:326). This potential lack of communication places a greater burden on the practitioner to ask appropriate questions and provide thorough and understandable explanations (Clark 1959:205; Lurie and Lawrence 1971:778–779; Quesada 1976:326).

Role of the Family

There can be little doubt that the sanctioning role of the Mexican-American family in health care exercises a pervasive influence throughout the entire course of the treatment process. As observed, consultation with family members is warranted following the initial diagnosis; it is also not unreasonable to suggest family consultations for extended treatment of chronic conditions if the clinician wishes to increase compliance.

Hospitalization, particularly for a prolonged period, may be resisted by Mexican Americans because it entails isolation from the ministrations and support of kinsmen and *compadres* (Saunders 1954:166; Clark 1959:231, 235; Schulman 1960:956; McLemore 1963; Madsen 1964a: 93). Additional institutional complications may arise when a Mexican American does become hospitalized, since members of this group expect and generally receive a great number of visitors (Clark 1959:231)— often considerably more than hospital administrators and other personnel feel is desirable for hospital routine. Yet patients resent having their families excluded from medical situations. The conflict between what patients and their families desire and need and what hospitals (often inflexibly) require may lead ultimately to a patient's leaving the hospital against medical advice (Lurie and Lawrence 1971:780).

Family roles and expectations condition attitudes to treatment in additional ways. Mexican-American males, for example, generally consider that sickness reflects moral weakness. Accordingly, disclosing illness to outsiders is felt to be a shameful and painful experience if a person possesses *dignidad* (Clark 1959:195). Moreover, it is very difficult for men to tolerate loss of authority or self-esteem before family members who regard them as *patrones*. In light of these self-evaluations and cultural expectations, it is not uncommon for male patients to discontinue treatment immediately following signs of symptom relief; that is, once the patient is capable of resuming normal activities, treatment is no longer viewed as socially acceptable (Quesada 1976:326). It is important to note that resumption of treatment is generally possible if someone the patient recognizes as an authority figure encourages him to continue. From the standpoint of health workers, it may therefore be important to explore a patient's network of relationships for such a person (for example, older males, *patrones, compadres*).

Patient Expectations and Compliance

Mexican Americans often expect quick and conclusive therapeutic results and consequently engage in peripatetic "shopping" among a variety of practitioners—both folk and modern. They also tend to move rather quickly through successive stages of referral and consultation with these multiple providers (Rubel 1966:175; Weaver 1970). This pattern is often indicated to clinicians by the "brown-bag syndrome"—that is, the patient appears in the examining room with a paper bag containing an assortment of medications acquired from previous consultations (S. Fisch, personal communication). Itinerant health-seeking behavior is frequently frustrating to biomedical practitioners, who place value on the continuity of care. It is important to recognize, however, that a patient's preoccupation with symptom relief may indicate a lack of information on the nature and consequences particularly of chronic diseases. Again, we emphasize the need for clinicians to acquaint patients thoroughly with the entire expected course of a disease so that quick cures will not be anticipated. In the case of many illnesses this not only serves an important educational function, it also may prepare patients to cope with unfamiliar technological interventions. Otherwise, such interventions remain unexpected and unexplained and may be viewed as sufficiently threatening to warrant withdrawal from treatment (Quesada 1976:325).

Dietary Practices and Adherence to Therapy

A number of cultural beliefs and practices have a potential bearing on problems of biomedical compliance. Dietary practices and their relationship to the hot/cold doctrine may be of significance in this regard. Particular attention is given to items of diet during pregnancy and the menstrual period. "Hot" foods such as chilies may be avoided during pregnancy, since they may be believed to affect the infant's health adversely in later life; "cold" or acid foods are to be avoided during the menstrual period, since they are thought to cause menstrual blood to congeal and later reappear as cancer (Clark 1959:122–123; Kay 1977: 153).

Among many Mexican Americans, the period of *la cuarentena* or *la dieta* (that is, 40 days postpartum) continues to be viewed as a sensitive time. New Mexican-American mothers often complain that they are served foods in the hospital that are "bad" for them because they are either too "hot" or too "cold." Such patients should therefore have a choice of dietary items so they can avoid these unacceptable foods (for example, pork, tomatoes, pickles, spinach, cucumbers) and not be forced to go hungry in order to avoid violating food taboos (Clark 1959:227; Kay 1977:155). The ideal postpartum diet for Mexican-American women consists of chicken, eggs, toasted tortillas and bread, milk, cereals, sweet rolls, and meats (other than pork).

For other patients, the difficulties of hospitalization can be made more tolerable by greater attention to the staples of the Mexican-American diet. For example, simple Mexican foods such as rice, pinto beans, tortillas, sausage, cheese, and chili sauce may be served more frequently (Clark 1959:227).

Finally, the widespread belief in the healing power of herbal remedies is another cultural element that physicians might use to enhance adherence to any biomedical treatment involving the necessity of high or regular liquid intake (for example, for infant diarrhea). Instead of suggesting water under such circumstances, the physician could recommend herbal tea, which would be more likely to prompt compliance and might also avoid problems of infection resulting from unboiled impure water (Clark 1959:226–227).

Conclusion

It is obvious that many of the factors affecting adherence to medical treatment are related to the socioeconomic circumstances of patients and are beyond the control of clinicians. However, by familiarizing themselves with the expectations and perceptions that Mexican Americans may bring to the treatment process, physicians can not only provide more satisfying care to their clients but greatly improve the success of biomedical treatment. Providers of medical care would do well to remember that care of the sick is embedded in the social relations and beliefs of a given people.

Recovery, Rehabilitation, and Death

Data on recovery and rehabilitation among Mexican Americans derive from a limited number of sources and are largely inferential (Clark 1959; Madsen 1964a, 1969; Rubel 1966; Weaver 1970). Hard data are not available on the impact of catastrophic illness among Mexican Americans, but existing evidence suggests that convalescence for members of low-income families tends to be abbreviated (Quesada 1976). It is impossible to determine the extent to which this phenomenon reflects economic constraints, which may force resumption of normal activities, or the effect of supportive mechanisms, which may actually accelerate recovery. There is little doubt, however, that during periods of illness, Mexican Americans have available a strong and cohesive natural support system in the form of the extended family (Madsen 1969; Keefe, Padilla, and Carlos 1979).

Although there is a dearth of empirical evidence concerning the actual process by which support is mobilized or activated, many Mexican Americans appear to be part of familial networks involving a well-defined set of shared values and normative expectations that are currently thought to enhance support through positive feedback. Not only do Mexican-American families define the individual as a valued and cared-for member of a viable social unit, they also implicate him in an ongoing network of mutual obligations, which reinforces these sentiments. Such nurturant interpersonal exchanges are generally conceded to moderate life stress, to have a salutary impact on health outcomes, and to play a protective role in life crises (Cobb 1976). In short, these factors suggest that Mexican Americans may be well equipped to deal with the emotional impact of serious social disruptions such as catastrophic illness and bereavement (Finlayson 1976; Walker, McBride, and Vachon 1977).

During periods of illness, it is typically the case that family members, relatives, and *compadres* relieve the afflicted person (especially women) of domestic chores and child-care duties, provide close and constant emotional support, and extend economic resources to carry the person through a period of incapacity (Clark 1959:190,194).

Although there are contradictory reports concerning the extent to which practices associated with the *cuarentena* (40-day postpartum period) persist (Clark 1959:226 228; Kay 1977:155), newly delivered mothers still tend to be the focus of much attention. Particular care is taken that they are not exposed to upsetting experiences. Friends, neighbors, and relatives visit, assist with home-care duties, and offer personal attention and social support.

In cases of serious illness, Mexican Americans inevitably choose to remain at home surrounded by the support and ministrations of the family. Hospitals are feared not only because they remove the individual from the family but also for a variety of other reasons—fear of the unknown, lack of understanding of reasons for treatment and hospital procedures, fear of discriminatory treatment, fear of affronts to modesty and individual dignity. These attitudes certainly suggest that physicians would do well to minimize the hospital stays of Mexican-American patients and to treat problems in the home to the maximum extent possible. Since the evidence concerning the advantages of longer periods of hospitalization following major surgical interventions is equivocal, the advisability of this approach is underscored.

Of considerable relevance to the process of recovery among many Mexican Americans is the close association between religion and sickness; for illness often becomes the occasion for propitiatory rituals. Whatever the material effects of folk healers may be, they clearly provide a powerful form of ritual reassurance which invokes the power of God in any outcome (Rubel 1966:172–178; Kiev 1968). Many Mexican-American homes contain altars where devotions are carried out before statues and images of the saints. Masses may be said in the home, devotional offerings and personal sacrifices made, and religious activities adopted in order to regain health. Vows of penance are offered to special saints in return for their intercession and commendation, and in some instances, conservative Mexican Americans may make pilgrimages to shrines in Mexico (Holland 1963:91–92; Kay 1977:120–123). Obviously, this emphasis on faith and religious conviction cannot be underestimated in the recovery process (see Frank 1961).

From the standpoint of modern medicine, there is little doubt that familism and a conservative world view can be a two-edged sword. Particularly during the diagnostic and treatment phases of medical intervention, these factors may limit or modify the form of care that clinicians might deem most appropriate. During the recovery phase, however, they clearly provide a form of social and psychological support that is generally impossible to offer in an institutional setting. Physicians are well advised to keep this fact in mind—particularly in their treatment of terminally ill patients. These elements of Mexican-American life provide a level of emotional reassurance and personal meaning that is too often underestimated by biomedical healers.

Concluding Remarks

Although social class, degree of acculturation, and involvement in relatively closed family or community networks all produce differences in health behavior among Mexican Americans, there are a number of general points that clinicians can keep in mind while treating members of this ethnic group.

Language Use

Because of the importance of language in treating the illness aspect of any sickness and the varying degrees of competence in English displayed by Hispanics, clinicians who regularly treat Mexican Americans should take steps to become bilingual. When this optimal course of action is impractical, the clinician should attempt to ascertain the patient's level of English comprehension in a way that is not threatening or demeaning to the patient. This can generally be accomplished during routine history taking, by asking the patient to describe the symptoms of any chronic or fatal illness reported for a close relative. If language is perceived to be a problem, resort to a translator will be necessary; preferably this translator will be someone who has accompanied the patient for that purpose or a person specifically trained in medical terminology.

Interaction Style

Several features of the interaction style of folk healers serve to underscore culturally important behaviors that deliverers of mainstream medical care might well emulate.

1. The clinician should act in a warm, personal way with patients and their families.
2. In treating poorer patients, the clinician should give thought to prescribing less expensive, though of course equally effective, medications and treatments when such alternatives are available.
3. Ample provision should be made to include the patient's family in therapeutic decisions. This implies that the clinician should be willing to discuss alternative treatments with family members.
4. To conform with the values of *dignidad* and *respeto,* the clinician might do better to suggest a course of action to a patient than to issue orders.
5. Little is gained for patient-practitioner rapport by the practitioner's blaming the patient for his illness.

Dealing with Folk Concepts of Illness

1. Since one cannot assume that a folk label is always applied to the same cluster of symptoms, the clinician must focus on a description of the symptoms rather than the diagnostic label when taking a history or eliciting the presenting problem.

2. Although patients may define and label diseases in conformity with biomedical notions, they may posit a different etiology for them and therefore treat them differently. As a result, it is often important for the clinician to elicit the patient's etiological concepts in order to explain a recommended regimen in a manner most likely for it to be followed.

3. Mexican Americans tend to view varicosities, fever, gastrointestinal symptoms, and nervous tension as being more serious than biomedical professionals do. Mainstream providers of care should therefore attempt to allay patients' anxiety when they present with these symptoms by describing the diagnosis and prognosis clearly and in detail.

4. Little medical benefit derives from a clinician's either ignoring or ridiculing a patient's folk diagnosis. The clinician should be prepared to answer questions about his diagnosis and to discuss the reasons for it, which may assist the patient in comparing the two types of diagnosis.

Diagnostic Examinations

In general, Mexican Americans' standards of modesty suggest that bodily exposure in a physical examination and discussions of sexual matters between the sexes be limited to what is essential for the situation. In addition, diagnostic tests that involve blood loss should be carefully explained, and the patient forewarned concerning the amount of blood that will be taken and what will be done with it.

Treatment

Because of the importance of the Mexican-American family in sanctioning and following through on a therapeutic regimen, it is important to include family members in discussions of diagnosis and treatment. In cases of chronic illness, it may be important to determine who the important authority figures in the family network are, in order to enlist their influence in fostering adherence to treatment. This is particularly relevant when treatment must persist in the absence of symptoms.

For some chronic conditions it may also be advisable to determine if the patient is simultaneously under folk treatment in order to learn if the medicines being used in the two therapies interact in any adverse way. It is useful for physicians, particularly those practicing in border states, to learn the pharmacological properties of locally used folk remedies.

Therapeutic diets for inpatients or outpatients should take into account both Mexican-American food preferences and beliefs about the particular therapeutic effects of different foods.

The Importance of Patient Education

Because Mexican Americans have by and large been marginal participants in the mainstream medical system, they have had little access to biomedical knowledge. For this reason, clinicians can have a significant impact by taking their educative role seriously. In particular, they should take care to inform patients about diagnostic tests, routine procedures of the health-care system, and prodromal symptoms of major treatable diseases.

Notes

We would like to acknowledge the helpful comments of Stanley Fisch, M.D., who read the chapter in draft form.

1. See Stern et al. (1975), however, who report a decline in age-adjusted mortality rates for diabetes among Mexican Americans in San Antonio, Texas.

References

ABAD, VICENTE, JUAN RAMOS, and ELIZABETH BOYCE. 1974. A Model for Delivery of Mental Health Services to Spanish-speaking Minorities. *American Journal of Orthopsychiatry* 44:584–595.

ACOSTA, PHYLLIS B., et al. 1974. Nutritional Status of Mexican-American Preschool Children in a Border Town. *American Journal of Clinical Nutrition* 27:1359–1368.

ADAMS, RICHARD, and ARTHUR RUBEL. 1967. Sickness and Social Relations. In *Handbook of Middle American Indians,* vol. 6, ed. Robert Wauchope. Austin: University of Texas Press.

AGUIRRE, LYDIA. 1978. Alternative Health Practices along the Western Texas Border. In *Modern Medicine and Medical Anthropology in the United States-Mexico Border Population,* ed. Boris Velimirovic. Pan American Health Organization Scientific Publication, no. 359.

AMERICAN PUBLIC HEALTH ASSOCIATION. 1974. *Minority Health Chart Book.* Washington, D.C.: U.S. Government Printing Office.

ARANDA, ROBERT G. 1971. The Mexican American Syndrome. *American Journal of Public Health* 61:104–109.

BACA, JOSEPHINE. 1973. Some Health Beliefs of the Spanish-speaking. In *Family-Centered Community Nursing,* ed. Adina M. Reinhardt and Mildred D. Quinn. St. Louis, Mo.: Mosby.

BRADFIELD, ROBERT B., and THIERRY BRUN. 1970. Nutritional Status of California Mexican Americans. *American Journal of Clinical Nutrition* 23:798–806.

BRADSHAW, BENJAMIN S., and FRANK D. BEAN. 1973. Trends in Fertility of Mexican Americans, 1950–1970. *Social Science Quarterly* 53:688–696.

BROOM, LEONARD, and ESHREF SKEVSKY. 1952. Mexican Americans in the United States: A Problem in Social Differentiation. *Sociology and Social Research* 36:150–158.

CAMPOS, DANIEL. 1978. Application of an Indirect Technique of Infant Mortality Estimation in Eleven South Texas Counties. M.P.H. thesis, The University of Texas School of Public Health, Houston, Texas.

CARDENAS, JOSÉ, CHARLES E. GIBBS, and ELEANOR A. YOUNG. 1976. Nutrition Beliefs and Practices in Primigravid Mexican-American Women. *Journal of the American Dietetic Association* 69:262–265.

CASILLAS CUERVO, LETICIA. 1978. Health and Culture in Urban Marginal Districts. In *Modern Medicine and Medical Anthropology in the United States-Mexico Border Population,* ed. Boris Velimirovic. Pan American Health Organization Scientific Publication, no. 359.

CERVANTES, ROBERT A. 1972. The Failure of Comprehensive Health Services to Serve the Urban Chicano. *Public Health Reports* 87:932–940.

CHASE, H. PETER, et al. 1971. Nutritional Status of Preschool Mexican-American Migrant Farm Children. *American Journal of Diseases of Children* 122:316–324.

CHENEY, CHARLES C., and GEORGE L. ADAMS. 1978. Lay Healing and Mental Health in the Mexican-American *Barrio.* In *Modern Medicine and Medical Anthropology in the United States-Mexico Border Population.* ed. Boris Velimirovic. Pan American Health Organization Scientific Publication, no. 359.

CLARK, MARGARET. 1959. *Health in the Mexican-American Culture.* Berkeley: University of California Press.

COBB, SIDNEY. 1976. Social Support as a Moderator of Life Stress. *Psychosomatic Medicine* 38:300–314.

COLES, ROBERT. 1970. *Uprooted Children: The Early Life of Migrant Farm Workers.* Pittsburgh: University of Pittsburgh Press.

COLLADO ARDÓN, ROLANDO. 1978. Rural Medical Care or Rural Organization for Health? In *Modern Medicine and Medical Anthropology in the United States-Mexico Border Population,* ed. Boris Velimirovic. Pan American Health Organization Scientific Publication, no. 359.

CRESON, D. L., CAMERON MCKINLEY, and RICHARD EVANS. 1969. Folk Medicine in Mexican-American Sub-Culture. *Diseases of the Nervous System* 30:264–266.

CURRIER, RICHARD.   1966.   The Hot-Cold Syndrome and Symbolic Balance in Mexican-American and Spanish-American Folk Medicine. *Ethnology* 3:251–263.

EDGERTON, ROBERT, and MARVIN KARNO.   1971.   Mexican-American Bilingualism and the Perception of Mental Illness. *Archives of General Psychiatry* 24:286–290.

EDGERTON, ROBERT, MARVIN KARNO, and IRMA FERNÁNDEZ.   1970.   *Curanderismo* in the Metropolis: The Diminished Role of Folk Psychiatry among Los Angeles Mexican Americans. *American Journal of Psychotherapy* 24: 124–134.

FABREGA, HORACIO.   1974.   *Disease and Social Behavior: An Interdisciplinary Perspective.* Cambridge, Mass.: MIT Press.

FABREGA, HORACIO, J. D. SWARTZ, and C. A. WALLACE.   1968.   Ethnic Differences in Psychopathology. *Journal of Psychiatry Research* 6:221–235.

FARGE, EMILE J.   1975.   *La Vida Chicana: Health Care Attitudes and Behaviors of Houston Chicanos.* San Francisco: Adam S. Eterovich.

————.   1978.   Medical Orientation among a Mexican-American Population: An Old and New Model Reviewed. *Social Science and Medicine* 12:277–282.

FINLAYSON, ANGELA.   1976.   Social Networks as Coping Resources. *Social Science and Medicine* 10:97–103.

FLORES, JOSÉ L.   1978.   The Utilization of a Community Mental Health Service by Mexican Americans. *International Journal of Social Psychiatry* 24:271–275.

FONNER, EDWIN, JR.   1975.   Mortality Differences of 1970 Texas Residents: A Descriptive Study. Master's thesis, the University of Texas School of Public Health.

FOSTER, GEORGE M.   1948.   *Empire's Children: The People of Tzintzuntzan.* Publications of the Institute of Social Anthropology, no. 6. Washington, D.C.: Smithsonian Institution.

————.   1953.   Relationships between Spanish and Spanish-American Folk Medicine. *Journal of American Folklore* 66:201–247.

FRANK, JEROME.   1961.   *Persuasion and Healing.* Baltimore: Johns Hopkins Press.

GALARZA, ERNESTO, HERMAN GALLEGOS, and JULIAN SAMORA.   1969.   *Mexican Americans in the Southwest.* Santa Barbara, Calif.: McNally and Loftin.

GILBERT, ARNOLD, and PAUL F. O'ROURKE.   1968.   Effects of Rural Poverty on the Health of California's Farm Workers. *Public Health Reports* 83:827–834.

GILLIN, JOHN.   1948.   Magical Fright. *Psychiatry* 11:387–400.

GONZÁLEZ, JOSÚE.   1978.   Language Factors Affecting Treatment of Bilingual Schizophrenics. *Psychiatric Annals* 8:68–70.

GREBLER, LEO, JOAN W. MOORE, and RALPH C. GUZMAN.   1970.   *The Mexican-American People: The Nation's Second Largest Minority.* New York: The Free Press.

HERNÁNDEZ, JOSÉ, LEO ESTRADA, and DAVID ALVÍREZ.   1973.   Census Data and the Problem of Conceptually Defining the Mexican-American Population. *Social Science Quarterly* 53:671–687.

HOLLAND, WILLIAM. 1963. Mexican-American Medical Beliefs: Science or Magic? *Arizona Medicine* 20:89–101.

HOPPE, SUE KEIR, and PETER L. HELLER. 1975. Alienation, Familism, and the Utilization of Health Services by Mexican Americans. *Journal of Health and Social Behavior* 16:304–314.

INGHAM, JOHN M. 1970. On Mexican Folk Medicine. *American Anthropologist* 72:76–87.

JACO, E. GARTLY. 1969. Mental Health of the Spanish Americans in Texas. In *Culture and Mental Health,* ed. Marvin Opler. New York: Macmillan.

————. 1960. *The Social Epidemiology of Mental Disorders: A Psychiatric Survey of Texas.* New York: Russell Sage Foundation.

JOHNSON, CARMEN A. 1976. Mexican-American Women in the Labor Force and Lowered Fertility. *American Journal of Public Health* 66:1186–1188.

JOHNSON, L. V., and MARC MATRE. 1978. Anomie and Alcohol Use: Drinking Patterns in Mexican-American Neighborhoods. *Journal of Studies on Alcohol* 39:894–902.

KARNO, MARVIN. 1966. The Enigma of Ethnicity at a Mental Health Clinic. *Archives of General Psychiatry* 20:233–240.

KARNO, MARVIN, and ROBERT B. EDGERTON. 1969. Perceptions of Mental Illness in a Mexican-American Community. *Archives of General Psychiatry* 20:233–238.

————. 1974. Some Folk Beliefs about Mental Illness: A Reconsideration. *International Journal of Social Psychiatry* 20:292–296.

KARNO, MARVIN, and ARMANDO MORALES. 1971. A Community Mental Health Service for Mexican Americans in a Metropolis. *Comprehensive Psychiatry* 12:116–121.

KARNO, MARVIN, ROBERT N. ROSS, and ROBERT A. CAPER. 1969. Mental Health Roles of Physicians in a Mexican-American Community. *Community Mental Health Journal* 5:62–69.

KAY, MARGARITA A. 1977. Health and Illness in a Mexican-American Barrio. In *Ethnic Medicine in the Southwest,* ed. Edward Spicer. Tucson: University of Arizona Press.

————. 1978. Parallel, Alternative, or Collaborative: *Curanderismo* in Tucson, Arizona. In *Modern Medicine and Medical Anthropology in the United States-Mexico Border Population,* ed. Boris Velimirovic. Pan American Health Organization Scientific Publication, no. 359.

———— 1979 Lexemic Change and Semantic Shift in Disease Names. *Culture, Medicine and Psychiatry* 3:73–94.

KEARNEY, MICHAEL 1978 *Espiritualismo* as an Alternative Medical Tradition in the Border Area. In *Modern Medicine and Medical Anthropology in the United States-Mexico Border Population,* ed Boris Velimirovic. Pan American Health Organization Scientific Publication, no. 359.

KEARNEY, MICHAEL, and DAVID RICHMAN. 1977. Transcultural Psychotherapy: Anglo Therapists and Mexican Patients (abstract). *Transcultural Psychiatric Research* 14:108–111.

KEEFE, SUSAN E., AMADO M. PADILLA, and MANUEL L. CARLOS. 1979. The Mexican-American Extended Family as an Emotional Support System. *Human Organization* 38:144–152.

KIEV, ARI. 1968. *Curanderismo.* New York: The Free Press.

KLEIN, JANICE. 1968. *Susto:* The Anthropological Study of Diseases of Adaptation. *Social Science and Medicine* 12:23–28.

KLINE, LAWRENCE Y. 1969. Some Factors in the Psychiatric Treatment of Spanish Americans. *American Journal of Psychiatry* 125:88–95.

LANTZ, EDITH L., and PATRICIA WOOD. 1958. Nutrition in New Mexican, Spanish-American, and "Anglo" Adolescents: Blood Findings, Height and Weight Data, and Physical Condition. *Journal of the American Dietetic Association* 34:145–153.

LARSON, LORA BETH, et al. 1974. Nutritional Status of Children of Mexican-American Migrant Families. *Journal of the American Dietetic Association* 64:29–35.

LEWIS, OSCAR. 1960. *Tepoztlán: Village in Mexico.* New York: Holt, Rinehart, and Winston.

LURIE, HUGH J., and GEORGE L. LAWRENCE. 1971. Communication Problems between Rural Mexican-American Patients and their Physicians. *American Journal of Orthopsychiatry* 42:777–783.

MACDONALD, ELEANOR J., and E. B. HEINZE. 1975. *Epidemiology of Cancer in Texas: Incidence Analyzed by Type, Ethnic Group, and Geographic Location.* New York: Raven Press.

MACKLIN, JUNE. 1974. Belief, Ritual, and Healing: New England Spiritualism and Mexican-American Spiritism Compared. In *Religious Movements in Contemporary America,* ed. Irving Zaretsky and Mark Leone. Princeton, N.J.: Princeton University Press.

———. 1978. *Curanderismo* and *Espiritismo:* Complementary Approaches to Traditional Mental Health Services. In *Modern Medicine and Medical Anthropology in the United States-Mexico Border Population,* ed. Boris Velimirovic. Pan American Health Organization Scientific Publication, no. 359.

MADSEN, WILLIAM. 1955. Hot and Cold in the Universe of San Francisco Tescospa, Valley of Mexico. *Journal of American Folklore* 68:123–139.

———. 1964a. *The Mexican Americans of South Texas.* New York: Holt, Rinehart, and Winston.

———. 1964b. The Alcoholic Agringado. *American Anthropologist* 66:355–361.

———. 1964c. Value Conflicts and Folk Psychotherapy in South Texas. In *Magic, Faith, and Healing,* ed. Ari Kiev. New York: The Free Press.

———. 1969. Mexican Americans and Anglo Americans: A Comparative Study of Mental Health in Texas. In *Changing Perspectives in Mental Illness,* ed. Stanley Plog and Robert Edgerton. New York: Holt, Rinehart, and Winston.

MARTÍNEZ, CERVANDO, and HARRY W. MARTIN. 1966. Folk Diseases among

Urban Mexican Americans. *Journal of the American Medical Association* 196:147–164.

MCCLAIN, CAROL. 1977. Adaptation in Health Behavior: Modern and Traditional Medicine in a West Mexican Community. *Social Science and Medicine* 11:341–347.

MCLEMORE, S. DALE. 1963. Ethnic Attitudes toward Hospitalization: An Illustrative Comparison of Anglos and Mexican Americans. *Social Science Quarterly* 43:342–346.

MEADOWS, ARNOLD, and DAVID STOKER. 1965. Symptomatic Behavior of Hospitalized Patients: A Study of Mexican-American and Anglo-American Patients. *Archives of General Psychiatry* 12:267–277.

MENCK, H. R., et al. 1975. Cancer Incidence in the Mexican American. *Journal of the National Cancer Institute* 55:531–536.

MOUSTAFA, A. TAKER, and GERTRUDE WEISS. 1968. Health Status and Practice of Mexican Americans. Study Project Advance Report no. 11, UCLA Graduate School of Business Administration.

MURRY, SISTER MARY JOHN. 1954. *A Socio-cultural Study of 118 Mexican Families Living in a Low-Rent Public Housing Project in San Antonio, Texas.* Washington D.C.: The Catholic University of America Press.

NALL, FRANK C., and JOSEPH SPEILBERG. 1967. Social and Cultural Factors in the Responses of Mexican Americans to Medical Treatment. *Journal of Health and Social Behavior* 8:299–308.

NEWTON, FRANK. 1978. The Mexican-American Emic System of Mental Illness: An Exploratory Study. In *Family and Mental Health in the Mexican-American Community*, ed. J. M. Casas and Susan E. Keefe. Los Angeles: Spanish Speaking Mental Health Research Center, UCLA, monograph 7.

O'NELL, CARL W., and HENRY A. SELBY. 1968. Sex Differences in the Incidence of *Susto* in Two Zapotec Pueblos: An Analysis of the Relationship between Sex Role Expectations and a Folk Illness. *Ethnology* 7:95–105.

PADILLA, AMADO M., and RENE A. RUIZ. 1973. *Latino Mental Health: A Review of Literature.* National Institute of Mental Health, DHEW Publication no. (HSM) 73–9143.

PADILLA, AMADO M., RENE A. RUIZ, and RODOLPHO ALVAREZ. 1975. Community Mental Health Services for the Spanish-Speaking Surnamed Population. *American Psychologist* 30:892–905.

PENALOSA, FERNANDO. 1967. The Changing Mexican Americans in Southern California. *Sociology and Social Research* 51:405–417.

PHILLIPUS, M. J. 1971. Successful and Unsuccessful Approaches to Mental Health Services for an Urban Hispano-American Population. *American Journal of Public Health* 61:820–830.

QUESADA, GUSTAVO M. 1973. *Mexican Americans: Mexicans or Americans?* Lubbock, Tex.: Southwestern Council of Latin American Studies.

———. 1976. Language and Communication Barriers for Health Delivery to a Minority Group. *Social Science and Medicine* 10:323–327.

QUESADA, GUSTAVO M., and PETER L. HELLER. 1977. Sociocultural Barriers to Medical Care among Mexican Americans in Texas: A Summary

Report of Research Conducted by the Southwest Medical Sociology Ad Hoc Committee. *Medical Care* 15:93–101.

QUESADA, GUSTAVO M., WILLIAM SPEARS, and PETER RAMOS. 1978. Interracial Depressive Epidemiology in the Southwest. *Journal of Health and Social Behavior* 19:77–85.

RICHARDSON, WILLIAM C. 1972. Poverty, Illness, and the Use of Health Services in the United States. In *Patients, Physicians, and Illness,* ed. E. Gartly Jaco. New York: The Free Press.

ROBERTS, ROBERT E., and CORNELIUS ASKEW, JR. 1972. A Consideration of Mortality in Three Subcultures. *Health Services Reports* 87:262–270.

ROBERTS, ROBERT E., and EUN SUL LEE. 1980a. The Health of Mexican Americans: Evidence from the Human Population Laboratory Studies. *American Journal of Public Health* 70:375–384.

———. 1980b. Medical Care Use by Mexican Americans: Evidence from the Human Population Laboratory Studies. *Medical Care* 18:266–281.

ROMANO, OCTAVIO. 1965. Charismatic Medicine, Folk-Healing, and Folk Sainthood. *American Anthropologist* 67:1151–1173.

RUBEL, ARTHUR J. 1960. Concepts of Disease in Mexican-American Culture. *American Anthropologist* 62:795–814.

———. 1964. The Epidemiology of a Folk Illness: *Susto* in Hispanic America. *Ethnology* 3:268–283.

———. 1966. *Across the Tracks: Mexican Americans in a Texas City.* Austin, Tex.: University of Texas Press.

RUBEL, ARTHUR J., and CARL W. O'NELL. 1978. Difficulties of Presenting Complaints to Physicians: *Susto* Illness as an Example. In *Modern Medicine and Medical Anthropology in the United States-Mexico Border Population,* ed. Boris Velimirovic. Pan American Health Organization Scientific Publication, no. 359.

SANDLER, ALAN P., and L. S. CHAN. 1978. Mexican-American Folk Belief in a Pediatric Emergency Room. *Medical Care* 16:778–784.

SAUNDERS, LYLE. 1954. *Cultural Difference and Medical Care.* Philadelphia: William F. Fell.

———. 1958. Healing Ways in the Spanish Southwest. In *Patients, Physicians, and Illness,* ed. E. Gartly Jaco. New York: The Free Press.

SCHREIBER, JANET M., and LORALEE PHILPOTT. 1978. Who Is a Legitimate Health Care Professional? Changes in the Practice of Midwifery in the Lower Rio Grande Valley. In *Modern Medicine and Medical Anthropology in the United States-Mexico Border Population,* ed. Boris Velimirovic. Pan American Health Organization Scientific Publication, no. 359.

SCHULMAN, SAM. 1960. Rural Healthways in New Mexico. *Annals of the New York Academy of Sciences* 84:950–958.

SCHULMAN, SAM, and ANNE M. SMITH. 1963. The Concept of "Health" among Spanish-speaking Villagers of New Mexico and Colorado. *Journal of Health and Human Behavior* 4:226–234.

SCRIMSHAW, SUSAN C., and ELIZABETH BURLEIGH. 1978. The Potential for the Integration of Indigenous and Western Medicines in Latin America and

Hispanic Populations in the United States of America. In *Modern Medicine and Medical Anthropology in the United States-Mexico Border Population,* ed. Boris Velimirovic. Pan American Health Organization Scientific Publication, no. 359.

SHELDON, PAUL M. 1966. Community Participation and the Emerging Middle Class. In *La Raza: Forgotten Americans,* ed. Julian Samora. Notre Dame, Ind.: University of Notre Dame Press.

STERN, MICHAEL P., et al. 1975. Affluence and Cardiovascular Risk Factors in Mexican Americans and Other Whites in Three Northern California Communities. *Journal of Chronic Diseases* 28:623–636.

TELLER, CHARLES H., and STEVE CLYBURN. 1974. Trends in Infant Mortality. *Texas Business Review* 48:1–7.

TORREY, E. FULLER. 1969. The Case for the Indigenous Therapist. *Archives of General Psychiatry* 20: 365–375.

———. 1972. *The Mind Game: Witchdoctors and Psychiatrists.* New York: Emerson Hall.

TREVINO, FERNANDO M., JOHN G. BRUHN, and HARVEY BUNCE, III. 1979. Utilization of Community Mental Health Services in a Texas-Mexico Border City. *Social Science and Medicine* 13A:331–334.

TROTTER, ROBERT T., and JUAN ANTONIO CHAVIRA. 1978. Discovering New Models for Alcohol Counseling in Minority Groups. In *Modern Medicine and Medical Anthropology in the United States-Mexico Border Population,* ed. Boris Velimirovic. Pan American Health Organization Scientific Publication, no. 359.

UHLENBERG, PETER. 1973. Fertility Patterns within the Mexican-American Population. *Social Biology* 20:30–39.

UNITED STATES DEPARTMENT OF COMMERCE, BUREAU OF THE CENSUS. 1976. Current Population Report, Population Characteristics. Persons of Spanish Origin in the United States: March 1975. Series P–20, no. 290.

UNITED STATES DEPARTMENT OF HEALTH, EDUCATION, and WELFARE. 1972. *Ten-State Nutrition Survey, 1968–1970 (V-Dietary).* Publication no. (HSM) 72–8133. Atlanta: Center for Disease Control.

UZZEL, DOUGLAS. 1974. *Susto* Revisited: Illness as Strategic Role. *American Ethnologist* 1:369–378.

VELIMIROVIC, BORIS, ed. 1978. *Modern Medicine and Medical Anthropology in the United States-Mexico Border Population.* Pan American Health Organization Scientific Publication, no. 359.

WALKER, GEORGE M. 1979. Utilization of Health Care: The Laredo Migrant Experience. *American Journal of Public Health* 69:667–672.

WALKER, KENNETH N., ARLENE MACBRIDE, and MARY L. S. VACHON. 1977. Social Support Networks and the Crisis of Bereavement. *Social Science and Medicine* 11:35–41.

WARNER, DAVID. 1978. Mexican-American Health Care in South Texas. LBJ School of Public Affairs, University of Texas (mimeographed).

WEAVER, JERRY L. 1969. *Health Care Service Use in Orange County, California: A Socioeconomic Analysis.* Long Beach Center for Political Research, California State University, Long Beach.

————. 1973. Mexican-American Health Care Behavior: A Critical Review of the Literature. *Social Science Quarterly* 54:85–102.

WEAVER, THOMAS. 1970. Use of Hypothetical Situations in a Study of Spanish-American Illness Referral Systems. *Human Organization* 29:140–154.

WECLEW, ROBERT V. 1975. The Nature, Prevalence, and Level of Awareness of *"Curanderismo"* and Some of Its Implications for Community Mental Health. *Community Mental Health Journal* 11:145–154.

WELCH, SUSAN, JOHN COMER, and MICHAEL STEINMAN. 1973. Some Social and Attitudinal Correlates of Health Care among Mexican Americans. *Journal of Health and Social Behavior* 14:205–213.

WOTEKI, CATHERINE E., ELLIOT WESER, and ELEANOR A. YOUNG. 1977. Lactose Malabsorption in Mexican-American Children. *American Journal of Clinical Nutrition* 30:470–475.

YANOCHIK-OWEN, ANITA, and MORISSA WHITE. 1977. Nutrition Surveillance in Arizona: Selected Anthropometric and Laboratory Observations among Mexican-American Children. *American Journal of Public Health* 67:151–154.

YOUNG, ALLAN. 1976. Some Implications of Medical Beliefs and Practices for Social Anthropology. *American Anthropologist* 78:5–24.

6
Navajos

STEPHEN J. KUNITZ AND JERROLD E. LEVY

Identification of the Ethnic Group

Definition and History of the Group

THE NAVAJO are an Athabaskan tribe, related to the Apache, who appear to have entered the American Southwest by the sixteenth century. The first traces of them are found in what is now northwestern New Mexico, from which point they moved south and west over succeeding centuries (Hester 1962). Originally a hunting and gathering society, the Navajo acquired knowledge of agriculture from the Pueblo Indians, particularly after many Pueblos joined Navajo groups following the Pueblo rebellion in 1680. From the Spaniards they acquired livestock, in particular sheep and horses but also cattle. Unlike many other Apachean groups, the Navajo did not slaughter and consume the sheep acquired in raids but used them to build up flocks of their own. By 1800 the shift to a pastoral economy was essentially complete (Hester 1962).

The transition to pastoralism made it possible for the Navajo to exploit areas that were marginal for agriculture and hunting, thus permitting them to move to lower elevations (for example, into the drainage systems of the Colorado and Little Colorado Rivers). Warfare, resulting from Navajo raiding of Spanish, Mexican, and Anglo-American ranches for livestock and slaves, and raiding of Navajo settlements in turn by these groups and by other Indians (notably Utes), served to push the Navajo westward as well (Kemrer 1974).

The most devastating campaign against the Navajo was led by Kit Carson in 1863 and resulted in the destruction of crops, livestock, and homes. After considerable loss of life, many Navajos capitulated and were incarcerated at the Bosque Redondo, New Mexico, from 1864 to 1868. In 1868 about 8,000 Navajos finally returned to a treaty reservation straddling what is now the Arizona–New Mexico border. If one estimates that about 2,000 people never went to the Bosque Redondo, there were approximately 10,000 Navajo on and near the reservation in 1868.

Recent Contact with American Health and Other Social Institutions

Over the next 60 years, until about 1930, the Navajo were allowed to live in relative peace. During the period 1869–1934 the reservation was expanded on several occasions, mostly into lands with marginal value to Anglo ranchers and other developers (Parman 1976). Though the land base thus increased to about 24,000 square miles during this period, the number of Navajo and their livestock expanded even more rapidly. This relatively rapid growth in the human population was probably due in large measure to the dispersed nature of Navajo settlement, which made epidemics of devastating magnitude far less likely than among their more densely settled neighbors, the Hopi (Kunitz 1974a). The results of this marked increase in human as well as herd population were the overgrazing of already marginal range land and a decline in the real value of livestock (Johnston 1966). Although government agents made unsuccessful efforts to improve the breed of sheep used by the Navajo (Kelly 1968), little else was done to relieve their problems.

The depression of the 1930s brought major consequences for the Navajo. An activist administration came to Washington concerned, among other things, with Indian problems and determined to do something about them. The range of the Navajo was severely overgrazed, and they were unable to sell their sheep because of the national economic situation. The Bureau of Indian Affairs under John Collier ordered that Navajo livestock be reduced, made efforts to improve the breed of sheep, and provided wage-paying jobs in the Civilian Conservation Corps (CCC) to make up for the loss of income from livestock.

Although CCC activities waned in the late 1930s, entry of the United States into World War II provided opportunities for the Navajo in both military service and war industries. Of a population of no more than 50,000 in 1940, approximately 3,600 Navajos entered the armed forces, and an estimated 10,000 left for employment outside the Reservation.

At the end of the war returning veterans and workers could find no employment on the reservation, the livestock economy was no longer viable, and severe weather made conditions even worse. Voluntary and government relief efforts were inadequate, and in 1950 the Navajo-Hopi Long Range Rehabilitation Act was passed. Over the next 10 years the money authorized under this act for roads, schools, and hospitals was all appropriated, whereas funding for business and economic development languished (TNY 1961).

HISTORY OF HEALTH CARE ON THE RESERVATION   Health care was to be provided to the Navajo as a treaty right when they returned to the reservation in 1868. Throughout the last part of the nineteenth and the early twentieth centuries, government-paid physicians were therefore stationed at various locations on the reservation to provide care without charge. A survey of health care on Indian reservations in the 1920s, however, implies that these physicians were badly paid, often poorly trained, and isolated without adequate facilities, and they were mainly furnishing acute rather than preventive care (Institute for Government Research 1928).

In contrast, during the 1930s efforts were made to provide care in a way that was sensitive to the needs and cultures of the particular Indian tribes for which the Bureau of Indian Affairs was responsible (Leighton and Leighton 1944). This was a difficult task, however, since funds were inadequate during the depression, and several hospitals were forced to close (Underhill 1963). In the 1940s cutbacks necessitated by World War II forced further curtailment of services, with the result that by 1949 the number of government hospitals was reduced to five, less than half the number located on the reservation some ten years earlier (Pijoan and McCammon 1949). The decline in manpower and facilities was reflected in a decline in hospitalizations: from about 9,000 in 1940 to about 6,600 in 1955. As population had increased substantially, the hospitalization rates dropped from 182.8 to 81.7 per 1,000 population (Kunitz and Temkin-Greener 1980).

Since 1955, when the responsibility for Indian health care was transferred from the Bureau of Indian Affairs to the U.S. Public Health Service, old hospital facilities have been replaced, more staff recruited, and new field clinics constructed. By 1973 there were 543 beds available on the reservation—475 in government hospitals, 23 in a mission hospital, and 45 in a hospital administered by project HOPE (Davis 1977). Compared to 1940, however, this total represents an absolute decline in the number of beds, during a period when the population increased almost threefold (from about 50,000 to 134,000 people). With improved access to facilities, the percentage of Navajo hospitalized per year has increased since 1955 and by the early 1970s was virtually the same as it had been 30 years earlier (approximately 18 percent in 1940 and 17.4 percent in 1972). The decline in the number of beds may in part be seen as a response to shortened hospital stays, due in no small measure to a decline in admissions of tuberculosis patients.

What has changed dramatically since 1940 are the rates of outpatient utilization. In 1974 Navajos had an estimated 3.9 outpatient visits per person per year, compared to only 0.9 in 1940 (Navajo Medical News 1940) and compared to 5.0 per person for the United States population (in 1973). Furthermore, in 1975 between 15 and 23 percent of Navajos (depending on the area sampled) had visited a physician within the month prior to the interview (Stewart and Muneta 1976; May et al. 1977). This marked increase in outpatient utilization in recent years may be attributed to improved transportation, rising educational levels among the Navajo, and increasing outreach activities by health-care providers.

General Demographic Picture of the Population

For various reasons the Navajo population has been notoriously difficult to enumerate. Factors such as the inaccessibility of many parts of the reservation, migration, language barriers, and inadequate recording of births and deaths until about the mid-1950s have contributed to inaccuracies in enumeration (Johnston 1966). A recent study, which attempted to match the tribal rolls with an actual census, showed that the rolls overestimated the number of Navajos, whereas past government-sponsored censuses are known to have underestimated it. The best estimate of the reservation population to date is one provided by the tribe's Office of Program Development in cooperation with the Bureau of the Census and the Bureau of Indian Affairs (U.S. Bureau of the Census 1977). This estimate places the on-reservation population of Navajos at 134,340 on July 1, 1975 (Faich 1977). The off-reservation Navajo population, located mainly in cities in California and the Southwest, was reported to be approximately 37,000 in 1970 (U.S. Bureau of the Census 1973).

Since 1950, the number of Navajos has increased at a rate of between 2.4 and 3.3 percent per annum (Johnston 1966:152). This impressive rate of growth is a reflection partly of improvements in health care and general standards of living, and partly of a continuing high fertility rate (approximately 31 per 1,000 in 1974). Some of the effects of this rapid population growth are as follows: first, the Navajo population today is a young one, with an estimated 43 to 46 percent below age 18; second, there are more people entering the labor force each year than there are jobs available; third, life expectancy has increased, though it is not clear by how much; and fourth, with a growing population, high unemployment, and high dependency, per capita income has declined in recent years, from $686 in 1969 to $567 in 1974 (in 1967 dollars). In contrast, comparable figures for the general United States population show an increase in per capita income from $2,283 to $2,991 during these years (Wistisen, Parsons, and Larsen 1975, vol. 2:4). It is noteworthy, too, that in 1974 the per capita income for Navajos was only 18.9 percent of the national figure.

Since several authors (Aberle 1969; Jorgensen 1971; Robbins 1975) have discussed in detail the peripheral situation of the Navajo and other Indian reservation populations in the national economy, we will make only two points in this regard. First, the unavailability of sources of steady income for the vast majority of the population (unemployment is estimated at between 50 and 60 percent) has worked to create what Aberle (1969) has called the "Navajo style." That is, reciprocity among extended kin continues to be the norm, because it permits income from a variety of unstable sources (welfare, occasional wage work, livestock, agriculture, the sale of craft items) to be distributed within the kin group. Second, the jobs that are available on the reservation are mainly in federal, state, local, or tribal governments, virtually all in human and social-service occupations (Kunitz 1977a). This fact has important consequences, especially in the health-care field (see the concluding section for further discussion).

An additional area in which considerable change has occurred over the past century is education. At present virtually all Navajo children of ages 6 to 18 are enrolled in school. That this has not been the pattern for long, however, is suggested by the fact that the median number of years of education for reservation Navajos aged 25 and above was only 4.1 in 1970, lower than the number for any other Indian reservation population (U.S. Bureau of the Census 1973).

Evaluation of the Existing Data

There are, broadly speaking, two kinds of information available on the characteristics of the Navajo population: community studies generally carried out by one researcher, and large-scale surveys of which the census is the most obvious example. We cannot describe here the many community studies that have been done on the reservation; for interested readers an extensive recent review is available (Henderson and Levy 1975). Likewise, we cannot discuss in detail the various large-scale surveys that have been done. It is sufficient to say here that several problems arise in connection with interpreting the available data. First, the census has consistently underenumerated the reservation population. Second, community studies often cannot be generalized to the entire population because there are significant regional variations. Third, surveys done for purposes other than the census (for instance, livestock ownership, employment status, health and housing conditions) may suffer from numerous difficulties including the lack of an adequate sampling frame; bias due to circular migration patterns, which may mean that some contributing members of a household are not included in the study; and definitions of household in a society where kin networks are still important. Fourth, epidemiological data are biased by the selectivity with which people use health-care facilities (the source of most such information) and the lack of postmortem examinations in many facilities, which may lead to the inaccurate assignment of cause of death in an unknown number of cases. And fifth, when field studies are done of various health conditions, they tend to be carried out in one or only a few communities, thus giving a potentially distorted picture of conditions throughout the reservation.

Sources of Intraethnic Diversity

There are a variety of sources of diversity within the Navajo population, each of which exerts a diversifying influence on health behavior and health status.

GEOGRAPHIC VARIATION   Studies of aggregate data have shown that areas on the eastern end of the reservation tend to have populations with higher levels of education and employment, better housing, and lower dependence on welfare and livestock raising than populations living on the western end. In addition, fertility rates (particularly among women in the later childbearing years) are higher among women in the west. Since the crude mortality rates are virtually the same all across the reservation, the result is a greater rate of population growth in the west than the east and higher rates of emigration from the former area as well. Indeed, though there are centers of wage-work activity on the western side of the reservation, it appears for the most part that this population may be characterized as more nearly residual (that is, less employable, less educated, and older) than the population in the east (Kunitz 1974b, 1977b, and unpublished data).

Field studies in a number of communities support the analyses of aggregate data. In general, rural areas have lost their young adult populations to wage work centers on the reservation, in border towns, or to cities elsewhere in the Southwest and California. The young people who remain tend to have lower educational levels than those who migrate, and the young women seem to have higher rates of fertility.

VARIATION IN DISTRIBUTION OF WEALTH   Another source of diversity within the Navajo population has to do with access to wealth in the traditional stratification system. The establishment of the reservation put an end to raiding and meant that young men could no longer acquire livestock and build up flocks in that manner. Furthermore, the period of stock reduction during the 1930s put an effective limit on the number of livestock that could be grazed in each land management district. The result was to crystallize the old system, in which some individuals and families had considerable amounts of stock and others had little or none. The members of the impoverished group were forced either to work outside the reservation or to become dependent on the wealthy families (Levy and Kunitz 1974). Of course, as population has grown but the amount of allowable livestock has remained essentially constant, even the traditionally wealthy families have become poorer and poorer; thus practically no Navajo can get by today on livestock alone, and pastoralists living in the hinterlands are dependent on welfare and occasional wage work to at least as great a degree as they are on their animals.

VARIATION IN SOCIAL ORGANIZATION   Differences in access to wage work by region and differences in outmigration rates have also created considerable variability in Navajo settlement patterns and social organization. During the early period of the reservation, two social rules helped create a distinctive Navajo social organization. The first demanded that after marriage a young couple take up residence with the bride's parents. This form of residence produced what is frequently called the camp, or matrifocal extended family, composed of a senior married couple, their unmarried children, and their married daughters with their spouses and children. Independent nuclear families occurred when new camps were first established or when the sons of older couples without daughters married and left home. The second social rule (matrilineal descent) stipulated that an individual belongs to the descent group, or clan, of his mother and that he should not marry into his own clan. These rules resulted in a tendency for contiguous areas of farming and grazing land to be occupied by extended families who were matrilineally related to each other. Communities were kin-based, with leaders representing the interests of kinsmen rather than those of status or occupation.

Population growth and consequent migration from one area of the reservation to another, however, has eroded the control of contiguous land areas by matrilineal kinsmen. Areas of the reservation in which wage work has replaced farming as an important basis for subsistence have become heterogeneous, with higher proportions of independent, single-household residence units. In 1972 single households accounted for as much as 87 to 90 percent of all residence units around the new electrical station near Page, Arizona. In more isolated areas such as Black Mesa, on the other hand, single households accounted for only 36 percent of all residence units (Callaway, Levy, and Henderson 1976), In all areas studied, however, the matrifocal extended family was still the most prevalent form of multihousehold residence units. The importance that residence in traditional kin settings plays in determining health and behavior will be discussed in subsequent sections.

RELIGIOUS VARIATIONS   Traditional Navajo religion is directed toward the maintenance of harmonious relationships between man, nature, and the supernaturals. Since illness is a major indicator of disharmony, Navajo religious ritual is predominantly health-oriented. During the twentieth century both Christianity and peyotism have gained large followings on the reservation, with implications for changing health concepts and behavior that have not yet been studied.

The peyote religion, now formally organized as the Native American Church, is a nativistic religion that began among the Kiowa and Comanche Indians of the south plains during the latter half of the nineteenth century and spread to the tribes of the plains, prairies, and Rocky Mountains. By embracing some central tenets of Christianity in an Indian ritual framework, it provides an Indian answer to the white man's religion.

Prior to the stock reduction period of the late 1930s, the Navajos showed little interest in the new religion, although the Utes, their neighbors to the north, had adopted it in the early part of the twentieth century. According to Aberle (1966), the stresses of stock reduction made the Navajos receptive during these years, and he documents the religion's rapid growth in those communities most affected by the reduction program. Peyotism has continued to exert an appeal and to spread across the reservation since that time.

In the areas where we have worked we detect two additional reasons for the continued popularity of the Native American Church. First, the decline of real income has made it more difficult for Navajo families to pay for the large traditional healing ceremonies that last from five to nine nights and involve hosting large numbers of guests. The peyote ceremony lasts only one night and is, in consequence, more economical than most Navajo ceremonies. Since it introduces no new beliefs about the causes of disease and denies none of the central Navajo beliefs, it is easy to use as a substitute for traditional ceremonies. In fact, we have found many families who utilize both forms of treatment.

Second, the years of apprenticeship necessary to master any of the major Navajo ceremonials make it impossible for young men with wage jobs to achieve status as traditional ceremonialists. The peyote ritual, which is performed on a single weekend night and is relatively easy to learn, is particularly suited to patients and practitioners who must conform to the demands of wage work. Young Navajos who do not have, or want, access to status in the non-Indian world find that becoming a peyote leader gives them status in their own community. It is our opinion that economic change has created a shortage of traditional ceremonialists which will become crucial during the next 10 years, despite the existence of a federally subsidized school for training ceremonialists which has been in operation for several years.

The same conditions that have promoted the growth of the Navajo Native American Church have also worked to make the fundamentalist

Christian denominations more popular. Missionary activities, begun by the Spaniards in the 17th century and continued by several Protestant denominations after the establishment of the reservation, never gained large numbers of converts prior to the stock reduction period. The mission church was always run by non-Indians, with the result that it was separate from Navajo community life. In recent years, however, the "camp church" has gained popularity because it has Navajo preachers who do not withdraw from their kin networks. In 1950, there were 36 organized congregations with pastors, two of whom were Navajo. In contrast, in 1978 there were 343 congregations, and 203 of these had Navajo preachers (DuBois 1978). The greatest growth has been among such evangelical groups as the Nazarenes, Pentecostals, and Baptists.

Currently, the Navajo Native American Church claims that 50 percent of the reservation population is peyotist. In areas where good survey research has been done, all Christian denominations combined account for 50 to 70 percent of the populations adjacent to new wage-work opportunities, where skilled workers have migrated into the area. The Navajo Native American Church accounts for 15 to 20 percent of the populations in more rural areas (not including people who combine peyotism with traditional religion) (Callaway, Levy, and Henderson 1976:57). These data, however, are from the western portion of the reservation and cannot be generalized to the more densely populated areas to the east, where peyotism first took root.

The point to be made is that diversity in religious practices is considerable, and although religious variations probably have important consequences for changing health beliefs and behaviors, no research to date has concentrated on this problem. Without detailed studies that connect religious belief to health behavior, we think it would be premature to use religious preference as an indicator of changed health behavior. Most accounts of the conversion experiences of Navajo adults that we have heard involve the use of Christian prayer or peyote either to cure a specific illness or to protect against witchcraft.

Epidemiological Characteristics

Biases in the Data

We have already discussed briefly the problems of enumerating the Navajo population. For epidemiological studies one needs both a denominator and a numerator, and the most basic numerator data are birth and death reports. However, birth and death certificates list place of residence (so residence on or off the reservation may be counted) but do not routinely note tribe. Thus, one must assume that an Indian birth occurring to a woman living in a Navajo Reservation community is in fact a Navajo birth. An unknown number of Indians of other tribes live and work on the reservation, however, and they would be included in these figures. Never-theless, in general the facts of birth and death have been increasingly adequately recorded over the past 20 years (Johnston 1966).

Although birth and death statistics are reasonably well recorded, the study of morbidity among Navajos does present some problems. Few sur-veys comparable to the National Health Interview Survey have been at-tempted; instead there have been studies of a variety of phenomena in single communities: for instance, nutritional status (Reisinger, Rogers, and Johnson 1972), general treated morbidity (McDermott et al. 1960), and alcohol use (Levy and Kunitz 1974). As noted previously, there are wide social, economic, and demographic variations across the reserva-tion, so generalizing from community studies such as these may cause considerable misunderstanding.

Most of the morbidity material that has been published is based on treated cases. Because the vast majority of care is provided by the U.S. Public Health Service, these data are in some respects very good. On the other hand, problems of access to and utilization of care make the inter-pretation of much of this material difficult. For example, the rates of several operative procedures (bilateral tubal ligation, therapeutic abor-tion, appendectomy, and cholecystectomy) vary with the distance of the patient's home from the hospital, and hospital reports of a variety of ac-cidents also correlate with the distance the accident victim lives from the hospital. Since there is no a priori reason to believe that cholecystitis, ap-pendicitis, and accidents of all sorts occur most frequently among people living close to a hospital, one must conclude that facility-based reporting of morbidity is seriously biased by accessibility of care.

Not only does access to care bias the morbidity data, but there appears to be some bias related to the characteristics of people who seek care. While we know of no really detailed studies of this problem, Levy has observed that young, traditional males may be less likely to seek care than any other segment of the population (unpublished data).

Major Causes of Mortality and Morbidity

Broadly speaking, the Navajo are experiencing a demographic and epidemiological transition similar to that which has been observed in many populations since the sixteenth century. However, unlike the ex-tended transition that took place in populations of western Europe, that of the Navajo has taken place over a relatively short period of time. The term "demographic transition" refers to the change populations are said to undergo in the course of "modernization," in which they move from a state of high mortality and fertility to one in which mortality has declined but fertility is still high, and then to a third phase in which both fertility and mortality are low. Population grows slowly if at all during the first phase, rapidly in the second phase, and slowly if at all in the third phase. It should be clear from our description of Navajo population growth that they are in the second phase, where mortality has declined much more rapidly than fertility.

The decline in mortality during this process, which has been called the "epidemiological transition" (Omran 1971), is the result of a decline in the incidence of epidemic infectious diseases. In consequence, the causes of mortality and morbidity that become of prime importance are those that are either man-made or degenerative in nature.

In regard to the decline in mortality, it is important to recall that vital data did not really become adequate until the mid-1950s. The available data (Johnston 1966:174; Morgan 1973; Kunitz 1976a:25) are nevertheless quite consistent in showing that mortality began to decline in the late 1940s and by the late 1950s reached its present low level of about 5.7 per 1,000 (Kaltenbach 1976). It is perhaps worth observing that the major reduction appears to have occurred before the Indian Health Service took over responsibility for the provision of medical care.

Concurrent with this drop in mortality rates has been a shift in causes of death. Table 6.1 shows the proportionate contribution to mortality of a number of diagnostic categories in the years 1954–1956 and 1965–1967. By 1954–1956 crude mortality rates had reached their present low level, but we can still observe the "epidemiological transition" in process from the slight increase in the importance of accidents, heart disease, and neoplasms and the decline in influenza and pneumonia, gastritis, and certain diseases of early infancy from the first to the second period.

Table 6.1 Leading causes of death among Navajos in Navajo Area, 1954–1956 and 1965–1967.

Cause of death	1954–1956 (%)	1965–1967 (%)
Accidents	16.8	22.9
Diseases of the heart	4.2	6.5
Malignant neoplasms	3.4	7.4
Influenza and pneumonia (excluding newborns)	14.2	8.1
Certain diseases of early infancy	9.6	7.4
Gastritis	10.5	5.6
All others	41.3	42.1
Total	100.0	100.0

Source: U.S. Public Health Service (1971:27).

Table 6.2, using slightly different diagnostic classifications, shows the proportionate contribution to mortality of the most important causes of death in the Navajo Area in 1974. It can be seen that accidents have increased dramatically over the earlier period, and that respiratory and gastrointestinal diseases have declined equally dramatically.

One point that should be made clear is the significance of the large category of unknowns. The category "symptoms and ill-defined conditions," which appears as the second leading cause of death in 1974 (table 6.2), is probably buried in the category "all others" in table 6.1. Unfortunately, the diagnosis of cause of death is still often not made accurately. Nonetheless, the data appear good enough to be able to support the statement that the epidemiological transition described above is in fact taking place among the Navajo and that man-made and degenerative diseases are increasing in both absolute and relative importance.

ACCIDENTS If we assume that the crude mortality rate in 1955 was 7.6 per 1,000 and that 16.8 percent of the deaths were due to accidents, then the accident mortality rate was 127 per 100,000. In 1974, 38.5 percent of Navajo deaths were due to accidents. If the crude rate was 5.7 per 1,000, then the accident mortality rate was about 223 per 100,000, an increase of almost 60 percent. Thus, over the past 20 years accidents

Table 6.2 Leading causes of death among Navajos in Navajo Area, 1974.

Cause	Percent	Number
Accidents	38.5	283
Symptoms and ill-defined conditions	20.7	152
Circulatory disorders	8.6	63
Mental disorders (alcoholism)[a]	5.6	41
Respiratory disorders	5.4	40
Digestive tract disorders	5.4	40
Infective/parasitic disorders	4.2	31
Neoplasms	4.2	31
Perinatal mortality	3.9	29
Genitourinary disorders	1.9	14
Endocrine, nutritional, metabolic disorders	1.5	11
Total	99.9	735

Source: Derived from Kaltenbach (1976).

a. The category "mental disorders" includes alcoholism. According to Kaltenbach (1976:18) all the Navajo Area deaths in this category were diagnosed as caused by alcoholism.

have increased both in absolute and relative importance as a cause of death.

Despite the fact that accidents have been the single most important cause of mortality among the Navajo for at least 20 years and account for more hospital days than any other cause but childbirth (Davis 1977), only two studies have been done of this particular phenomenon. One study of hospital records in 1966–1967 showed that the accidental death rate of the Navajo was 104.2 per 100,000, 1.8 times greater than the rate for the United States population (58.0 per 100,000). The death rate for Navajo males was 160.6 per 100,000, as opposed to 48.9 for females (relative risk 3.3). Navajo males aged 25 through 34 had the highest incidence of accidents, but males above the age of 65 had the highest death rate from accidents. Motor vehicle accidents were responsible for almost half (48.2 percent) of the accidental deaths but accounted for only about 2 percent of the total number of accidents recorded (Brown et al. 1970). It should be emphasized that this study was based on hospital records; thus people who died before reaching the hospital would not have been included, which probably accounts for the lower reported rate than we have calculated for both 1955 and 1974 on the basis of death certificates.

Using data collected somewhat earlier than those cited above, the second study (Omran and Loughlin 1972) analyzed the pattern of accidents affecting the residents of one rather isolated Navajo community in the years 1957 through 1962. Accidental deaths (10 in all) were responsible for 15.4 percent of all deaths, and "the leading cause of accidents were domestic injuries, followed by injuries due to sharp instruments that the average Navajo uses in every day life" (Omran and Loughlin 1972: 17). The authors also suggest that psychosocial factors as well as environmental hazards were significant in causing the accidents in their sample: "As a people in transition, the Navajos exhibit many insecurities and inabilities to cope with their changing way of life. This has resulted in a great deal of stress, violence, alcoholism, undisciplined children and social maladjustment. It is generally assumed that the relatively high rate of accidents associated with alcohol and violence is symptomatic of deeper seated social disorders among the Navajos. Drinking was associated with at least five of the fatal accidents, and with the more serious injuries, especially those inflicted by others, as well as a number of motor vehicle accidents" (Omran and Loughlin 1972:18).

More recent data published by the Indian Health Service indicate that alcohol use is associated with some categories of accidents, but it is less clear that the accidents are caused by alcohol. Table 6.3 shows the proportion of accidents of different types that were, in the estimation of the attending professional, alcohol-related. Unfortunately, we do not have

Table 6.3   Alcohol-related accidents[a] as a percentage of total accidents among Navajos in Navajo Area, 1972.

Type of accident	Alcohol-related (%)
Motor vehicle	19.5
All other	2.3
Falls	2.1
Cutting, piercing objects	3.2
Suicide attempts	17.9
Injuries purposely inflicted by others	28.7

Source: U.S. Public Health Service (1973).
a. Treated on an outpatient basis.

data gathered in a comparable way from non-Navajo populations with which to compare these figures.

Apart from the two studies mentioned earlier, additional material on mortality and morbidity from accidents comes from the Indian Health Service and is based on data having the limitations discussed above. Community studies on the reservation that would attempt to assess risk factors, such as the number of miles driven per year, have not been carried out. Some data collected for other purposes (Wistisen, Parsons, and Larsen 1975; Callaway, Levy, and Henderson 1976), however, suggest that the number of miles Navajos drive is substantial. Many families may drive a vehicle between 20,000 and 30,000 miles per year, for instance.

A recent study of motor vehicle accidents based on police reports from the reservation indicates that fatal accidents declined between 1973 and 1975, partly as a result of lower speed limits. It also showed that Indian drivers involved in fatal accidents are often without valid licenses, and in single-car accidents have often been drinking (Katz and May 1979). The decline in accidents is confirmed by a study of hospitalization patterns between 1972 and 1978 (Kunitz and Temkin-Greener 1980).

Without additional data beyond those reported by the Indian Health Service, it is difficult to get a true picture of the accident phenomenon or to have much confidence in the explanations commonly offered for the high and increasing mortality rates that have been observed. Explanations usually revolve around notions such as stress, social disorganization, and anomie, but so far other risk factors such as number of miles driven, highway conditions, and quality of vehicles have not been assessed, so the relative contributions of these factors cannot yet be sorted out.

ALCOHOLISM   According to the 1974 data reported by Kaltenbach (1976), alcoholism accounted for more than 5 percent of deaths among

Navajos. As is the case with accidents, alcoholism is more significant among males than females, the proportionate contribution to mortality being 7 and 2 percent respectively. As with accidents, too, psychosocial stress caused by acculturation and deprivation is often said to be the most important explanatory variable. And, as with accidents, there is reason to believe that this explanation is not entirely adequate.

In a series of previous studies (Levy and Kunitz 1974; Kunitz and Levy 1974) we have observed that patterns of drinking behavior as well as mortality rates from alcoholic cirrhosis, suicide, homicide, accidents, and crude mortality differ among tribes. These differences are not random but appear to be related to differences in ecological adaptation, social organization, and social control (Kunitz 1976b). A detailed discussion of these studies is beyond the scope of this chapter, but it is important to point out here that Navajos do not have mortality rates from alcoholic cirrhosis that are significantly different from the national average. And though public intoxication is not infrequent, one must be careful not to label such drinkers as alcoholics without careful workups.

The definition of alcoholism is a difficult one. If it is defined partially by its economic consequences, then relatively small amounts of money (in middle-class terms) spent on drinking may bring about measurable harm to a family whose income is 18 percent of the national average. If it is defined by its impact on the automobile accident rate, one might wonder what would be the rate if prohibition were not in effect on the reservation and people could therefore drink at home instead of in border towns from which they are likely to drive home drunk. Finally, it is not entirely clear to us that the highly visible groups of men engaged in drinking are alcoholics in the sense that we usually mean it when we think of alcoholism in the larger society. Many of these men may go for long periods of time without drinking and without craving alcohol; and when they do drink, it may be the result of peer pressure. Moreover, usually in their late thirties or early forties most Navajo men who have been known as heavy drinkers—many having experienced the unpleasant symptoms of alcohol withdrawal after occasional prolonged bouts—either give up their drinking entirely or become much more moderate. (This fact explains, we think, the success reported by several disulfiram treatment programs on the reservation.) Among relatively well educated Navajos, the prevailing pattern of alcohol consumption appears to approximate the styles found in the larger American society: an occasional drink (usually beer) at home after work and on weekends, or subdued drinking in a cocktail lounge in a border town.

Though men are undoubtedly the ones who drink the most among Navajos, relatively few of them are what we would class as true alcoholics. Among women who drink, however, it appears to us that the proportion who may be classified as alcoholics is much higher than it is among men. Furthermore, unlike the men, women who are chronic drinkers are often social isolates and are labeled as deviants by the community (Levy and Kunitz 1974:78).

Although many see alcoholism as the most significant health problem of the Navajo, we believe that much drinking behavior may be inappropriately diagnosed as alcoholism. Faced with the results of automobile accidents in which alcohol is involved, health-care workers understandably wonder whether they should attempt to do something about heavy drinking. It appears to us, however, that the most observable and most common form of drinking is so intimately related to patterns of Navajo child rearing, to many traditional values, to peer group solidarity, and to mechanisms of social control that only as the society continues to undergo major changes will group drinking begin to be altered.

HEART DISEASE   We have seen in table 6.2 that heart disease is much less significant at present as a cause of mortality among the Navajo than are accidents. The figures are somewhat misleading, however, because deaths from rheumatic (infectious) and ischemic processes (such as coronary artery disease) have been included in the heart disease category. Numerous investigators have attempted to explain the low rates of ischemic heart disease among Indians in general and the Navajo in particular (Hesse 1964; Maynard, Hammes, and Kester 1967; Sievers 1967). These studies have usually been concerned with exploring the exposure of populations to a variety of factors thought to be associated with the risk of developing coronary artery disease in the general United States population.

Such risk factors as hypercholesterolemia, hypertension, cigarette smoking, physical activity, dietary patterns, acculturation, and social mobility have been considered. Navajos and other Indians have been found to have low serum cholesterol, even though some investigators are of the opinion that their diet is high in saturated fats (Page, Lewis, and Gilbert 1956; Abraham and Miller 1959; Fulmer and Roberts 1963; Comess, Bennett, and Burch 1967). It has been suggested that perhaps Navajos metabolize cholesterol in such a fashion that it is excreted in the bile, which would explain the high prevalence of cholesterol gallstones observed by Small and Rapo (1970). Hypertension is infrequent among reservation residents but is more common among migrants in urban areas and may be increasing among reservation populations as well (Cohen 1953; Clifford et al. 1963; Alfred 1970; Reisinger, Rogers, and Johnson 1972:75; Strotz and Shorr 1973; Destafano, Coulehan, and Wiant 1979). Cigarette smoking is not common (Sievers 1968). Most Navajos engage in physical activity, at least to a moderate extent. The low rate of ischemic heart disease has also been attributed in part to low levels of psychosocial stress (Streeper et al. 1960; Fulmer and Roberts 1963; Sievers 1967).

It is puzzling that for the same tribe, high accident rates have been attributed to high levels of stress and low coronary heart disease rates to low levels of stress. This paradox should make one wary of invoking "stress" as a causative factor when other explanations fail, although it is possible that psychosocial factors are important in the etiology of both accidents and ischemic heart disease. In the case of heart disease, however, such factors may interact with a variety of physiological characteristics that take a long time to manifest themselves and that are of no importance in the etiology of accidents. In other words, psychosocial factors may be necessary conditions in the etiology of both accidents and ischemic heart disease, but in the case of accidents they may be more nearly sufficient as well.

CANCER Death rates from cancers of all types have generally increased among American Indians but are still lower than in the general United States population (Smith, Salsbury, and Gilliam 1956; Smith 1957; Creagan and Fraumeni 1972). Certain specific cancers do occur more frequently among Indians, however; for example, death rates from cancer of the gallbladder and bile duct are higher among Indians, presumably as a result of the higher prevalence of gallstones.

There is some controversy concerning the relative importance of carcinoma of the cervix among Indians (including the Navajo) and non-Indians. Some studies find the rates among Indians to be lower than, or the same as, rates in the general population (Bivens and Fleetwood 1968; Jordan et al. 1972), whereas other studies find the rates to be higher (Creagan and Fraumeni 1972; Dunham, Baillar, and Laquer 1973). The differences may be due primarily to the different methods used in calculating the rates: the lower rates were calculated from hospital statistics on the proportion of positive Pap smears among Indian and non-Indian patients, whereas the higher rates were calculated from mortality data. The differences might be explained if Indians, for whatever reason, were less thoroughly screened and were therefore more likely to die from this cancer. However, it is not clear that this is the case. Since Indian women appear to engage in sexual relations at a relatively early age, one of the risk factors in carcinoma of the cervix may be present. It would not be surprising, therefore, if the rates were found to be at least as high as those in the general United States population.

The incidence of lung cancer is lower among Indians than among non-Indians (Sievers and Cohen 1961; Creagan and Fraumeni 1972). The lower rate is probably due to the facts that Indians smoke less than non-Indians, live in rural settings with clean air, and do not engage in occupations that expose them to carcinogens. The only documented cases of lung cancer among the Navajo are said to have been found among former uranium miners (A. Val-Spinosa, personal communication). It appears likely that Navajos and other Indians will show an increase in carcinomas to the extent that their life-styles and smoking habits change and they participate more actively in American economic life.

INFANT MORTALITY   Navajo infant mortality has in general declined over the past generation or two (table 6.4). Hadley's estimate (1955) of 139 infant deaths per 1,000 live births in the early 1950s probably represents in itself a considerable reduction since the pre-World War II era, when the rate may have been more than 200 per 1,000 live births, as it was among the Hopi at the time (Kunitz 1974a).

Though Navajo infant mortality has been reduced dramatically in recent years, it is still higher than in the general United States population. Moreover, the rate is quite variable from one part of the reservation to another (Kunitz 1976a). Factors such as use of prenatal care (Iba, Niswander, and Woodville 1973; Brenner, Reisinger, and Rogers 1974), birth weight (Rosa and Resnick 1965), feeding patterns and nutritional status of the infant (Darby et al. 1956; French 1967; Van Duzen et al. 1969; Reisinger, Rogers, and Johnson 1972), and complicated pregnancies (Brenner, Reisinger, and Rogers 1974), are all related to infant mortality. It is likely that most improvements in the future will result from improved living conditions, usually associated with higher economic status, rather than from improved medical care (Oakland and Kane 1973).

CHILD HEALTH   Nutritional deficiencies in children are still significant on the Navajo Reservation. Overt protein-calorie malnutrition was reported from the western end of the reservation as late as the 1960s but is virtually unknown on the eastern end (Wolf 1961; Van Duzen et al.

Table 6.4 Navajo infant mortality rates

Date	Rate per 1,000 live births	Area	Source
1949–1951	139.4	Reservation-wide	Hadley 1955
Late 1950s	70.0	Many Farms	McDermott, Deuschle, and Barnett 1972
Early 1970s	37.0	Fort Defiance	Brenner, Reisinger, and Rogers, 1974
1970	31.5	Reservation-wide	USPHS 1971

1969:1398). Throughout the reservation, however, Navajo children are found to be smaller and lighter than non-Indian age-mates (Van Duzen et al. 1969; Reisinger, Rogers, and Johnson 1972). Borderline malnutrition may even have a measurable influence on the ability to learn skills necessary in school and elsewhere (Moore, Silverberg, and Read 1972).

Compounding nutritional deficiencies are problems related to chronic otitis media (middle ear disease). An enormous literature has developed on this condition as it is related to learning disorders among the Navajo in particular and American Indians and Alaska natives generally (Brody 1964; Brody, Overfield, and McAlister 1965; Johnson 1967; Reed, Struve, and Maynard 1967; Zonis 1968; Jaffe 1969; Ling, McCoy, and Levinson 1969; Maynard 1969; Gregg et al. 1970; Reed and Dunn 1970; Maynard, Fleshman, and Tschopp 1972; Rossi 1972). Though chronic otitis media does not necessarily result in deafness in adulthood, it may lead to difficulties in language acquisition among affected children and thus may have a measurable impact on school performance. Growing interest in this problem is an additional indication of the passage of the Navajo population into the later stages of the epidemiological transition, where concern for problems related to morbidity rather than mortality becomes increasingly important.

MATERNAL MORTALITY It is worth noting that one of the leading causes of death among Navajo women as recently as the early 1940s was maternal mortality (estimated by Leighton and Kluckhohn (1948) to be about 1,000 per 100,000 live births). By the early 1970s the rate had dropped to about 30 per 100,000 live births, still somewhat higher than the national rate of 24.2 (Slocumb and Kunitz 1977). The factors contributing most importantly to maternal mortality at present are (1) toxemia of pregnancy, which has a higher incidence and case-fatality rate than in the general United States population and reflects inadequate prenatal preventive care; and (2) hemorrhage, which appears to be related to a high prevalence of anemia among women in the childbearing years, as well as to inadequate blood banking facilities at many of the hospitals serving the Navajo.

Concepts of Disease and Illness

Despite the fact that Navajos utilize many different kinds of treatment for illness, including modern medicine, curers from neighboring tribes, peyote ceremonies, Christian ministers, and on occasion, faith healers, there has been remarkably little incorporation of these foreign ideas into the traditional Navajo belief system about disease and its causes. This can be attributed, we believe, to two facts: (1) the healing system is sacred, representing the very core of Navajo religion, and (2) the aim of healing ceremonies is to remove the causes of disease, not to alleviate symptoms. This leaves the patient free to seek relief by any means available to him. In consequence, we feel justified in discussing the traditional belief system without considering influences that other systems may exert upon it. Utilization of other medical systems does not necessarily imply a corresponding change in concepts on the part of the patient. Individuals do change, however, and the extent to which Navajo health beliefs have changed and are changing is an area that must be investigated empirically.

Etiology of Disease

According to traditional Navajo belief, disease may be contracted by "soul loss," "intrusive object," "spirit possession," "breach of taboo," and "witchcraft." Specific agents may cause disease by one or more of these means.

SOUL LOSS   The notion of soul loss is not directly related to the causation of specific diseases. Yet there is reason to believe that the concept is important to the Navajo. The soul, or "wind" as it is most often called, enters the body soon after birth and forms the individual's basic personality. At death the soul leaves the body and proceeds to the afterworld. Faintness and suffocation are signs that the wind-soul is leaving the body and signal the final stage of an illness. The child's first laugh indicates that the soul has become attached to the body; prior to this time, the infant may die easily. During old age the soul is, once more, loosely attached, and death at this time is considered natural. The ghosts of the very old and of infants are not thought to be potent causes of disease, while those of people who die while the wind-soul is well attached are thought to be potent etiological agents.

INTRUSIVE OBJECTS   A disease-causing agent may be injected into the body by a special form of witchcraft, which has been termed "wizardry" by Kluckhohn (1944). This form of witchcraft is said to have been borrowed in the nineteenth century from the Pueblos, among whom it is relatively prominent. Neither wizardry nor its cure, the Sucking Way, is central to Navajo healing belief and practices. The Sucking Way is said to have been borrowed from the Chiricahua Apaches (Haile 1950). Emaciation, together with pain in the part of the body where the object has lodged, is indicative of wizardry.

SPIRIT INTRUSION   Spirit intrusion, or possession, involves the displacement of the wind-soul by the spirit of a dangerous being, most often a supernatural. Kaplan and Johnson (1964) maintain that possession is the central concept of disease causation among the Navajo and relate it to what they assert is a predisposition for Navajo mental illnesses to be hysterical in nature. Though there are no quantitative data available to either support or deny this assertion, several observations are in order. When Navajos talk about actual cases—how a specific illness was contracted by a particular individual—they never mention spirit intrusion. On the other hand, the recorded myths of healing ceremonies and the ceremonialists with whom we have discussed this matter describe the principal diseases in terms of possession. The myth of the Evil Way chant, for example, tells how the supernatural known as Coyote sent his ghost into the hero in order to "witch" him (Haile 1950). When a person is possessed by the mythical Gila Monster, his arms begin to shake, a sign that he has the gift to diagnose illness by "hand trembling" (Wyman 1936). It is possible that lay people do not know the myths in sufficient detail to be cognizant of the role spirit possession plays. More likely, however, the tendency to avoid implicating spirit possession results from a desire to avoid anxiety-provoking diagnoses. It may be less threatening to hear that one has inadvertently stepped on a coyote track than to learn that one is possessed by Coyote himself.

BREACH OF TABOO   Some form of breach of taboo is the most frequently reported kind of diagnosis among the Navajo. Breach of taboo includes not only the commission of prohibited acts like incest but also coming into contact with a "dangerous" object. For example, sibling incest is thought to cause the signs of a generalized seizure. In this instance the breach of a major taboo is involved, and some degree of volition is implied. However, the Navajo also call this disease "Moth sickness" and believe that the moth is the principal etiological agent. The original act of incest is said to have been committed by the Butterfly People in the mythical past, who became "like moths who fly into the fire," twisting and convulsing. Today, a human with seizures may be diagnosed as suffering from "Moth sickness" because he behaves like a moth, but it is not necessary that actual incest be committed.

By virtue of sympathetic magic (that is, like causes have like effects, and objects once in contact with each other retain each other's properties), diseases may also be contracted through inadvertent contact with an etiological agent. Thus, Moth sickness may also be contracted if a real moth, which shares the properties of the mythical Moth, touches a person. Although no volition on the part of the individual is involved, this occurrence is a breach of taboo because disease-causing objects or beings are considered "dangerous," and one should have no contact with anything that is dangerous.

In some instances, the responsibility for breaking a taboo may lie with someone other than the afflicted. Thus, a pregnant woman may breach a taboo and cause her child to become ill later in life. In addition, a witch can make a person come into contact with a dangerous object in order to make him ill. In the example of Moth sickness, a witch can either cause the victim to touch a moth or cause the victim's mind to go "wild" so that he will become like a moth. In this event the person will ultimately commit incest and develop seizures.

WITCHCRAFT   Witchcraft is another frequently mentioned means of contracting disease. We have already mentioned the form of witchcraft that Kluckhohn has labeled "wizardry." In his monograph on the subject he discusses three other types: witchery, sorcery, and Frenzy Witchcraft (Kluckhohn 1944).

Witchery, the primary form of Navajo witchcraft, is mentioned in the creation myth as being originated by First Man and First Woman. Witches are associated with the dead and with incest, two of the most dangerous etiological agents. To qualify as a witch, a person is believed to have to kill a close relative, especially a sibling. In the myths, male witches invariably live in incestuous unions with one of their daughters. Some informants claim that the witch-initiate must eat part of a murdered relative's body. The effective means of working witchery is by touching the victim with a powder made from corpse flesh, thus bringing him into contact with a "dangerous" etiological agent. Most often, witches transform themselves into wolves, coyotes, or dogs but also into bears, owls, foxes, and crows in order to travel undetected. Witchery mirrors and is the evil opposite side of Navajo religion. Not only is witchery based on the two great "dangers," incest and death, but witches band together and perform their own ceremonials using chants, sand paintings, body paintings, and masks. Since "corpse powder" is brought into contact with the victim, it is not surprising that the signs of witchery are the same as those of ghost sickness, fainting and unconsciousness.

Sorcery is closely associated with witchery, and sorcerers participate in the witchery ceremonials. Sorcerers use spells to work their evil. The sorcerer must have a bit of the victim's personal excreta (hair, nails, feces, and so on) over which he casts his spell. Even in this instance, however, breach of taboo is involved, since the parts of the victim's person are most often buried near a lightning-struck tree or a grave, which are "dangerous." Personal excreta and clothing still retain properties of the victim, and because like causes produce like results, what is done to them is also done to the victim.

Frenzy witchcraft is primarily love magic, though it is also used in trading, gambling, and hunting. The master of this form of witchcraft uses a concoction made from datura in much the same way as corpse powder is used in witchery. The datura plant contains scopolamine and hyoscyamine and produces hallucinations, dissociative reactions and, in some instances, coma when ingested. According to Navajo belief, the victim has only to be touched by the concoction, although smoking or ingesting it bring about the same results. When women are bewitched in this manner, they "go out of their minds," run around in circles, and sometimes may tear off their clothes or fall to the ground and lose consciousness. The aim is to make the woman lose her senses and run away from human habitation in a state of sexual frenzy so that the witch can catch and seduce her. When this witchcraft is used in gambling against men, the victim goes out of his mind, gambles recklessly, and loses his wealth to the witch.

Even though witches may be said to cause disease, it is important to remember that they are really manipulating the etiological agents that cause disease. Though a person is said to be "witched," he is thought to have the disease caused by the etiological agent with which he came into contact and should have the appropriate ceremony for that particular agent. Because witchery is so prevalent and because it uses corpse powder, the ceremonial that cures ghost sickness is said to be particularly good against witchcraft in general.

ETIOLOGICAL AGENTS   According to Navajo beliefs, almost anything can cause disease. Even beneficent deities may be a source of illness if approached improperly. Wyman and Kluckhohn (1938) note that Navajos recognize four classes of etiological agents: animals, natural phenomena, healing ceremonies, and evil spirits. The discussion will be confined to those etiologies that are the most frequently diagnosed or are considered the most "dangerous."

1. *Animals.* Wyman and Kluckhohn (1938:14) obtained a list of animals that cause illness from an elderly informant which included 10 mammals, 7 reptiles, 12 birds, and all fish. To this should be added at least 7 insects (Wyman and Bailey 1964). The most frequently invoked beings in this class are the bear, coyote, porcupine, snake, eagle, moth, ant, long-horned grasshopper, and camel cricket. In light of the fact that datura can cause illness, as can any plant used for ceremonial purposes, this class might be thought of as including sentient beings of all sorts.

2. *Natural phenomena.* The most common causes of illness in this class are lightning and whirlwinds. Water, hail, and the earth itself are mentioned less often. Lightning is generalized to include all things that are long, slender, and move in a zigzag motion—for example, arrows and snakes. In Navajo belief there are many kinds of wind, both beneficent and "dangerous," among which whirlwinds are especially destructive. It is interesting that the two most frequently used healing ceremonials, the

Wind and Shooting (Lightning) Way chants, not only protect against a broad array of symptoms but also overlap in the domain of causal agents.

3. *Ceremonials.* Any ceremonial can cause illness. All powerful forces are "dangerous," so when the Holy People (beneficent deities) are present during a ceremony a person may be affected. People who become ill in this way are said to have the same illness the ceremonial is said to cure. Transgressions of taboos associated with ceremonials (for example, the prohibition against cohabitation during and after the proceedings) can cause illness.

4. *Evil spirits.* Ghosts of the dead are prominent in this category. The belief that a ghost can affect the living deleteriously is a common and probably ancient belief among North American Indians. The Navajo believe that any contact with the corpse, the house where death has occurred, places once occupied by the ancients (for example, the Pueblo ruins), and even old artifacts will cause ghost sickness. A variety of mythical monsters are also included in this class, although diagnoses involving them are rare at present.

IMPLICIT ETIOLOGIES In the opinion of most observers, disease is classified by etiological agent. Each healing ceremony is known by the causal factors it is thought to cure. At the same time, however, there appear to be some operational classifications that are somewhat separate from the explicit formalization of Navajo disease theory. The implicit classification of disease by symptom will be discussed in the following section, although it is relevant to point out here that some of the most prominent symptoms tend to be associated with some of the more "dangerous" etiological agents such as bear, coyote, moth, and ghosts.

Navajos also recognize that some diseases are contagious, although this may be a post-contact development since there are no etiologies that are thought specifically to cause such maladies. Distinctions made between white disease and Navajo diseases have been noted in the literature and will be discussed in the following section.

Social Contexts for Discussion of Nosology and Etiology

To our knowledge, no systematic observations have been made of the contexts in which discussion of nosology takes place; nor do we know for certain how debate between Navajos of different persuasions proceeds when white observers are not present. The discussion that follows is based entirely on our personal experience.

It is our impression that discussion between family members concerning the relative merits of Christianity or peyotism is restrained and does not take the form of debate, as one might expect. When peyotism first came to the communities in which Levy worked in the early 1960s, the younger Navajos who considered themselves peyotists did not argue the matter with their parents. Such arguments were seen as attacks on the religion of the parents, which led to bad feelings. Instead, the younger Navajos would persuade their parents to attend a peyote meeting after traditional ceremonies had failed to help a family member. Ultimately, even families of ceremonialists would attend a meeting. Christians view peyotism as a competing form of religion rather than as a medical system and do not consider it as an option.

Family discussions concerning the benefits of modern medicine, in our experience, do not argue the relative merits of concepts but rather focus on the tangible success of various treatments. Younger, more educated Navajos often try to explain concepts such as germ theory to their elders. The traditional Navajos are interested to hear of these strange ideas but do not conceive of them as competing with their own beliefs. White belief is good for whites, and Navajo belief is good for Navajos; they are two distinct phenomena. The traditional Navajo attitude is that exchange of knowledge is good, but attacking another person's beliefs (for example, in witches) is impolite and uncouth.

Occasionally, physicians have tried to convince their Navajo patients that the traditional ceremonies are ineffective and perhaps even dangerous. Since the communication was always one-sided, one could hardly call these instances discussions. Prominent ceremonialists sometimes gather together to discuss religious and medical matters, but we have never been present at such gatherings.

Learning Medical Concepts and Intraethnic Variation

Because Navajo religion is remarkably complex, it is not surprising to find considerable differences between the young and the old and between the layman and the professional in respect to knowledge of medical concepts. The typical traditional Navajo learns from childhood which taboos must be observed to avoid illness. Just how these taboos derive from the myths of the healing ceremonies is not always well understood by the layman, however. We found repeatedly that many Navajo patients did not know why a ceremonial was performed for them beyond the fact that the diagnostician had recommended it. Some families had more medical knowledge than did others, which seemed to be a result of the presence of a ceremonialist in the extended family. As a rule, the children of ceremonialists learned more about medical matters than other children.

To learn a major ceremonial can take as long as eight years of apprenticeship. Most ceremonialists specialize in only one or two complete ceremonies and know the short forms of several others. The shift to a wage-work economy has made it almost impossible for most young men to find time to learn the ceremonials. To date, increased transportation and a growing network of paved roads have permitted ceremonialists to serve a larger number of patients. It is possible, however, that there will be an acute shortage of knowledgeable ceremonialists in another 10 years.

Virtually all Navajo children attend school and are exposed to some basic modern ideas of disease causation. In addition, Navajos come into contact with whites in a variety of contexts. Health information is disseminated by the Indian Health Service, and increasing numbers of Navajos are choosing careers in the health professions. There is no doubt that the general level of biomedical understanding is changing, although there are no published studies to date that assess levels of understanding in different segments of the Navajo population.

It is important to note that the traditional healing system persists with a remarkable internal consistency across a reservation the size of West Virginia, and that the ceremonies and normative beliefs are practically identical with those documented at the turn of the century. Individuals may cease to believe in the old ways, but to date there is little evidence to suggest that traditional Navajo beliefs have changed by incorporating new concepts of curing techniques. Adair and Deuschle (1970:33) quote a prominent Navajo politician and ceremonialist as saying that there are diseases which (1) the Navajos cannot cure but white physicians can, (2) both physicians and ceremonialists can cure, and (3) only Navajo ceremonialists can cure. In our opinion it would be erroneous to infer from this public statement that Navajo ceremonialists currently have a new category called "white diseases" which they recognize and for which they recommend modern therapy. The example most often mentioned is tuberculosis, which the Navajo have come to learn can be cured by INH therapy. However, tuberculosis is not a condition that can be diagnosed by Navajo methods, and we have never encountered a patient who was diagnosed as having either a white disease or tuberculosis.

We do observe a growing acceptance of modern medicine among the Navajo, based on its demonstrated effectiveness. Neither ceremonialists nor their patients are averse to seeking treatment from physicians. It has not always been so, however. Prior to the introduction of antibiotics and INH therapy for tuberculosis, modern medicine did not cure an impressive number of tuberculosis or pneumonia patients. The Navajo regarded the hospitals and sanitoriums as "houses of death," where it was almost certain the patient would contract ghost sickness. However, Navajo acceptance of the hospital has changed as the rate of cure has improved, with the result that today a ceremonialist may tell a patient to do what the white doctors say rather than telling him to stay away at all costs. Today virtually all Navajos utilize modern medicine, although this change in attitude and behavior does not imply a change in the traditional system itself.

Since peyotists and Christians both accept witchcraft as a major cause of disease, it is our impression that education is a better predictor of changed health concepts than religious affiliation per se. At the same time, however, it must be pointed out that the more educated Navajos tend to be Christian, peyotists, or unaffiliated. And there are several Navajos of our acquaintance who have a college education but who still attend ceremonials occasionally.

Becoming Ill

Classification and Understanding of Symptoms

As demonstrated in the previous section, Navajos tend to classify diseases by cause rather than symptoms. In consequence, it is difficult to determine precisely the role symptoms play in diagnosis, a subject we will discuss in the next section. It is important to note here that no Navajo disease is known by the symptoms it produces or by the part of the body it affects. There is, for instance, no disease like "wandering of the uterus" (hysteria) or "the falling sickness" (epilepsy). Rather, Navajos refer to their illnesses by the agents thought to cause them (bear sickness, porcupine sickness) or by the ceremonials used to cure them ("that which is treated by the Shooting Chant"). Because the traditional health culture does not rely on a knowledge of symptoms in the diagnostic process, Navajo patients often have difficulty understanding the purpose of history taking and the physical examination, a circumstance that often leads to misunderstanding in the clinical setting.

Nevertheless, Navajos do recognize that they are ill by the discomfort they experience, and there is little reason to believe, as many physicians have suggested, that Navajos are poor observers (Leighton and Kennedy 1957). Landar (1967) has shown that the language of pain is sophisticated, and it is our experience that symptoms are well described and that Navajos are good historians when it is made clear to them why a physician needs to have a good history of their condition.

Wyman and Kluckhohn (1938) have noted a loose association between etiological agents and symptoms. A single cause may produce any of several symptoms and, conversely, a single symptom may be caused by any of several etiological agents. Several diagnoses and treatments may be tried before the correct one is determined, and chronicity of symptoms itself seems to be an important factor in diagnosing and classifying illness. Nevertheless, certain groups of healing ceremonies do appear to be associated with certain symptoms and not others, while several ceremonies appear to be good for a broad range of symptoms.

The question remains, however, whether patients are actually diagnosed and treated according to their symptoms or according to more random, magical, or social considerations. For, if informants believe that certain ceremonies are good for certain symptoms, they also maintain that a given ceremony will be used because of a specific etiological agent, regardless of the symptoms. Thus, the Shooting Way may be considered especially good for bodily aches and pains, but it will also be used for treatment of insanity if the illness is diagnosed as being caused by lightning or snakes. Remarkably little quantitative research has been done to answer this question by correlating reported symptoms with native diagnoses and treatments for any sizable number of patients.

One study has attempted to determine the degree to which Navajos distinguish various types of epileptic seizures from one another, whether epileptic seizures are distinguished from hysterical seizures (conversion reactions), and whether seizure patients actually receive the native diagnoses and treatments that Navajo informants claim are especially effective in curing these symptoms (Levy, Neutra, and Parker 1979 and in press; Neutra, Levy, and Parker 1977). This last aspect of the study will be discussed in greater detail in the following section, although it is relevant to point out here that various symptoms and signs associated with seizures were indeed found to be significantly related to the kinds of treatment instituted. With regard to differential diagnosis of seizure states, Navajo tradition gives a prominent position to (1) the signs of the grand mal seizure, which are said to be caused by sibling incest; (2) the signs of the psychomotor seizure or any bout of irrational behavior that culminates with the patient falling to the ground with loss of consciousness (such episodes are attributed to a form of witchcraft); and (3) unilateral convulsions, shaking, or trembling, which are thought to indicate the gift of "hand trembling," the major method of diagnosing disease. Whether less startling signs and symptoms than those of epilepsy also determine diagnoses must be determined by further research, however.

Tolerance for Symptoms

Virtually no organized investigations have been undertaken in the area of tolerance for pain or tolerance of different symptoms by the Navajo. Over the years, the clinical experience of numerous physicians has indicated that, in general, Navajos tend to define themselves as sick according to the degree of pain they experience rather than by the appearance of symptoms per se. In addition, Navajos appear to be more stoic than white patients (Leighton and Kennedy 1957). In our opinion there is no evidence to suggest that the threshold of pain is higher among the Navajo, although this has been suggested by some physicians working on the reservation. It seems more likely that poor people who lead harsh lives find that seeking treatment is costly and not to be undertaken lightly. Since most conditions are self-contained, Navajos tend to put up with ailments that cause little discomfort and do not impair function. In consequence, although the presence of disease may be recognized, treatment may not be sought by a person until the pain is great and he cannot function adequately. Prior to reaching this state, most Navajos tend not to talk about their pain to family members in order not to worry them. Navajos who live close to a hospital and thus avoid the costs of transportation tend to use the services of a physician more frequently.

There is some reason to believe that "mental" disorders are of special concern to Navajos. "Mind loss" manifested by fainting, dissociative reactions, and seizures is thought to be the final stage of most, if not all, diseases. In fact, many Navajo informants have told us that they recognized they were ill when they experienced anxiety-provoking dreams that had no obvious cause. However, the question of whether there is less tolerance for such symptoms by the Navajo (in the sense that they promote earlier treatment or provoke more anxiety than would be occasioned by other symptoms) is moot.

Extremes of behavior appear to signal the need for psychiatric treatment (Kaplan and Johnson 1964). In 1962 and 1963, Levy interviewed most of the schizophrenic patients seen in the Tuba City hospital (N = 16). Despite the facts that these patients did not exhibit overt violence and that few were diagnosed as paranoid, the admission records of the male patients contained accounts of violence. During the interview, however, patients and families maintained that actual violence had not taken place but that treatment had been sought because they feared violence might occur if something were not done to avert it. Patients would say something like, "I was afraid I might hurt my wife and children." It would seem that expressing a potential for violence signals the need for treatment more effectively than other, more typical symptoms of schizophrenia. In contrast to male schizophrenics, females were brought to hospital after they had become so withdrawn that they could no longer cook for their families or, as was sometimes mentioned, do their weaving. Hallucinations, delusions, and disorientation were rarely described as presenting symptoms by families at the time of admission.

A number of congenital malformations like cleft palate appear to be negatively labeled by the Navajo community; others, like supernumerary digits and congenital hip displacement, excite no comment (Adair and Deuschle 1970). The high prevalence of these last two disorders probably accounts for their greater acceptance. Twin births are disvalued and are thought to be caused by promiscuity as well as chance. The survival rate of twins among the Navajo has been shown to be poor, even taking into account the tendency for twins to be born prematurely (Levy 1964a). The hermaphrodite, on the other hand, occupied a valued position (Hill 1935), at least until recently.

Due to the belief that generalized seizures are caused by sibling incest, epileptic patients in many instances lead difficult lives. In one study, for example (Levy, Neutra, and Parker 1979), female epileptics were found to have records of social problems such as incest, promiscuity, illegitimate births, and heavy drinking significantly more often than did hysterical females with conversion reactions that looked like seizures (p = .01 by Fisher's Exact Test). When incest, rape, and illegitimate births were considered alone, the difference was still significant (p = .04). None of the 10 female "hysterics" had these problems, whereas 4 of the 10 female epileptics did. In fact, 3 of the epileptics in the Tuba City Service Unit had actually committed sibling incest. These cases occurred in less wealthy and somewhat disorganized families. More wealthy, traditional families reared their epileptic children in isolation to protect them from community censure, and these children did not have problems of the sort described. Ten of the 11 male epileptics for whom there was adequate information had problems with alcohol. Four of these were prone to violence, and one had committed sibling incest. Because drinking is prevalent among Navajo males generally and because there was only one male "hysteric" in the study, we cannot tell for certain whether these problems are more prevalent among male epileptics than would be expected.

The seizure patients in the Tuba City Service Unit sample were followed for a period of 11 years (1964–1974). During this period, 4 of the 11 epileptics died from unknown or unnatural causes: suspected suicide, 1; exposure after drinking, 2; cause undetermined, 1. All but the suspected suicide were females. It is our impression that these deaths are unusual even for epileptics, but we have no hard data for comparative purposes from other cohorts of epileptics in other populations. Only one "hysteric" died during this period, and this was from old age. The only epileptics who avoided social problems were those reared in isolation and the very acculturated ones who were well maintained on medication.

Discussion of Symptoms

No research has been done on how Navajos discuss their symptoms within the family, larger kin group, or community. Although we know that families sometimes make a diagnosis without consulting a diagnostician, the very fact that traditional methods of diagnosis do not utilize symptoms indicates that such discussions may not be a routine matter. Prior to being diagnosed, Navajos have a number of expressions they use to indicate the degree of discomfort they feel (Leighton and Kennedy 1957; Werner 1963, 1965; Levy 1964b). Werner and Levy maintain that these expressions, though incorporating terms for aches and fever, do not imply the presence of any specific type of pain. Leighton and Kennedy, on the other hand, believe that "feeling bad all over" indicates the presence of one of a small number of disease syndromes which the authors do not identify. Our guess is that most often, a person will express the degree of pain experienced rather than the specific symptoms, unless there is obvious trauma like a broken leg.

Nevertheless, as the data from the epilepsy study suggest, observable signs are discussed. It is also reasonable to assume that in matrifocal households, daughters will feel free to discuss their own and their children's symptoms with their mothers and maternal aunts. Although we know that problems of patient management are discussed in the family setting, we do not know whether symptoms are discussed in the same way. Husbands and wives are often reticent to discuss health matters with each other when they involve "women's problems." Kunitz (1976c) has found that there is remarkably little communication among female kinsmen concerning birth control and female sexuality. In sum, though Navajos learn about disease, and symptoms do not go completely undiscussed, patterns of communication are not known to outside investigators.

When we compare what we know of the role symptoms play in the process of seeking help among the Navajo with what has been reported for the poor in general (McKinlay 1975), we find some strong similarities due to poverty and some differences due to culture. The poor in general are reported to react to pain, rather than to any specific symptom—as do the Navajo. Economic considerations tend to make health concerns take low priority. At the same time, however, the Navajo appear to be sensitive to symptoms such as violence and irrationality in much the same way that various ethnic groups in the general population seem to react more quickly to certain symptoms than to others.

Health Behavior of Nontraditional Navajos

The discussion thus far has dealt exclusively with traditional Navajo patients. Yet between 20 and 37 percent of male household heads, and higher proportions of their spouses, were found to be Christian in areas surveyed by the Lake Powell Research Project, and between 4 and 18 percent were peyotists (Callaway, Levy, and Henderson 1976). Furthermore, the Navajo population is more educated now than it has ever been. While it is important to know how acculturation affects health behavior, there are no studies that actually compare traditional with nontraditional Navajos. On the behavioral level, however, some obvious general statements may be made: Christians, more educated Navajos, and those reared away from the reservation as a rule do not use traditional Navajo healing ceremonies. What changes have occurred in the perception of symptoms among these groups is not known.

Peyotists present themselves as two groups: those who claim to be peyotists only and those who claim adherence to both peyotist and traditionalist religions. Our impression is that definitions of disease and symp-

tom perception are not radically different between peyotists and traditionalists if level of education is controlled. The peyotist, however, will rely
on peyote leaders both for diagnosis and for treatment, despite the fact
that the cause and understanding of the malady are often expressed in
traditional terms.

Coping with Illness outside the Mainstream Medical System

Treatment within the Family

FAMILIAL ROLE RESPONSIBILITIES   Mothers are responsible for
the care of their infants and young children. Both parents are responsible
for their minor children in general. Adults are responsible for the care of
their aged parents, and close kinsmen are relied upon to help implement
decisions by providing economic support. Although these general statements sound much like the role responsibilities of the white American
middle class, there are some important differences. The most obvious one
is the degree of autonomy given to individuals, even to relatively young
children. White health workers are often nonplussed when, after asking
whether a child is following a prescribed course of treatment, for example,
the mother says, "Why don't you ask him?" A field health nurse once
asked Levy what she ought to do in a case that involved an 11-year-old
boy with an incurable condition, who would not take his medication and
whose mother insisted it was the boy's choice. After following advice to
talk directly with the boy, the nurse was surprised to find that he had an
adequate understanding of his illness and that his decision not to take
medication was a reasonable and intelligent one. According to the patient,
he had decided to discontinue medication and to face almost certain
death because continuing to come to the hospital and being restricted in
his activities worked considerable hardship on his mother and, in effect,
took food out of the mouths of his brothers and sisters. It pained him to
see his mother neglect his younger siblings because of her concern for
him, and he felt that since there was no hope for a cure in any case, it was
best for all concerned that the family return to a normal state as soon as
possible.

Physicians and nurses have often commented on the fact that Navajo
parents seem remarkably unaware of their children's symptoms and appear uncaring and callous. We do not think this attitude is due either to a
conscious extension of the idea that it is up to each individual to decide
when he is ill or to any lack of concern and affection for children; rather,
we think it has something to do with the tendency for poor people living
in harsh conditions to react only to the most obvious signs in others and
to considerable pain of their own. We have had occasion to discuss this
idea with a few articulate Navajo women, all of whom said that they just
do not react and sometimes hardly notice when their children have run-

ning noses, coughs, fevers, diarrhea, or loss of appetite. They only become concerned when the child can hardly move—despite the fact that they are good observers of their own symptoms. It is quite clear, however, that this pattern is changing as more and more mothers are educated and have more contact with whites.

HOME TREATMENT   Various plants are thought to be good for treating a large variety of symptoms. Navajos who have a knowledge of these plants and who are able to obtain them will utilize them much as the general population uses aspirin, Kaopectate, or any other popular over-the-counter remedy. Many of these plants have been identified (Elmore 1944; Wyman and Harris 1951), but little research has been done on the actual effectiveness of these remedies. It is our impression that over-the-counter remedies, readily available at trading posts and cash-and-carry stores, are rapidly superseding the old herbal remedies.

Traditionally many Navajos had mastered the art of setting bones and cauterizing wounds. Currently, however, these conditions are almost invariably treated at a hospital or clinic. Heat treatment was and still is used for aches, pains, swelling, and broken bones. The affected part is placed over a pit of hot coals and covered with blankets. However, this form of treatment is also being superseded by modern medical practices. The sweat bath remains popular as a home treatment for a large variety of symptoms; it is also the primary means of bathing when there is no running water and is of ceremonial importance as a means of ritual purification. Emetics are used during ceremonies but not as home remedies unless a family member is a ceremonialist or herbalist.

We have not detected any pattern of preference for treating some symptoms at home but not others; nor is there enough knowledge about the prevalence of home treatments, their benefits, or their dangers for any general statements to be made at this time.

RELEASE FROM ROLE RESPONSIBILITIES   The issue of a person's release from role responsibilities during illness is another area in which our knowledge is deficient. Our impression is that the autonomy allowed each individual in deciding when he is ill and when he needs treatment permits him to withdraw from his role responsibilities prior to diagnosis and treatment. We have already mentioned, however, that the cessation of functions is in itself a sign of the need for treatment and that most people tend to continue their routine activities until discomfort is quite severe.

The physician's recommendation that a patient be cared for at home and remain relatively inactive places a considerable burden on the family. Initially there is a mobilization of resources to care for the invalid; children may be kept home from school to help out and efforts made to obtain transportation so the patient can return to the hospital for follow-up treatments. If the condition does not improve, however, family resources dwindle and the education of the child kept home from school suffers. At this point the family is likely to ask that the patient be kept in hospital, or frequently the family may slacken its efforts, especially when the patient is elderly or an infant. All too often these behaviors are interpreted by physicians as evidence of indifference or irresponsibility.

Lay Consultation and Referral

Little is known about the topic of lay consultation and referral. Though there is no doubt that considerable discussion about health problems takes place within the nuclear and extended family and, frequently, within the wider kin network, actual patterns of consultation have not been accurately ascertained. As a general rule, adults seem to be able to define when they are ill and need treatment and are also able to decide which form of treatment they require. However, adult heads of extended families have the final decision when large outlays of money are involved.

Nonmainstream Medical Care outside the Home

As mentioned previously, there is a strong tendency for Navajos to use both native and modern therapies for the same illness because of the belief that modern medicine removes symptoms, while Navajo medicine cures the illness itself. Although we do not have detailed studies of Christians and peyotists, it is our impression that Christians will use modern medicine in conjunction with prayer to aid in obtaining a cure, while peyotists are more like the traditionalists in the way they combine or select one form of treatment over another.

In order to appreciate some of the reasons Navajos might have for seeking modern medical treatment, it is important to understand what is involved in arranging for a ceremonial cure. Although a Navajo may decide he is ill in much the same way as white Americans do, the path from perception of illness to treatment is a complex one. Ideally, a diagnostician such as a hand trembler or a star gazer will be called upon to determine the cause of the ailment. The diagnostician, aided by a relatively simple ritual, depends on what he "sees" or "hears" while in a trance to learn the nature of the causal agent. Once this is done, the appropriate healing ceremony may be contracted for with the ceremonialist or "singer." More than 75 ceremonies have been identified among the Navajo. Though most are used to remove the cause of an existing illness, some, notably the Blessing Way chants, are used for the prevention of illness, maintaining and attracting the forces of beauty and harmony. (These preventive ceremonies have been omitted from our tabulations of cures provided to patients throughout the chapter.) Ideally, a ceremony should be performed four times before a cure is assured. Since most ceremonies cannot be performed during the summer months, considerable time may pass between diagnosis and ceremonial treatment. Traditionally, herbalists have been utilized for the alleviation of symptoms during the periods of waiting. The cost of paying for the services of several professionals and for four ceremonies is considerable, especially today when real income is declining and stock holdings are restricted. Therefore, self-diagnosis and use of physicians who do not charge fees are common practices.

CHOICE OF TREATMENT A study conducted in the 1960s (Levy 1962b) provides some information about the kinds of symptoms for which various forms of treatment were utilized. In a group of kinsmen comprising 106 persons of all ages who lived some 20 miles from an Indian Health Service Hospital, 77 decisions were made over a two-year period either to seek or not to seek treatment for symptoms recognized by the patient (or a responsible adult in the case of minor children) as indicating the presence of illness. Of the 77 instances of recognized illness, only 10 resulted in a decision not to seek treatment outside the home. This remarkably high proportion (87 percent) of decisions to seek medical help from professionals, whether native practitioners or physicians, may be an artifact of the research design, which allowed subjects to define the point at which illness occurred rather than asking about the appearance of symptoms.

Five of the ten decisions not to seek any treatment were made by mothers for infants or young children. There was one case of general malaise (later diagnosed as a mild iron deficiency after the child was taken to the hospital), two cases of upper respiratory infection, and two cases of measles. In one family measles had broken out, and the older sibling (age 13) had been taken to the hospital; the younger children, aged 3 and 4, had not been seen by a physician because the symptoms did not appear to the mother as acute as those of the older brother.

Among adults, one instance of upper respiratory infection went untreated, and two instances of diarrhea were treated with "pills" that were obtained from a trading post and could not be identified. An adult with vague pains decided against treatment, and an elderly, asymptomatic woman who knew she had come into contact with lightning and needed a ceremonial was overruled by her granddaughter, who was the head of the extended family and felt the family did not have the resources to contract for a five-night ceremonial.

After decisions against seeking treatment were excluded, there were 67 instances involving an initial choice to seek either native or modern forms of treatment. In 32 instances (48 percent), only modern medical care was utilized. Twenty-six decisions (39 percent) involved utilizing both native healers and physicians, while only 9 (13 percent) involved the exclusive use of native practitioners. Modern treatment was utilized for fractures, lacerations, and childbirth significantly more often than for all other problems combined (table 6.5). Fainting, vague symptoms, and culturally defined illnesses without symptoms were never treated by physicians alone. From this we infer that bodily injury from accidents, along with childbirth, tend to be viewed as "natural" occurrences which do not, in themselves, require ceremonial cure. In the population studied, physicians appear to have supplanted herbalists, who formerly treated these kinds of conditions.

In addition to the Navajo ceremonialist, native healers from neighboring tribes are sometimes utilized. The people in our sample lived within easy driving distance of several Hopi villages. The Hopi are thought to be powerful witches who utilize the method of shooting an object into a victim, and Hopi healers are thought to be experts at curing this as well as other forms of witchcraft. Of 35 instances in which non-Western healers were used, five involved the use of Hopi practitioners exclusively. In one case Hopi and Navajo treatments were used conjointly, and in another Hopi treatment was combined with a visit to the hospital. Hopi treatments were what are known as "sucking" cures. They involve, in addition to "seeing" the cause of the illness, the process of "sucking" the intrusive object from the patient's body.

Since the 1960s when this study was conducted, the activities of peyotist and fundamentalist Christian missionaries have increased greatly in the area occupied by the study population. Between 1956 and 1960,

Table 6.5 Use of physicians and native practitioners for self-defined illness among 106 Navajos over a two-year period.

Symptoms and conditions	Number seeking treatment		
	Physician only	Native only	Both
Childbirth and trauma[a]	23	0	7
All others[b]	9	9	19

$X^2 = 19.6$; df = 2; p = .001.

a. Childbirth; prenatal and postnatal complications and examinations; fractures; lacerations; contusions.

b. Problems of the respiratory system including tuberculosis, pneumonia, and upper respiratory infections; muscle and joint pain including arthritis; deafness; crippling, including congenital hip displacement; blindness (cataracts); rashes, sores, abscesses including impetigo; diarrhea; faints; conditions ultimately diagnosed as diabetes, prostate infection, thrombosis, urinary tract infection, measles, and chicken pox; vague complaints and malaise; "lightning contamination" (no symptoms) and nightmares.

no peyote ceremonies were performed for individuals in the population studied. Between 1961 and 1965, although the number of native treatments for the group remained the same, 78 percent were peyote ceremonies. Economic factors and the growing shortage of qualified ceremonialists were the major reasons for this increased reliance on peyote ritual cures (Levy and Kunitz 1974:129). The general point to be made here is that the use of alternative ceremonial treatments varies from community to community and also varies over time within a community.

In a survey of hospital use in two populations conducted in the early 1960s (Levy 1962a), we found that the major variable influencing the frequency of hospital use was distance from the hospital. The closer a population lived to the hospital, the greater was the frequency of use. These findings have been replicated by research conducted in the 1970s (Davis and Kunitz 1978). By 1965, there were no individuals in the populations studied who had never used modern medicine.

SYMPTOMS AND KINDS OF TRADITIONAL CEREMONIALS USED The study of seizure disorders mentioned earlier provides data on the relationship between symptoms and their treatment by different traditional ceremonies (Levy, Neutra, and Parker 1979). Data were gathered from 11 epileptics, 7 of whom had conversion reactions in addition to their epileptic convulsions, and from 9 patients with conversion reactions that looked like seizures. The ceremonies performed for these 20 subjects were documented from the time of onset to the time of the initial interview. (An additional 5 epileptics and 1 "hysteric" had had no ceremonies performed for them, while 3 epileptics and 1 "hysteric" were acculturated and relied only on nontraditional forms of treatment.) The profile of ceremonies obtained was then compared with the ceremonies performed over a five-year period for two groups of Navajos, one rural and the other living near a government settlement. This "control" group of 208 persons of all ages displayed a broad array of typical health problems ranging from upper respiratory tract infections and gastrointestinal problems to gallbladder disease. None of them had had seizures or suffered from any behavioral disorder.

Seizure patients and controls alike utilized ceremonies such as the Shooting Way and the Wind Way, which are thought to be good for a wide variety of symptoms. Both groups used the Evil Way chant with some frequency, a ceremony thought to be good for fainting and anxiety attacks but not for seizures or insanity. More than 90 percent of all ceremonies performed for patients in the control group were in this class of popular ceremony, whereas only 60 percent of all ceremonies performed for the seizure patients were in this category. Both groups used ceremonies like the Night Way and the Plume Way, which are expensive, and the rare

Earth and Beauty Ways. These ceremonies comprised from 5 to 6 percent of the total for both groups. None of these ceremonies is thought to be good for seizures, but they are especially noted for their effectiveness against head ailments, abdominal pains, and joint inflammation and swelling. Both controls and seizure patients used Life Way and Flint Way, which are used for injuries and chronic disorders of all sorts (seizure patients, 4 percent; controls, 2 percent). An important finding was that no ceremonies thought to be good specifically for seizure-like behavior (Coyote Way, Hand Trembling Way, Frenzy Witchcraft Way, Moth Way, Mountain Top Way, and various minor ceremonies like the Twirling Basket ritual) were utilized by the control group whereas 30 percent of all ceremonies performed for the seizure patients were of this type. The differences between the two groups in respect to the use of healing ceremonies were significant and led to the conclusion that symptoms and signs are of some importance in determining the appropriate traditional treatments, at least in the domain investigated.

The chronicity of symptoms also seems to be an important factor in influencing the methods used to treat disease. In the study on seizure disorders, 9 of 11 epileptics with grand mal seizures who had ceremonial treatment ultimately used ceremonies thought to be good especially for generalized seizures. None of the 3 patients with conversion reactions that emulated generalized seizures had these sings performed for them. The difference between the two groups was significant (p = .03 by Fisher's Exact Test). The epileptic patients, regardless of seizure type, received the treatments that were appropriate for their seizures significantly more often than did the hysterical patients (p = .01 by Fisher's Exact Test). We do not think these differences are due to an ability to distinguish accurately between an epileptic seizure and a conversion reaction but to the fact that epileptic seizures persisted for years, whereas the conversion reactions were more transient. Seizure-specific ceremonies were only resorted to after a number of other ceremonies had been tried, even though some epileptics were diagnosed as needing such a ceremony soon after the onset of their seizures. Whether less startling signs and symptoms than those of epilepsy are used to determine treatment with sufficient frequency to offset the tendency to try several treatments (and thus produce statistically significant associations between symptoms and treatments) is not known, and further research must be conducted on this subject.

To date there are insufficient data to determine whether ceremonial cures have either a beneficial or a deleterious effect on any specific diseases. The Navajo predilection for using modern and traditional therapy conjointly indicates that poor utilization of services is less the result of adherence to native beliefs than of difficulties of access to hospitals and poor communication between patients and medical personnel.

Encounters with Mainstream Medical Practitioners

Settings

Earlier in the chapter we described the changing patterns of contact Navajos have had with a variety of institutions of the dominant society, most notably with the health-care system as it has evolved on the reservation. We have shown that the number of outpatient visits is lower for Navajos on the average than for the general United States population. On the other hand, average annual rates of hospitalization and average length of hospital stay are essentially the same for Navajos as for the general United States population, though patterns of discharge diagnoses differ. Navajos have higher rates of hospitalization related to childbearing, accidents, and infectious and parasitic diseases, and lower rates for neoplasms, circulatory disorders, and both gastrointestinal and genitourinary diseases (Davis and Kunitz 1978). We have also shown that distance from the facility is perhaps the single most important variable explaining utilization. We must now ask what the facilities are like at which Navajos receive the bulk of their medical care.

The Indian Health Service (IHS) has divided the reservation into eight service units (or catchment areas), most of which have hospitals located in them and all of which have a variety of field clinics staffed either full time or part time (figure 6.1). Staffing patterns vary and may include paraprofessionals, nurses, or physicians. The same is true in clinics located within hospitals, except for the fact that these all have physicians working in them.

The hospital clinics have many of the same characteristics as those found in urban hospitals serving poor people: they tend to be crowded, waiting times are often prolonged, there is no real appointment system, and there is commonly a language barrier between patient and physician. Such problems persist, despite the efforts of many conscientious health-care workers to change them, because manpower is scarce and the growth of facilities has not kept up with the growth of population. For instance, the physician-population ratio in 1977 was between 1 per 1,316 and 1 per 1,122 on the reservation, compared to 1 per 604 in 1974 in the nation generally.

Similar problems exist on the inpatient services as well. Though several new facilities have been built since the IHS assumed responsibility for care on the reservation in 1955, some of the facilities still in use are old, outmoded, and unsafe (Adkinson and Vienna 1974). In 1973, 25 percent of the beds in one of the hospitals were closed due to lack of personnel, primarily nurses (McKenzie 1974). In 1976 the IHS hospital in Winslow was closed because it was outmoded and unsafe; it is due to be replaced.

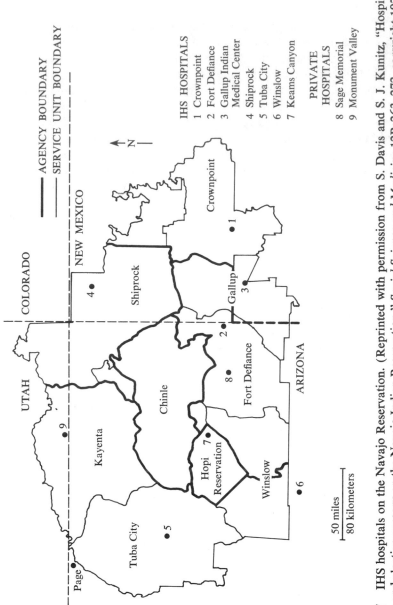

Figure 6.1 IHS hospitals on the Navajo Reservation. (Reprinted with permission from S. Davis and S. J. Kunitz, "Hospital utilization and elective surgery on the Navajo Indian Reservation," *Social Science and Medicine* 12B:263–272, copyright 1978, Pergamon Press, Ltd.)

Finally, with the termination of the doctor draft, the IHS has had difficulty getting physicians to staff many of its facilities. This has been less
of a problem on the Navajo reservation than elsewhere, but even here
it is no longer possible to fill all the available positions. Moreover, the
failure to retain a significant proportion of physicians longer than a year
or two means that painfully learned lessons must constantly be relearned.
Since there are scarcely any Navajo physicians, the IHS will continue to be
dependent on transient non-Indian physicians for years to come. The
solution would appear to be to develop a cadre of highly trained Navajo
medical interpreters and paraprofessional health-care providers, who
could not only give some care themselves but could serve to educate the
new non-Navajo physicians who enter the Service each year. Occasional efforts to accomplish this have occurred from time to time since
at least the 1930s, but without notable or lasting success (see, for example, Adair and Deuschle 1970).

Expectations in the Medical Encounter

The Navajo ceremonialist is an older person who has spent years
learning the rituals in which he specializes. The Navajo diagnostician
relies on magical power to make a rapid diagnosis, rather than on a review
of symptoms. In contrast, modern physicians on the Navajo reservation
are young and question patients carefully to obtain a history and description of their symptoms. As a result, Navajo patients get the impression
that white doctors are inexperienced and do not know what they are
doing. Navajo ceremonialists and diagnosticians build their reputations in
their home communities, whereas the IHS physician is an unknown person who comes from a distant place, spends about two years among the
Navajo, and then leaves before he really comes to understand his patients. Navajos are disappointed in and resentful of this type of doctor-
patient relationship, and many are convinced that white physicians come
to the reservation as a part of their education to practice on Navajo
patients before settling permanently among their own people.

Navajos complain bitterly about the long hours spent getting to a hospital and the hours spent waiting to see a doctor, which are terminated by
only a few minutes of actual contact with the physician (Kane and Kane
1972). Poor interpreting between Navajo and English, rude treatment
from Navajo health personnel, and a tendency for physicians to be conservative in prescribing medications are also major complaints made by
Navajo patients.

Although the language barrier has long been recognized by the IHS,
remarkably little has been done to alleviate the problem. There are no
Navajo personnel specifically trained and employed as medical interpreters. Early efforts to train such personnel (Levy 1964b; Adair and

Deuschle 1970) have not been continued by the IHS. In consequence, simple misunderstandings that could easily be avoided continue to plague the treatment process. One of the major findings of the early training programs was that translating lexical items is less important for good communication than the transmission of concepts. Once the intent of a physician is well understood by an interpreter, the message can be put into Navajo despite the fact that exact lexical correspondences may not exist. The foundation for all such translations of concepts rests on a good knowledge of the similarities and differences between the Navajo and modern medical systems. What physicians may take to be self-evident is most often not well understood by interpreters and is also strange and foreign to patients. A speaking knowledge of English cannot be taken as indicating the knowledge of either the logic of biomedicine or the principles of cause and effect utilized by Navajo health practitioners.

Navajo patients respond positively to attempts to communicate clearly and well. In particular, they appreciate being treated as adults who can make mature decisions when in possession of the pertinent facts.

During the years immediately following World War II, when tuberculosis and infectious diseases generally were prevalent on the reservation, the introduction of antibiotics (notably penicillin and isoniazid) produced dramatic results. The Navajo came to expect liberal prescription of these "wonder" drugs by physicians, which confirmed and perhaps helped to shape their view of the physician as an alleviator of symptoms rather than one who can cure the underlying cause of disease. Presently, many Navajo patients still expect to receive injections for any and all complaints and do not understand the reasons for the current tendency for physicians to be more conservative in their use of these medications. Again, careful explanation is appreciated, and with good interpreting new understanding can be attained.

Interactional Norms

Norms of social interaction among the Navajo include respect for the aged, extreme modesty between the sexes, avoidance of argument, and a quiet demeanor generally. The tendency for whites to talk excessively and to be impatient with periods of silence goes against the grain. Common courtesy is most often sufficient to put a Navajo patient at his ease, and Navajos, recognizing that physicians operate in a different manner, can put up with physical examinations when the reasons for them are well explained and when handling of the body is done gently. The hearty approach achieves less than a quiet manner and a gentle touch.

Acceptance of Medical Diagnosis

We have already discussed Navajo ideas of disease causation. How the physician diagnoses a condition is often of less interest to the patient than how he proposes to treat it, as long as the physician does not suggest that his explanation is superior to that of traditional ceremonialists. Most patients are interested to know how the physician perceives their condition. Acceptance of a diagnosis is not essential for adequate compliance, however.

Adherence to Biomedical Treatment

Studies of Compliance

Very few studies are available on the adherence of Navajos to therapeutic regimens prescribed by medical practitioners. Most of those that have been done relate to the effectiveness of contraceptive use. The work of Slocumb, Kunitz, and Odoroff (1975, 1979) reviews much of this material in detail and provides recent data as well. Though the studies differ in methodology, they generally indicate that Navajos are less effective in their use of family planning than many other populations. Continuing use of intrauterine devices is 40 percent at three years, which is comparable to what has been observed in several other populations both in the United States and elsewhere. However, continuing use of oral contraceptives is 12 percent at three years, which is lower than what has been reported in any other population. The incidence of complications and side effects does not explain the lack of success with oral contraceptives, since the most common reason invoked for discontinuance is "personal." Several factors appear to be important: the general incongruence between the professional culture of the providers of care and the pronatalist beliefs of many Navajos; pressure from family members exerted on a woman not to use contraception; low educational attainment; the difficulty of getting to clinics for the refill of prescriptions; and the lack of outreach workers in family planning programs.

Another study of compliance, which was carried out by the staff of the Cornell–Many Farms project in the late 1950s and early 1960s, involved the use of Frejka aprons for the treatment of children found to have hip abnormalities short of complete dislocation. (Congenitally dislocated hips are a relatively common abnormality among the Navajo and several other American Indian tribes.) It was observed that virtually none of the families used the prescribed aprons for several reasons: first, dislocated hips were not regarded as unusual or necessarily an aesthetic disadvantage; second, dislocated hips did not prevent people from carrying out tasks common in Navajo society; and third, cradle boards were in common use in the Many Farms community at the time, and the apron was not compatible with this means of child care (Barnett and Rabin 1970).

A second study at Many Farms on the compliance with an isoniazid regimen for the treatment of tuberculosis estimated that "approximately 75 percent of the people managed their chemotherapy satisfactorily; an additional 10 percent did so if they were regularly prodded and supervised; and approximately 15 percent of the group, for one reason or another, could not be relied upon to do their part" (McDermott et al. 1960:283).

Several studies have also been carried out involving the use of disulfiram in alcohol treatment programs (Ferguson 1968; Savard 1968; Levy and Kunitz 1974). In general, it appears that clients in these programs do not take their medication in the way prescribed, many stopping treatment almost immediately after discharge from hospital. Nonetheless, follow-up interviews indicate that a high proportion of these patients have either stopped or markedly reduced their alcohol consumption. The explanation advanced is that for many Navajos alcohol use is seen as something foreign to the individual, or rather as behavior that is appropriate at one stage of life but not at another. Admission to the hospital and the taking of the drug provided a focus around which drinking could stop. The effect of the drug was not to condition people to become ill when they thought of using alcohol (the original rationale for its use) but was more like a placebo, the effect of which was perceived to be similar to an antibiotic that eradicated whatever it was that had caused excessive drinking in the first place.

Noncompliance with modern medical regimens should not necessarily be interpreted as rejection of modern medicine by Navajos because of a preference for the traditional system. Levy (1962b) found that failure to follow native medical advice was just as frequent as failure to follow the advice of a physician. However, refusals to comply with native advice reflected the low priority given to the aged and infants when large expenses were required to have the ceremony performed, whereas refusals to comply with modern medical advice reflected Navajos' distrust of surgery and their negative feelings about leaving home for protracted treatment in a tuberculosis sanatorium.

Subcultural and Familial Influences

Freidson has proposed a typology in which the two dimensions are "lay culture" and "lay referral systems" (1970:293). The term "lay culture" refers to the degree to which the laymen in a population have a set of beliefs and knowledge that are similar to or different from those of the professional health-care workers who provide them service. The term "lay referral system" refers to the structure of relationships in which laymen are embedded; such networks of relationships may include friends, kin, or both. Such individuals may be part of a very dense network characterized by intense relationships with a variety of people, or they may be relatively isolated and uninvolved with kin and friends.

Freidson has suggested that when lay and professional cultures are congruent and when lay referral systems are dense and extended, health-care utilization will be high, since the family or friends (or both) act to move the person needing care into the treatment system. On the other hand, when lay referral systems are dense and extended but the lay and professional cultures are not congruent, the family or friends will keep the person out of the professional treatment system. In a study of the use of contraception, for example, it was observed that dependence on kin among the Navajo did seem to be related to the prevalence of contraceptive use: the more dependent on kin the informant was, the less likely she was to be a contraceptive user (Kunitz and Tsianco, in preparation).

In several contexts it has been found that an understanding of Navajo social organization may improve compliance. Most often, physicians deal with patients on an individual basis. However, a patient's decision to comply with medical advice is often reversed after consultation with relatives who were not included in the original conference but whose cooperation is important for the successful completion of the course of treatment.

Despite regional variations found in Navajo patterns of settlement and social organization, the most prominent residence unit after the independent nuclear family is the matrifocal extended family. The married women in this residence group provide the core of the extended family because they are united by ties of blood, while the inmarrying males have no common bonds. As mentioned earlier, kin networks beyond the extended family are comprised of matrilineal kin. Thus, the extended family will live in the neighborhood of the senior woman's sisters and female matrilateral parallel cousins,[1] who are themselves heads of extended families. These matrilineally related women are the core of an enduring decision-making network.

After noting the number of decisions made for others by heads of extended families when treatment required mobilization of considerable resources (Levy 1962b), the Navajo Health Education Project included all adult members of the patients' extended families in educational conferences concerning elective surgery. Such conferences were invariably constructive, and the mutually agreed upon regimen was adhered to. Noting also that the Field Health Program kept "family" folders which included only the nuclear family, Levy contacted the extended families of school children found to have positive skin tests in a tuberculosis screening program conducted in the schools (Levy 1962c, 1963). Because an extended family includes the children of several matrilineally related women married to men with different surnames, children living in the same residence group, who may be exposed to the same disease source, will be listed in separate family folders with no indication that they live together. Not only was this method of contacting whole extended families a more efficient means of discovering tuberculosis contacts, it also elicited cooperation from relatives of the children who were asked to come in voluntarily for x-rays.

As we have already pointed out, modern medicine is viewed by the Navajo as a means to alleviate symptoms rather than to cure the disease itself. Because, in our opinion, this is a major source of incongruence between the lay (Navajo) and professional (Anglo) health cultures, many if not most of the problems of compliance can be derived from this attitude. The Navajo way of saying "doctor" is "bearer of medicines"; this approximates the expression for the traditional herbalist and does not imply the status given to the Navajo ceremonialist. Hospital is expressed as "where medicine is made," and the outpatient clinic is "where medicine is applied." It is significant, we believe, that the process of removing or protecting against illness is not referred to. In accordance with this observation, we find Navajos eagerly accepting all treatments in Anglo settings that involve rapid alleviation of symptoms, the repair of lacerations and broken bones, and procedures that make childbirth more comfortable. However, diagnostic procedures are usually not well understood, and surgery is frequently resisted (Mico 1962).

It is important to stress that this perception of modern medicine is not immutable, dictated by unchanging cultural definitions; it has a history grounded in real experience. Prior to the second World War, the hospital was known as the "house of death," and Navajos saw little that was good in modern medical practice. The postwar years saw the introduction of antibiotics. The tangible benefits of drug therapy were accepted, and Navajo perceptions adjusted to the new reality. Currently, the lay culture is undergoing considerable change. Not only is the general level of education rising rapidly, but the lay referral system includes an ever-growing number of persons who have benefited from and have positive attitudes toward surgery and long-term therapies of various sorts. The physician practicing on the reservation today should be less concerned about combating specific beliefs or "superstitions," and should instead devote his energies to creating a good doctor-patient relationship based on mutual respect and the kind of communication that permits the development of a more congruent lay referral system.

Dietary Patterns

There is some evidence that the nutritional status of the Navajo has improved over the past generation. Frank cases of marasmus and kwashiorkor, which were occasionally seen on the western end of the reservation as recently as the 1960s (Wolf 1961; Van Duzen et al. 1969), are no longer present. And in a study of a Navajo community carried out in 1968–1969 (Reisinger, Rogers, and Johnson 1972), it was noted that some measures of nutritional status had improved since a similar study conducted 15 years previously. Clinically observable forms of malnutrition were rare in both studies, but subclinical and borderline cases still were found to exist. According to Reisinger, Rogers, and Johnson, "Frank, specific malnutritional states were not often found in the younger portion of the population by clinical or laboratory examination. However, low serum levels of specific nutrients were observed in portions of the adult population, though clinical signs of specific nutritional deficiencies were not found. Marginal iron deficiency was demonstrated in all age groups by the high prevalence of low serum iron and low transferrin saturation values. Several older adults also showed low levels of Vitamin C and total protein" (1972:88). It was concluded that "all age groups might benefit from increased dietary iron; children and old persons from increased total calories; and adults from increased protein and ascorbic acid" (1972:89). Subsequently, Slocumb and Kunitz (1977) noted that the higher than expected rate of postpartum hemorrhage observed among Navajo women might be due in part to their high prevalence of iron deficiency anemia.

Factors that inhibit adequate dietary intake among the Navajo are economic, physiological, and cultural in nature. Extreme poverty, distance from food stores, lack of electricity, and the decline of the livestock industry combine to make it difficult for Navajos in most parts of the reservation to obtain a wide variety of foods, though surplus commodities provided by the Department of Agriculture have ameliorated this situation to some extent. There are some complications, however. Research among other Indian groups (Nelson 1969; McCracken 1971; Harrison 1975) indicates that it is most likely that a high proportion of Navajos have a lactase deficiency. This makes it difficult to get school-age children to consume dairy products, even when powdered milk is made available to compensate for the lack of refrigeration. In addition, Navajos, in common with most peoples, have some pronounced food preferences. Many Navajos feel that hospital meals are tasteless, for example. Mutton, which is the only meat eaten with relish, is rarely obtainable in the hospital or from food stores. Several items provided by the surplus commodities program are discarded by many Navajos, including powdered milk, pinto beans, farina, canned butter, noodles, and peanut butter. Exactly why a taste for these foods has not developed is not known.

Navajos divide food into two categories: "strong" and "weak." "Strong" foods promote health and are the traditional foods of the nineteenth century reservation: mutton, game animals, and perhaps Indian corn, fried bread, and potatoes. These tastes are changing, however, since fewer and fewer families have access to mutton and Indian corn on a daily basis. The most frequently mentioned "weak" food is milk. The aged may drink goats' milk and infants drink mothers' milk, but these are not considered fit foods for adults. Families who raise and butcher their own livestock, whether sheep or cattle, eat virtually all parts of the animal and have a rich source of nutrients, whereas those who must buy their meat in stores do not get organ meat or bone marrow. The decline of the livestock industry has created problems for which adequate solutions have not yet been found.

Recovery, Rehabilitation, and Death

Coping with Chronic Illness, Terminal Illness, and Death

Navajos believe that the spirits of the dead are dangerous and cause illness when the living come into contact with them. Thus, the dead are buried hurriedly, at some distance from human habitation and with no ceremony. Those who handle the corpse must have a ritual of purification performed before they can resume normal activities. If death should occur in the home, traditional Navajos will abandon the dwelling and move to a new location. In the past, the terminally ill were frequently kept in shelters constructed at some distance from the home to minimize the risk of such contamination. Today, most Navajos are willing to have the terminally ill spend their last days in hospital and for the Indian Health Service to handle all burial arrangements. Missionaries have also been allowed to conduct burial services so that the family could avoid contact with the corpse.

The problem of coping with chronic illness is a relatively new one for the Navajo. Increasingly, as medical care improves, older people are surviving with chronic disabilities, which puts considerable economic strain on most families. Before the advent of modern medical programs few Navajos survived to old age, and those who did were relatively healthy and able to perform some domestic functions, especially caring for young children. As a result, old people were not a serious economic burden and were respected and valued. Today these values are difficult to live up to, and new ways of caring for the aged and chronically ill are emerging. The tribe has considered establishing nursing homes on the reservation, for example (Levy 1967).

Chronic disabilities in general are coped with by each family as best they can. When ceremonials are found to be ineffective, the case is often given up as hopeless. Some families are able to keep someone at home to help the long-term patient feed himself and be comfortable; other families frequently must leave patients unattended for varying periods of time. Children are often observed helping the blind and the crippled get around.

We have already discussed the fact that long-term treatment under a physician's care often places economic burdens on the family that cannot be sustained for long periods of time. Poor compliance is most often the final outcome. Many conditions such as congenital hip displacement, crippling in general, deafness, blindness, and the like may simply be ignored. Routine care for the chronically ill, which might easily be managed in a home with running water, electricity, and telephone service, is all too often a difficult task for Navajo families. It is remarkably difficult to maintain minimal sanitary conditions in most Navajo homes. Because of these conditions, it is often wise to have the home evaluated by paramedical personnel to determine whether care can be adequately provided. Moreover, it is imperative that the adults in the extended family understand what will be required of them to achieve successful maintenance. Considering the difficulties involved in getting to the hospital on short notice, these relatives should have a thorough understanding of the signs and symptoms that indicate the need for a return visit to the hospital.

A pervasive problem related to the care of the chronically ill is that of taking medications properly. Diabetics are frequently not well cared for at home, for example. The reasons for this problem are complex and not well understood in specific cases, however, and we have no easy solutions to offer.

Concluding Remarks

In the opening section of this chapter we pointed out that the peripheral position of the Navajo in the national economy has had several important consequences for both their health and their medical practices. One was the continuing adaptive significance of the extended kin network for the redistribution of income when its sources are multiple and fluctuating; we have seen that this situation has some impact on the way health services are used. A second consequence is that the economic situation of the Navajo has had a major impact on the epidemiological and demographic patterns that we have described. A third consequence, to which we alluded briefly, was the impact on employment opportunities that such an economy creates. It is to this third issue that we will address ourselves in this section.

Unemployment rates on the Navajo Reservation are estimated to be between 50 and 60 percent. Of the people who are employed in the wage economy, between 65 and 70 percent work in the service sector as employees of either the federal, state, local, or tribal government (Kunitz 1977a). This situation is clearly a result of the lack of employment opportunities in other economic sectors as well as treaty obligations which mandate that the government provide health and educational services to Indians. Several important consequences flow from this situation.

First, Indian young people are often exhorted to get an education so they may come back to the reservation to serve their people. Since most job opportunities on the reservation are in the service sector, most Indian college graduates have majored in one of the service oriented fields such as education, social work, nursing, or—increasingly—premedical subjects. Furthermore, most of the Indian professionals to whom they are exposed work in service occupations. Thus, the available role models and the educational system itself conspire to channel young people into these fields.

Second, as a result of the War on Poverty, many "new careers in human services" were created as a means of both providing employment in poor communities and bringing about community organization. This was no less true on Indian reservations than it was in urban ghettos. Because service fields are labor-intensive and because there are real and pressing conditions that need to be dealt with, there is always room for more service workers. Moreover, from the perspective of the larger society it is appropriate to have indigenous workers dealing with social problems on a case-by-case basis rather than dealing with the larger institutional problems that may be the root causes of the problems faced by Indian communities. Whether it is good, in the long run, for Indians to see alcohol use, for instance, as a personal disease problem rather than a phenomenon with larger causes is of course another matter.

Though it is reasonable to maintain that many services are necessary because of the real needs and problems of the population, the converse is also true. Thus, not only may services arise in response to problems, but phenomena may be defined as particular kinds of problems as a result of the development and institutionalization of particular human and social services (Kitsuse and Cicourel 1963). For example, the prevalence, significance, and causes of such phenomena as drinking, suicide, homicide, and accidents may differ from one tribe to another in consistent ways depending on ecological adaptation, social organization, and personality structure (Levy and Kunitz 1974; Kunitz 1976b). Service workers, however, tend to impose on patients, clients, and communities their own interpretations of these behaviors, interpretations that may or may not be adequate explanations of what is occurring. Indeed, Navajo health workers have been shown to view problems from a perspective closer to that of the non-Indian professionals with whom they work than to that of the community they are said to represent (Kane and McConatha 1975).

The fact that Navajos have been disproportionately employed in the service area rather than other sectors of the local economy does not mean that they have had the most prestigious positions or that they have saturated the available jobs. As a result of both poor educational opportunities in the past and resistance from non-Indian professionals, their positions have generally been in the lower levels of the bureaucracy (see May 1977, for example, on the Indian Health Service). Adair and Deuschle (1970) have described the resistance of public health nurses to the full use of Navajo health visitors because of the perceived threat to their own positions.

Recent legislation has led to preferential hiring of Indians by federal agencies dealing with Indians, in particular the Bureau of Indian Affairs and the Indian Health Service of the U.S. Public Health Service. This means that, especially as educational attainments increase, a higher proportion of jobs at higher levels will be occupied by Indians. In many respects this is clearly desirable. On the other hand, as we have shown elsewhere (Kunitz 1977a), even if all wage and salaried positions on the reservation in 1974 (totaling 20,140) had been occupied by Navajos, 62.6 percent of the employed would still have been in human and social services; that is, the economy would still have been structured as it is at present.

Assuming that employment opportunities do not grow significantly in other sectors of the reservation economy, what are the implications of the continued dependence on the service sector, particularly as job opportunities for Indians continue to expand as a result of the legislation mentioned above?

First, non-Indian professionals are likely to find increasingly that they must deal with Navajos as equals and often as superiors. For many this may be a difficult adjustment, particularly if they believe that their Navajo co-workers are not adequately trained but have been promoted for political reasons. There seems to be some feeling that this situation is indeed developing, and it appears that a few non-Indian health professionals are already seeking transfers from the reservation for this reason. If this does turn out to be the case, it may be just as well for the Navajo. However, until sufficient trained Navajo manpower is available, there is the possibility that some disruption in services might occur. The problem may be exacerbated if (as in many former colonies) jobs are filled on the basis of characteristics other than professional qualifications—something that is especially likely to happen in a kin-based society.

Second, with sources of employment concentrated in the health, education, and welfare bureaucracies, future Navajo executives of these agencies will wield considerable influence over aspects of life that are not necessarily within their realms of expertise—a situation in which non-Navajos now find themselves. Unlike the present incumbents of these jobs, however, who have no personal stake in reservation political and economic life, Navajos in these positions may well find themselves intimately involved in tribal politics, for better or worse. Indeed, this has begun to happen already. The present tribal chairman first came to public attention as the director of the Office of Navajo Economic Opportunity, and one of his major challengers in the 1978 Primary was a prominent Navajo physician holding a high-ranking position in the Indian Health Service. It may happen, therefore, that the service bureaucracies will become even more politicized than they are at present, with consequences that we are unable and unwilling to predict.

Finally, as we have noted throughout, the reservation does not exist in a political or economic vacuum. The service sector, supported by federal dollars, is the single most important source of earned and unearned income. During the 1960s there was a sense of optimism about the possibilities of substantial economic improvement on the reservation. Since the late 1960s (with administrations in Washington whose watchword, especially in the health field, has been cost containment), the earlier feeling of optimism has dissipated. Indeed, in an economy whose very base is federal support of human and social service bureaucracies, the concern with controlling the costs of health care may be felt particularly intensely. A major source of cash in the local economy may gradually provide less money than in the past, and jobs in service agencies may become even harder to obtain and more valuable than they were in the past (though this situation may be mitigated for a time by Indian preference in hiring). Furthermore, innovations in the delivery of services may become less and less likely, as bureaucrats strive to maintain what they have. With a continuing increase in population occurring at the same time as health services remain constant, the providers of care will be under increasing pressure to handle problems hurriedly. Job dissatisfaction may increase, hastening the turnover among highly trained, non-Navajo personnel and adding to the problems of giving adequate care. Finally, it is not inconceivable that the government will begin to reassess the degree of its commitment to provide health care by reexamining the original treaties made at the start of the reservation period. The picture for Navajo health care, at least in the near future, is not a happy one.

Note

1. Matrilateral parallel cousins are the offspring of one's mother's sisters.

References

ABERLE, D. F.   1966.   *The Peyote Religion Among the Navaho.* Chicago: Aldine.

————, 1969.   A Plan for Navajo Economic Development. In *Toward Economic Development for Native American Communities,* a compendium of papers submitted to the Subcommittee on Economy in Government of the Joint Economic Committee of the U.S. Congress. Washington, D.C.: U.S. Government Printing Office.

ABRAHAM, S., and D. C. MILLER.   1959.   Serum Cholesterol Levels in American Indians. *Public Health Reports* 74:392–389.

ADAIR, J., and K. W. DEUSCHLE.   1970.   *The People's Health: Medicine and*

Anthropology in a Navajo Community. New York: Appleton-Century-Crofts.

ADKINSON, F. K., and D. VIENNA. 1974. Testimony on Indian Health Care before the Permanent Subcommittee on Investigations of the Committee on Government Operations, U.S. Senate, 93rd Congress. Washington, D.C.: U.S. Government Printing Office.

ALFRED, B. 1970. Blood Pressure Changes among Male Navaho Migrants to an Urban Environment. *Canadian Review of Sociology and Anthropology* 7:189–200.

BARNETT, C., and D. RABIN. 1970. Collaborative Study by Physicians and Anthropologists: Congenital Hip Disease. In *The People's Health,* ed. J. Adair and K. W. Deuschle. New York: Appleton-Century-Crofts.

BIVENS, M. D., and H. O. FLEETWOOD. 1968. A 10-Year Survey of Cervical Carcinoma in Indians of the Southwest. *Obstetrics and Gynecology* 32:11–16.

BRENNER, C., K. S. REISINGER, and K. D. ROGERS. 1974. Navajo Infant Mortality, 1970. *Public Health Reports* 89:353–359.

BRODY, J. A. 1964. Notes on the Epidemiology of Draining Ears and Hearing Loss in Alaska with Comments on Future Studies and Control Measures. *Alaska Medicine* 6:1–4.

BRODY, J. A., T. OVERFIELD, and R. McALISTER. 1965. Draining Ears and Deafness among Alaskan Eskimos. *Archives of Otolaryngology* 81:29–33.

BROWN, R. C., B. S. GURUNANJAPPA, R. J. HAWK, and D. BITSUIE. 1970. The Epidemiology of Accidents among the Navajo Indians. *Public Health Reports* 85:881–888.

CALLAWAY, D. G., J. E. LEVY, and E. B. HENDERSON. 1976. The Effects of Power Production and Strip Mining on Local Navajo Populations. Bulletin no. 22 of the Lake Powell Research Project. Los Angeles: Institute of Geophysics, University of California.

CLIFFORD, N. J., J. J. KELLY, T. F. LEO, and H. R. EDER. 1963. Coronary Heart Disease and Hypertension in the White Mountain Apache Tribe. *Circulation* 28:926–931.

COHEN, B. M. 1953. Arterial Hypertension among Indians of the Southwestern United States. *American Journal of Medical Sciences* 225:505–513.

COMESS, L. J., P. H. BENNETT, and T. A. BURCH. 1967. Clinical Gallbladder Disease in Pima Indians. *New England Journal of Medicine* 277:894–898.

CREAGAN, E. T., and J. F. FRAUMENI. 1972. Cancer Mortality among American Indians, 1950–1967. *Journal of the National Cancer Institute* 49.959–967.

DARBY, W. J., C. G. SALSBURY, W. J. McGANITY, H. F. JOHNSON, E. B. BRIDGE-FORTH, and H. R. SANDSTEAD. 1956. A Study of the Dietary Background and Nutrition of the Navajo Indian. *Journal of Nutrition* 60 (suppl.):3–85.

DAVIS, S. 1977. Hospitalization and Elective Surgery on the Navajo Indian Reservation. M. S. thesis, Department of Preventive Medicine and Community Health, University of Rochester, Rochester, N.Y.

DAVIS, S., and S. J. KUNITZ. 1978. Hospital Utilization and Elective Surgery on the Navajo Indian Reservation. *Social Science and Medicine* 12B:263–272.

DESTAFANO, F., J. L. COULEHAN, and M. K. WIANT. 1979. Blood Pressure Survey on the Navajo Indian Reservation. *American Journal of Epidemiology* 109:335–345.

DUBOIS, J. 1978. Navajos Are Coming to Jesus. *Navajo Times,* July 27, B 8–9.

DUNHAM, L. J., J. C. BAILAR, III, and G. L. LAQUER. 1973. Histologically Diagnosed Cancers in 693 Indians of the United States, 1950–1965. *Journal of the National Cancer Institute* 50:1119–1127.

ELMORE, H. 1944. *Ethnobotany of the Navajo.* Albuquerque: University of New Mexico Press.

FAICH, R. G. 1977. A Reapportionment Plan for the Navajo Tribal Council. Window Rock, Arizona: Research and Statistics Division, Office of Program Development, The Navajo Tribe.

FERGUSON, F. N. 1968. Navaho Drinking: Some Tentative Hypotheses. *Human Organization* 27:159–167.

FREIDSON, E. 1970. *Profession of Medicine.* New York: Dodd, Mead.

FRENCH, J. G. 1967. Relationship of Morbidity to the Feeding Patterns of Navajo Children from Birth through Twenty-four Months. *American Journal of Clinical Nutrition* 20:375–385.

FULMER, H. S., and R. W. ROBERTS. 1963. Coronary Heart Disease among the Navajo Indians. *Annals of Internal Medicine* 59:740–764.

GREGG, J. B., J. P. STEEL, S. CLIFFORD, and H. E. WERTHMAN. 1970. A Multidisciplinary Study of Ear Disease in South Dakota Indian Children. *South Dakota Journal of Medicine* 23:11–20.

HADLEY, J. N. 1955. Health Conditions among Navajo Indians. *Public Health Reports* 70:831–836.

HAILE, B. 1950. *Legend of the Ghostway Ritual in the Male Branch of Shootingway and Sucking Way in Its Legend and Practice.* St. Michaels, Ariz.: St. Michaels Press.

HARRISON, G. G. 1975. Primary Adult Lactase Deficiency: A Problem in Anthropological Genetics. *American Anthropologist* 77:812–835.

HENDERSON, E. B., and J. E. LEVY. 1975. Survey of Navajo Community Studies. Lake Powell Research Project Bulletin no. 6. Los Angeles: Institute of Geophysics, University of California.

HESSE, F. G. 1964. Incidence of Disease in the Navajo Indian. *Archives of Pathology* 77:553–557.

HESTER, J. J. 1962. *Early Navajo Migrations and Acculturation in the Southwest.* Papers in Anthropology, no. 6. Santa Fe, N. Mex.: Museum of New Mexico Press.

HILL, W. W. 1935. The Status of the Hermaphrodite and Transvestite in Navaho Culture. *American Anthropologist* 37:273–279.

IBA, B. Y., J. D. NISWANDER, and L. WOODVILLE. 1973. Relation of Prenatal Care to Birth Weights, Major Malfunctions, and Newborn Deaths of American Indians. *Health Services Reports* 88:697–701.

INSTITUTE for GOVERNMENT RESEARCH. 1928. *The Problem of Indian*

Administration, technical director L. Meriam. Baltimore: Johns Hopkins Press.

JAFFE, B. F. 1969. The Incidence of Ear Diseases in the Navajo Indians. *Laryngoscope* 79:2126–2134.

JOHNSON, R. L. 1967. Chronic Otitis Media in School Age Navajo Indians. *Laryngoscope* 77:1990–1995.

JOHNSTON, D. F. 1966. *An Analysis of Sources of Information on the Population of the Navaho.* Bureau of American Ethnology, Bulletin no. 197. Washington, D.C.: U.S. Government Printing Office.

JORDAN, S. W., R. L. SOPHER, C. R. KEY, D. BRYLINSKI, and J. HUANG. 1972. Carcinoma of the Cervix in Southwestern American Indian Women. *Cancer* 29:1235–1241.

JORGENSEN, J. G. 1971. Indians and the Metropolis. In *The American Indian in Urban Society,* ed. J. O. Waddell and O. M. Watson. Boston: Little, Brown.

KALTENBACH, C. 1976. Health Problems of the Navajo Area and Suggested Interventions. Window Rock, Ariz.: Navajo Health Authority.

KANE, R., and R. KANE. 1972. Determination of Health Care Expectations among Navajo Consumers: Consumers in a Federal Care System. *Medical Care* 10:421–429.

KANE, R. L., and P. D. McCONATHA. 1975. The Men in the Middle: A Dilemma of Minority Health Workers. *Medical Care* 13:736–743.

KAPLAN, B., and D. JOHNSON. 1964. The Social Meaning of Navajo Psychopathology. In *Magic, Faith and Healing,* ed. A. Kiev. New York: Free Press of Glencoe.

KATZ, P. S., and P. A. MAY. 1979. Motor Vehicle Accidents on the Navajo Reservation, 1973–1975. Window Rock, Ariz.: Navajo Health Authority.

KELLY, L. C. 1968. *The Navajo Indians and Federal Indian Policy.* Tucson: University of Arizona Press.

KEMRER, M. F. 1974. The Dynamics of Western Navajo Settlement, A.D. 1750–1900: An Archaeological and Dendrochronological Analysis. Ph. D. dissertation, Department of Anthropology, University of Arizona, Tucson.

KITSUSE, J., and A. CICOUREL. 1963. A Note on the Use of Official Statistics. *Social Problems* 11:131–139.

KLUCKHOHN, C. 1944. *Navajo Witchcraft.* Papers of the Peabody Museum of American Archeology and Ethnology, vol. 22, no. 2. Cambridge, Mass.: Harvard University.

KUNITZ, S. J. 1974a. Factors Influencing Recent Navajo and Hopi Population Change. *Human Organization* 33:7–16.

———. 1974b. Navajo and Hopi Fertility, 1971–1972. *Human Biology* 46:435–451.

———. 1976a. The Relationship of Economic Variations to Mortality and Fertility Patterns on the Navajo Reservation. Lake Powell Research Project Bulletin no. 20. Los Angeles: Institute of Geophysics, University of California.

———. 1976b. Fertility, Mortality, and Social Organization. *Human Biology* 48:361–377.

————. 1976c. A Survey of Fertility Histories and Contraceptive Use among a Group of Navajo Women. Lake Powell Research Project Bulletin no. 21. Los Angeles: Institute of Geophysics, University of California.

————. 1977a. Underdevelopment and Social Services on the Navajo Reservation. *Human Organization* 36:398–404.

————. 1977b. Economic Variation on the Navajo Reservation. *Human Organization* 36:186–193.

————. (in preparation). A Multivariate Analysis of Navajo Hospital Utilization.

KUNITZ, S. J., and J. E. LEVY. 1974. Changing Ideas of Alcohol Use among Navaho Indians. *Quarterly Journal of Studies on Alcohol* 35:243–259.

KUNITZ, S. J., and H. TEMKIN-GREENER. 1980. Changing Patterns of Mortality and Hospitalized Morbidity on the Navajo Indian Reservation. Working paper, Department of Preventive, Family, and Rehabilitation Medicine, University of Rochester School of Medicine, Rochester, N.Y.

KUNITZ, S. J., and M. TSIANCO. (in preparation). Kinship Dependence and Contraceptive Use in a Sample of Navajo Women.

LANDAR, H. 1967. The Language of Pain in Navajo Culture. In *Studies in Southwestern Linguistics: Meaning and History in the Languages of the American Southwest,* ed. D. Hymes and W. E. Bittle. The Hague: Mouton.

LEIGHTON, A. H., and D. A. KENNEDY. 1957. Pilot Study of Cultural Items in Medical Diagnosis: A Field Report (mimeographed).

LEIGHTON, A. H., and D. C. LEIGHTON. 1944. *The Navaho Door: An Introduction to Navaho Life.* Cambridge, Mass.: Harvard University Press.

LEIGHTON, D. C., and C. KLUCKHOHN. 1948. *Children of the People.* Cambridge, Mass.: Harvard University Press.

LEVY, J. E. 1962a. Some Trends in Navajo Health Behavior. Window Rock, Ariz.: USPHS, Division of Indian Health (mimeographed).

————. 1962b. Medical Decision Making in a Navaho Outfit: Preliminary Report. Ethnologist's report, Tuba City, Arizona, USPHS Indian Hospital (mimeographed).

————. 1962c. The Influence of Social Organization on Behavioral Response to a Health Activity. Ethnologist's report, USPHS, Division of Indian Health, Window Rock, Arizona (mimeographed).

————. 1963. Tuba City Case Finding Program, July, 1962. Ethnologist's report, attachment 1:2, Tuba City, Arizona, USPHS Indian Hospital (mimeographed).

————. 1964a. The Fate of Navajo Twins. *American Anthropologist* 66:883–887.

————. 1964b. Interpreter Training Program. Window Rock, Ariz.: USPHS Division of Indian Health (mimeographed).

————. 1967. The Older American Indian. In *Older Rural Americans,* ed. E. G. Youmans. Lexington: University of Kentucky Press.

LEVY, J. E., and S. J. KUNITZ. 1974. *Indian Drinking: Navajo Practices and Anglo-American Theories.* New York: Wiley-Interscience.

LEVY, J. E., R. NEUTRA, and D. PARKER. 1979. Life Careers of Navajo Epileptics and Convulsive Hysterics. *Social Science and Medicine* 13B:53–66.

———. (in press). Hand Trembling, Frenzy Witchcraft and Moth Madness: A Study of Navajo Seizure Disorders. Tucson: University of Arizona Press.

LING, D., R. H. McCOY, and E. D. LEVINSON. 1969. The Incidence of Middle Ear Disease and Its Educational Implications among Baffin Island Eskimo Children. *Canadian Journal of Public Health* 60:385–390.

MAY, P. A. 1977. Health Manpower Survey. Window Rock, Ariz.: Navajo Health Authority (mimeographed).

MAY, P. A., D. W. BROUDY, M. YELLOWHAIR, K. BATTESE, and M. HUDSON. 1977. Final Report: Comparative Health Services Evaluation Project. Window Rock, Ariz.: Navajo Health Authority (mimeographed).

MAYNARD, J. 1969. Otitis Media in Alaskan Eskimo Children: An Epidemiologic Review with Observations on Control. *Alaska Medicine* 10:93–97.

MAYNARD, J., J. K. FLESHMAN, and C. F. TSCHOPP. 1972. Otitis Media in Alaskan Eskimo Children. *Journal of the American Medical Association* 219:597–599.

MAYNARD, J. E., L. M. HAMMES, and F. E. KESTER. 1967. Mortality Due to Heart Disease among Alaskan Natives, 1955–1965. *Public Health Reports* 82:714–720.

McCRACKEN, R. D. 1971. Lactase Deficiency: An Example of Dictary Evolution. *Current Anthropology* 12:479–517.

McDERMOTT, W., K. DEUSCHLE, J. ADAIR, H. FULMER, and B. LOUGHLIN. 1960. Introducing Modern Medicine in a Navajo Community. *Science* 131:197–205, 280–287.

McDERMOTT, W., K. W. DEUSCHLE, and C. R. BARNETT. 1972. Health Care Experiment at Many Farms. *Science* 175:23–31.

McKENZIE, T. 1974. Testimony on Indian Health Care before the Permanent Subcommittee on Investigations of the Committee on Government Operations, U.S. Senate, 93rd Congress. Washington, D.C.: U.S. Government Printing Office.

McKINLAY, J. B. 1975. The Help Seeking Behavior of the Poor. In *Poverty and Health: A Sociological Analysis* (revised ed.), ed. J. Kosa and I. K. Zola. Cambridge, Mass.: Harvard University Press.

MICO, P. 1962. Navajo Perception of Anglo Medicine. Berkeley, Calif.: University of California; Educational Resources Information Center, Arlington, Virginia, ED036383.

MOORE, W. M., M. M. SILVERBERG, and M. S. READ, eds. 1972. *Nutrition, Growth and Development of North American Indian Children.* DHEW Publication no. (NIH) 72–26. Washington, D.C.: U.S. Government Printing Office.

MORGAN, K. 1973. Historical Demography of a Navajo Community. In *Methods and Theories of Anthropological Genetics,* ed. M. H. Crawford and P. L. Workman. Albuquerque: University of New Mexico Press.

NAVAJO MEDICAL NEWS. 1940. Report of Navajo Medical Service, September 28, p. 1. Window Rock, Ariz.: Bureau of Indian Affairs.

NELSON, H. 1969. Navajos, Milk: What Causes Them To Be Incompatible. *Los Angeles Times,* January 13, p. 2.

NEUTRA, R., J. E. LEVY, and D. PARKER. 1977. Cultural Expectations Versus Reality in Navajo Seizure Patterns and Sick Roles. *Culture, Medicine, and Psychiatry* 1:255–275.

OAKLAND, L., and R. L. KANE. 1973. The Working Mother and Child Neglect on the Navajo Reservation. *Pediatrics* 51:849–853.

OMRAN, A. R. 1971. The Epidemiologic Transition: A Theory of the Epidemiology of Population Change. *Milbank Memorial Fund Quarterly* 49:509–538.

OMRAN, A. R., and B. LOUGHLIN. 1972. An Epidemiologic Study of Accidents among the Navajo Indians. *Journal of the Egyptian Medical Association* 55:1–22.

PAGE, I. H., L. A. LEWIS, and J. GILBERT. 1956. Plasma Lipids and Proteins and Their Relationship to Coronary Disease among Navajo Indians. *Circulation* 13:675–679.

PARMAN, D. L. 1976. *The Navajos and the New Deal.* New Haven: Yale University Press.

PIJOAN, M., and C. S. McCAMMON. 1949. The Problem of Medical Care for Navajo Indians. *Journal of the American Medical Association* 140: 1013–1015.

REED, D., and W. DUNN. 1970. Epidemiologic Studies of Otitis Media among Eskimo Children. *Public Health Reports* 85:699–706.

REED, D., S. STRUVE, and J. MAYNARD. 1967. Otitis Media and Hearing Deficiency among Eskimo Children: A Cohort Study. *American Journal of Public Health* 57:1657–1663.

REISINGER, K., K. D. ROGERS, and O. JOHNSON. 1972. Nutritional Survey of Lower Greasewood, Arizona Navajos. In *Nutrition, Growth and Development of North American Indian Children,* ed. W. M. Moore, M. M. Silverberg, and M. S. Read. DHEW Publication no. (NIH) 72–26. Washington, D.C.: U.S. Government Printing Office.

ROBBINS, L. 1975. The Impact of Industrial Developments on the Navajo Nation. Lake Powell Research Project, Bulletin no. 7. Los Angeles: Institute of Geophysics and Planetary Physics, University of California at Los Angeles.

ROSA, F., and L. RESNICK. 1965. Birth Weight and Perinatal Mortality in the American Indian. *American Journal of Obstetrics and Gynecology* 91:972–976.

ROSSI, D. F. 1972. Hearing Deficiency in Pueblo Indian Children. *Rocky Mountain Medical Journal* 69:65–69.

SAVARD, R. J. 1968. Effects of Disulfiram Therapy on Relationships within the Navajo Drinking Group. *Quarterly Journal of Studies on Alcohol* 29:909–916.

SIEVERS, M. L. 1967. Myocardial Infarction among Southwestern American Indians. *Annals of Internal Medicine* 67:800–807.

————. 1968. Cigarette and Alcohol Usage by Southwestern American Indians. *American Journal of Public Health* 58:71–82.

SIEVERS, M. L., and S. L. COHEN. 1961. Lung Cancer among Indians of the Southwestern United States. *Annals of Internal Medicine* 54:912–915.

SLOCUMB, J. C., and S. J. KUNITZ. 1977. Factors Affecting Maternal Mortality and Morbidity among American Indians. *Public Health Reports* 92:349–356.

SLOCUMB, J. C., S. J. KUNITZ, and C. L. ODOROFF. 1979. Complications of IUD and Oral Contraceptives among Navajo Indians: Implications for the Provision of Services. *Public Health Reports* 94:243–247.

SLOCUMB, J. C., C. L. ODOROFF, and S. J. KUNITZ. 1975. The Use-Effectiveness of Two Contraceptive Methods in a Navajo Population: The Problem of Program Dropouts. *American Journal of Obstetrics and Gynecology* 122:717–726.

SMALL, D. M., and S. RAPO. 1970. Source of Abnormal Bile in Patients with Cholesterol Gallstones. *New England Journal of Medicine* 283:53–57.

SMITH, R. L. 1957. Recorded and Expected Mortality among the Indians of the United States with Special Reference to Cancer. *Journal of the National Cancer Institute* 18:385–396.

SMITH, R. L., C. G. SALSBURY, and A. G. GILLIAM. 1956. Recorded and Expected Mortality among the Navajo, with Special Reference to Cancer. *Journal of the National Cancer Institute* 17:77–89.

STEWART, T. J., and A. MUNETA. 1976. Final Report: Comparative Health Services Evaluation Project. Window Rock, Ariz.: Navajo Health Authority (mimeographed).

STREEPER, R. B., R. U. MASSEY, G. LIU, C. H. DILLINGHAM, and A. CUSHING. 1960. An Electrocardiographic and Autopsy Study of Coronary Heart Disease in the Navajo. *Diseases of the Chest* 38:305–312.

STROTZ, C. R., and G. I. SHORR. 1973. Hypertension in the Papago Indians. *Circulation* 48:1299–1303.

T.N.Y. 1961. The Navajo Yearbook, vol. 8. Window Rock, Ariz.: The Navajo Agency, Bureau of Indian Affairs.

UNDERHILL, R. M. 1963. *The Navajos*. Norman, Oklahoma: University of Oklahoma Press.

U.S. BUREAU OF THE CENSUS. 1973. Census of Population: 1970. Subject Reports, Final Report PC (2)–1F, American Indians. Washington, D.C.: U.S. Government Printing Office.

————. 1977. Report on the findings of special enumeration population register match for three chapters of Navajo Reservation. Washington, D.C.: U.S. Department of Commerce (mimeographed).

U.S. PUBLIC HEALTH SERVICE. 1971. Indian Health Trends and Services, 1970 edition. PHS Publication no. 2092. Washington, D.C.: Indian Health Service, Office of Program Planning and Evaluation, Program Analysis and Statistics Branch.

————. 1973. Ambulatory Patient Care Services: Injuries, Navajo Area. Window Rock, Ariz.: Navajo Area Indian Health Service (mimeographed).

VAN DUZEN, J., J. P. CARTER, J. SECONDI, and C. FEDERSPIEL. 1969. Protein and Calorie Malnutrition among Pre-School Navajo Indian Children. *The American Journal of Clinical Nutrition* 22:1362–1370.

WERNER, O.   1963.   Navajo Medical Vocabulary (manuscript).

————.   1965.   Semantics of Navaho Medical Terms: I. *International Journal of Medical Linguistics* 31:1–17.

WISTISEN, M. J., R. J. PARSONS, and A. LARSEN.   1975.   A Study to Identify Potentially Feasible Small Businesses for the Navajo Nation. Provo, Utah: Center for Business and Economic Research, Survey Research Center, Brigham Young University.

WOLF, C. B.   1961.   Kwashiorkor on the Navajo Indian Reservation. *Henry Ford Hospital Medical Bulletin* 9:566–571.

WYMAN, L. C.   1936.   Origin Legend of Navajo Divinatory Rites. *Journal of American Folklore* 49: 134–142.

WYMAN, L. C., and F. L. BAILEY.   1964.   *Navajo Indian Enthnoentomology.* Albuquerque: University of New Mexico Press.

WYMAN, L. C., and S. K. HARRIS.   1951.   *The Ethnobotany of the Kayenta Navaho.* Albuquerque: University of New Mexico Publications in Biology, 5.

WYMAN, L. C., and C. KLUCKHOHN.   1938.   *Navajo Classification of Their Song Ceremonials.* American Anthropological Association Memoir, 50.

ZONIS, R. D.   1968.   Chronic Otitis Media in the Southwestern American Indian. *Archives of Otolaryngology* 88:40–45.

7

Mainland Puerto Ricans

ALAN HARWOOD

Identification of the Ethnic Group

IN 1898, AT THE CLOSE of the Spanish-American War, the island of Puerto Rico became part of United States territory. Although formal relations between the United States government and the islanders have changed a number of times in the ensuing years, Puerto Rico's proximity to the mainland and its political ties with the United States not only have made the migration pattern of this ethnic population different from that of other immigrants but also have affected the way in which migrants have been incorporated into mainland society.

A Cautionary Note on the Demographic Data

In the absence of almost any other sources, one must rely on the U.S. Bureau of the Census and the Department of Labor for most demographic data on Puerto Ricans. These sources are conspicuously flawed, however, both by their inaccuracy and their noncomparability. Inaccuracy in the census has been uncovered mainly by comparing Census Bureau statistics with figures compiled either by other agencies or by different methods. Such comparisons have consistently revealed undercounts of the Puerto Rican population, sometimes as large as 30 percent, particularly for males and school-age children (Harwood 1970; Wagenheim 1975:6–7; Korns 1977).

Noncomparability, the second problem with Census Bureau statistics on Puerto Ricans, derives from changes that have occurred in the Bureau's way of classifying this ethnic group. In the 1950 and 1960 censuses, the

category "Puerto Rican" included only people either born in Puerto Rico
or with one or more parents born on the island. To avoid the underenumeration that obviously resulted from that classification (because of the
omission of Puerto Ricans whose ancestors resided on the mainland for
three or more generations), the 1970 census gathered data on the place of
birth of the respondent and his self-attributed "origin" or "descent."
Although the new format avoided the particular underenumeration problem posed by earlier censuses, the changed definition of ethnic membership renders analysis of long-term population trends exceedingly difficult
(U.S.Commission on Civil Rights 1976:2).

Migration Patterns

Although Puerto Rican migration to the continental United States
began in the nineteenth century, a sizable influx of islanders to the mainland occurred only after World War II. Today the Puerto Rican population
of the continent (defined as all people born either in Puerto Rico or to
parents on the island) numbers approximately 1.8 million (U.S. Bureau of
the Census 1978:5). This population is predominantly urban (79 percent
residing in central cities, 16 percent in periurban areas) and is concentrated in nine states (New York, New Jersey, Illinois, California, Pennsylvania, Connecticut, Florida, Massachusetts, and Ohio).

Though the destination of most Puerto Rican immigrants has been
cities, the more affluent and better educated have also located in suburbs
(Wagenheim 1975:11). In addition, an average of 20,000 seasonal laborers come to the continent annually (mainly under special contracts
supervised by the Office of the Commonwealth of Puerto Rico) to work
on farms located principally in the Northeast and Middle West (U.S.
Commission on Civil Rights 1976:31). About 10 percent of these laborers remain on the continent at the expiration of their contracts and
either move to major cities or settle in towns near the farming areas where
they have worked (Fitzpatrick 1971:15–20). An estimated 30,000 to
40,000 of these workers, however, have entered the migrant labor pool
and constitute a highly mobile segment of the continental Puerto Rican
population (Wagenheim 1975:5).

Because Puerto Ricans have been United States citizens since 1917 and,
as such, have been free to move between the island and the mainland
without legal or political restriction, the migration pattern of this ethnic
group has been marked by a singular degree of bidirectionality. This
movement between island and mainland, facilitated by relatively low
transportation costs, involves not only short-term visits to kinsmen (both
periodically and during times of crisis) but also long-term population
shifts in adjustment to the relative demands for labor on the island and the
continent (Fitzpatrick 1971:14–15; U.S. Commission on Civil Rights

1976:26–30). A major consequence of high mobility between the island and the mainland is a tendency for Puerto Ricans to reject an assimilationist adaptation to American society in preference to a bicultural mode of existence (Rodríguez 1975).

The most recent shift in Puerto Rican migration patterns has occurred as a result of declining economic conditions on the continent during the 1970s. This decline has caused a net outmigration of Puerto Ricans from the mainland, the first since the depression of the 1930s (U.S. Commission on Civil Rights 1976:30). A concomitant of this outmigration is that for the first time births, rather than immigration, have become the predominant source of population increase among continental Puerto Ricans. Furthermore, with a fertility rate approximately 20 percent higher than that of the United States urban white population (Sweet 1974:104), continental Puerto Ricans now consist almost equally of those born on the mainland and those born on the island (U.S. Commission on Civil Rights 1976:41).

Demographic Profile

In keeping with the purposes of this volume, I shall discuss only those demographic characteristics of continental Puerto Ricans that clearly impinge on health and medical care. The interested reader may wish to consult Maldonado-Denis (1972:302–324), Wagenheim (1975), and the U.S. Commission on Civil Rights (1976) for more detailed analyses of Puerto Rican demography.

In spite of the aforementioned problems with the available demographic data on Puerto Ricans, several characteristics of this population are still clearly discernible. First, and most obviously, the Puerto Rican population on the mainland is young. Compared to a median age of 28.6 for the total United States population in 1975, the median age for mainland Puerto Ricans was only 19.4. Furthermore, while 37 percent of all United States inhabitants were 21 years old or less, fully 53 percent of continental Puerto Ricans were 21 or under.

Correspondingly, Puerto Rican families on the continent tend to be in the expansion phase of the domestic cycle—44 percent with children under age 6 and 76 percent with children under 18 (Wagenheim 1975:12, 1972 figures). In addition, Puerto Rican families are larger than average for the nation as a whole: in 1972 20 percent of Puerto Rican families had four or more children, whereas only 9 percent of all U.S. families were that large (U.S. Commission on Civil Rights 1976:39).

In addition to being youthful, the Puerto Rican population on the continent is poor. Compared to the median family income of $16,009 for the nation as a whole in 1978, the median for Puerto Ricans was only $7,972, the lowest of any Hispanic group (U.S. Bureau of the Census 1978:10).

Furthermore, in March, 1978, 11.8 percent of Puerto Ricans in the working force were reported as being unemployed (U.S. Bureau of the Census 1978:8). Indeed, the economic position of Puerto Ricans on the continent appears to be getting worse. In 1959, before the War on Poverty, the median income of Puerto Rican families was 71 percent of the national median; in 1974 it had fallen to 59 percent, and in 1977 to 49 percent (U.S. Commission on Civil Rights 1976:52; U.S. Bureau of the Census 1978:10). Furthermore, in 1977 the incomes of 39 percent of all Puerto Rican families were below the poverty level—twice the percentage of other Hispanic groups and more than four times the percentage for non-Hispanics (U.S. Bureau of the Census 1978:10).

The low incomes of Puerto Rican families are related to two factors, both of which also influence the health and medical care of this population. The first of these factors is the high percentage of female-headed families (29 percent in 1972, compared to 12 percent for the nation). Although this proportion probably represents an overcount because of the underenumeration of Puerto Rican males in the census, the lower earning power of women nevertheless means that families headed by women generally have lower incomes than intact families and thus depress the average income for the group. The second factor related to the low income of Puerto Rican families is the general lack of occupational skills and work experience among those in the working force, particularly among the island-born segment of the population (U.S. Commission on Civil Rights 1976:66). One of several causes of this lack of occupational skills (and a population characteristic that relates to medical-care issues as well) is the relatively low educational level of Puerto Ricans. In 1970 the median number of school years completed by all adults in the United States over the age of 24 was 12, while the median for Puerto Ricans was 8.6 (Wagenheim 1975:83).

This characterization of mainland Puerto Ricans as poor and unskilled must be tempered, however, with an appreciation of the variation that exists within the ethnic collectivity. Thus, in spite of pervasively low incomes, more than three-quarters of Puerto Rican families on the continent are economically self-sufficient (U.S. Commission on Civil Rights 1976:8); moreover, 16 percent of Puerto Rican families earned between $10,000 and $14,999 a year in 1977, and some 24 percent earned $15,000 or more (U.S. Bureau of the Census 1978:10). Approximately a third of Puerto Ricans have completed high school (U.S. Bureau of the Census 1978:7), and more than 6 percent are employed in professional, technical, or administrative jobs (1978). Although this economic and educational variation within the Puerto Rican population does not invalidate the central tendencies discussed above, it does influence the generalizability of some of the findings on health and medical practices among Puerto Ricans, as will be seen in the section on evaluation of the data.

The Puerto Rican Family

Any discussion of sociocultural factors in Puerto Rican health care must begin with a description of the family. For, even though changes in traditional kin relationships have occurred in adaptation to urban, industrial life (Murillo-Rohde 1976), the extended family continues to be the mainstay of Puerto Ricans in time of trouble.

The preferred residence pattern among Puerto Ricans is for a couple to establish a separate domicile at the time of marriage, while continuing to maintain close ties to the kin networks of both spouses. These networks may involve not only biological kin but also affines and *compadres*.[1] As described by the sociologist Lloyd Rogler,

> The system incorporates the nuclear family into the extended family, because mutual help criss-crosses blood and affinal relationships. Mutual help, in fact, has the force of a sacred, obligatory norm: it is sustained by the double edge of guilt and gratitude. That is, not to help a relative in need evokes feelings of sinful guilt; in turn to be helped by a relative induces feelings of gratitude. The norm applies through time because the person is bound permanently to his or her family of origin; and it applies through space, because relatives who are separated by geographical distance behave in accordance with the norm. (1978:250)

Thus, in a time of crisis—be it illness, a legal difficulty, or financial trouble—the extended family will mobilize its often limited economic but immense psychological resources for the aid of the afflicted person. In health matters, this means that the patient is usually surrounded by a large "therapy-managing group" (Janzen 1977), which helps to interpret the problem, advises and assists the patient in seeking care, and nurses the sick. This group serves as a major support to both sick people and their immediate relatives and may usefully be drawn into the planning and management of patient care, as will be discussed later.

Another aspect of the Puerto Rican family that figures importantly in matters of health care is the traditional sexual division of labor within the nuclear family. In this division of functions, the woman is the homemaker as well as the caretaker of the children and the sick; the man is the economic provider and ultimate authority. Although there is evidence that this traditional role allocation is changing with the entry of more women into the labor force (Padilla 1958:101–160; Torres-Matrullo 1976:710–711), the fact remains that Puerto Rican women with children under age 18 still participate in the continental labor force to a significantly smaller degree than either white or black women (30 percent among Puerto Ricans, compared to 49 and 59 percent among whites

and blacks respectively) (U.S. Commission on Civil Rights 1976:62–
63). These women with young children remain at home and continue to
play the key role in organizing and overseeing the health care of the
Puerto Rican family. It is they with whom most health professionals interact, and it is therefore they who provide the major link between the
family and the subculture of biomedicine.

Evaluation of the Existing Data

Four kinds of sources, of varying quality, provide information on
the health and medical care of Puerto Ricans in the continental United
States.

1. Vital statistics and studies of specific diseases or health problems constitute
   the major sources of epidemiological data.
2. Survey data—which mainly focus on the topics of perceived health status,
   recalled incidents of morbidity, the use of medical facilities, and attitudes
   toward health and medical care—are of two types. The first is the relatively
   large-scale survey which specifically includes in the sample either Puerto
   Ricans or Hispanics identified as predominantly Puerto Rican (for example, Suchman 1964; Blue Cross–Blue Shield 1975); the second type,
   most examples of which are unpublished, is the small-scale survey, often
   carried out in the target area of a health center located in a Puerto Rican
   community (Harwood 1970; Johnson 1972).
3. Programmatic or descriptive articles (and occasionally books) on the medical delivery system provide information on special problems or modifications in mode of delivery that are relevant to a Puerto Rican clientele
   (Cohen 1972; Marcos et al. 1973; Kaplan and Roman 1973).
4. Finally, community studies place health and medical data on Puerto Ricans
   in a broader sociocultural context. Some of these studies are general in
   nature but treat health and medicine in considerable detail (for example,
   Padilla 1958); others focus specifically on health issues (Berle 1958; Garrison 1972, 1977b).

I carried out a study of the last type in a low-income area of New York
City between 1968 and 1970. Because this research (called the Health
Center Study for purposes of this chapter) constitutes a relatively major
source of data for this review of Puerto Rican health care, a brief summary of its methods will be given here. (For more detailed material on
the research setting, sample, and methods, see Harwood 1977:6–33).

As the name implies, the Health Center Study was carried out in affiliation with one of the many neighborhood health centers funded by the
Office of Economic Opportunity in the late 1960s. The area in which the
Center was established consisted of 42 square blocks, the boundaries of
which were defined by two "Health Areas" of the New York City Department of Health. These areas had been targeted for increased medical
service because of their poor showing on various health indices (Wise

1968:298; Harwood 1977:7). At the time of the study the residents of the area numbered approximately 45,000, about 36 percent of whom were Puerto Rican or other Hispanics.

The research, which was funded by the Carnegie Corporation of New York, took place in 11 multifamily tenement buildings in the area. The buildings were selected randomly, with the added proviso that at least 60 percent of the households in each building consented to participate in the project. Over the course of approximately a year, researchers from the area (whom I had trained in techniques of participant observation, formal interviewing, and process recording) visited the study buildings nearly every day and looked in on each household at least once every two weeks. The researchers' basic task was to observe both health maintenance practices (diet, use of medicines and herbs, and so on) and illness behavior in their natural setting. Some information (for example, on diet, medicines kept in the home, the classification of diseases) was elicited through formal interviews. Other data were collected through observation of behavior as it unfolded, with further elucidation of these observations through immediate or subsequent questioning of the participants. Researchers recorded these data in daily process notes.

Over the course of the study, 79 Puerto Rican households participated in the project for periods of from 1 to 13 months.[2] The sample households were in general poor (40 percent earned below the established poverty line for the time), predominantly Puerto Rican–born (94 percent of all household heads), and little educated (the median number of years of schooling for adults over age 24 was seven, with high school graduates comprising only 17 percent). Though several households could be considered middle-class in terms of their aspirations and the usual socioeconomic indicators, there were too few in this range to provide an adequate portrayal of the effects of class on health and medical practices. Thus, although some variation in beliefs and behavior can be traced to educational and income differences within the sample, data from the Health Center Study derive almost entirely from low-income, working-class Puerto Ricans.

Limitations of the Data and Sources of Intraethnic Diversity

A survey of some 70 books and articles of all four types enumerated at the beginning of this section reveals that while much of the research on the health of continental Puerto Ricans is quite recent (within the past 10 years), most investigations have focused on urban areas (87 percent of 68 studies), and 65 percent deal exclusively with New York City residents. Moreover, only a very few (3 percent) treat cities outside the East Coast. Although this attention on urban, East Coast Puerto Ricans quite accurately reflects the predominant residence pattern of the ethnic group, it is important to recognize that we have little information about the health and medical practices of certain other important sectors of the mainland Puerto Rican population—specifically, the migrant workers and the new, generally more affluent suburbanites.

The range of intraethnic variation, even within the urban population, is not well represented in the existing data. Like the Health Center Study, about half the research reports that were surveyed focus on low-income urbanites. The other half (mostly studies using survey techniques), however, do sample more widely from various income groups. Aside from income, other variables contributing to intraethnic diversity among Puerto Ricans have been largely ignored in health studies; these variables include education, place of birth, and extent of migration back and forth between the island and the mainland.

In sum, most of the data on Puerto Rican health and medical practices that will be reviewed in this chapter derive from low-income, urban samples. Although these samples are certainly useful in representing the modal continental Puerto Rican, it is unfortunate that we do not have adequate information on sources of intraethnic diversity in health and medical practices such as income, education, migration history, and degree of acculturation. Where information on this diversity is available, however, it will be provided.

Epidemiological Characteristics

Nature of the Data

As mentioned earlier, vital statistics and medical articles on specific diseases or health conditions are the two main sources of epidemiological data on continental Puerto Ricans. The only comprehensive analysis of vital statistics for continental Puerto Ricans comes from New York City (Alers 1978) and will necessarily constitute an important source of information for this chapter.[3]

In general, several notable limitations characterize vital statistics for continental Puerto Ricans. Most importantly, because of the nature of government record-keeping systems, the various institutions that gather health statistics define "Puerto Rican" differently. On the one hand, infant mortality, birth, and prematurity rates are calculated using a definition of Puerto Rican based on parental birthplace; mortality rates, on the other hand, define as Puerto Rican only those born on the island (Alers 1978:1).[4] This record-keeping anomaly not only makes comparison difficult but also often makes calculated rates questionable, because the appropriate denominator figure has not always been used. In addition, because the Puerto Rican population is comparatively young, vital statistics are relatively uninformative unless comparisons with the general population are controlled for age. Beyond these special limitations, the usual problems with regard to all morbidity data also prevail—namely, the bias introduced by their being derived typically from treated cases.

Studies of specific diseases or health conditions, the second source of epidemiological data on Puerto Ricans, either focus on Puerto Ricans specifically or include them as part of a larger sample. Very few of these studies concern the migrant labor sector of the Puerto Rican population, and the data, like other health information on this ethnic group, derive almost exclusively from low-income, urban samples (usually clinic patients).

In providing data on Puerto Rican health and disease in this section, I will first review the fragmentary information on migrant workers and then present the findings on mortality and morbidity for urban populations. Although the data from the two populations are being separated in this way, it is important to recognize that they are not mutually exclusive and that migrants often spend part of the year in continental cities and towns. The findings on migrants should, however, serve to alert urban physicians to the importance of discovering whether their new patients participate in migrant labor so that they may screen more thoroughly for the special problems of this group.

Health Status of Puerto Rican Migrant Workers

The rare health studies of migrant workers that focus specifically on Puerto Ricans provide a very inadequate picture of the general health status of this population. Only scattered data on vitamin deficiencies, occupational hazards, and dental health are available.

An analysis of circulating vitamins in blood samples from 409 adult Puerto Rican migrant farmworkers revealed deficiencies in vitamins B_6, B_{12}, and A, as well as probable deficiencies in biotin and nicotinate (Quinones et al. 1976).[5] Evidence from dietary reports of an adequate intake of fruits and vegetables and higher than average levels of circulating riboflavin, pantothenate, and β-carotene made the finding of vitamin A deficiency both unexpected and unexplained.

A small subsample of this same farmworker population ($N = 12$) was also tested for exposure to organophosphate pesticides, which are powerful inhibitors of acetylcholinesterase activity in the nervous system. Six of the workers tested were found to have plasma cholinesterase activity on the low end of the normal range, and four other workers were below the lower limit of normal activity (Bogden, Quinones, and El Nakah 1975).

The only other study of Puerto Rican migrants (in Massachusetts) focuses on dental health and concludes, as one might expect, that the population is undertreated (Gluck et al. 1972).

Major Causes of Mortality among Urban Puerto Ricans

The data to be reported in this section come mainly from Alers's study (1978) of mortality and selected morbidity patterns of Puerto Ricans in New York City. In the absence of comparable data from other places, it is difficult to judge how representative these figures are. One can reasonably suppose, however, that mortality from homicide and drug dependence is likely to be higher in New York City than elsewhere, but that disease-caused mortality probably differs little from other East Coast cities, where Puerto Ricans are also predominantly poor and live in substandard housing.

INFANT AND MATERNAL MORTALITY   For some 20 years, since the figures were first recorded in 1950, the rate of infant mortality for Puerto Ricans in New York City was intermediate between the rates for whites and those for nonwhites. This same pattern was also observed in Philadelphia in 1971 (Osofsky and Kendall 1973:113). Since 1974, however, white and Puerto Rican rates in New York City have ranged from 15.2 to 17.7 deaths per 1,000 live births annually and, except for 1977, have not differed significantly from one another. A similar downward trend in mortality is observable for maternal deaths starting in 1975, when the Puerto Rican rate also began approximating that for whites (Alers 1978: 12). Although the causes for the decline in these two sources of mortality are not completely clear, it is likely that both higher levels of education among Puerto Rican women of childbearing age and increased and improved prenatal and obstetrical services to low-income populations have played a role.

ACCIDENTS, HOMICIDE, AND DRUG DEPENDENCE   Table 7.1 presents data from the period 1969–1971 on the eight major causes of death for Puerto Rican–born New Yorkers of all ages combined, as well as for the following age groups separately: under 15, 15–44, 45–64, and 65 and over. The table also compares mortality rates of the Puerto Rican–born with those of the total New York City population.

One notes immediately that whereas the total mortality rate for Puerto Rican–born New Yorkers was considerably lower than that for all New York residents, young Puerto Ricans (those under age 45) died at a much higher rate than the same age cohort in the general population. Furthermore, the chief causes of death for the Puerto Rican–born in this age range were not diseases but accidents, homicide, and drug dependence. Together these causes accounted for 39 percent of all deaths in this age group. Moreover, the rates for these causes were in almost every case nearly twice the rates for the general population. If this pattern of mortality continues, as the now youthful Puerto Rican population moves in-

Table 7.1 Average annual mortality rates for chief causes, Puerto Rican–born and total populations, New York City, 1969–1971.

| Chief causes in rank order[a] | Puerto Rican–born population | | Total population | | |
	Average annual rate[b]	%	Average annual rate	%	Rank
All ages					
Heart diseases	152.4	25.3	440.2	39.6	1
Malignant neoplasms	94.4	15.6	225.1	20.2	2
Cirrhosis of the liver	45.4	7.5	36.5	3.3	5
Cerebrovascular disease	35.0	5.8	78.4	7.1	3
Accidents	29.3	4.9	27.8	2.5	7
Influenza and pneumonia	20.5	3.4	44.5	4.0	4
Other diseases of digestive system	17.7	2.9	29.4	2.6	6
Diabetes mellitus	17.7	2.9	25.4	2.3	8
All other	191.3	31.7	204.7	18.4	
Total	603.7	100.0	1,112.1	100.0	—
Under 15 years					
Accidents	22.3	28.0	12.5	22.5	1
Malignant neoplasms	10.3	13.0	10.1	18.2	2
Influenza and pneumonia	8.0	10.1	4.8	8.7	4
Congenital anomalies	6.3	7.9	5.5	10.0	3
Homicide	4.6	5.8	1.8	3.3	6
Diseases of nervous system	2.9	3.6	2.6	4.7	5
Bronchitis, emphysema, and asthma	1.7	2.2	1.0	1.6	8
Heart disease	1.1	1.4	1.0	1.9	7
All other	22.3	28.0	15.2	27.5	—
Total	79.5	100.0	55.5	100.0	—
15–44 years					
Homicide	58.3	18.9	28.5	11.3	2
Drug dependence	37.9	12.3	23.2	9.2	5
Cirrhosis of the liver	30.0	9.7	24.6	9.7	4
Accidents	24.9	8.1	17.7	7.0	6
Malignant neoplasms	22.7	7.3	34.6	13.7	1
Heart disease	21.5	7.0	26.7	10.5	3
Cerebrovascular disease	7.8	2.5	8.1	3.2	7
Other diseases of digestive system	7.1	2.3	7.3	2.9	8
All other	98.0	31.9	82.4	31.9	—
Total	308.1	100.0	253.2	100.0	—

Table 7.1   continued.

Chief causes in rank order[a]	Puerto Rican–born population			Total population		
	Average annual rate[b]	%		Average annual rate	%	Rank
45–64 years						
Heart disease	303.8	28.7		465.8	36.6	1
Malignant neoplasms	224.7	21.2		361.0	28.3	2
Cirrhosis of the liver	120.1	11.3		84.0	6.6	3
Cerebrovascular disease	62.9	5.9		64.9	5.1	4
Accidents	39.5	3.7		26.5	2.1	8
Diabetes mellitus	36.9	3.5		29.1	2.3	7
Other diseases of digestive system	35.0	3.3		35.7	2.8	5
Influenza and pneumonia	29.4	2.8		31.1	2.4	6
All other	206.3	19.6		175.3	13.8	—
Total	1,058.6	100.0		1,273.3	100.0	—
65+ years						
Heart disease	1,832.6	41.7		2,644.3	48.4	1
Malignant neoplasms	813.2	18.5		1,032.0	18.9	2
Cerebrovascular disease	410.7	9.3		495.5	9.1	3
Influenza and pneumonia	214.3	4.9		244.4	4.5	4
Diabetes mellitus	201.3	4.6		144.0	2.6	6
Other diseases of digestive system	146.1	3.3		144.7	2.6	5
General arteriosclerosis	110.4	2.5		118.4	2.2	7
Accidents	68.2	1.6		92.6	1.7	8
All other	595.7	13.6		547.3	10.0	—
Total	4,392.5	100.0		5,463.0	100.0	—

Source: Adapted from Alers (1978:6, 8, 10).

a. The eight leading causes of death are arranged in order of importance for Puerto Ricans.

b. Rates are per 100,000 U.S. Census (New York City) population.

creasingly into early adulthood, the demands on public medical services for treatment of accidents, homicide, and drug abuse will increase. Rather than waiting to treat these afflictions medically, it would seem both efficient and humane for health professionals, as citizens, to begin exerting political pressure to remedy the causes of these problems through social, legal, economic, and educational measures.

MORTALITY FROM DISEASE   Table 7.1 reveals two notable differences in disease-caused mortality for the Puerto Rican–born and total New York City populations in the under-15 age group. First, mortality rates for five respiratory diseases (excluding tuberculosis, which is not included in Alers's tables) were appreciably higher for Puerto Rican–born children than for the general pediatric population. This pattern undoubtedly accounts in part for the considerable concern Puerto Rican parents demonstrate with regard to respiratory ailments. The second noteworthy difference in death rates in the under-15 age group was the significantly higher rate attributable to "other" causes among the Puerto Rican–born population (22.3 compared to 15.2 per 100,000). This finding suggests a higher mortality rate from diseases not routinely seen in general pediatric practice.[6]

In the older age groupings, it is striking that the rankings of the major causes of death for the Puerto Rican–born population and the total New York City population are quite similar in the age ranges over 44 but notably dissimilar in the 15–44 age range, where, as we have already observed, traumata and drugs were the major killers of Puerto Ricans. Two diseases, diabetes mellitus and cirrhosis of the liver, constitute exceptions to the general similarity in rankings by cause for older Puerto Ricans, however. Both these diseases result in higher mortality rates among the Puerto Rican–born population—diabetes among persons over the age of 44, and cirrhosis in the entire 15–64 age range.[7]

Although heart disease and malignant neoplasms ranked as the two major killers in both the Puerto Rican–born and total populations over age 44, mortality rates from both these causes were markedly lower among the Puerto Rican–born. With regard to malignancies, however, the generalized death rates recorded in table 7.1 mask differentials in rate by type of malignancy that are relevant to Puerto Ricans. An analysis of 99 percent of the cancer deaths that occurred among New York City residents in the period 1949–1951, for example, revealed that Puerto Ricans had significantly different mortality rates from those of whites of the same sex for cancers of several sites (Seidman 1970). Specifically, Puerto Rican males had 62 percent lower mortality from cancer of the lungs but 20 percent higher mortality from cancer of the stomach. And while Puerto Rican women had 40 percent lower mortality from cancer of the colon and 56 percent lower mortality from cancer of the breast, their death rates from cancers of the uterine cervix and corpus were significantly higher (221 percent and 129 percent respectively; p − .01).

Though it seems safe to say that these differentials in cancer mortality reflect group differences in not only morbidity but also medical treatment, no studies could be located that specifically attempted to explain the observed variations. A number of related findings are suggestive, however. For example, a study of coronary heart disease which compared nearly

25,000 males of ages 45 to 64 in Framingham (Mass.), Honolulu, and the San Juan area reported that among the San Juan males there were proportionately fewer smokers than in the other two cities and that the Puerto Ricans who did smoke consumed fewer cigarettes (Gordon et al. 1974:332–333). If one assumes a similar pattern of tobacco consumption among Puerto Rican males in New York City, then the lower mortality from lung cancer may well be due to a lower prevalence of the disease itself, related in turn to lower levels of exposure to the major etiological agent.

High mortality rates among Puerto Rican women for the two types of uterine cancer, however, seem to require contrasting explanations. Stewart and his colleagues (1966) report a very high incidence of cervical cancer among Puerto Rican women in New York City (105.7 per 100,000, compared to 4.1 for Jews and 15.0 for non-Jewish whites) but a low incidence of cancer of the uterine corpus (7.3 per 100,000, compared to 13.1 for non-Jewish whites and 15.6 for Jews). The high mortality among Puerto Rican women from cancer of the cervix would therefore seem to reflect a higher rate of morbidity for the disease as compared to New York whites, whereas the death rate from cancer of the corpus would seem, in contrast, to reflect deficiencies in detection or treatment, or both. In spite of these suggestive findings, detailed studies of the differential mortality and morbidity rates for cancers of various sites among Puerto Ricans are clearly necessary and, if performed comparatively, may well provide insights into the general causes of these diseases.

SUICIDE   A study of attempted and completed suicides among Puerto Ricans, blacks, and whites, age 18 and over, in East Harlem (New York City) for the years 1968 through 1970 (Monk and Warshauer 1974) reveals that Puerto Ricans of both sexes attempted suicide at rates at least twice those of either blacks or whites of the same sex (table 7.2). Puerto Rican males also completed suicide at a higher rate than any other sex or ethnic category, while the rate of completion for Puerto Rican females fell below that of all categories except black females. Nonbarbiturate drugs were used most often in suicide attempts; jumping was the most common method for completed instances. A clinical analysis of suicide attempts among 93 Puerto Ricans admitted to a public hospital in New York City suggests that these acts are primarily unpremeditated, impulsive, and accompanied by a temporary loss of awareness (Trautman 1961:77–78).

In the Monk and Warshauer study no relationship could be established between either attempted or completed suicide and such demographic variables as marital status, place of birth, length of residence in New York City, or socioeconomic area of residence within East Harlem. The

Table 7.2 Annual age-adjusted rates (per 100,000) of attempted and completed suicide among persons 18 and over in East Harlem by ethnic group and sex.

Suicide	Males			Females		
	Puerto Rican	White	Black	Puerto Rican	White	Black
Attempted	348.0	175.7	149.8	604.0	220.2	208.0
Completed	44.5	31.5	29.6	17.5	32.5	10.7
Ratio— attempted : completed[a]	9:1	5:1	5:1	14:1	5:1	19:1

Source: Adapted from Monk and Warshauer (1974:338).
a. Ratio is based on numbers, not rates (Monk, personal communication).

only variable tested that did bear some relation to completed suicide was residence in public housing, where rates for both men and women were less than half those of people living elsewhere.

Although Monk and Warshauer present a strong argument for the validity of their data (1974:341–343), questions concerning the causes and the generalizability of their findings still remain. With regard to causes, Monk and Warshauer rather vaguely suggest migration, poverty, and "how [Puerto Ricans] react to the emergency of self-injury" as factors related to the high attempt rates in their sample (1974:344). Although Trautman (1961) describes more persuasively how these three factors contributed to the suicide attempts he observed, the absence of any control data on poor migrants who do not commit suicide still leaves the question of causality essentially unanswered. With regard to the generalizability of Monk and Warshauer's findings, it is safest not to extrapolate their East Harlem suicide rates to other urban areas until the causes are better understood.

Morbidity in Three Urban Populations

Although the importance of morbidity data in planning health services has long been recognized (White 1967), the problems of securing these data have usually precluded their use. We are therefore fortunate in having access to three unpublished studies of morbidity among Puerto Ricans (the Health Center Study in New York City, the Health Ecology Project in Miami, and the Quirk Middle School Project in Hartford). Unhappily, however, these studies utilized different methods of data collection and are therefore not strictly comparable.[8] Nevertheless, if the findings (table 7.3) are examined with caution, they do provide some insight into the principal symptoms and conditions common to urban

Table 7.3 Most common symptoms and acute and chronic conditions of Puerto Ricans in three urban areas.

	Hartford	Miami	New York City	
	Children and teenagers[a] (N = 80)	Adults and children combined[b] (N = 129)	Adults[c] (N = 96)	Children and teenagers[c] (N = 98)

Symptoms and percentage experiencing the symptom	No information[d]	1. Fever 61
		2. Cough 43
		3. Aches and pains 35
		4. Loss of appetite 30
		5. Hoarseness 27
		6. Upset stomach, vomiting, nausea 26
		7. Nervousness 19
		  Diarrhea 19
		8. Tiredness 18
		9. Breaking out or itching of skin 16
		10. Shortness of breath 15
			1. Pain 31
			2. Stomachache, upset stomach 14
			3. "Nerves" (*nervios*) 6
			  No appetite 6
			  Headache 5
			4. Hoarseness (*ronquera*) 5
				1. Fever 14
				2. Rash 12
				3. Cough 10

Acute conditions and prevalence per 100 persons	No information	1. *Gases* (fullness, bloating, pain in abdominal area) 21 2. Colds, flu, virus[e] 11	1. Colds, influenza, tonsillitis, sore throat 70 2. "*Asma*"[t] 17 3. Accidental lacerations, burns, etc. 14 4. Bronchitis, pneumonia, "*fatiga*"[t] 10 5. Foot problems (corns, ingrown toenail, infected nail, etc.) 7 6. Diarrheal disease 5	1. Colds, influenza, tonsillitis, sore throat 93 2. Accidents (fractures, burns, lacerations, etc.) 26 3. "*Asma*"[t] 16 Intestinal virus or other diarrheal disease 16 4. Bronchitis, pneumonia, "*fatiga*"[t] 13 5. Childhood diseases (measles, mumps, chicken pox) 10 6. Earache 6

Chronic conditions and prevalence per 100 persons						
1. Dental problems	35	1. Nervous trouble	15	1. Allergies	9	1. Asthma	4
2. Parasites (including *Schistosoma*, hookworm, *Trichuris*, *Giardia*, and minor infections)g	32	2. Allergy	11	2. Diabetes	7	2. Tuberculosis	3
3. Skin problems (eczema, acne, etc.)	19	3. High or low blood pressure	7	3. Arthritis	5	Parasites	3
4. Obesity	18	Varicose veins	7	4. Drug dependence	4	Allergies	3
5. Vision problems	16	Back/spine trouble	7	Hypertension	4		
6. Positive urine	15	4. Asthma	5	"Heart condition"	4		
7. Dysmenorrhea	11	Serious eye trouble	5	Asthma	4		
Positive tine test	11	5. Heart trouble	4				
8. Hearing problem	6	Speech difficulty	4				
Dysuria	6						
Asthma	6						
Scoliosis	6						

Sources: For Hartford data, Hispanic Health Council (n.d.:30–31); for Miami data, Weidman (1978:325–448); for New York City data, research data of the Health Center Study.

a. Age range 10–15.

b. Of the total Miami sample, 68 percent were under 20 years of age.

c. Persons 18 years and over are considered adults; those under 18, children or teenagers. The adults ranged from 18 to 81 years of age, with a median of 32.5 years. Children ranged from one month to 17 years, with a median of 9 years.

d. Although some of the problems listed under "chronic conditions" are symptoms or signs (e.g., dysuria, positive urine), they have not been listed as "symptoms" in the table because they were not elicited from laity but discovered on clinical examination.

e. Complete tabulation of acute conditions not provided in research report.

f. For a discussion of the meanings of the terms *asma* and *fatiga* in this context, see note 10.

g. N = 60.

Puerto Ricans on the continent. Because of the varying methods by which the data were collected, the recorded prevalence rates are less informative than their rank ordering, and the precise figures are included only to give a clearer indication of the relative frequencies of symptoms or conditions *within* each study population.

Given that certain differences among the findings undoubtedly derive from the contrasting methods used, the similarity in rank ordering of the most prevalent symptoms and conditions is noteworthy. Indeed, the similarity to morbidity patterns in the general population is also striking (U.S. Department of Health, Education, and Welfare 1978).[9] Despite this similarity, however, three sets of conditions with high prevalence among the Puerto Rican samples deserve special comment: (1) the group consisting of respiratory symptoms, acute respiratory infections, and *fatiga* or *asma;*[10] (2) symptoms of upset stomach, nausea, and diarrhea, with accompanying evidence (from the Hartford and New York City studies) of parasitosis; and (3) asthma, allergies, and skin problems.

RESPIRATORY CONDITIONS   Upper respiratory infections deserve particular attention in the Puerto Rican population in light of three facts: the higher mortality rates from respiratory diseases among Puerto Rican–born children; evidence of a much higher incidence of rheumatic fever in Puerto Rican children than in either black or white children (Brownell and Bailen-Rose 1973); and the considerable anxiety about respiratory infections observed among Puerto Rican parents in the Health Center Study. Several important observations may be drawn from these facts. First, the anxiety of Puerto Rican parents over upper respiratory infections does not seem to be misplaced: their children in fact run higher risks of dying from respiratory diseases and of contracting other serious, related conditions like rheumatic fever. Second, although the reason given by many Puerto Rican parents for their anxiety over respiratory problems may not be accepted by the medical profession (namely, that there is a direct, sequential relationship between minor, uncured upper respiratory infections and more serious respiratory diseases like tuberculosis and pneumonia), the relationship they allude to may itself be empirically valid, though explicable by different means (that is, lowered resistance to streptococcal diseases from repeated upper respiratory infection and overcrowded living conditions). For the clinician, the practical implications of these facts are as follows: (1) to exercise particular care in diagnosing respiratory infections and in following up suspicious indications in Puerto Rican children, and (2) to deal directly with parents' anxieties as well as counseling them on the importance of follow-up visits.

CONDITIONS OF THE DIGESTIVE SYSTEM   In examining the data in table 7.3, one notes both the high ranking of gastrointestinal symptoms and conditions and a rate of parasitic infection in a sample of elementary school pupils as high as 32 percent. For comparative purposes, the results of four additional parasite surveys among inner-city, predominantly poor continental Puerto Ricans are presented in table 7.4.

Although several wide discrepancies exist among the findings of some of the studies, a number of rather consistent indicators of risk emerge. In all studies the highest rates appeared among Puerto Rican–born subjects and in the age range of school children (5- to 6-year-olds) through young adults (24- to 36-year-olds). Among the continental-born, the prevalence of parasites, as one might expect, was consistently higher among those who had visited Puerto Rico at some time in their lives, although low rates of infection with *Trichuris, Giardia, Entamoeba coli,* and *Endolimax nana* were also observed in children who had never been to the island (Winsberg et al. 1975:528–529; Hargus et al. 1976:928–929). The Hartford study (reported in table 7.3) also found that children with parasites tended to be the offspring of parents with lower levels of education than children without parasites (Schensul et al. 1978:22).

The implications of these findings for the clinician and health planner, however, are moot—in part because the prevalence studies are so few in number, but mainly because the information on the long- and short-term effects of subclinical infection from various parasites is virtually nil (especially in nonendemic areas). Without this information and additional prevalence studies, it becomes difficult to develop a clear policy on screening (Bernick 1978:43–45) or even treatment for parasites.

Given this absence of adequate information (and the improbability, for political reasons, of instituting a mass screening program), the clinician would be well advised to consider routine stool examinations for those patients most at risk (as described above) and, in keeping with current opinion among parasitologists (for example, Brown 1975:341), to treat all cases of infection, provided a safe and effective chemotherapeutic agent exists.[11] General consultation with a parasitologist familiar with the epidemiology of the particular population coming for treatment would also be advisable. It is important to emphasize, however, that there is no basis for attributing the problem of parasitosis to the majority of continental Puerto Ricans or for precipitously interpreting gastrointestinal symptoms as indicative of this problem.

ASTHMA, ALLERGIES, AND SKIN PROBLEMS   Although consideration of the epidemiology and etiology of asthma, allergies, and skin problems is beyond the scope of this book, these conditions nevertheless warrant special mention here in view of both their high rank ordering among the disorders recorded in table 7.3 and the paucity of special studies directed to

Table 7.4 Prevalence rates of parasitosis among continental Puerto Ricans.

Study and sample	Schistosoma mansoni (%)	Trichuris trichiura (%)	Hook-worm (%)	Giardia lamblia (%)	Strongyloides stercoralis (%)	Ascaris (%)	Entamoeba histolytica (%)	One or more parasites		
								Puerto Rican born (%)	Continental born (%)	Total (%)
Kagan, Rairigh, and Kaiser 1962 (N = 103 male adults)	28[a] 44[b]	—	—	—	—	—	—	—	—	—
Winsberg et al. 1974 (N = 412 adults and children)	21.6[a]	c	c	c	c	0	—	—	—	—
Winsberg et al. 1975 (N = 358 adults and children)	—	13.9	6.6	3.9	1.7	0	0	28.2	4.2	18.6
Hargus et al. 1976 (N = 129 elementary school children)	—	34.9	5.4	24.0	0.8	3.9	2.3	80.7	30.6	54.3

a. Based on recovery of eggs through rectal biopsy.
b. Based on intradermal test.
c. Reports prevalence rate of 19.6 percent for hookworm, *Trichuris*, *Strongyloides*, and *Giardia* combined.

understanding their prevalence in the Puerto Rican population. (A notable exception to this dearth of special studies is the demonstration by Alcasid and her associates (1973) that bronchial asthma in 131 predominantly Puerto Rican patients had no significant correlation with intestinal parasitism.) Though studies of these three afflictions among lower socioeconomic groups in general are certainly relevant to comparable Puerto Rican populations, the importance of social and psychological factors in the genesis of these conditions argues, in addition, for special investigation of their etiology and treatment in Puerto Rican families.

Miscellaneous Diseases or Conditions of Particular Relevance to Puerto Ricans

DRUG ABUSE The disproportionate number of drug-related deaths among Puerto Rican-born New Yorkers in the 15- to 44-year age bracket (see table 7.1) prompts a brief review of the scant information that is available on narcotics addiction in this ethnic group. In 1974 (the most recent statistics from the New York City Narcotics Registry available to me) the incidence of narcotics addiction among "Hispanics" (about two-thirds of whom were Puerto Rican, according to the census definition of the term) was 508 per 100,000 population, compared to rates of 773 for blacks and 132 for whites (Alers 1978:24).[12] This pattern of incidence, intermediate between blacks and whites, has been consistent since the first publication of addiction figures for New York City (Newman et al. 1974; Alers 1978:26).

To view drug abuse solely in terms of mortality and incidence, however, totally neglects its relationship to the social life of real people. Yet, apart from an unpublished study by Fitzpatrick (1975), little information on this crucial aspect of the phenomenon exists. The Fitzpatrick study, based on in-depth interviews with 50 addicts and 50 non-addicts of Puerto Rican ethnicity in New York City, reports a drug-use pattern that is different from the "drug culture" usually described in the literature for addicts from the general population (1975:2–5). According to the study, Puerto Rican addicts are not generally isolated from kin and community and have not developed an esoteric subculture of drug use. Indeed, many people in the community from which Fitzpatrick's sample of addicts was drawn knew the procedures for drug use, and the study reports quite widespread consumption of drugs (including "hard" drugs) in social situations involving non-addicts and "successful addicts" (that is, those who held jobs sufficiently well paying to support their habit and perhaps a family as well). As a rule, Puerto Rican peer groups segregated addicts only for involvement in other illegal activities or after apprehension by the police. Since police reports constitute a sizable input of names to the Narcotics Register (Alers 1978:23, 25), official statistics on Puerto Rican addicts thus derive mainly from those "problem cases" whom the community has isolated.

In spite of this reported integration of drug use into the New York Puerto Rican subculture, one cannot ignore the negative effects of drug abuse on the health and social life of Puerto Rican communities. Not only are there high rates of drug-related deaths, but "problem addicts" are a major source of distress to residents of poor neighborhoods, where they are feared not only as robbers and burglars but also as incendiaries, who squat in unrented apartments or abandoned buildings and burn fires for light and heat, often carelessly. Furthermore, though Puerto Rican family and extended-kin ties may be important in preventing addiction (Fitzpatrick 1975:2, 109–110), the psychological toll on many parents from worrying about the possibility of their children becoming addicts is considerable (Health Center Study observations). Families with an addicted member often experience both a financial drain from supporting their kinsman's habit and disruptive conflicts over how best to deal with the addict. Given these problems, it is no wonder that Puerto Ricans consistently rank drugs as the foremost health problem of their communities (Alers 1978:71–73; Health Center Study, structured interviews).

To add to this sense of calamity about drug abuse, there is also widespread doubt among Puerto Ricans that the available treatment programs do much good—a sentiment that is in fact supported by empirical evidence (Snarr and Ball 1974). To improve treatment methods for Puerto Rican addicts, Fitzpatrick and his co-workers have tentatively suggested that both the addict's extended kin and, when possible, his mother should be involved in the therapeutic program, too (1975:109–111).

THE "PUERTO RICAN SYNDROME" (*Ataques*)   Although the Spanish word *ataque* may be used, like its cognate "attack" in English, to refer to the sudden onset of any ailment (as in *ataque de corazón,* heart attack, or *ataque epiléptico,* epileptic attack), it is most commonly used to refer to a sudden partial loss of consciousness, accompanied by either clonic or tonic seizures and at times by screaming, tearing of clothing, or foaming at the mouth. Such attacks may last from a few minutes to as long as four days (Berle 1958:159) and terminate as suddenly as they began. This form of *ataque* may be further qualified in Spanish as being *de nervios* (of nerves) and has entered the medical literature as the "Puerto Rican syndrome" (Berle 1958:158–162; Fernández-Marina 1961; Mehlman 1961; Rothenberg 1964).

Precise prevalence statistics for the syndrome are unavailable. However, *ataques* appear to be more common among women than men and more characteristic of the lower than the upper socioeconomic classes. An *ataque* may be a culturally approved or expected behavior at certain times and places, or it may be an idiosyncratic response to a nexus of personal life experiences.

Culturally appropriate times and places for *ataques* include occasions when a show of grief is called for (such as funerals) and when one has either witnessed or received news of a shocking event, particularly one affecting a loved one (Padilla 1958:115). While not necessarily approved, ataques are also expected from some women when they do not get their own way or when they are faced with an act of aggression they cannot otherwise stop (Garrison 1977a:388–389). In these contexts, the *ataque* is a "culturally recognized, acceptable cry for help or an admission of inability to cope, and family and friends are required by norms of good behavior to rally to the aid of the *ataque* victim and relieve the intolerable stresses" (Garrison 1977a:389).

Other instances of *ataque,* however, occur unpredictably and are more idiosyncratic and endogenously determined. They may be understood according to folk theory as a spiritual disturbance (Garrison 1977a; Harwood 1977:74–75), or in a psychiatric framework as hysterical dissociation in the face of unacceptable, angry, or aggressive impulses (Fernández-Marina 1961; Rothenberg 1964). People who suffer this type of attack may be brought to a medical facility for emergency care and later referred to a psychiatrist or spiritist (or both) for treatment, depending on the attending clinician's recommendation and the beliefs of the victim and his close associates.

It is important for the clinician to recognize that only victims of the second, more idiosyncratic form of *ataque* are likely to present in the medical setting. In addition, the clinician should be aware that there are culturally acceptable spiritual healers for these forms of *ataque,* whose goals and treatment methods parallel in many respects those of mental health professionals (Garrison 1977a:441–444; Harwood 1977:188–199). Furthermore, treatment of an *ataque* victim by a mental health professional may subject the sufferer to the stigmatizing label of being *loco* (crazy), while treatment by a spirit medium allows the victim to sustain the nonstigmatizing diagnosis of *nervioso* (nervous) or *enfermo de los nervios* ("nerve-sick") (Rogler and Hollingshead 1965; Garrison 1977b)

In consequence of these facts, it is advisable for the clinician to probe the beliefs of the victim and his family concerning the causes of the *ataque* and to ascertain how they intend to deal with the sufferer, if follow-up care seems indicated. If the clinician determines that the family and victim interpret the *ataque* as spiritually caused and intend to pursue therapy with the appropriate modality, it is probably best not to press psychiatric treatment. For, although no controlled studies comparing the outcomes of orthodox psychiatric and spiritist modes of treatment are available, it is likely that treatment within the cultural idiom and milieu of the sufferer is at least as effective as that provided by a psychiatric facility. (Additional information on spiritist theories of illness and spiritist treatment methods will be found in the sections on concepts of disease and nonmainstream sources of care respectively.)

RUBELLA   Several studies (reviewed in Vaeth 1974) have revealed a considerably lower level of immunity to rubella among Puerto Rican adults than prevails in the general population. Puerto Rican rates range from a low of 49 percent for a sample of Puerto Rican female medical students to a high of 65 percent for a cohort of Puerto Rican army recruits. These figures compare to a level of immunity of approximately 90 percent in samples from the general United States adult population. In view of this evidence of low levels of immunity among Puerto Ricans and the adverse consequences of rubella in pregnant women, routine rubella titers for all Puerto Rican females of childbearing age without a history of the disease are advisable. Rubella vaccine should then be administered as needed.

SARCOIDOSIS   A study of 311 clinic patients with biopsy-confirmed sarcoidosis indicates that Puerto Ricans (N = 54) tend to present for treatment at an earlier stage of the disease than either blacks or whites, largely because of a propensity among Puerto Rican women for the disease to start with a bothersome eruption of erythema nodosum (Teirstein, Siltzeach, and Berger 1976). As a consequence of early presentation, the prognosis for Puerto Rican sufferers of sarcoidosis is generally good, although the course of this disease is variable.

SYSTEMIC LUPUS ERYTHEMATOSUS AND SERUM GAMMA GLOBULIN LEVELS   Among Puerto Rican females in the New York City area, the average annual incidence rate for systemic lupus erythematosus (SLE) has been observed to be intermediate between the rates of black and white females (Lee and Siegel 1976). Although the SLE rates were not found to correlate with quality of housing, domiciliary crowding, or duration of residence in New York City, they do parallel the rank ordering of serum gamma globulin levels found in healthy members of the three groups. The meaning of this finding in terms of the etiology of SLE is unclear, however (Siegel et al. 1965). Elevated serum gamma globulin levels for Puerto Ricans do not seem to be related to place of birth (Puerto Rico or New York) or, among the Puerto Rican–born population, to length of residence in New York. Consequently, Siegel and his co-workers suggest a genetic cause for the observed group differences (1965:719).[13] In the absence of any clear understanding of the relationship between SLE and elevated serum gamma globulin levels, the main clinical import of this research is the suggestion by Siegel and his colleagues (1965:720) that the upper limit of normal for serum gamma globulin be set at a higher level for Puerto Ricans. (They suggest a value of 1.8 gm for a confidence interval of 95 percent under the laboratory conditions and procedures of their study.)

Summary

In reviewing the chief causes of mortality and morbidity among Puerto Ricans, one can scarcely avoid the conclusion that many of the major "medical" problems of this ethnic group are in large part the outcome of class inequalities. One must acknowledge, for example, the important effects of a depressed economic and social position in the etiology of such major causes of mainland Puerto Rica mortality and morbidity as homicide, drug dependence, childhood influenza and pneumonia, parasitic infections, allergic conditions, and pesticide and lead poisoning (Alers 1978:27–29).[14] To some extent this conclusion is biased by the derivation of much of the epidemiological data from low-income, urban populations, as mentioned earlier. However, since most Puerto Ricans on the mainland are in fact poor and urban, this conclusion cannot be ignored or dismissed. It is also noteworthy that as strongly as class factors shape the epidemiological picture of Puerto Ricans as a group, they do not completely override the important effects of ethnic heritage and subculture (for example, on particular patterns of suicide and drug use, tropical sources of infection and reinfection, and the culture-specific syndrome *ataque*).

Concepts of Disease and Illness

Theories of Disease Etiology

The following sections will describe several theories of disease causality that derive from folk, popular, and biomedical traditions and are shared among various sectors of the Puerto Rican population. The discussion does not exhaust all the theories used by Puerto Ricans but covers the ones that have significant implications both for communication between Puerto Ricans and biomedical healers and for adherence of Puerto Ricans to medical regimens.

THE HOT/COLD (HUMORAL) THEORY   Widely disseminated throughout the Latin world, the hot/cold theory of disease rests on the assumption that a healthy body is somewhat "wet" and "warm" and that disease is a deviation from this state. Some diseases are conceived as a deflection from health in the direction of a "cold" (*frío*) condition, and some toward a "hot" (*caliente*) one. These deflections may be produced by sudden changes in body temperature or by the ingestion of immoderate amounts of foods and other substances, which are also classified as "cold" or "hot." Table 7.5 presents the classification of major diseases or bodily states, foods, medicines, and herbs as observed among Puerto Ricans in the Health Center Study in New York City (Harwood 1971a). As the table indicates, the Puerto Rican cultural variant of the hot/cold system contains an intermediate category, *fresco* ("cool"), which is applied to both foods and medications but not to diseases or bodily states.

Therapy in this hot/cold system consists of treating "cold"-classified states with "hot" foods and medications, and "hot" states with "cool" (*not* "cold") substances. To follow the theory, one should also avoid ingesting "cold" or "hot" substances when one is in a parallel physical state. The theory also provides a way to mitigate the unwanted effects of "hot" foods and medications by a procedure known in Spanish as *refrescando el estómago* ("refreshing or "cooling" the stomach). This procedure, a kind of neutralization process, consists of ingesting a "cool"-classified substance simultaneously with a "hot" one. As we shall see in the section on adherence to treatment regimens, this principle of neutralization can be a useful aid to the clinician in managing treatment regimens involving "hot" medicines or foods.

It is important to note that although the terminology of hot/cold therapeutics suggests that it is based on temperature, the thermal state in which foods and herbal remedies are taken is not in fact relevant. White beans served straight off the fire, for example, are considered "cold," whereas iced beer, because of its alcoholic content, is considered "hot." Thus, foods and other ingested substances are thought to produce "cold" or "hot" conditions of the digestive tract depending on their classification in the hot/cold system, rather than on their thermal state when eaten.

Temperature does play a role in the system, however, with regard to ideas about the etiology of certain diseases. Thus, "cold" diseases of the joints, muscles, or respiratory tract are believed to be caused by a chill that may occur when a person moves from heated to unheated surroundings. Colds, for example, are commonly attributed to drafts or to going outside with insufficient clothing, and arthritic pain in the fingers is often ascribed to switching the hands suddenly from hot to cold water.

CONCEPTS OF MENTAL ILLNESS   Although this book does not focus on psychiatric issues, it is nevertheless important to indicate briefly the major concepts held by Puerto Ricans about mental problems and their etiology, not only for their own general relevance to clinical practice but also as an introduction to spiritist theories of disease etiology.

Research on the topic of Puerto Rican concepts of mental illness (Rogler and Hollingshead 1965; Lubchansky, Egri, and Stokes 1970;

Gaviria and Wintrob 1976; Garrison 1977a; Harwood 1977) is remarkably consistent in indicating a clear distinction in Puerto Ricans' thinking between the concepts *locura* ("insanity," "craziness") and *nervios* ("nerves"; also referred to as *enfermedad de los nervios,* "sickness of the nerves"). *Locura,* on the one hand, refers to unpredictable behavior, often without regard for self-preservation; on the other hand, *nervios* may, in its "manic" aspect (*manía*), include such symptoms as chronic agitation, inability to concentrate, or pacing, and crying or silent brooding in its depressive manifestation. While "nerves" may be treated with rest, a change of scene, medication, or talking, sufferers of *locura* are stigmatized and thought to require physical restraint and confinement (Rogler and Hollingshead 1965). Both conditions, however, may be attributed to organic, situational (see the discussion of "stress" below), or spiritual factors working either alone or in combination (Gaviria and Wintrob 1976; Harwood 1977:77). Whether spiritual factors are implicated in particular cases of *nervios* or *locura* depends somewhat on the nature of the sufferer's symptoms but also on his beliefs and those of close associates.

SPIRITIST ETIOLOGICAL THEORIES   Most Puerto Ricans of various Christian persuasions conceive of human beings as consisting of two aspects: a finite, physical body and an eternal, nonmaterial spirit. Many Puerto Ricans also believe that the disembodied spirits of both deceased and divine beings play an active role in influencing the circumstances and behavior of the living. Only some Puerto Ricans, however, seek out spiritist mediums to diagnose and influence spiritual interventions in their own and others' lives. Estimates of the proportion of Puerto Ricans who do so vary from 30 to 40 percent in samples of the general population to more than 90 percent in samples from psychiatric clinics (Garrison 1977b: 99–100).

In accordance with a cosmology that posits both material and spiritual aspects of humanity, spiritist theories basically rely on the following three causes to explain disease: material factors, the disembodied spirits of divine or deceased humans, and the activities of living humans. Each of these causes may operate alone or in combination.

Material causes of illness include everything from hot/cold foods and drafts to germs and organic brain damage. That is, spiritist believers may espouse a range of theories concerning the etiology of material complaints, and all evidence indicates that believers in spirits and spirit communication attribute most somatic symptoms, at least initially, to these material causes and thus turn to medical facilities as the first source of care (Garrison 1977b:71–72, 101–104, 158–159; Harwood: 1977:74–77, 204–206). Since spiritists believe that a troubled spirit can contribute to

Table 7.5 Puerto Rican hot/cold classifications.

Category	*Frío* (cold)	*Fresco* (cool)	*Caliente* (hot)
Illnesses and bodily conditions	Arthritis Colds and upper respiratory symptoms (including asthma) *Empacho*[a] Menstrual period Muscular spasm (*pasmo*) Pain in the joints Upset stomach (*frialdad del estómago or frío en el estómago*)	None	Constipation Diarrhea Rashes Tenesmus (*pujo*) Ulcers
Medicines and Herbs	None	Bicarbonate of soda Linden flowers (*flor de tilo*) Mannitol (*maná de manito*) Mastic bark (*almácigo*) $MgCO_3$ (*magnesia boba*) Milk of magnesia Nightshade (*yerba mora*) Orange-flower water (*agua de azahar*) Sage	Anise Aspirin Castor oil Cinnamon Cod-liver oil Iron tablets Penicillin Rue (*ruda*) Vitamins

Foods

Avocado	Barley water	Alcoholic beverages
Bananas	Bottled milk	Chili peppers
Coconut	Chicken	Chocolate
Lima beans	Fruits	Coffee
Sugar cane	Honey	Corn meal
White beans	Raisins	Evaporated milk
	Salt cod (*bacalao*)	Garlic
	Watercress	Kidney beans
		Onions
		Peas
		Tobacco

Source: Adapted from A. Harwood, "The hot-cold theory of disease: Implications for treatment of Puerto Rican patients," *Journal of the American Medical Association* 216:1153–1158, copyright 1971, American Medical Association.

a. Characterized by nausea, vomiting, and/or diarrhea, mainly in children, *empacho* is attributed to an obstruction in the stomach or intestines caused by either a bolus of undigested food or saliva swallowed by a teething baby.

a material problem, however, people with medically diagnosed and treated somatic conditions (particularly those that are chronic or terminal) may also seek the services of a spirit medium to help them with the spiritual aspect of their illness. (See the section on becoming ill for further discussion of the symptoms that lead people to suspect a spiritual etiology for problems.)

Ideas concerning the spiritual causation of illness involve relationships between disembodied and incarnate spirits (that is, the living). According to spiritist belief, every person receives a guardian angel at birth, and perhaps additional helpers (*protecciones* or *guías*) at various times in life, to assist in maintaining his well-being and to advise in making right decisions. In addition to these spirits, who influence the living toward good behavior and higher spiritual goals, there are other, "little-elevated" spirits, who can influence people in adverse ways. These spirits can operate either on their own to cause people problems in life or at the instigation of the living, who may enlist them in acts of sorcery (*brujería*) against their enemies. In short, spiritual causes of illness or other problems may be seen as involving either purely spiritual agents or a combination of spiritual and human executors. The kinds of treatment that are instituted for such problems will be examined more closely later in the chapter.

Mal de Ojo (EVIL EYE)   The concept of the "evil eye" is used to explain the sudden onset in children of anything from mild discomfort to severe chronic illness or even death. Accepted as fact by nearly 70 percent of the mothers in the Health Center Study, this concept attributes children's problems to the inordinate attentions of an adult, usually a casual acquaintance rather than a close associate of the child's family. The adult is typically described as having praised or admired the child excessively or having secretly coveted him. To dispel any possibility of causing harm, an adult who has shown particular attention to a child blesses him during or at the close of the interaction with the phrase, "*¡Diós le [la] bendiga!*" ("God bless him [her]!"). Children may also wear charms made of jet (*azabache*) or coral, which are believed to serve as protection against the evil eye and are thought to shatter if the child falls under its influence.

Mal Humor   The concept of *mal humor* can be used in a variety of senses. In addition to signifying an angry disposition (similar to its direct English equivalent, "bad humor"), *mal humor* is also used to describe a congenital condition "of the blood," which is manifested in its carriers by chronic skin problems (for example, acne, boils, cuts that do not heal readily). Menstruating women may also be described as having *mal humor,* and they are believed to cause babies to come down with diarrhea if they handle them. *Mal humor* is thus both a source of affliction for its possessors and a contaminant for infants. Although both senses of the concept are widely known, the latter belief is treated by many as an old wives' tale, while the former receives more general credence.

"Virus" Although the "virus" has taken its place alongside drafts and chills as a cause of colds in the explanatory system of many Puerto Ricans, the precise referent of the term is vague or nonexistent for most of its users. Judging from the contexts in which "virus" is used, the idea almost surely derives from the mass media rather than from biomedical sources. Some people, for example, describe what they perceive to be the symptoms of "virus colds" as contrasted to chill-caused colds, often in the very terms used by advertisements in the mass media (Health Center Study). However, there is almost no consistency among informants in the criteria they use to distinguish the two concepts. For some people "virus" has also replaced or been added to "hot" foods as an etiological agent for diarrhea and other intestinal disorders.

"Stress" Although the actual word "stress," or its Spanish equivalent, is not generally heard in discussions of the causes of illness, several commonly used phrases readily equate with the popular meaning of this term in English. These phrases include "bad times" (*malos ratos*), "suffering" (*sufriendo*), "too many problems" (*demasiados problemas*), and "worry" (*preocupación*). These situational factors are deemed responsible for *nervios,* high blood pressure, and in some instances for other organic conditions as well, since a troubled mind is generally thought to precipitate physical ills (Padilla 1958:280–281; Murillo-Rohde 1976: 177; observations in the Health Center Study).

Popularized biomedical theories The biomedical concepts of disease most utilized by lay Puerto Ricans are germ theory, parasitic infection, and "allergy." (The term "allergy" has been placed in quotation marks to indicate that the concept is incompletely understood by most users of the term. Thus, although common allergens are widely recognized as such, the basic theory of allergic reactions is not generally understood.) It is significant that for many less educated people, biomedical concepts are used for conditions that have been diagnosed at some time in a family member or associate. In talking about such conditions, people often attribute their knowledge of the cause to a medical professional who has explained the etiology clearly. Sometimes, however, when the clinician has not explained the etiology fully, a dietary or behavioral restriction that has been prescribed in treating a disease is taken as its cause. (For example, walking upstairs may be seen as the "cause" of high blood pressure, sugar as the "cause" of diabetes.) Thus, biomedical professionals are directly and importantly responsible for the degree to which patients and their associates comprehend and employ biomedical concepts of causation correctly.

Classification of Illnesses

In a task administered as part of the Health Center Study, 11 adults were asked to sort 105 terms for diseases and bodily conditions into groups that they considered "went together."[15] Analysis of the responses revealed that eight principles of classification serve to sort all the terms into major classes and subclasses (table 7.6).

Clearly, all eight principles also serve in biomedicine for classifying diseases, symptoms, and professional specialties. The relative frequencies with which various principles are used by laymen and by medical personnel undoubtedly differ, however. In addition, although the classificatory principles used may be the same, in some cases both the terms linked by a particular principle and the meanings attached to specific terms may be quite different. A number of these differences that were verified as having

Table 7.6 Principles used by Puerto Rican respondents to classify diseases and bodily conditions.

Principle of classification	Example	Number of respondents (N = 11)
Part of the body afflicted	Diseases of the bones, heart; intestinal diseases	11
Sequential development (i.e., diseases or bodily conditions linked in a sequence, such that failure to cure one condition is said to bring on the next)	"If a person does not take care of a cold, bronchitis develops; and from bronchitis comes pneumonia."	10
Common cause	Parasitic diseases; "illnesses caused by bites"	8
Taxonomy	Types of cancer or tuberculosis	7
Common victims	Diseases of women, of children	6
Common effects	Paralytic diseases	5
Contagion	Contagious diseases	4
Chronicity	Chronic diseases	1

Source: Health Center Study.

more general currency among Puerto Ricans in the study have noteworthy implications for the health care of this population.

Before discussing these implications, however, it is important to point out that the sorting task, as well as subsequent discussions with the larger sample of Puerto Rican adults, revealed that among the vast majority of the sample the understanding of anatomy, the assignment of most conditions and diseases to an appropriate organ or organ system, and the knowledge of the symptoms of common optic and major respiratory diseases (tuberculosis, pneumonia) all conformed with the views of contemporary biomedicine. Moreover, most of the Puerto Ricans in the sample were conversant with major tropical diseases and parasites, and at least a third of the 11 respondents in the sorting task provided biomedically congruent definitions for rather abstruse terms such as pleurisy, urticaria, aneurysm, eclampsia, and leukemia. The following discussion of conceptual differences between the understandings of Puerto Rican laymen and those of biomedical professionals must therefore be viewed in the context of a considerable degree of conceptual congruence that also exists. It is also important to note that the degree of congruence is markedly greater, according to our data, for people with a year or more of secondary education.[16]

TERMS OR CONCEPTS CAUSING PROBLEMS IN COMMUNICATION   Terms for diseases or symptoms may engender difficulties in communication between patients and medical professionals if (1) the terms mean something different to patients and professionals, (2) the terms are ambiguous in the patient's native language, or (3) the terms refer to diseases with strong emotional connotations. Each of these possible sources of difficulty may influence Puerto Ricans' interactions with medical personnel.

1. Table 7.7 provides a list of terms that are likely to cause communication problems between professionals and laymen. Some of these terms (such as *falfayota* and *golondrinos*) are dialectal usages in Puerto Rican Spanish and may therefore cause problems in comprehension for speakers of other dialects. Other terms (such as *raquitis*, "rickets," *alta* and *baja presión*, "high" and "low blood pressure") involve nonbiomedical theories of disease and therefore require further explication.

Five out of the 11 people who participated in the Health Center Study's sorting task identified *raquitis* ("rickets") as tuberculosis in children. Further discussion with these people and other adults in the study indicated that the equation of these two diseases is based on their common association with poor nutrition. Because tuberculosis is widely feared among Puerto Ricans, the clinician would do well to forestall parents' fears by informing them clearly about the nature of rickets and its consequences if a child should be diagnosed with this condition.

Table 7.7 Potentially misunderstood Spanish terms for diseases or physical conditions.

Spanish term	English gloss
Acidez en el (*or* del) estómago	Stomach acidity, sour taste in mouth and throat after eructation
Alta presión	High blood pressure[a]
Anemia en los huesos	Literally, anemia in the bones, considered by many to be a form of tuberculosis
Asma	Asthma, can also refer to shortness of breath from any cause[a]
Ataque de alferecía	Convulsions in infants, thought to be caused by sudden fright (*susto*)[a]
Ataque cerebral	Stroke
Ataque de nervios	Nervous attack[a]
Baja presión	Low blood pressure[a], anemia
Catarro	"Cold," usually refers to one localized in the chest[a]
Ceguera	Conjunctivitis, any inflammation of the eye with exudate
Deficiencia en la sangre	"Weak blood," blood deficiency
Empacho	Upset stomach, nausea, attributed to a bolus of food in the intestine
Falfayota (*also* farfayota)	Mumps
Fatiga de ahogo	Asthma[a]
Fiebre palúdica	Malaria, sometimes used to refer to yellow fever
Flujo	Discharge, flow, particularly from vagina
Glándulas	Glands, swollen salivary glands
Golondrino	Small underarm tumor or cyst, said to occur in multiples
Jaqueca	Very bad headache, sometimes accompanied by nausea; migraine
Mala circulación	Bad circulation, may be caused by *sangre gruesa* (q.v) .
Nube en los ojos	Cataract
Orisma (aneurisma)	Aneurysm
Pasmo	Spasm of clonic or tonic variety, particularly facial paralysis. Thought to be caused by chills or drafts.[a]

Table 7.7 continued.

Spanish term	English gloss
Quebraduras	Hernia
Raquitis (mo)	Rickets; tuberculosis in children
Resfriado	Cold, usually refers to one localized in the nose
Reuma	Rheumatism, used as a synonym for arthritis
Sangre gruesa	Literally, "thick blood," blood overly rich in red corpuscles, polycythemia
Sapo	Thrush
Septicemia	"Pus" or "poison" in the blood, often associated with leukemia
Soplo en el corazón	Heart murmur
Tuberculosis en los huesos	Tuberculosis of the bone, sometimes equated with rickets (*raquitis*)

Source: Health Center Study.
a. See text for further explanation.

Ideas about blood pressure and other blood conditions vary considerably within the Puerto Rican population. In the Health Center Study sample, *alta presión* ("high blood pressure") was generally interpreted either as too much blood or, less often, as blood high in hemoglobin. The latter condition was alternatively labeled *sangre gruesa* ("thick blood") by some people, although 10 of the 30 adults with whom *sangre gruesa* was discussed claimed not to know this term at all. *Baja presión* ("low blood pressure"), on the other hand, was widely understood among the study population to mean "weak blood" (*sangre débil*), that is, blood low in hemoglobin. Thus for some Puerto Ricans (approximately a third of the study sample), either *alta presión* or *sangre gruesa* is closest in meaning to the medical term "polycythemia" and contrasts with *baja presión* which approximates the biomedical term "anemia." Although few people in the Health Center Study thus share the biomedical understanding of what high blood pressure is, many were nevertheless aware of etiological factors correlated with the condition (for example, overweight; "stress," as defined above; kidney problems). In view of these findings, a careful explanation of blood pressure would seem warranted for many Puerto Rican patients.

2. Two sets of terms—*catarro-resfriado* and *asma-fatiga*—may present problems in communication with medical professionals, largely because they have variant meanings to different Spanish speakers. In such a case,

when one may not be quite sure of a speaker's meaning in his native language, translation is likely to compound the unclarity even further.

Both *catarro* and *resfriado* are used to label the common cold. However, speakers of Puerto Rican Spanish differ in their usage of these terms: some use them synonymously and claim there is no difference between the two; others, however, use *resfriado* to refer to a cold in the nose or head, and *catarro* for a cold in the chest; still others make this distinction between the location of symptoms but use exactly the opposite terms for doing so. Because of these variations, a Spanish speaker may be unsure of the precise symptoms his interlocutor is referring to and may need to ask for further clarification—a procedure that the clinician might profitably carry over into the medical setting. Furthermore, it is important to note that in rendering both *catarro* and *resfriado* simply as "cold" in English, a translator may obscure information that the Spanish speaker has provided about the location of respiratory symptoms.

A similar though somewhat more complex situation prevails with the words *asma* and *fatiga* in Puerto Rican Spanish. Although the majority of people use these terms synonymously, they may use them to label different symptoms. Thus for some, the two terms are used to refer to shortness of breath accompanied by wheezing; for others, however, the terms are used to refer simply to shortness of breath, regardless of cause. In the Health Center Study a number of people spoke of themselves or others as having *asma* or *fatiga* when they gasped for air after having climbed stairs or exerted themselves in any way. (Some of the people so described had medically diagnosed cardiovascular conditions.) Other Spanish speakers (about a third of the Health Study sample) do not use the terms *asma* and *fatiga* synonymously at all. For these people *fatiga* is an acute condition, accompanied by wheezing, a cough, and high fever, whereas *asma* refers to a chronic condition, characterized by shortness of breath and wheezing. Because of the wide range of meanings attached to these two terms, the clinician might well probe for further clarification if either term should be reported in a history or as a symptom.

3. In addition to the terms mentioned above, there are a number of others that may present communication problems, not because of their meanings, however, but because of their emotional connotations—particularly the emotions of fear and disgrace. Probably the two most feared diseases among Puerto Ricans are cancer and tuberculosis—the former because it is regarded as incurable, and the latter because it is contagious. The fear attached to these diseases may cause people to delay seeking medical help for symptoms associated with them and may also inhibit discussion with the physician of their suspected or actual diagnosis.

A sense of disgrace, the other major emotional impediment to communication with medical personnel, is most often attached to venereal disease[17] and *locura* ("insanity") in Puerto Rican culture. Because tuberculosis is viewed as contagious and its victims are likely, therefore, to be shunned by neighbors and kin, this disease carries a certain stigma as well.[18] If a person should contract one of these stigmatized ailments, close relatives are likely to report to neighbors, children, or more distant kin that the sick person is suffering from a different, nonstigmatized ailment. Some of the substituted ailments have gained sufficient currency to function as euphemisms for stigmatized diseases. "Anemia," for example, often refers to tuberculosis. This social practice is relevant for medical care in that patients may be unable to provide an accurate family medical history because they do not in fact know that a close relative has either had or died of a stigmatized illness, particularly if they were children at the time the person was ill.

EFFECTS OF DIFFERENT MODES OF CLASSIFICATION   "Sequential development" (see table 7.6) is the principle of classification most likely to produce instances in which the understandings of some Puerto Ricans are at variance with those of medical professionals. (This principle posits that a disease or condition develops out of a prior condition if the latter is not cured.) The variance comes from the layman's linking conditions or diseases in a sequence which, in the biomedical view, does not occur.

The Health Center Study isolated three developmental sequences which are not considered valid biomedically but which were posited by varying numbers of Puerto Ricans. The most commonly accepted of these sequences (by 23 out of 28 adults in the study) is that ulcers (of both the skin and the gastrointestinal tract) lead to cancer. The other two sequences, that untreated venereal disease can lead to tuberculosis and that a vaginal discharge (*flujo*) can turn into cancer, were less widely accepted (by only about one-quarter of the adults in the study). It is noteworthy that in all three of these instances the subsequent disease is more deadly, and thus more feared by patients, than the first. In practical terms, it may therefore be wise for the clinician who diagnoses the first condition to probe the patient's understanding of what may develop, in order to allay any unwarranted fears of more serious consequences.

Another developmental sequence that is very prevalent in many Puerto Ricans' thinking about disease links together various respiratory ailments, all of which are classified as "cold" in the humoral theory of disease. In its most elaborate form the sequence posits that a cold (usually *catarro* is the Spanish word used in this context) may lead to influenza, which may lead to bronchitis, which may lead ultimately to pneumonia. In simpler versions, influenza and bronchitis may be eliminated from the series, thus approximating it more closely to the biomedical view. An additional sequence, also stemming from hot/cold theory, predicates either a cold (*catarro*) or bronchitis, persistent and uncured, as a forerunner of chronic asthma.[19] This sequence is related to an idea that any cold-classified symptom (cough, stomach pain, joint pain) may become chronic if the sufferer is further exposed to a chill or eats cold-classified foods. The verb *pasmarse* is used to describe this eventuality, as in the statement, *Cuando tenía ronquera, tomé jugo de china y me pasmé,* which best translates as, "When I was hoarse with a cold, I drank orange juice and became chronically hoarse." These beliefs about the sequential development of progressively more serious "chill-caused" respiratory diseases provoke considerable concern among Puerto Ricans who live in substandard, inadequately heated housing.

ARCHAIC CONCEPTS AND IDIOMS   Although some Puerto Ricans consider a number of the concepts discussed previously as archaic (for example, the hot/cold theory, the evil eye, *sangre gruesa*), research in the Health Center Study revealed that these concepts are far from extinct. The concepts "weak womb" (*matriz débil*) and *alferecía,* however, were very widely considered moribund and were encountered among only a handful of women, mostly over age 45.

A *matriz débil* ("weak womb") is thought to leap about in the abdominal cavity in search of something "hot." In doing so, it may rise into the gastric region and is believed capable of choking the victim unless it is treated by a "hot" remedy. Although this condition is generally treated by either home remedies or lay curers (see the section on nonmainstream care), the clinician may encounter an elderly woman who describes similar symptoms.

Although most Spanish-English dictionaries translate *alferecía* as "epilepsy," it is clearly distinguished from epileptic attacks (*ataques epilépticos*) in Puerto Rican Spanish. *Alferecía* refers instead to convulsions in babies, thought to be a reaction to fright (*susto*) brought on by loud noises or other startling occurrences. Although this concept was generally considered an "old wives' tale" and was not widely used in the Health Center population, clinicians should be aware of it in order to avoid using *alferecía* as a translation for epilepsy.

Pain in the lower back or kidney region is often referred to as *la cintura abierta.* Although this phrase translates literally as "open waist," it does not in fact imply any such etiology and functions simply as an idiom referring to a lower-back problem.

Intraethnic Variation in Concepts

Although clearly it would be clinically useful to provide a formula by which health-care providers could predict which Puerto Rican patients were most likely to hold what beliefs about disease classification and etiology, this is not now possible with the data at hand. Additional studies, using samples that included a broader geographic and socioeconomic cross section of the Puerto Rican population, would be necessary to provide reasonably accurate predictions. To cope with this indeterminacy, the clinician should be aware of diagnoses, treatment regimens, and other aspects of the medical encounter that are likely to be influenced by beliefs about disease, in order to know when to explore an individual patient's views in some detail.

Notwithstanding this caveat about the current limitations of our ability to predict individual patients' beliefs, the Health Center Study does suggest that the most reliable indicator of Puerto Ricans' health beliefs is educational attainment. Completion of at least one year of high school seems to differentiate with reasonable probability between adherence to popularized and more orthodox biomedical theories and adherence to hot/cold or other folk theories of disease.

It is important to point out, however, that the relationship between education and belief is more subtle than just a simple correlation. First, beliefs and values by their very nature are subject to complex situational determinants that often make highly accurate prediction about either verbal statements or actions very difficult. Thus, for example, we have observed among the more educated some individuals who verbally disparage the hot/cold theory but who, when ill, use remedies from this system, remembered from childhood.

Furthermore, more educated people may also apply biomedical theories erratically to different diseases. For example educational attainment seems to correlate nicely with adherence to biomedical concepts for explaining childhood diseases. Thus, among the 32 adults in the Health Center Study who were questioned about the causes of measles, mumps, chicken pox, and whooping cough, the 8 who attributed these diseases to germs or contagion had a median educational attainment of 9 years, whereas the 24 adults who attributed the diseases to chills or seasonal changes in temperature or who said they did not know the causes had a median educational attainment of only 5 years. When the same 32 adults, plus 5 others from the study, were questioned about the etiology of colds, however, the relationship between educational background and beliefs was not so apparent. Thirty people (with a median educational attainment of 6 years and a range of 0 to 11 years) attributed the cause of colds to agents or behaviors implied by the hot/cold theory (for example, "change in temperature," "not wearing a sweater when it's cold," "bare feet on a cold floor"), 3 (with educational attainments of 1, 5, and 8 years) to contagion ("contact with a person who has a cold," "dust [polvo] that one breathes in the street"), and 4 (with educational attainments of 4, 7, 8, and 10 years) to both hot/cold agents and contagion. Ideas about the causes of asthma reflected a similar lack of correlation and educational attainment: of 28 adults, 7 (with a median educational attainment of only 3 years) attributed this condition to various allergens (dog or cat hair, dust, pollen, and so on), while 19 (with a median educational attainment of 5 years) attributed it to an old, uncured cold, dampness, or chill; and 2 people (with educational attainments of 5 and 10 years) attributed it to both sets of factors. In sum, although completion of at least one year of high school predicts with some reliability a general tendency to apply popular or biomedical rather than folk concepts, it may fail to predict actual behavior and beliefs about specific diseases or conditions.

The reason for the incomplete abandonment of folk medical theories (especially the hot/cold theory) by more educated people seems to rest with two facts. First, although hot/cold and biomedical therapies differ in their basic premises, the behavior they imply is probably more similar than antipathetic. Thus, the use of penicillin for rheumatic fever, aspirin for relief of colds or arthritic pain, and dietary restrictions for ulcer patients are therapeutic interventions that comport equally with both etiological systems. The two systems, in other words, are in many cases not in competition. A second reason for the retention of hot/cold and other folk theories seems to rest in the indeterminacy of biomedical theory itself. The notion that germs cause colds, tuberculosis, and so on still leaves open the question of why only some individuals contract these diseases when the germs are known to be omnipresent. Because biomedicine has traditionally lacked a theory of the healthy person and what contributes to individual well-being, concepts such as the hot/cold balance, "worry," the equation of body weight with health, and other theories have filled this important gap in health beliefs for Puerto Ricans. Only recently has the biomedical emphasis on prevention begun to provide concepts that can replace these older folk ideas.

Becoming Ill

In a set of classic articles, Zola (1964, 1966, 1973) discussed variations in the way symptoms are evaluated by several American ethnic groups. Briefly, he found two basic styles of presenting complaints: one, a narrow focus on specific organic dysfunctions (typical of Irish ethnics); and the other, a more global presentation of a variety of malfunctions (common among Italians). While the Puerto Rican pattern seems closer to the Italian one in many respects, Puerto Ricans also focus on certain specific symptoms and areas of the body for evaluating physical discomfort.

Attention to Symptoms

On various health-status inventories Puerto Ricans on both the mainland and the island consistently reported more psychiatric and somatic symptoms than did other American ethnic groups (Dohrenwend and Dohrenwend 1969; Haberman 1970, 1976; Weisenberg et al. 1975: 125; Weidman 1978:336ff.); they also reported more such symptoms than 610 ostensibly healthy New Yorkers of varying backgrounds (Garrison 1977b:table 16). Since evidence indicates that the inventories used in these studies do not reflect actual morbidity so much as "perceived health status" (Suchman and Phillips 1958, Pasamanick 1962, Kole 1966, for the Cornell Medical Index; Dohrenwend and Dohrenwend 1969:57–94, Haberman 1976, for the 22-item Langner list developed for the Midtown Manhattan Study), the results of these studies may best be used to identify symptom clusters that are most salient to Puerto Ricans in evaluating their health status.

In brief, the inventories indicate that the following somatic irregularities receive particular attention in evaluating health among Puerto Ricans: fever, respiratory problems (see Weidman 1978:321), fatigue, loss of appetite or weight, hoarseness, and (in women) urogenital problems. In addition, responses to the inventories imply a greater propensity among Puerto Ricans, as compared to other American groups, to express distress freely in terms of not only somatic but also psychological symptoms (Dohrenwend and Dohrenwend 1969:81–88; Weisenberg et al. 1975). This observation is complemented by evidence that Puerto Rican nurses are more prone to infer high psychological distress in medical patients than their professional counterparts from other countries—specifically Japan, Taiwan, Thailand, and the continental United States (Davitz, Davitz, and Higuchi 1977). It is also the case, moreover, that Puerto Ricans of varying educational and occupational levels interpret psychological symptoms as "illness" significantly less frequently than members of other ethnic groups of comparable class background (Guttmacher and Elinson 1971).

It is important to point out that the dichotomy between somatic and psychological symptoms appears not to be drawn as rigidly in the popular Puerto Rican subculture as it is in the general American or biomedical subcultures. Indeed, Puerto Ricans are very likely to associate physical symptoms with psychosocial causes (Murillo-Rohde 1976:177). For example, suffering and worry are thought to cause pains in the chest around the heart and throat as well as difficulty in breathing. They are also said to damage the nerves (Padilla 1958:280 281, 287) and to cause generalized aches and pains (*achaques*) (Padilla 1958:280–281, 283–284, 287).

Thus, in many ways Puerto Ricans' view of illness is fundamentally holistic or truly psychosomatic and therefore at variance with the prevailing physicalistic conceptions of biomedicine (Engel 1977). Indeed, one might suggest that the reason Puerto Ricans are often seen by health professionals as suffering from psychosomatic ills is that out of a fundamentally different cultural conception of illness, they do indeed present themselves in this way. To the extent that Puerto Ricans are then "diagnostically dismissed" or referred to psychiatrists, they have become the victims of a cultural discrepancy between their own views of illness and those of biomedicine; their problems have not in fact been addressed.

Interpreting Symptoms

Although symptoms may be *understood* in terms of the hot/cold, popularized biomedical, spiritist, and other explanatory frameworks described earlier, they are most likely to be *acted upon* in terms of their perceived seriousness, persistence, and incapacitating effects. Certain symptoms (for example, fever, blood loss, respiratory problems) are considered inherently serious, however, and generally result in remedial action, often medical consultation. Several nonsomatic symptoms may be interpreted as being specifically spiritual in origin by those who accept this theory of causality and are then referred to an appropriate folk specialist for further consultation. (See the following section for a discussion of spiritist therapy.)

Most other symptoms, however, depend for their evaluation not so much on any notion of their inherent seriousness as on the sex, age, and role responsibilities of the sufferer. Thus, although wives and mothers talk about their symptoms a great deal, they generally do not consider them serious enough to require action unless the condition persists or becomes incapacitating. Men, on the other hand, tend to deny symptoms altogether but do respond to them when they interfere with work or some other habitual activity.

The task of evaluating the seriousness of symptoms and recommending a course of action generally falls upon women. Children and husbands turn to their mothers and wives respectively, although some married men still prefer the opinion of their mothers when feeling ill. Women confer with female relatives or friends about their own symptoms and those of their families. Relatives and neighbors who work in medical settings or have had any kind of nursing training are especially sought for their opinions, particularly in situations in which the symptoms are feared to be serious. When a child evidences symptoms, a grandmother or a great-aunt may assume the role of diagnostician and will be heeded out of respect for her age, even when the mother does not entirely agree with the recommended course of action.

Implications for Clinical Practice

Given the relative openness with which Puerto Ricans express both emotional and physical concerns, the clinician may, after taking a standard history, be confronted with a relatively long and (from a professional viewpoint) perplexingly diffuse set of symptoms for evaluation. In coping with this situation, the clinician should, however, be cautious in making psychiatric diagnoses, not only because the number and kinds of psychiatric symptoms reported by Puerto Ricans are quite clearly culturally conditioned (Dohrenwend and Dohrenwend 1969:79–93, 169–170; Haberman 1976) but also because the evidence is persuasive that cultural and linguistic factors do bias the diagnosis and hospitalization of Hispanic patients (Rendon 1976:118–120; Alers 1978:16–21). An appropriate medical workup should also precede any attempt to diagnose reported physical symptoms as "psychosomatic."

Though reports of somatic symptoms should generally be taken as valid and handled medically until there is adequate justification for treating them psychologically, it is true that certain symptoms tend to function for Puerto Ricans as verbalizations for a general feeling of malaise rather than as actual descriptions of physical sensations. Thus, since a normal, healthy body is assumed not to become chronically tired or devoid of the desire for food, the sufferer who complains of either fatigue or loss of appetite or weight may only wish to convey vague feelings of physical or psychological unease. In addition, reports of menstrual irregularity may be a way of expressing general malaise or physical impairment, since menstruation is believed to keep women healthy by ridding the body of "unclean" or "waste" blood (Scott 1975:107–108). When any of these symptoms are reported, therefore, deeper inquiry into the meaning the patient assigns to them is warranted.

The fact that women are the main evaluators of symptoms and the ones who make preliminary diagnoses and decisions about treatment implies that they are likely targets for health education. Since female relatives and friends also consult one another about symptoms and, if possible, seek out acquaintances with formal health-care training, information might best be disseminated along such preexisting channels. This would mean training more Hispanic health-care professionals who could act as information sources in the community.

Coping with Illness outside the Mainstream Medical System

Nonmainstream medical care is defined here as all health care provided outside a professional medical setting—that is, in the home, the local pharmacy, or the dispensary of a folk healer. These sources of care may be used prior to, in conjunction with, or subsequent to consultation with mainstream health professionals. This section will discuss the kinds of treatment offered by these various sources of care, the sequence in which they may be used, and their possible benefit or harm to the sufferer and his kin.

Medical Care in the Home and Family: Health Maintenance

For many Puerto Ricans, "to be strong, to have good color (pink cheeks), to be plump, and to have no pains" are the signs of good health (Padilla 1958:278). To maintain this state, three activities are deemed important: eating right, keeping warm, and keeping clean (Health Center Study; Weidman 1978:311–312).

DIETARY PATTERNS   "Eating right" entails taking sufficient food to feel full and maintain a constant body weight, which is often higher than medically recommended levels (particularly for women).[20] Furthermore, loss of weight or appetite is seen as one of the most important signs of illness, as mentioned previously.

Puerto Ricans generally follow a three-meal-a-day pattern of food consumption, often with the addition of several snacks during the day.[21] For adults breakfast usually consists of coffee that is about half milk, taken with bread and butter; for children eggs or cereal are also provided. Although children and working adults often adopt the more general American pattern of a sandwich for lunch, the midday and evening meals are by preference substantial and consist of rice, a variety of beans, and often meat and salad. Milk consumption is high among both children and adults (a finding reported by Sanjur, Romero, and Kira 1971 for a rural mainland population and supported by Lieberman 1979 and my own urban data). Although some nutritionists have expressed concern over the underconsumption of iron (Browering et al. 1978) and green vegetables by continental Puerto Ricans (Torres 1959:352; Sanjur, Romero, and Kira 1971:1325), the diet is generally considered adequate in essential nutrients (Yohai 1977:274; Bowering et al. 1978).

An additional component of what many Puerto Ricans consider to be a healthful diet are tonics (*tónicos*), the most popular of which are eggnogs and *malta* (a commercially manufactured beverage made from caramel, a small quantity of malt extract, and sugar). These tonics are consumed for added strength and energy, particularly by children who appear pale or underweight and by pregnant and postpartum women. Tonics (and vitamins) are also believed to stimulate the appetite. This use of high-calorie substances as appetite stimulants, as well as the preference for two substantial meals a day, underscores the importance of weight maintenance in Puerto Ricans' conception of good health.

KEEPING WARM   In agreement with popular Western concepts, many Puerto Ricans see respiratory ailments as being directly related to chills and drafts. (See the earlier discussion of illness classification.) As a result, they tend to bundle infants and children warmly in winter and to keep windows closed. The substandard housing conditions under which many poor Puerto Ricans in the northern United States live, where heating is often problematic during the winter months, means that parents are unable to provide the warm living conditions for their children which are considered necessary to good health. This failure, together with the additional health hazards and outright discomfort of poor housing, has led many Puerto Ricans to consider housing development and renovation as a logical and necessary concomitant of preventive medicine (Harwood 1971b; Alers 1978:77).

Care of the Sick in the Home

CARETAKERS   Just as women tend to act as diagnosticians for all family members, so, too, do they act as caretakers to the sick. When the woman of the household is herself ill, or when the amount of care required for a family member is more than the wife/mother can handle alone, female relatives of the wife or husband often assist. *Comadres*[22] and a few close neighbors may help out as well. During the period of observation 24 of the 79 households in the Health Center Study either provided or received substantial help from other households during either pregnancy or an illness episode. In these circumstances kinswomen or *comadres* assisted one another with child care, shopping, and other household chores, as well as actual nursing care.

CONDITIONS LIKELY TO BE TREATED AT HOME   Among the families in the Health Center Study, no chronic symptoms or conditions were treated exclusively within the home. Among acute conditions, colds (unless accompanied by a high fever), "virus," diarrhea, "nervous attacks" (*ataques de nervios*), minor burns and cuts, and minor muscular pains were all more likely to be treated at home than by any outside source of care. On the other hand, influenza, headache, upset stomach, children's diseases (mumps, chicken pox, measles), earache, and hoarseness were handled in the home about as frequently as they were taken outside it for care. Other acute conditions (coughs, sore throat, fever, major injuries, and chest or back pains) were more commonly taken to outside sources for treatment—practices that are consistent with the diagnostic importance of fever and respiratory ailments as indicators of serious illness for members of this ethnic group.

TREATMENTS RENDERED IN THE HOME   Table 7.8 lists by functional categories the herbal and over-the-counter preparations found in 36 of the 79 households that participated in the Health Center Study.[23] The tabulation underestimates the prevalence of herbal use, however, since these substances are generally not kept in stock but are procured as needed

Table 7.8 Frequency of occurrence of nonprescription (herbal and over-the-counter) medicines in 36 Puerto Rican households.

Type of medication	Percentage of households with one or more such medication[a] (N = 36)
Balms, essences, and liniments	100
Alcohol, *alcoholado*[b], or *Alcoholado Relámpago*[c]	100
Agua florida	6[d]
Assorted liniments (Ben-Gay, Sloan's, mutton tallow, etc.)	25
Analgesics (aspirin, Bufferin, etc.)	92
Medicines for upper respiratory infections	89
Vicks VapoRub	56
Cough syrups	42
Medicines for sore throats (gargles, medicated lozenges, etc.)	14
Nose drops or spray	8
Medicines for digestive disorders	53
Antacids and other medication for upset stomach (Pepto-Bismol, Gelucil, star anise)	39
Laxatives	25[e]
Vitamins, tonics, and other food supplements	17
First aid supplies (antiseptics, Band Aids, etc.)	14
Medicines for rashes and other skin conditions	8
Eyewash	6

Source: Health Center Study.

a. Percentages reported for subcategories of medication do not equal total percentage because some households stocked more than one type.

b. *Alcoholado* is a 70% solution of rubbing alcohol.

c. *Alcoholado Relámpago* is a 70% isopropyl alcohol solution mixed with oil of eucalyptus, oil of pine, menthol, and camphor.

d. The percentage of households that stock *agua florida,* an essence used for headaches and for spiritist practices, is without doubt underestimated here, since this substance is not considered a "medicine" by many and therefore may not have been produced in answer to the researchers' request to see all medications in the household.

e. The most commonly used laxative was milk of magnesia.

either from an herb shop (*botánica*) or from relatives in Puerto Rico. Most of the remedies listed are used both for conditions treated exclusively in the home and, in conjunction with prescribed medication, for those illnesses treated simultaneously outside it. Balms and liniments, herbal teas, aspirin, milk of magnesia, and Pepto-Bismol are preparations that respondents considered "traditional" home remedies (*remedios caseros*). Headache compounds and Vicks VapoRub, on the other hand, were purchased as a result of advertisements in the mass media. Buffered aspirin and certain antacids (for example, Gelusil) were generally recommended by a doctor or nurse.

Most over-the-counter preparations are administered symptomatically in conformity with popular American standards—that is, commercial cough syrups for coughs; aspirin for headaches, fever, and muscular pain; and so forth. Cathartics, however, may be taken as treatment for any acute condition to rid the body of infection (Padilla 1958:287). In addition, one-third of the 36 families in the study used cathartics on a regular, though infrequent basis to "clean" the system. The dosing intervals varied from once a month to once a year, and the most common recipients were children and the elderly.

One patent medicine, Vicks VapoRub, approaches the status of a panacea for Puerto Ricans. It is used for a far wider range of ailments than recommended on the label (for example, for asthmatic attacks, backache, muscular pain, headache, and earache); it may also be taken internally, either alone or in tea, for a "congested" (*apretado*) chest.

Several herbal and over-the-counter preparations are quite routinely administered in conformity with the hot/cold theory of disease etiology. For example, the preferred remedy for upset stomach and constipation (both "hot" conditions) is "cool"-classified milk of magnesia rather than either castor oil, which is "hot," or other commercial cathartics, whose categorization in the hot/cold system is less clear. Similarly, "hot" children's diseases involving rashes, like measles and chicken pox, are treated with special "cool" preparations (for example, raisins soaked in milk) to "bring out the rash." For treating colds, however, "hot"-classified substances (such as cod-liver oil, ginger, or oregano tea) are preferred, and certain emetic or cathartic syrups (*jarabes*), concocted of mainly "hot" but also some "cool" substances, are also often administered, particularly to children. Reputedly serving to remove accumulated phlegm from the digestive tract, the most common of these syrups, *los siete aceites* (the seven oils) consists of honey, ipecac, cod-liver oil, almond extract, castor oil, oil of eucalyptus, and the "oil" of an egg (the clear residue after the white has been beaten until fluffy). Herbal teas and infusions (*tés* or *tisanas*) may also be used as part either of hot/cold therapeutics or of a less systematic tradition of herbal treatment. (See the section on herb shops below.)

A highly important aspect of Puerto Rican home treatment is the use of massage with a variety of balms and alcohol compounds (see table 7.8, which attests to the ubiquity of these medications in the home). This form of treatment may be used not only for specific symptoms (cough, headache, fever, or muscular and joint pains) but also for nonspecific "aches and pains," lassitude, or "nerves." Indeed, giving a rubdown (*dar un sobo*) to an ailing person epitomizes the caring relationship between close kin and undoubtedly serves important psychological functions for not only the sick but also their caretakers.

To provide some indication of the frequencies with which different kinds of medications are administered in treating an ailment commonly handled within the home, table 7.9 itemizes the treatments used for 46 cases of influenza that occurred during an epidemic in the winter of 1969 (Health Center Study data). Every influenza victim received at least one remedy, and almost half were treated with at least two. As can be seen, remedies from both the popular and folk health traditions are used.

USE OF MEDICATION PRESCRIBED FOR OTHERS   Although it is quite common for people to save prescription medicines for their own use in the event that they experience the same symptoms again, 14 pairs of individuals in the Health Center Study were also involved in at least one instance of borrowing prescription medicines. Most commonly the pairs were women who were close friends and neighbors. The conditions for which medications were borrowed include "nerves" (for which tranquilizers were taken), asthma, abdominal or stomach pain, hay fever, earache, and "vaginal pain." Three pairs of women were involved in regular transfers of medication, one for "ulcers" (self-diagnosed) and two for "nerves."

Table 7.9   Home treatment by Puerto Ricans of 46 cases of influenza (1969).

Kind of treatment	Cases treated[a]	
	No.	%
Aspirin	25	54
Tea	17	37
Massage (VapoRub or alcohol)	9	20
Home botanical (syrups or infusions)	6	13
Juice or other liquid	3	7
"Penicillin" injection[b]	2	4
Prescription medicine left from earlier ailment	2	4
Over-the-counter tonic or cough syrup	2	4

Source: Health Center Study.

a. Since some cases were treated with more than one remedy, the treatments total 66 instead of 46, and the sum of the percentages does not equal 100.

b. One of these injections was administered by a physician during an office visit, the other at home by the sick person's sister, who was a nurse. Whether the substance injected was actually penicillin was not confirmed.

Though socially these transfers of medication clearly serve to enhance relationships of reciprocity and trust by demonstrating the willingness of one party to assist the other in time of distress, medically their effects are somewhat more difficult to assess. Thus, even though two instances of borrowing resulted in drug reactions, the ill effects were not serious enough to warrant medical attention and were sufficiently frightening to the protagonists to prevent further borrowing. In other instances, the medications were inappropriate for the borrower's ailment but were not harmful in themselves. In only one instance (the chronic borrower of medicine for "ulcers") did the practice have a clearly negative effect in delaying presentation for medical diagnosis of the condition.

Lay Referral for Care outside the Home

As chief diagnosticians and caretakers, Puerto Rican women play a key role in the lay referral network. Positive and negative experiences with lay and professional sources of care are routinely discussed among kinswomen and neighbors, and participants in the Health Center Study agreed very closely as to which hospitals and outpatient facilities were best for different services. Thus, except for the most isolated families, when the decision to seek care outside the home is reached, the range of appropriate facilities is usually already known. The choice of which facility to attend in any given instance, however, is conditioned by a number of factors. As discussed in the previous section, symptoms constitute a major factor, although considerations of cost and distance may override judgments about the best facility based on the sufferer's symptomatology.

Because of women's greater knowledge of health-care facilities and their accepted role as caretakers of the sick, the wife/mother is generally the most influential family member in deciding where to go for care outside the home. However, the husband in his role as provider may alter her decision when considerations of cost are an issue. Adult children exert strong influence in convincing ailing elderly parents to go for treatment outside the home (Tallmer 1977:94–95; Health Center Study observations).

Nonmainstream Care outside the Home

Studies of Puerto Ricans' usage of health-care facilities (Padilla 1958:284; Garrison 1977b:158; Weidman 1978:269, 272; Lieberman 1979; Health Center Study observations) report with notable uniformity a primary reliance on mainstream biomedical care. Nevertheless, in certain circumstances, determined mainly by symptoms and cost, care may also be sought either in the first instance or secondarily from pharmacists, herb shops (botánicas), spiritists (espiritistas and santeros), curanderos, or evangelical faith healers.

PHARMACISTS AS SOURCES OF CARE   Like people of any ethnic background, Puerto Ricans often turn to a pharmacist for diagnostic assistance
for digestive and mild respiratory complaints. These requests for diagnostic advice usually result in the purchase of an over-the-counter preparation, which is typically recommended by the druggist with the admoni-
tion that the customer see a doctor if the symptoms persist. Some
neighborhood pharmacies are also known to sell drugs without prescription to recognized customers. These stores typically supply either refills,
when the customer does not wish to spend the time or money to return to
the doctor, or self-prescribed medications, the uses for which are common
knowledge (for example, penicillin). Hispanic pharmacies are the main
providers of certain patent medicines popular in Latin America (such as
Serebrina la Francesa, a bromide used for menstrual cramps, and *Emul-
sión Jiménez,* a mixture of cod-liver oil and ipecac extract used for
coughs), as well as of substances used in traditional forms of treatment
(for example, *Alcoholado Relámpago* or mannite, used as a "cooling"
agent in the hot/cold system of therapy). Some "American" pharmacies
in Hispanic neighborhoods also stock these items.

HERB SHOPS (*Botánicas*) AS SOURCES OF CARE   Found in most Hispanic neighborhoods, *botánicas* are patronized for both herbal and spiritist
remedies, and customers vary as to whether they use them for only one
or both of these systems of therapy.[24] In keeping with their caretaker role,
women tend to be the major buyers of botanicals; they are also the principal users. (In addition to Hispanics, the clientele of herb shops often
also include West Indians and American blacks.)

Apart from their use in spiritist treatment, which will be discussed below, *botánicas* are patronized mainly for "nerves" (*los nervios*) and for
digestive, respiratory, rheumatic, and genitourinary symptoms. Thus, the
complaints for which these herb shops are used parallel closely the problems taken to pharmacies. In general, people with a secondary-school education or people raised on the mainland use only pharmacies for these
complaints; others may patronize one source of care or the other, depending on their knowledge of a remedy for the particular complaint.
Botanicals may also be used conjointly with medically prescribed regimens or, as a last resort, after medical treatment has been considered a
failure.

Deriving from both Native American and European traditions, the most
commonly administered botanicals include orange-flower water (*agua
de azahar*) and linden tea (*tilo*) for "nerves"; peppermint (*yerba buena*),
star anise (*anís estrella*), and chamomile (*manzanilla*) teas for digestive
disorders; and fomentations or poultices concocted of substances such as
flaxseed, mustard, and ginger for rheumatic and lower back pains. Since

herbal medicine is largely a pragmatic art, however, individuals often have their own idiosyncratic pet remedies.

Except for a few laxative substances—for example, *pasote* (*Chenopodium* spp.) and licorice (*Glycyrrhiza glabra*)—most of the commonly used botanicals are probably of little pharmacological benefit.[25] However, a number of them, although rarely used, may be harmful: members of the genera *Artemisia* (wormwood, mugwort; Spanish, *ajenjo, artemisa*), *Kalmia* (laurel; Spanish, *laurel*), and *Sanguinaria* (bloodroot; Spanish, *correguela* or *sanguinaria*).

SPIRITISTS AS SOURCES OF CARE   Spiritist healers are mediums—that is, people who are said to be capable of giving over their bodies to incorporeal spirits so that these spirits can communicate with the living. Spiritists work in a group, which is headed by the medium reputed to have the strongest powers of contacting and controlling spirits. The group may meet regularly either in the head medium's house or in special ritual quarters called a *centro*. These *centros*, located in storefronts, the back rooms of *botánicas*, or the basements of apartment buildings, are commonplace in Hispanic neighborhoods.

Surveys have indicated that approximately one-third of all Puerto Rican adults seek help from a spiritist at some time in their lives (Lubchansky, Egri, and Stokes 1970:313; Garrison 1972:256–257). These spiritist consultations most frequently occur under a number of conditions (Garrison 1977b:162–163; Harwood 1977:74–76): (1) when people experience certain symptoms that are indicative in psychiatric nosology of intrapsychic problems (for example, insomnia, suicidal urges, repeated nightmares, unaccountable crying or silent brooding, fugue states, or unpredictable, repeated *ataques*); (2) interpersonal problems, often associated with life transitions (for example, puberty, the beginning years of marriage, menopause); (3) medically diagnosed chronic or terminal conditions (for example, asthma, cancer), for which patients may come under joint medical and spiritual treatment; and (4) somatic complaints which a physician has been unable to either diagnose or treat to the patient's satisfaction.

Occasionally, too, a person will turn to a medium with a medically undiagnosed but feared somatic symptom (for example, when cancer may be implicated). Because spiritism accepts both material and spiritual causes of problems, spiritists in such circumstances often treat the "spiritual cause" and recommend consultation with a physician for treatment of the "material cause" (Harwood 1977:75–77). All available evidence indicates that spiritists do *not* compete with physicians in treating medically manageable organic diseases (Garrison 1977b:158–159; Harwood 1977:204–206).

Most spiritist clients receive short-term, crisis-oriented treatment, which entails three elements: (1) diagnosis of the problem in sociospiritual terms (that is, in terms of both the client's social relationships and the intervention of spirits in his life), (2) procedures for ridding the client of noxious spiritual influences and for improving his relationships with beneficent spiritual protectors, and (3) direct counseling concerning social relationships and personal attitudes. These activities may take place in private sessions between the medium and client, in family groups, or in large groups at *centro* meetings. The second aspect of treatment mentioned above generally involves a regimen of prayer, performance of certain rites for pertinent spirits, and the use of herbal preparations. Clients are provided with prescriptions, which are filled at *botánicas,* for the substances required in these activities.

A relatively small percentage of spiritist clients receive long-term treatment. These clients are generally people who present to the spiritist with serious and persistent psychological symptoms, such as fugue states, suicidal feelings, repeated *ataques,* or a combination of these conditions. Basically the treatment involves these clients in a prolonged relationship with a mediumistic group, during which they learn to control their symptoms (interpreted as spirit intrusions) and to use the ability to be possessed by spirits in order to help others similarly afflicted. (Since this volume concerns primarily medical rather than psychiatric issues, I shall not discuss in greater detail either spiritist treatment methods or their implications for the psychotherapeutic care of Puerto Rican patients. The interested reader can consult Rogler and Hollingshead 1961, 1965; Koss 1970; Seda 1973; Garrison 1977a, 1977b; Harwood 1977. The medical implications of spiritist practices will, however, be discussed in the final part of this section.)

Curanderos AS SOURCES OF CARE *Curandero* (*curandera,* feminine) is a generic term, applied to a variety of healers who treat a narrow range of conditions, generally by means of botanicals and massages but occasionally also by cupping (*ventosas*). Before the dispersion of biomedical services throughout Puerto Rico, these healers were important providers of care to the sick. On the mainland today, however, they treat only dislocations, *empacho* (a form of indigestion), and the same mild digestive, respiratory, and rheumatic complaints that are also treated with pharmaceuticals or herbs. Some *curanderas,* who were formerly lay midwives (*comadronas*) in Puerto Rico, may also administer various kinds of massage to pregnant women and, before the legalization of abortion, were sometimes patronized for this service as well. Based on observations in the Health Center Study, however, *curanderos* are little used today, except for the treatment of *empacho* and occasionally for muscular or articular conditions that have proved refractory to medical therapy.

Empacho is indigestion attributed to a bolus of food obstructing the intestines. Teething babies are also purported to fall victim to a kind of *empacho* caused by swallowing saliva. The condition is indicated by nausea, vomiting, mild fever, loss of appetite, diarrhea, pains in the stomach or abdomen, or a combination of these symptoms. Classified as a "cold" condition, *empacho* is distinguished from indigestion caused by "hot" foods, which produces a burning sensation in the stomach. Because of its classification, *empacho* may be treated at home with either a "hot" cathartic (generally castor oil) or occasionally a "cool" one (milk of magnesia). In children, however, the condition is frequently treated by a neighborhood *santiguador* (*santiguadora,* feminine), a kind of *curandero* who specializes in the treatment of both this condition and *matriz débil* ("weak womb," discussed earlier). The *santiguador* massages the victim's abdomen to dislodge the obstruction, and after it "falls," he makes the sign of the cross (*santiguar*) and prays over the spot where the obstruction formed. The healer may also administer a cathartic.

EVANGELICAL FAITH HEALERS AS SOURCES OF CARE   Although statistics on Protestant church membership are not available for all Puerto Ricans on the mainland, several surveys carried out in New York City in the 1960s indicate that between 6 and 11 percent of the Puerto Rican population of that city is affiliated with a Protestant church (Fitzpatrick 1971:128; Garrison 1974:301–302). Of this proportion, by far the largest number belong to the Pentecostal denomination. Although Puerto Rican Pentecostals and other evangelical Protestants practice healing by laying on of hands, Garrison observed no differences in medical usage patterns between samples of Pentecostal and Catholic Puerto Ricans in the South Bronx (1974:319 320). Though the health implications of evangelical healing among Puerto Ricans have not been studied specifically, one can nevertheless infer from Garrison's data that these practices supplement medical intervention, rather than substituting for it.

Implications of Nonmainstream Medicine for Mainstream Medical Care Delivery

1. The available data reveal that by and large the nonmainstream sources of health care utilized by Puerto Ricans are not in direct competition with medical services. Home treatment with pharmaceutical or botanical products is provided for mild complaints, which are referred for medical attention should they persist, incapacitate, or eventuate in symptoms considered serious (for example high fever). When a decision is reached to take a somatic complaint outside the home for treatment, the overwhelming choice of Puerto Ricans in the first instance is mainstream medicine. Alternative sources of care are used secondarily when mainstream medicine has failed to provide symptom relief that is satisfactory

to the patient or when mainstream medical care has controlled the somatic symptoms but has failed to handle attendant psychosocial problems satisfactorily.

2. Puerto Ricans closely associate somatic symptoms with psychosocial distress. For this reason, attention to both these aspects of the illness experience is particularly important in treating this ethnic group. The administration of herbal teas, massage, and other non-mainstream kinds of treatment is part of the way in which the family and other associates of the ailing person deal with the crucial psychosocial aspect of illness (leaving aside whatever organic effects these medicaments may possibly have). To demonstrate an understanding of the importance of this aspect of patient care, the clinician might well discuss with the patient and his family in a nonjudgmental fashion the curative efforts they are making and, when these treatments are not contraindicated, express appreciation and support for their actions. Willingness to support the family's efforts in this regard are productive not only of trust but probably also of compliance with the medical regimen. Expressions of appreciation and reinforcement of the family's role in patient care do not, of course, absolve the clinician from dealing personally with psychosocial aspects of the patient's experience. Specific ways in which the clinician can attend to these aspects of the treatment of Puerto Rican patients will be discussed in the following section.

3. Spiritist beliefs and spiritist *centros* serve a number of psychological and social functions in the Puerto Rican community at large (Harwood 1977:179–184), and their utilization in crisis intervention and psychotherapeutic treatment has been well described. It is also important, however, to recognize their role in the treatment of organic disease. Thus, when treating patients with chronic and terminal illnesses, spiritists may assist in managing attendant emotional and interpersonal issues; and when consulted about feared somatic symptoms, they have been observed to prepare clients for medical consultation by allaying fears and recommending medical attention.

In treating a chronically ill or terminal patient, the clinician might therefore explore in a nonjudgmental way whether the patient is seeing a spiritist and, if indicated, consult with the spiritist on management and other therapeutic issues. (Since devout Roman Catholics and Pentecostals regard spiritism as "Devil's work" and may be insulted at the suggestion that they are consulting a medium, the clinician should first establish the patient's religious bent by inquiring whether he either attends Mass regularly or belongs to a Pentecostal church.) In addition, health facilities in Hispanic areas might encourage local spiritists to continue recommending clients for medical treatment and provide them with information on the early signs and symptoms of somatic diseases that provoke anxiety for their target population and also have a high probability of cure if detected early.

4. Mainstream health-care providers should be aware that when they tell a Hispanic patient after a thorough physical examination that they can find nothing wrong and drop the matter there, it is tantamount to referring the patient to some form of nonmainstream medical treatment. For, as long as the patient feels ill, care will be sought. Furthermore, the seemingly uncaring attitude of the medical provider will reinforce any tendency on the patient's part to use mainstream medicine episodically.

Encounters with Mainstream Medical Practitioners

The particular sources of mainstream medical care used by Puerto Ricans depend more on socioeconomic factors and the structure of the delivery system than on any distinctive cultural features of this ethnic group. Their usage patterns therefore resemble those of other urban minorities of comparable socioeconomic status. Once Puerto Ricans enter a medical setting, however, cultural influences (for example, on interactional norms, expectations about the goal of medical treatment, and so on) do become significant in determining the outcomes of these encounters. Both of these topics, usage patterns and cultural influences on medical encounters, will be considered in this section. The discussion will focus on urban Puerto Ricans rather than their rural compatriots, who receive much of their care under the Migrant Health Program of the Public Health Service.

Settings for Delivery of Mainstream Medical Care

Except under certain conditions discussed below, Puerto Ricans receive their medical care primarily in public or voluntary, rather than private, medical facilities (Erhardt, Nelson, and Pakter 1971:2247; Okada and Sparer 1976:168; Alers 1978; Schensul et al. 1978; Weidman 1978:257; Health Center Study data). The major determinants of this usage pattern are the greater cost of private medical care and the longer distances usually necessary to travel to private physicians because of their scarcity in Hispanic neighborhoods (Alers 1978:44–55). Moreover, since only a small proportion of physicians in low-income areas have hospital affiliations, people who suspect that they have serious ailments go directly to hospital facilities, knowing that the private physicians they might occasionally use would have to refer them there anyway.[26]

EMERGENCY ROOMS AS SOURCES OF CARE Evidence from various eastern cities indicates that the principal point of entry to mainstream medical care for lower-income Puerto Ricans is the hospital emergency room (Podell 1973:1121; Schensul et al. 1978:8–9; Lieberman 1979).

Although patients themselves are typically blamed for this "misuse" of the delivery system, in fact it is the structure of the system itself that probably accounts most for the pattern of usage. Because emergency services permit nonscheduled visits, often require shorter waiting times than outpatient departments and are generally accessible by public transportation, they most closely approximate the convenience factors of private care for people who cannot afford it. These cost and convenience factors, coupled with the difficulty of arranging medical visits because of work and childcare responsibilities, seem to account for the importance of emergency rooms in the medical care of Puerto Ricans.[27]

The Health Center Study data indicate, however, that when a Hispanic-oriented neighborhood health center is available to Puerto Ricans as a central source of care, hospital emergency room use tends to approximate more closely the medical conception of "real" emergency situations. Thus, Puerto Rican households that were registered for care at the Health Center were observed to utilize hospital emergency rooms mainly for life-threatening situations (poisoning, severe lacerations or bruises, broken bones, animal bites, pain around the heart) as well as for certain symptoms regarded as "serious" by this population (high fevers in children, asthmatic attacks, unexplainable fainting spells, pain or vomiting with sudden onset, and conditions that had gone untreated until patients were in severe discomfort and distress).

USE OF OUTPATIENT FACILITIES   Data from southern New York State reveal that of all ambulatory services, pediatric and obstetrical clinics receive heaviest use by Hispanics (Alers 1978:40). This utilization pattern stands to reason in view of the youthfulness of the population. In other respects, however, usage of outpatient clinics by Hispanics does not differ appreciably from that of other white and black users with one exception: mental health services. Most statistics (typically from urban areas) indicate that Puerto Ricans use these services much less than do groups of comparable poverty and minority status (Abad, Ramos, and Boyce 1974:590–91), although utilization can be increased when programs are made more relevant to the needs and culture of this ethnic group (Lehmann 1970; Cohen 1972; Abad, Ramos, and Boyce 1974; Normand, Iglesias, and Payn 1974). Despite these efforts, however, both the prevalence of culturally different conceptions of the etiology of mental illness, as discussed earlier, and the stigma of psychiatric treatment will undoubtedly continue to make mental health clinics unpopular with Puerto Ricans.

USE OF PREVENTIVE SERVICES   Mainland Puerto Ricans have typically been reported to eschew such preventive services as prenatal care

(Chase and Nelson 1973:33), routine physical examinations (Weidman 1978:299–304), and well-child physicals (Podell 1973). Since income and education have been found to predict the utilization of preventive services quite accurately (Bullough 1972; Hershey, Luft, and Gianaris 1975:845), and since none of the usage studies of preventive care involving Puerto Ricans have, to my knowledge, controlled for both income and education, the cause of Puerto Ricans' patterns of preventive care seems more likely to be their generally low income and educational levels than any special cultural attitudes and preferences.[28]

One might also argue that low usage of two of the three preventive services studied (routine adult and well-child physicals) is perfectly rational behavior because they would be of negligible influence on the health status of this population, given not only the controversial evidence on the value of annual physicals for adults (Whitby et al. 1974; Delbanco 1976) but also their irrelevance to the major causes of mortality for the under-45 segment of this population (accidents, homicide, drug dependence, and acute infectious diseases; see table 7.1 for a complete presentation of these data). Thus, Puerto Ricans as a group should not be reproached for their failure to use preventive services; it is more likely that greater impact on their health levels would come from changes in the economic and social circumstances that are more directly responsible for their utilization habits and disease prevalences.

UTILIZATION OF PRIVATE PRACTITIONERS Working people, for whom a short waiting time is often more important than cost, are most likely to use private practitioners. In general, however, low-income Puerto Ricans, because of the cost and distance factors mentioned above, use private practitioners only under special circumstances (unless the practitioner is known to accept Medicaid without question).[29] Thus, physicians in private practice may be patronized either when confidentiality is a priority (for example, for a urogenital problem) or when an injection has been denied as treatment at a public facility and is thought to be the most effective remedy for the patient's ailment. Spanish-speaking physicians are particularly sought for treatment whenever the condition requires considerable explanation or is believed to be something that an "American" doctor has not sufficiently understood and therefore treated inadequately. In short, low-income Puerto Ricans consult physicians in private practice mainly after undergoing treatment at a public facility which they have considered unsatisfactory.

Expectations in the Medical Encounter

In discussions among participants in the Health Center Study, both before and after medical consultations, Puerto Rican patients expressed three criteria for evaluating a medical encounter as favorable. The first criterion is that the patient must receive a "good" physical examination, whether the visit is for diagnostic purposes or for follow-up. The examination must include some procedure in which the practitioner comes into physical contact with the patient (for example, by listening to the patient's chest or heart, or by taking his blood pressure). In addition, it must include an explanation of how recommended laboratory tests relate to the patient's symptoms. This explanation is particularly important with regard to blood tests, since many Puerto Ricans in the Health Center Study expressed the belief that laboratories take far more of this vital fluid than is necessary. Well over half the adults in the study maintained that part of the blood was not used for tests at all but was retained or sold by hospitals and clinics for transfusions. Many also claimed to feel weak after giving more than three tubes of blood and expressed anxiety over the quantity lost for tests.

The second criterion for judging a medical encounter, as expressed by Puerto Ricans in the Health Center Study, is that the patient should receive an explanation for what is wrong, preferably from the physician (see Padilla 1958:295 for an expression of the same opinion). The explanation must include an intelligible exposition of the diagnosis. Some people, however, preferred not to know the disease if it were fatal. In addition to an explanation of the diagnosis, participants in the Health Center Study also expected a clear explanation of the treatment regimen—particularly how any activity restrictions are related to the disease and how medication is to be used.

In discussing their desire for explanations, patients reasoned that they went to a physician because of his special training and professional expertise, and the explanation was therefore part of the doctor's job. Moreover, it is important for clinicians to realize that because patients are likely to discuss their conditions with relatives and friends, any biomedical explanations given by the physician will be passed on to others and thus have a multiplier effect educationally. Indeed, the major source of biomedical understandings of disease, according to the Health Center Study, is explanations provided by health professionals and shared by patients with members of their social networks.

The third criterion for judging medical encounters is that the practitioner show concern for the patient. Since this criterion has a great deal to do with interactional norms, it will be discussed in the following section.

Interactional Norms in the Medical Setting

CROSSING THE LANGUAGE BARRIER   Because of the ease with which Puerto Ricans can go back and forth between the island and the mainland, many retain Spanish as their first and sometimes only language.[30] Even those who can manage many situations in English often find it difficult to get their feelings across or to express the precise nuances of meaning they wish to convey when reporting symptoms. Consequently, a large number of Puerto Ricans feel more comfortable and thus prefer using Spanish in medical encounters. Since some people do prefer English, however, and may be offended by the assumption that they are only able to communicate in Spanish, it is important to leave the choice of language, as far as practicable, to the patient. This is best accomplished by a direct question like "Do you prefer using Spanish or English when talking with me?"

Optimally, the clinician who regularly treats Spanish-speaking patients should know the language, although use of a prestigious dialect may make some Puerto Rican patients self-conscious about their speech and consequently more reserved. Because of the scarcity of bilingual physicians, however, either translators or medical phrase books are typically employed to surmount the language barrier. Of the two, translators are probably preferable, since they do not restrict doctor-patient communication to the sparse vocabulary of the phrase book and thus allow for a dialogue in which statements concerning the illness aspect of the patient's problem can be qualified, clarified, and negotiated. The main drawback with translation, of course, is that it depends so heavily on the competence of one person to render meanings accurately. This problem can be mitigated, however, by selecting translators carefully and providing training for those who do the job regularly.

Although it may go without saying, translators should never be enlisted from among strangers assembled in a waiting room, since this practice constitutes a breach of confidentiality in the eyes of most Puerto Ricans. In general, it is also best to avoid using a patient's child as translator, since urogenital and other functions that are considered taboo subjects between parents and children may have to be discussed. A particularly awkward situation might also develop if a child should have to translate a communication censuring the parent's behavior.

If the patient brings an adult relative or friend into the consulting room to act as translator, this probably indicates the patient's confidence in his companion, although it does not necessarily establish the person's competence as a translator of anatomical and medical terms. For many purposes, however, the services of these close associates of the patient will be adequate, since the intimacy between the two will at least allow for a free exchange of information on that end of the dialogue. To improve the quality of the translation, however, the clinician might provide the following kind of instruction to the patient's companion: "Try to use your friend's own words when you tell me what he is saying. If you don't understand quite what he means by a particular word or phrase, discuss it until you have a clearer idea. Do the same with me; don't hesitate to ask me to explain what I say more clearly."

For most health workers who regularly act as translators, a short training program to heighten their skills in translation techniques and medical vocabulary is usually appropriate. In addition to standard vocabulary, instruction should cover words that have variant meanings in Puerto Rican Spanish (for example, *fatiga*) as well as terms (for example, *sangre gruesa*) that must be understood within the context of cultural concepts of disease etiology.[31] (See the section on concepts of illness for a discussion of relevant words and concepts.)

INTERPERSONAL BEHAVIOR   In addition to competence, Puerto Ricans expect health professionals to demonstrate that they care for their patients as individuals, not just as exemplars of a disease.[32] This expectation relates to the close association Puerto Ricans perceive between disease and the sufferer's psychosocial circumstances. It also relates to two important Hispanic values concerning interpersonal interaction: personalism (Mumford 1973:769) and *respeto* (Mumford 1973:770, Murillo-Rohde 1976:177).

To act personalistically requires that one attend to one's interlocutor as a person before getting down to the manifest purpose of an encounter. In other words, efficiency becomes secondary to the establishment of rapport. Although this order of priorities reverses that generally followed by health professionals, personal attention is important in putting Puerto Rican patients at ease and in making them feel less intimidated by the authority of the physician. Two simple and culturally expected procedures for enhancing personalism in doctor-patient interactions are for the physician to shake hands with the patient both at the beginning and end of an interview and to maintain eye contact with the patient during conversations. Listening to the patient's description of what is wrong before asking questions also communicates personal regard.

The Spanish word *respeto* not only covers such aspects of the English word "respect" as deference to authority and due regard for the value of the individual, it also encompasses proper attention to the formalities of interpersonal behavior. Respeto is overtly taught as a value to children from about the time they learn to walk, and its centrality to all interpersonal interactions makes it relevant to social encounters in the medical setting as well.

With regard to deference, *respeto* implies attentiveness and obedience to people who are older, more educated, or higher in social status than oneself. Because patients in general are of lower educational and socioeconomic status than their physicians, Puerto Rican patients, to demonstrate proper respect, will usually listen to a physician's advice or explanations without comments or questions, even if they would like to ask them. Because this behavior is not conducive to an effective therapeutic alliance, the physician must openly encourage Puerto Rican patients to ask questions, but he should do this in a manner that does not impugn their intelligence (since this would demonstrate a lack of *respeto* on the clinician's part). Phrasing the encouragement to ask questions in personalistic terms would, however, constitute a mark of respect. For example, the physician might say, "Because I want to understand your problems better, I would like you to ask me any questions you have about what I say."

With regard to the aspect of *respeto* that involves attention to the formalities of interaction, Puerto Rican adults as a rule expect physicians to act in a manner consistent with their education and authority. More specifically, this expectation requires the physician to demonstrate his knowledge by explaining tests and diagnoses in an intelligible but noncondescending manner. In addition, the clinician should avoid excessive informality (for example, calling an adult by his first name), which may be interpreted as a lack of regard for the patient's dignity.[33] To demonstrate *respeto,* a clinician may also be expected to dress in a white coat or conservative street clothes.

INTERACTION BETWEEN THE SEXES Although sex roles are changing among Puerto Ricans, traditional Latin concepts of male and female behavior still prevail, particularly among those raised on the island (Torres-Matrullo 1976:716). According to traditional concepts, women are ideally chaste, submissive, and domestic, while men are strong, sexually aggressive, and footloose. These concepts can influence practitioner-patient relationships, particularly when the participants are of opposite sex.

Puerto Rican men, for example, are reluctant to consult a woman clinician, especially for a urogenital problem, and Puerto Rican women avoid gynecological examinations by male health practitioners. As a result (and because there are relatively few female gynecologists), Puerto Rican women tend to avoid gynecological appointments for routine care and consent to vaginal examinations only when experiencing symptoms. Thus, primary care programs with a predominantly Puerto Rican clientele should make special efforts to have female gynecologists, physicians' assistants, and nurse practitioners on the staff. (See also Montijo 1975:476–477, for a consideration of this issue in psychotherapeutic relationships.)

The Family in Medical-Care Settings

When a person falls seriously ill, the extended family typically mobilizes to help. This may entail going to the hospital or clinic to be with the sick person or with the immediate family while they await the outcome of the medical examination or treatment procedure. To show this kind of concern is very important for Puerto Rican family solidarity, and without it a seriously ill patient may feel abandoned in time of need. Since hospital rules generally forbid large numbers of visitors on inpatient wards or in the emergency room and thus contravene a family's expectation of being with the patient, the excluded family members may become agitated over the situation. Hospital personnel should therefore be alert to recognize the family and their special concern by keeping them informed of the patient's condition. A courteous explanation of hospital rules and why they are necessary will also assist the family in accepting their inability to be with the patient.

Since Hispanic inpatients generally find hospital meals quite different from their normal cuisine, family members often bring them food from home. If the patient is under dietary restrictions, they should be explained to the family. Otherwise, however, the practice should be permitted for both the patient's and the family's peace of mind.

Etiological Concepts and Reactions to Medical Diagnosis

The effects of Puerto Rican nosological concepts on discussions of disease with health practitioners were discussed earlier in the chapter. However, etiological concepts also influence many Puerto Ricans' reactions to medical diagnoses. Because many Puerto Ricans feel that stress and psychosocial problems are intimately related to disease, these factors must be dealt with as part of treatment. Unless this aspect of illness receives attention, the patient is likely to view the practitioner as uncaring and the treatment as insufficient.

The principal ally a health professional has in treating stress and psychosocial aspects of a Puerto Rican's disease is the patient's family. Therefore, efforts to explain the medical situation and to relieve sources of stress should include significant family members, not all of whom may actually live in the same household with the patient. Persons significant in patient care can usually be identified from among those who visit an inpatient frequently or who accompany an outpatient on medical visits. Optimally, the health professional should assemble these people with the patient for a discussion of the family situation. In low-income families substandard housing, job insecurity, fear for the safety of the children, and other realities of slum life will constitute important topics for this discussion. Rather than simply referring the family to an appropriate social-service worker or agency, the health professional can enhance his therapeutic relationship with the family by demonstrating concern about these problems and attempting to understand their specific implications for the patient's medical condition.

Summary

The organizational arrangements of emergency rooms and hospital outpatient clinics often make it exceedingly difficult for health-care workers to interact in a personal and caring manner with patients and especially their families (Strauss 1969; Dutton 1978). Therefore, the striking paradox about Puerto Ricans' involvement with mainstream medical services is that their prevailing poverty disposes them to use mainly those facilities that are least prepared to provide both the kind of interpersonal relationships and the concern for psychosocial concomitants of disease that this ethnic group considers crucial to health care.

The creation of neighborhood health centers, the training of Puerto Rican paraprofessionals (family health workers, physicians' assistants, and so on), and the reorganization of hospital outpatient departments have all helped to resolve this paradox. Yet further efforts toward resolution must be made by training more Puerto Ricans of low-income background as nurses and physicians. For, like most people in the United States, Puerto Ricans by and large perceive these professionals as the most valued sources of medical care and so prefer to receive treatment from them. Moreover, medically trained Puerto Ricans, because of their early socialization within the ethnic subculture, are more likely to provide the desired personalism, respect, and concern for Hispanic patients in the cultural idiom they readily understand. This is not to say, of course, that health professionals of other backgrounds cannot provide quality medical care to Puerto Ricans, too. They must recognize, however, that special efforts are necessary to master the interpersonal skills and psychosocial awareness that will ensure a better fit between their expertise and the expectations for quality care held by many Puerto Rican patients.

Adherence to Biomedical Treatment

Although a plethora of variables have been found to correlate with patient compliance in general (for recent reviews, see Becker and Maiman 1975; Sackett and Haynes 1976; Schmidt 1977), a number of these variables have particular relevance for Puerto Rican patients. In addition to these general variables, there are a number of specific beliefs and attitudes held by Puerto Ricans that also influence their conformity to medical regimens. Before discussing these various influences on patterns of compliance among Puerto Ricans, however, it is important to point out that a certain degree of undercompliance with medical regimens is probably healthy for people who receive the kind of episodic, impersonal care that many Puerto Ricans experience in emergency rooms and outpatient clinics. For, in situations where follow-up may be minimal and dosage explanations impaired by language problems and other sources of faulty communication between physicians and patients (Svarstad 1976), a tendency to undermedicate or to discontinue medication at the first hint of possible side effects may be the wisest course of action.

General Factors Influencing Adherence to Medical Advice

Although there are no experimental data specifically on Puerto Ricans' compliance with medical regimens, data from similar low-income, clinic populations reveal two factors that seem particularly relevant to this ethnic group. The first of these factors is the demonstrated importance of family support in increasing compliance with regimens, especially for chronic ailments (Heinzelmann and Bagley 1970; Oakes et al. 1970). Because Puerto Rican families tend, as a cultural practice, to assume an important role in the care of ailing members, their enlistment in the treatment regimen is particularly appropriate.

The second factor that has been demonstrated to enhance conformity with medical advice is the nature of the doctor-patient relationship—specifically, aspects such as warmth, continuity of care, explanations of both the disease and the treatment regimen, release of tension in the encounter, and feedback from the physician (see, for example, Davis 1968, 1971; Korsch, Gozzi, and Francis 1968; Francis, Korsch, and Morris 1969; Howard et al. 1970; Finnerty, Mattie, and Finnerty 1973; Becker, Drachman, and Kirscht 1974; Aiken 1976; Haynes 1976). Since these are features that Puerto Ricans tend to expect from medical encounters anyway, their contribution toward enhancing compliance would seem to be particularly important for this ethnic group.

Specific Attitudes toward Physicians and Medication that Affect Compliance

MEDICATION AND ITS ADMINISTRATION   As a general rule, most Puerto Ricans prefer to receive medication by injection rather than orally, since the former method is known to be quicker-acting (Padilla 1958: 295; Health Center Study). As a holdover from earlier treatment practices, moreover, many Puerto Ricans expect penicillin injections for colds, fever, or "flu" and in these cases will visit private physicians who reportedly administer the desired medication. Some Puerto Ricans who have received "liver extract" injections on the island for "tiredness" or "weakness" also seek and apparently receive this type of treatment from private physicians.

Oral medications are often taken symptomatically. Effective dosages may be increased if symptoms worsen, or medication may be discontinued when symptoms disappear and then resume when they occur. These patterns often result from inadequate or inconsistent instruction by physicians (Svarstad 1976; Health Center Study data), but they are supported by a general feeling that medication is to be used only when one is feeling ill. By and large, Puerto Ricans tend to be wary of overdosing with prescription medication. This is particularly true of psychotropic drugs (popularly called "nerve pills"), which are thought to be addictive. Furthermore, physicians who frequently dispense this form of medication are often criticized as "pushers."

HOT/COLD BELIEFS AND COMPLIANCE WITH MEDICAL REGIMENS   Four kinds of compliance problems have been observed to occur among patients who follow the directives of hot/cold therapy (Harwood 1971b; see table 7.10). In managing these problems, the physician may attempt to alter the patient's behavior by invoking the authority of medical opinion in support of the prescribed regimen or by providing a nonjargonistic biomedical explanation for the treatment. An alternative approach, one that is particularly appropriate for elderly or less acculturated patients, is to work within the hot/cold system to achieve the desired therapeutic goal. Ways of doing this will be described in the following section.

In many instances hot-cold therapeutics comport with and may therefore reinforce standard treatment practices. For example, penicillin as therapy for rheumatic fever fits the logic of the system, because the joint pains that accompany this disease mark it as "cold" and thus make "hot" penicillin an acceptable medication. The use of aspirin for upper respiratory infections or relief of arthritic pain similarly accords with both therapeutic schemata. In addition, bland diets restrict intake of many "hot" foods and thus coincide with humoral notions of proper therapy for ulcer patients. Indeed, although hot/cold and biomedical therapeutics differ in their basic premises, the behavior they imply is probably more similar than antipathetic. One may even conjecture that the viability of the hot/cold system is founded to some extent on this agreement between the two systems of health behavior.

SURGICAL TREATMENT   Surgery as a form of treatment is taken very seriously, and patients commonly seek a second opinion before submitting to it (Health Center Study). Many people who have had an organ removed are called by the special term *operado* and regarded as delicate for some time (Padilla 1958:290).

CONFLICTS BETWEEN MEDICAL AND SPIRITIST FORMS OF THERAPY   Although most nonmainstream forms of treatment are administered concurrently with medical regimens, spiritist healers occasionally advise discontinuing medical therapy, particularly with psychotropic drugs (Mumford 1973:773; Harwood 1977:203). Their rationale for doing this is that psychotropic medication is regarded as undermining one of their own therapeutic modalities (*desarollo,* "development"), which is designed to sharpen clients' mental facilities and powers of concentration. Although such advice may not be common (see Garrison 1977b:129), it is worth checking on compliance with those psychiatric patients who are simultaneously seeing a spiritist.

Suggestions for Fostering Adherence to Treatment

The foregoing data suggest a number of procedures that clinicians can follow to increase the likelihood of Puerto Rican patients' following medical advice.

1. Include members of the family in explaining a diagnosis and treatment regimen, particularly when the regimen involves changes in lifestyle. Involvement of the woman or women who cook for the household is essential if dietary changes are being recommended.

2. When a patient has used Spanish in the medical interview, all therapeutic instructions (including the information on bottles of prescription medicines) should also be written out in Spanish and discussed with the patient in that language. This will not only ensure that the instructions are more intelligible to the patient but will also permit him to ask questions about them. Furthermore, in keeping with Puerto Ricans' expectations of good medical practice, the reasons for each instruction should be explained. Otherwise, out of *respeto,* the patient may agree outwardly with the clinician's advice but intend not to follow through on the recommendations.

3. Prescribing clinicians should follow up on treatment regimens themselves. This should be done not only in the interests of continuity, which has been shown to increase compliance, but also in response to Puerto Ricans' expectations of securing the clinician's personal concern.

4. Although hot/cold theory is part of the cultural repertoire of many Puerto Ricans, individuals vary not only in the degree to which they give it credence and model their behavior by it, but also to a lesser extent in the particular foods and medications they assign to the "hot," "cool," and "cold" categories. The clinician must therefore determine for each patient individually: (1) whether his condition and the proposed regimen are conceptualized in terms of the hot/cold framework, and (2) whether this conceptualization will affect the therapeutic outcome.

Since Puerto Ricans who are more acculturated to mainstream American behavior patterns are less likely to espouse the hot/cold theory than those who are less acculturated, one can usually assume that patients with such indicators of acculturation as a secondary school education or parents born on the United States mainland will not evaluate their physical conditions, foods, or medications in terms of the theory. (Without knowing the theoretical basis for their behavior, however, they may still use home remedies dictated by the hot/cold system.)

For all other Puerto Rican patients, it is in the interests of effective therapy to determine the extent to which hot/cold beliefs will limit the acceptability of a proposed treatment regimen. This task is best accomplished by posing questions which indicate the clinician's awareness of the belief system but which do not imply any judgment of it. A useful approach might be to employ the following probe (with substitutions that are appropriate to the particular situation for all bracketed words): "Some of my patients who suffer from [joint pains], like the ones you've been having, tell me that these [pains] are [frío], and they do not eat [frío] foods because of them. Have you been doing that?"

To discover how a patient classifies a particular medicine or food that is pertinent to the prescribed regimen, a helpful question (again with appropriate substitutions) might be: "When I have told some of my other patients to eat [bananas and dried fruits], they have told me that these foods are [frío]. Do you think so, too?"

With Spanish-speaking clinicians these probes should of course be rendered in Spanish. In medical delivery systems where Spanish-speaking staff translate for physicians or work closely with families, they should be made aware of those diseases and treatment regimens for which hot/cold beliefs pose problems in compliance so that they can handle these problems appropriately with patients. Table 7.10 suggests solutions to the four major compliance problems that arise out of the hot/cold system. The clinician should note that in working with patients within this therapeutic framework, the concept of "neutralization" (discussed in the section on concepts of disease and illness) is very useful. In addition, when recommended biomedical therapy agrees with humoral conceptions, the clinician might well point this out to the patient as a way of reinforcing the proposed regimen.

5. Clinicians treating Puerto Rican patients in the emergency room should not suggest that they go to their own physicians for follow-up care. Since most Puerto Ricans (like many urbanites today) do not have a family physician, this suggestion really refers the patient nowhere and virtually guarantees no follow up. In situations when it is important for patients to be seen again, the emergency room staff should therefore find out where they can go for subsequent appointments. If possible, they should also arrange the first appointment and provide written statements of what follow-up care is needed, so the patients can take these instructions with them to the appointment (Center for Human Resources Planning and Development et al. 1977).

6. To combat the tendency to take medicines symptomatically, clini-

Table 7.10 Management issues with Puerto Rican patients who follow hot/cold theory.

General problem	Example	Recommended solution within hot/cold framework
Patient fails to take prescribed medication or eat recommended foods because they directly contradict notions of good therapy within hot/cold framework.	Pregnant women avoid "hot" foods and medications to prevent their babies from being born with a rash or red skin. As a result, they do not take prescribed iron or vitamin supplements.	When patient rejects "hot" substances, use neutralization principle.[a] When patient rejects "cool" medication, use an alternative drug not classified in the hot/cold system.
Patient on maintenance dose of a "hot" medication stops therapy when he experiences a "hot" symptom. Patient on maintenance dose of a "cool" medication stops therapy when a "cold" symptom develops.	Patient on prophylactic program of penicillin stops therapy when he experiences diarrhea or constipation and may discontinue therapy entirely to prevent a recurrence.	With "hot" medications, follow neutralization principle[a] and advise patients to take them with a "cool" substance. With "cool" medications, use a drug not classified in the hot/cold system or prescribe an equivalent "hot" drug until the "cold" symptom subsides.
Patient discontinues "hot" or "cold" foods in a dietary regimen if symptoms within the same category develop.	Patients on diuretics who are told to eat dried fruits, oranges, and bananas (all "cold" or "cool" foods) as sources of potassium will stop these foods should "cold" symptoms develop. Since these symptoms include menstruation, women are most at risk.	For any dietary recommendation, provide options from all three categories of the hot/cold system. (For example, "hot" cocoa or peas might also be suggested as sources of potassium).
Substances traditionally used to "refresh" the stomach (that is, to neutralize "hot" foods) may be harmful in themselves.	To protect babies from developing rashes or other "hot" symptoms from formula made with evaporated milk, some mothers add "cool" $MgCO_3$ or mannitol to the bottle, often in quantities sufficient to cause diarrhea.	Stress use of harmless "cool" additives (barley water, fruit juice) in place of potentially harmful ones.

Source: Harwood (1979).
a. See text, section on concepts of disease and illness, for explanation of "neutralization."

cians should take special pains to explain the reasons why long-term medication is necessary for a patient's condition. In cases of chronic illness, patient compliance can also be enhanced by continuous close supervision, as well as by greater compliance by the clinician with the patient's expectations of good therapy (Haynes 1976).

Recovery, Rehabilitation, and Death
Role of the Family in Chronic and Terminal Illness

The extended family comes prominently into play during instances of incapacitating long-term or terminal illness. These situations are critical not only for showing family solidarity but also for repaying elders or other kinsmen for the care they provided in the past. These situations are also times when the comparatively easy trip between Puerto Rico and the mainland exerts an important influence on patient care, since relatives can come to the mainland to help nurse a bedridden kinsman, or the invalid can travel to Puerto Rico to recuperate or die among relatives there. In short, Puerto Ricans in general prefer caring for seriously sick family members at home, rather than abandoning them to nursing homes.

Diagnosis of a chronic but not seriously incapacitating condition often provides the impetus for an elderly person to move nearer to one of his married children (usually a daughter, who may have moved to another section of the city at the time of marriage). If the sick person still has a living spouse, the couple will generally take an apartment in the vicinity of the child; if the elderly parent is alone, however, he may move into the child's household. Extended kin may also offer this kind of care to psychiatric patients after they have been released from the hospital, although, because of the stigma attached to mental illness, patients may need group support in order to contact their kin before release (Rodríguez 1971).

For the clinician, both the mobility of patients in time of serious illness and the family's readiness to undertake patient care have important implications for arranging treatment.

1. Mobility means that the clinician should ensure that medical records are made available to chronic patients who intend to move. Patients should be informed of the importance of these records for continuity of care, as well as the necessary procedures for obtaining them.

2. The readiness of families to provide care to the seriously sick means that they are a tremendous resource, but they often must be assisted in their efforts. Because the generally low incomes of mainland Puerto Ricans produce considerable financial and psychological burdens on caretakers, the services of visiting nurses and part-time homemakers should be enlisted to help families in their attempts to keep seriously incapacitated kinsmen out of nursing homes.

3. Chronically ill elderly patients who move either near or into the

home of one of their children may need special help in adjusting to their new situations. As a result of relocating to a new neighborhood late in life, they may feel disoriented or fearful and therefore become overly dependent on their children. In spite of the good intentions of everyone involved, such overdependence frequently produces a strain in family relations. The services of a homemaker to help orient the patient to the new neighborhood may therefore be indicated for a short time after the move.

Resuming Normal Roles after Sickness

Since financial support of the family is traditionally considered the male role, unemployment for reasons of illness is particularly difficult for men to accept (Padilla 1958:257–259). A disabled man's feelings of inadequacy for not fulfilling his traditional responsibilities may also be exacerbated if his wife should begin to work, and more traditional women may even refuse jobs in order not to undermine their husbands' self-respect (Berle 1958:78–80). Although this situation is becoming increasingly rare as conceptions of marital roles change, special help for disabled or chronically ill males in finding less taxing employment or in adjusting to their disabilities may be necessary.

For some devout Puerto Ricans, resumption of normal activities after an illness may be accompanied by the performance of religious rituals. In particular, women (of almost any formal religious affiliation) may make a promise (*promesa*) to a saint or the Deity to perform such rituals if either they or a family member survives a serious illness or operation. The rituals may include attending religious services daily for a specified period and wearing a distinctive sash (*cordón*), decorated with pompons, in the color associated with a saint and perhaps also a plain dress of the same color. When such *promesas* are made by the sick themselves, the rituals can provide psychological support in the transition back to a normal life.

Death and Dying

Many Puerto Ricans who are nominally Roman Catholic turn to a priest only for major life passages, such as baptism, marriage, or death. Hospital staff should therefore be aware that a hospital call by a priest may incite considerable alarm in a patient, who may interpret the visit as an indication that he is near death. When appropriate, reassurance to the contrary by either the staff or the priest himself may be necessary. Protestants, on the other hand, usually expect their ministers to visit them when they are ill. However, hospitals may deny special visiting privileges to those clergy who head small storefront churches. In the interest of patients' sense of well-being, hospitals might extend these privileges to such nonestablishment clergy.

As a patient nears death, family members will gather to be with one another and to say their farewells to the dying person. Many Puerto Ricans believe that a person's spirit will not be free to enter the hereafter if he dies with something important left unsaid. Therefore, the dying often wish to converse with particular relatives or friends to complete their relationships with them. Because of the importance of this custom, many Puerto Ricans do not wish to spend their last days in a hospital, where access to kin and friends may be limited; or they may consent to hospitalization only after they have spoken to all intimates first. Many would prefer to die in Puerto Rico, where close kin may be living and where dying at home is more accepted.

In view of these beliefs, humane treatment of the dying would entail a more lenient attitude on the part of hospitals in allowing visitors to remain with gravely ill Puerto Rican patients. Clinicians should also be aware of the importance of informing either the patient or a close kinsman when an illness is terminal so that necessary communications can be completed in time. Awareness of these beliefs may also help the clinician to understand the hesitancy with which many Puerto Ricans face final hospitalization. Finally, hospital staff should realize that survivors may be particularly upset if a kinsman suddenly loses consciousness or dies precipitously, since in such cases death may have come before the victim has settled his affairs.

Conclusion

Clinicians who care for Puerto Rican patients by and large treat the somatic effects of social and economic inequality. As we have seen, low income, substandard housing, and poorly designed medical services contribute significantly to both the epidemiology and medical usage patterns of this ethnic group. While substantial improvement in the health and medical care of continental Puerto Ricans will thus come primarily from changes in the social and economic structure of this country, the fact still remains that most medical care is delivered, and undoubtedly will continue to be delivered, in face-to-face encounters among patients, their families, and clinicians. In these encounters Puerto Ricans' cultural conceptions of illness and treatment, their language preferences, their habitual patterns of social interaction, and their expectations of medical care are all pertinent to the therapeutic outcome. The clinician who is aware of these factors and can perceive their relevance to the individual patient is thus better able to respond to both the patient and his family in a culturally appropriate, caring manner.

Concise suggestions for dealing with significant sociocultural issues in

Puerto Rican patient-care have been provided on the foregoing pages. Mastering the skills of recognizing and responding appropriately, however, requires conscious attention on the part of the clinician to the total social context of treatment. The burden on the clinician who wishes to treat the patient and not just his disease is great, but the reward for both patient and clinician will be commensurate.

Notes

The Health Center Study, selected findings of which are reported in this chapter, was supported by a grant from the Carnegie Corporation of New York. I would also like to acknowledge the helpful comments of Ramón Vélez, M.D., who read the chapter in draft form.

1. *Compadrazgo* ("co-parenthood") refers to the mutual relationship between a child's parents and his godparents. The term *compadre* is used to refer to either man in such a relationship, and *comadre,* to either woman; both men and women jointly are called *compadres.* Although the rights and obligations entailed in *compadrazgo* vary in different classes and in different Latin American societies, assistance in time of trouble is a general feature of the relationship.

2. This variation in participation was due to high mobility in the area and subsequent refusals from some of the original participants. The median duration of participation, however, was eight months, so the data from most households are quite comprehensive.

3. New York is one of the few locations in the continental United States to record health statistics for Puerto Ricans as a routine procedure. Other states or cities with large Puerto Rican populations are usually able to retrieve vital statistics for Puerto Ricans on request, at least in years for which the data are stored on computers.

4. Efforts have been made in recent years to change the forms for birth and death certificates in all states to include an entry on "ethnic heritage." If this change is widely adopted, vital statistics on ethnic groups need no longer be based solely on place of birth.

5. For a relevant discussion of vitamin B_{12} deficiency in the differential diagnosis of pernicious anemia and tropical sprue in patients from the Caribbean area, see Meyers, Schweitzer, and Gerson (1977).

6. In-depth analysis of these "other" causes of infant and child mortality is strongly recommended, since this information would undoubtedly assist pediatricians who routinely treat Puerto Rican children by identifying serious but rare diseases that are likely to afflict this population.

7. Although high mortality among Puerto Ricans from cirrhosis of the liver is consistent with evidence of high rates of "implicative" or "suspicion-arousing" drinking among males in this ethnic group (Haberman and Sheinberg 1967), the survey questions on which these rates have been based are in my view culturally biased and of totally undemonstrated validity.

8. Briefly, the methods used in the three studies were as follows. The Hartford study (Hispanic Health Council n.d.; Schensul et al. 1978) was based on physical examinations of 80 teenage students of the Quirk Middle School who

were "new arrivals" from Puerto Rico. Data on the students' families were also gathered to permit examination of the interrelationships between physical findings and family background. The Miami project surveyed the health status and "health cultures" of five ethnic groups—Bahamians, Haitians, southern blacks, Cubans, and Puerto Ricans (Weidman 1978). The data on symptoms and conditions derive from a questionnaire administered to one member of each of 25 Puerto Rican households that were enrolled in a comprehensive health program run by the Department of Pediatrics, University of Miami. Each respondent reported the presence or absence of symptoms and medical conditions listed in the questionnaire among every household member during the previous 12 months. By sampling from a pediatric program, the study necessarily omitted both childless and, to a large extent, elderly families (Weidman 1978:330–331, 380). The New York City data derive from the Health Center Study described earlier in this chapter. The information on symptoms and conditions comes from households that participated in that study continually for at least seven months ($N = 39$ households, median period of observation, 12 months; range, 7–13 months). All symptoms and conditions were either observed directly by the researchers or reported to them by participants within one to two weeks of their occurrence. Since no significant differences were found in the rank ordering of symptoms or conditions in households observed in the study for different periods of time, the data were combined for purposes of presentation here.

9. In the general population the rank order of incidence of the five major categories of acute conditions is as follows: respiratory conditions, injuries, all other acute conditions, infective and parasitic diseases, and digestive system conditions (U.S. Department of Health, Education, and Welfare 1978: 10). In general the rates reported by the National Center for Health Statistics are higher than those of the studies discussed here, but again the studies are not strictly comparable, since the methods of data collection are different and the national figures describe incidence, whereas those reported above are for prevalence.

10. The acute conditions labeled *fatiga* or *asma* in table 7.3 were either acute respiratory infections (accompanied by shortness of breath and fever and termed *fatiga* by the sufferers or their caretakers) or isolated instances of shortness of breath or wheezing which had never been clinically diagnosed as asthma.

11. Findings on the self-limiting character of tropical parasitic infections in temperate climates have been conflicting. For example, Winsberg and her colleagues (1975:529) observed a marked decline in rates of both trichuriasis and hookworm in her sample after three years' residence on the continent. However, Hargus and his co-workers found duration of residence to effect little change in prevalence (1976:292).

12. For a brief summary of the many shortcomings of these data, see Alers (1978:23–25).

13. If gamma globulin production were a polygenic trait, as is likely, then the intermediate position of Puerto Rican serum levels between those of largely African-derived and European-derived groups would be expected, given

the mixed racial heritage of many Puerto Ricans. Since the Puerto Rican samples were not separated by racial background in the reported studies, it is impossible to tell, however, if a predictable variation exists within the Puerto Rican population. In speculating in this fashion it must of course be remembered that serum gamma globulin levels are only partly determined by genetic factors.

14. Although both blacks and Puerto Ricans in New York City share the same risk factor for lead poisoning—old, dilapidated housing (Graef 1977: 123, 128)—the incidence among Puerto Rican children under age 6 is less than half that for black children of comparable age (Guinee 1972:286). No studies investigating this ethnic difference could be located, however.

15. Toward the end of the Health Center Study, I asked 9 female and 2 male adults from different households in the sample to sort, classify, and talk about a set of 105 terms for diseases and physical conditions which had been mentioned or discussed in natural contexts during the participant-observation research over the previous year. The 11 respondents were chosen from among the families that had been most cooperative in the research and are representative of the study population in their range of age and educational backgrounds. Though the original discussions of these 105 terms had already provided considerable understanding of their meanings and uses, the sorting procedure permitted an examination of the relationships people perceived among different diseases and physical conditions as well as a further appreciation of people's understandings of the diseases and conditions themselves, because the exercise provided an opportunity for isolating dimensions of contrast between and among terms. To ascertain the generality of certain classifications and meanings of terms which were revealed by the sorting procedure, additional open-ended inquiries on specific points were conducted among adults in the remaining sample families. (The number of additional inquiries varied for different terms, although the total numbered around 30. The exact numbers will be reported where relevant.)

The results of this study constitute the basis for my discussion of disease classification, although there are of course limitations to the data. Besides representing only a small and relatively narrow socioeconomic, educational, and residential sector of the Puerto Rican population, the data suffer from the effects of boredom on the part of the participants entailed in the time-consuming procedure of sorting so many terms; of interruptions occasioned by the demands of normal household routines; and of observer efforts to expedite the procedure and to record the large quantity of information produced. On the other hand, these are, as far as I know, the only data on disease classification that have been gathered from any Puerto Rican population even this systematically and that are verifiable in the light of observational data gathered in the study on how concepts are used in natural settings. Thus, with due caution and the resolve to report only those findings judged most reliable, I present the research here. Furthermore, because of the nature of this volume, only those findings that have practical implications for health-care delivery will be discussed.

16. Several older studies of laymen's understandings of biomedical concepts

of disease (Suchman 1964; Klerman, Jones, and Hull 1966) indicated that Puerto Ricans were the "least informed" among the ethnic groups with which they were compared. In the Health Center Study, a differential in the same direction as compared to blacks who participated in the study was also noted, although the margin of difference was not striking. The greater knowledge that Puerto Ricans demonstrated in the Health Center Study was undoubtedly due both to the passage of time and, more importantly, to the difference in research methods of the two studies (Suchman used a structured questionnaire, whereas the Health Center Study used direct observation and open-ended questions).

17. Venereal disease is a taboo subject, particularly among women and between men and women, as a result of the Puerto Rican moral code which enjoins virginity on unmarried women and sexual fidelity on wives but allows considerable sexual latitude to males. According to such a code, a woman, to have a venereal infection, must have either committed an immoral act or contracted the infection from her husband. In either case, the matter is not easily discussed: in the first instance, the disease becomes an admission of immorality and in the second, a wife's confronting her husband with the infection may be interpreted as an illegitimate attempt on her part to control his sexual behavior.

18. These attitudes toward tuberculosis, described by Berle in the 1950s (1958:148–156), seemed little changed in 1970 (Health Center Study observations), in spite of the replacement of long periods of hospitalization by medication at home as the preferred mode of treatment.

19. Since asthma frequently presents initially as a chronic, nonproductive cough, often exacerbated at night, the idea that asthma derives from an "old cold" is understandable as an explanation for this symptom, which may indeed resemble the symptomatology of a lingering cold (Ramon Velez, personal communication).

20. Nutritional studies in Puerto Rico have indicated that 22 to 38 percent of Puerto Rican women in various age and socioeconomic categories are obese by continental American standards (Fernández et al 1968:653; Fernández-López, Burgos, and Asenjo 1969). No comparable nutritional studies could be found for Puerto Ricans on the mainland.

21. Information on diet was gathered among New York City Puerto Ricans during the Health Center Study by either observing meals or by recording recalls of food intake daily over a period of one week from all residents in 12 households in the sample. A reliability check on this information was performed by gathering daily intakes for most of the same households at least one other time during the course of the study. These data comport well with information reported for Boston (Yohai 1977) and urban Connecticut (Lieberman 1979), and the findings are probably applicable to urban-dwelling, mainland Puerto Ricans in general. Research on the diets of migrant workers, however, indicates significant differences from the pattern described here (Quinones et al. 1976).

22. See note 1 for an explanation of this term.

23. These data were collected near the end of the observation period in the Health Center Study. Researchers asked the chief caretakers in 41 house-

holds in which they were working to show them all medicines (prescription, over-the-counter, and herbal) that were in the house and, for the latter two types, to explain where they got them, who used them, for what purpose and how often they were used, when they were last used, and where they had heard about the medication. Table 7.8 omits data on five households which the researchers suspected gave incomplete information on over-the-counter and herbal preparations.

24. The data in this section come from the 79 households of the Health Center Study and from observations in a local *botánica*, made on 11 days in July, 1968, by Stanley Fisch, M.D. During approximately 35 hours of participant-observation Dr. Fisch recorded 22 transactions, identifying each purchaser and user by age and sex, the complaint for which the herbs were sought, and the manner in which they were to be used. I would like to thank Dr. Fisch for making this information available to me.

25. I am grateful to J. Worth Estes, M.D., of the Department of Pharmacology, Boston University School of Medicine, for evaluating the possible efficacy of the list of 56 botanicals and their uses compiled by Dr. Fisch. Dr. Fisch's list comprised the entire stock of one neighborhood *botánica*. *Botánicas* in the *Barrio* (Spanish Harlem), however, maintain more complete and generally fresher inventories.

26. With regard to cost of services as a determinant of usage patterns, it is important to note that a higher proportion of Hispanic than either black or white users of outpatient departments and emergency rooms in the southern New York region, at any rate, pay for treatment themselves rather than using either Medicaid or Blue Cross reimbursements (Alers 1978:39). Since figures on the average cost of this treatment are not available (it can range as low as 50 cents), this finding does not negate the general importance of expense in determining the utilization practices of Puerto Ricans. Nevertheless, it does suggest some special factors operating in the usage patterns of this ethnic group which bear further investigation.

27. Utilization figures from southern New York State (Alers 1978:40), which reveal that Hispanics more than either blacks or whites visit walk-in and screening clinics in hospital outpatient departments, further support the proposition that services that do not require appointments appeal strongly to this population.

28. A number of investigators have attributed Puerto Ricans' medical usage practices to various sociocultural features—for example, a "parochial" social organization and "popular" health orientation (Suchman 1964), previous experience with Public Health Clinics in Puerto Rico, saints cults (*santerismo*), or language barriers (Weidman 1978:300–301). However, since the data are insufficiently clear that Puerto Ricans' usage patterns for preventive services are in fact distinct from groups of comparable income and education, it seems unnecessary in my opinion to invoke these special cultural explanations.

29. In a study of the effects of Medicaid on the usage patterns of a sample of medically well-provided welfare recipients in New York City, Olendzki (1974) found that Puerto Ricans, in contrast to both whites and blacks, increased their utilization after Medicaid. In view of Alers's observation, dis-

cussed in note 26, that Puerto Ricans use Medicaid as the means of payment in public facilities far less than black or white patients, it seems logical to conclude that Medicaid reimbursement has supported Puerto Ricans' use of private practitioners.

30. According to the most recent (and doubtless outmoded) figures available (1969), 83 percent of all Puerto Ricans on the continent reported Spanish as their first language, and 72 percent reported it as the language usually spoken in the home (quoted in Wagenheim 1975:86, from U.S. Census Bureau figures). While thus favoring Spanish for intimate and domestic conversation, most mainland Puerto Ricans also know English. In the same 1969 survey, 69 percent reported an ability to read and write the language, although only 56 percent of women over 25 years of age claimed to do so. Since women usually take charge of the family's medical needs, language differences clearly play a role in medical encounters.

31. Although linguistic issues in psychotherapy with bilingual patients are not directly within the purview of this volume, a number of interesting contributions on this subject have been made with regard to Spanish speakers (see, for example, Sabin 1975; Marcos and Alpert 1976; and particularly Bluestone, Bisi, and Katz 1969, on the use of translators in psychotherapeutic evaluations and therapy). An important study of language in psychiatric evaluation (Marcos et al. 1973) is directly relevant to this book, however, since preliminary screening of psychiatric patients often occurs in medical clinics. The study indicated that bilingual patients (who were interviewed twice —once in Spanish, their first language, and once in English) were judged much more seriously ill on the basis of their English interviews than their Spanish ones. Moreover, the differences in evaluation were largely due to certain speech mannerisms, which were considered psychopathological in the English interview and were in fact problems of second-language mastery. Although the sample size in the study was small (N = 10), the results nevertheless suggest that in situations where psychopathology is suspected in a bilingual medical patient, preliminary evaluation would be made more accurately in Spanish.

32. In preparing this section and the following one on the family, I would like to acknowledge the aid of a useful training package for health professionals, "The Americans: Boricuas," developed by the Human Resources Development Trust (B.C.P.O. Box 3006, East Orange, N.J. 07019). The package includes a film, audio tapes, and a manual, designed to provide pertinent cultural information on Puerto Ricans.

33. First names, preceded by the honorific Don for males or Doña for females, may, however, be used as a sign of respect for the elderly.

References

ABAD, VICENTE, JUAN RAMOS, and ELIZABETH BOYCE. 1974. A Model for Delivery of Mental Health Services to Spanish-speaking Minorities. *American Journal of Orthopsychiatry* 44:584–595.

AIKEN, LINDA H. 1976. Chronic Illness and Responsive Ambulatory Care.

In *The Growth of Bureaucratic Medicine,* ed. David Mechanic. New York: Wiley.

ALCASID, MARIA LOURDES, et al. 1973. Bronchial Asthma and Intestinal Parasites. *New York State Journal of Medicine* 73:1786–1788.

ALERS, JOSÉ OSCAR. 1978. *Puerto Ricans and Health: Findings from New York City.* Hispanic Research Center Monograph Series, Fordham University, Monograph no. 1.

BECKER, MARSHALL H., ROBERT H. DRACHMAN, and JOHN P. KIRSCHT. 1974. A New Approach to Explaining Sick-Role Behavior in Low-Income Populations. *American Journal of Public Health* 64:205–216.

BECKER, MARSHALL H., and LOIS A. MAIMAN. 1975. Sociobehavioral Determinants of Compliance with Health and Medical Care Recommendations. *Medical Care* 13:10–24.

BERLE, BEATRICE BISHOP. 1958. *80 Puerto Rican Families in New York City: Health and Disease Studied in Context.* New York: Columbia University Press. (Reprinted 1975, Arno Press.)

BERNICK, KATHRYNE. 1978. Issues in Pediatric Screening. In *Children's Medical Care Needs and Treatments.* Report of the Harvard Child Health Project, vol. 2. Cambridge, Mass.: Balinger.

BLUE CROSS–BLUE SHIELD. 1975. *Who Uses Ambulatory Care Services?* American Cancer Society Report no. 3, New York.

BLUESTONE, HARVEY, RICARDO BISI, and ARTHUR J. KATZ. 1969. The Establishment of a Mental Health Service in a Predominantly Spanish-speaking Neighborhood of New York City. *Behavioral Neuropsychiatry* 1:12–16.

BOGDEN, JOHN D., MARK A. QUINONES, and AHMED EL NAKAH. 1975. Pesticide Exposure among Migrant Workers in Southern New Jersey. *Bulletin of Environmental Contamination and Toxicology* 13:513–517.

BOWERING, JEAN, et al. 1978. Infant Feeding Practices in East Harlem. *Journal of the American Dietetic Association* 72:148–155.

BROWN, HOWARD W. 1975. *Basic Clinical Parasitology* (4th ed.). New York: Appleton-Century-Crofts.

BROWNELL, KATHARINE DODGE, and FRANCES BAILEN-ROSE. 1973. Acute Rheumatic Fever in Children. *Journal of the American Medical Association* 224:1593–1597.

BULLOUGH, BONNIE. 1972. Poverty, Ethnic Identity and Preventive Health Care. *Journal of Health and Social Behavior* 13:374–359.

CENTER for HUMAN RESOURCES PLANNING and DEVELOPMENT, et al. 1977. The Americans: Boricuas. Multimedia training manual. Human Resources Development Trust, East Orange, N.J.

CHASE, HELEN C., and FRIEDA G. NELSON. 1973. A Study of Risks, Medical Care, and Infant Mortality: III. Education of Mother, Medical Care and Condition of Infant. *American Journal of Public Health* 63.11 (Suppl.): 27–40.

COHEN, RAQUEL E. 1972. Principles of Preventive Mental Health Programs for Ethnic Minority Populations: The Acculturation of Puerto Ricans to the United States. *American Journal of Psychiatry* 128:1529–1533.

DAVIS, MILTON S. 1968. Variation in Patients' Compliance with Doctors' Advice: An Empirical Analysis of Patterns of Communication. *American Journal of Public Health* 58:274–288.

———. 1971. Variation in Patients' Compliance with Doctors' Orders: Medical Practice and Doctor-Patient Interaction. *Psychiatry in Medicine* 2:31–54.

DAVITZ, LOIS L., JOEL R. DAVITZ, and YASUKO HIGUCHI. 1977. Cross-cultural Inferences of Physical Pain and Psychological Distress. *Nursing Times* 73.15:521–523, 73.16:556–558.

DELBANCO, THOMAS L. 1976. The Periodic Health Examination for the Adult: Waste or Wisdom? *Primary Care* 3:205–214.

DOHRENWEND, BRUCE P., and BARBARA S. DOHRENWEND. 1969. *Social Status and Psychological Disorder: A Causal Inquiry.* New York: Wiley-Interscience.

DUTTON, DIANA B. 1978. Explaining the Low Use of Health Services by the Poor: Costs, Attitudes, or Delivery Systems? *American Sociological Review* 43:348–368.

ENGEL, GEORGE L. 1977. The Need for a New Medical Model: A Challenge for Biomedicine. *Science* 196:129–136.

ERHARDT, CARL L., FRIEDA G. NELSON, and JEAN PAKTER. 1971. Seasonal Patterns of Conception in New York City. *American Journal of Public Health* 61:2246–2258.

FERNÁNDEZ, NELSON A., et al. 1968. Nutritional Status in [a] Puerto Rican Slum Area. *American Journal of Clinical Nutrition* 21:646–656.

FERNÁNDEZ-LÓPEZ, NELSON A., JOSE C. BURGOS, and CONRADO F. ASENJO. 1969. Obesity in Puerto Rican Children and Adults. *Boletín de la Asociación Medical de Puerto Rico* 61:153–157.

FERNÁNDEZ-MARINA, R. 1961. The Puerto Rican Syndrome: Its Dynamics and Cultural Determinants. *Psychiatry* 24:79–82.

FINNERTY, FRANK A., JR., EDWARD C. MATTIE, and FRANCIS A. FINNERTY, III. 1973. Hypertension in the Inner City: Analysis of Clinic Dropouts. *Circulation* 57:73–75.

FITZPATRICK, JOSEPH P. 1971. *Puerto Rican Americans: The Meaning of Migration to the Mainland.* Englewood Cliffs, N.J.: Prentice-Hall.

———. 1975. Puerto Rican Addicts and Non-Addicts: A Comparison. Institute for Social Research, Fordham University, New York City (manuscript).

FRANCIS, VIDA, BARBARA M. KORSCH, and MARIG J. MORRIS. 1969. Gaps in Doctor-Patient Communication: Patients' Response to Medical Advice. *New England Journal of Medicine* 280:535–540.

GARRISON, VIVIAN. 1972. Social Networks, Social Change and Mental Health among Migrants in a New York City Slum. Ph.D. dissertation, Department of Anthropology, Columbia University.

———. 1974. Sectarianism and Psychosocial Adjustment: A Controlled Comparison of Puerto Rican Pentecostals and Catholics. In *Religious Movements in Contemporary America,* ed. Irving I. Zaretsky and Mark P. Leone. Princeton, N.J.: Princeton University Press.

————. 1977a. The "Puerto Rican Syndrome" in Psychiatry and *Espiritismo*. In *Case Studies in Spirit Possession,* ed. Vincent Crapanzano and Vivian Garrison. New York: Wiley.

————. 1977b. Doctor, *Espiritista* or Psychiatrist: Health-Seeking Behavior in a Puerto Rican Neighborhood of New York City. *Medical Anthropology* 1.2:65–180.

GAVIRIA, MOISES, and RONALD M. WINTROB. 1976. Supernatural Influence in Psychopathology: Puerto Rican Beliefs about Mental Illness. *Canadian Psychiatric Association Journal* 21.6:361–369.

GLUCK, GEORGE M., et al. 1972. Dental Health of Puerto Rican Migrant Workers. *Health Service Reports* 87:456–460.

GORDON, TAVIA, et al. 1974. Differences in Coronary Heart Disease in Framingham, Honolulu, and Puerto Rico. *Journal of Chronic Diseases* 27:329–344.

GRAEF, JOHN. 1977. Lead Poisoning. In *Children's Medical Care Needs and Treatment.* Report of the Harvard Child Health Project, vol. 2. Cambridge, Mass.: Balinger.

GUINEE, VINCENT F. 1972. Lead Poisoning. *American Journal of Medicine* 52:283–288.

GUTTMACHER, SALLY, and JACK ELINSON. 1971. Ethno-Religious Variation in Perception of Illness: The Use of Illness as an Explanation for Deviant Behavior. *Social Science and Medicine* 5:117–125.

HABERMAN, PAUL W. 1970. Ethnic Differences in Psychiatric Symptoms Reported in Community Surveys. *Public Health Reports* 85:495–502.

————. 1976. Psychiatric Symptoms among Puerto Ricans in Puerto Rico and New York City. *Ethnicity* 3:133–144.

HABERMAN, PAUL W., and JILL SHEINBERG. 1967. Implicative Drinking in a Household Survey: A Corroborative Note in Subgroup Differences. *Quarterly Journal of Studies on Alcohol* 28:538–543.

HARGUS, E. P., et al. 1976. Intestinal Parasitosis in Childhood Populations of Latin Origin. *Clinical Pediatrics* 15:927–929.

HARWOOD, ALAN. 1970. Family-Centered and Comprehensive Care at the Martin Luther King, Jr. Neighborhood Health Center (unpublished report). (Printed, with modifications, as part of the *Dr. Martin Luther King, Jr. Health Center Fourth Annual Report,* pp. 151–169. Bronx, New York: Dr. Martin Luther King, Jr. Health Center.)

————. 1971a. The Hot-Cold Theory of Disease: Implications for Treatment of Puerto Rican Patients. *Journal of the American Medical Association* 216:1153–1158.

————. 1971b. Housing and Health in the Area of the Dr. Martin Luther King, Jr. Health Center. In *Nutrition and Human Needs,* part 4. Housing and Sanitation Hearings of the U.S. Senate Committee on Human Needs, 91st Congress. Washington, D.C.: U.S. Government Printing Office.

————. 1977. *Rx: Spiritist As Needed: A Study of a Puerto Rican Community Mental Health Resource.* New York: Wiley.

————. 1979. Ethnicity and Clinical Care: Puerto Ricans. *Physician Assistant and Health Practitioner* 3:71–74.

HARWOOD, ALAN, and MARCIA SORCINELLI. 1978. Leading Causes of Death among Puerto Rican–born New Yorkers under Age 15 (manuscript).

HAYNES, R. BRIAN. 1976. A Critical Review of the "Determinants" of Patient Compliance with Therapeutic Regimens. In *Compliance with Therapeutic Regimens,* ed. David L. Sackett and R. Brian Haynes. Baltimore: Johns Hopkins University Press.

HEINZELMANN, FRED, and RICHARD W. BAGLEY. 1970. Response to Physical Activity Programs and Their Effects on Health Behavior. *Public Health Reports* 85:905–911.

HERSHEY, JOHN C., HAROLD S. LUFT, and JOAN M. GIANARIS. 1975. Making Sense Out of Utilization Data. *Medical Care* 13:838–854.

HISPANIC HEALTH COUNCIL. n.d. Report on Activities (manuscript).

HOWARD, KAY, et al. 1970. Therapeutic Style and Attrition Rate from Psychiatric Drug Treatment. *Journal of Nervous and Mental Diseases* 150:102–110.

JANZEN, JOHN. 1977. *The Quest for Therapy in the Lower Zaire.* Berkeley: University of California Press.

JOHNSON, LOUISE A. 1972. *East Harlem Community Health Center.* New York: Mt. Sinai School of Medicine.

KAGAN, I. G., D. W. RAIRIGH, and R. L. KAISER. 1962. A Clinical, Parasitological and Immunologic Study of Schistosomiasis in 103 Puerto Rican Males Residing in the United States. *Annals of Internal Medicine* 56:457–470.

KAPLAN, SEYMOUR R., and MELVIN ROMAN. 1973. *The Organization and Delivery of Mental Health Services in the Ghetto: The Lincoln Hospital Experience.* New York: Praeger.

KLERMAN, R. V., J. G. JONES, and M. C. HULL. 1966. Puerto Ricans in a Small U.S. City. *Public Health Reports,* U.S. Department of Health, Education and Welfare, 81:369–376.

KOLE, DELBERT M. A. 1966. A Cross-cultural Study of Medical-Psychiatric Symptoms. *Journal of Health and Human Behavior* 7:162–173.

KORNS, ALEXANDER. 1977. Coverage Issues Raised by Comparisons between CPS and Establishment Employment. *Proceedings of the Social Statistics Section, American Statistical Association, 1977.*

KORSCH, BARBARA M., ETHEL K. GOZZI, and VIDA FRANCIS. 1968. Gaps in Doctor-Patient Communication: Doctor-Patient Interaction and Patient Satisfaction. *Pediatrics* 42:855–871.

KOSS, JOAN. 1970. Terapéutica del sistema de una secta en Puerto Rico. *Revista de Ciencias Sociales* (Rio Piedras) 14:259–278.

LEE, S. L., and M. SIEGEL. 1976. Systemic Lupus Erythematosus: Epidemiological Clues to Pathogenesis. In *Infection and Immunology in the Rheumatic Diseases,* ed. D. C. Dumonde. Oxford: Blackwell.

LEHMANN, STANLEY. 1970 Selected Self-Help: A Study of Clients of a Community Social Psychiatry Service. *American Journal of Psychiatry* 126:1444–1454.

LIEBERMAN, LESLIE SUE. 1979. Medico-nutritional Practices among Puerto

Ricans in a Small Urban Northeastern Community in the United States. *Social Science and Medicine* 13B:191–198.

LUBCHANSKY, ISAAC, GLADYS EGRI, and JANET STOKES. 1970. Puerto Rican Spiritualists View Mental Illness: The Faith Healer as Paraprofessional. *American Journal of Psychiatry* 127.3:312–321.

MALDONADO-DENIS, MANUEL. 1972. *Puerto Rico: A Socio-historic Interpretation,* trans. Elena Vialo. New York: Vintage. (Originally published as *Puerto Rico: Una interpretación histórico-social,* Mexico City, 1972.)

MARCOS, LUIS R., et al. 1973. The Language Barrier in Evaluating Spanish-American Patients. *Archives of General Psychiatry* 29:655–659.

MARCOS, LUIS R., and MURRAY ALPERT. 1976. Strategies and Risks in Psychotherapy with Bilingual Patients: The Phenomenon of Language Independence. *American Journal of Psychiatry* 133:1275–1278.

MEHLMAN, R. 1961. The Puerto Rican Syndrome. *American Journal of Psychiatry* 118:328.

MEYERS, SAMUEL, PHILIP SCHWEITZER, and CHARLES D. GERSON. 1977. Anemia and Intestinal Dysfunction in Former Residents of the Caribbean. *Archives of Internal Medicine* 137.2:181–186.

MONK, MARY, and M. ELLEN WARSHAUER. 1974. Completed and Attempted Suicide in Three Ethnic Groups. *American Journal of Epidemiology* 100:333–345.

MONTIJO, JORGE. 1975. The Puerto Rican Client. *Professional Psychology* 6:475–477.

MUMFORD, EMILY. 1973. Puerto Rican Perspectives on Mental Illness. *Mt. Sinai Journal of Medicine* 40:768–779.

MURILLO-ROHDE, ILDAURA. 1976. Family Life among Mainland Puerto Ricans in New York City Slums. *Perspectives in Psychiatric Care* 14.4:174–179.

NEWMAN, R. G., et al. 1974. Narcotic Addiction in New York City: Trends from 1968 to mid-1973. *American Journal of Drug and Alcohol Abuse* 1:53–66.

NORMAND, WILLIAM C., JUAN IGLESIAS, and STEPHEN PAYN. 1974. Brief Group Therapy to Facilitate Utilization of Mental Health Services by Spanish-speaking Patients. *American Journal of Orthopsychiatry* 44:37–42.

OAKES, THOMAS W., et al. 1970. Family Expectations and Arthritis Patient Compliance to a Hand Resting Splint Regimen. *Journal of Chronic Diseases* 22:757–764.

OKADA, LOUISE M., and GERALD SPARER. 1976. Access to Usual Source of Care by Race and Income in Ten Urban Areas. *Journal of Community Health* 1:163–174.

OLENDZKI, MARGARET C. 1974. Medicaid Benefits Mainly the Younger and Less Sick. *Medical Care* 12:163–172.

OSOFSKY, HOWARD J., and NORMAN KENDALL. 1973. Poverty as a Criterion of Risk. *Clinical Obstetrics and Gynecology* 16:103–119.

PADILLA, ELENA. 1958. *Up from Puerto Rico.* New York: Columbia University Press.

PASAMANICK, BENJAMIN. 1962. Prevalence and Distribution of Psychosomatic Conditions in an Urban Population According to Social Class. *Psychosomatic Medicine* 24:352–356.

PODELL, LAWRENCE. 1973. Health Care of Preschool Children in Families on Welfare. *New York State Journal of Medicine* 73:1120–1123.

QUINONES, MARK A., et al. 1976. A Preliminary Study of Circulating Vitamins in a Puerto Rican Migrant Farm Population in New Jersey. *American Journal of Public Health* 66:172–173.

RENDON, MARIO. 1976. Transcultural Aspects of Mental Illness among Puerto Rican Adolescents in New York. In *Youth in a Changing World: Cross-Cultural Perspectives on Adolescence.* The Hague: Mouton.

RODRÍGUEZ, CLARA. 1975. A Cost-Benefit Analysis of Subjective Factors Affecting Assimilation. *Ethnicity* 2:66–80.

RODRÍGUEZ, ISMAEL D. 1971. Group Work with Hospitalized Puerto Rican Patients. *Hospital and Community Psychiatry* 22:219–220.

ROGLER, LLOYD. 1978. Help Patterns, the Family, and Mental Health: Puerto Ricans in the United States. *International Migration Review* 12:248–259.

ROGLER, LLOYD H., and AUGUST B. HOLLINGSHEAD. 1961. The Puerto Rican Spiritist as a Psychiatrist. *American Journal of Sociology* 67:17–21.

———.1965. *Trapped: Families and Schizophrenia.* New York: Wiley.

ROTHENBERG, A. 1964. Puerto Rico and Aggression. *American Journal of Psychiatry* 120:962–970.

SABIN, JAMES E. 1975. Translating Despair. *American Journal of Psychiatry* 132:197–199.

SACKETT, DAVID L., and R. BRIAN HAYNES, eds. 1976. *Compliance with Therapeutic Regimens.* Baltimore: Johns Hopkins University Press.

SANJUR, DIVA, EUNICE ROMERO, and MARIAN KIRA. 1971. Milk Consumption of Puerto Rican Preschool Children in Rural New York. *American Journal of Clinical Nutrition* 24:1320–1326.

SCHENSUL, STEPHEN L., et al. 1978. Hispanic Health Research Project. Summary Project Report: The First Six Months, January–July, 1978 (manuscript).

SCHMIDT, DAVID D. 1977. Patient Compliance: The Effect of the Doctor as a Therapeutic Agent. *Journal of Family Practice* 4:853–856.

SCOTT, CLARISSA. 1975. The Relationship between Beliefs about the Menstrual Cycle and Choices of Fertility Regulating Methods within Five Ethnic Groups. *International Journal of Gynaecology and Obstetrics* 13:105–109.

SEDA, EDUARDO. 1973. *Social Change and Personality in a Puerto Rican Agrarian Reform Community* Evanston, Ill., Northwestern University Press.

SEIDMAN, HERBERT. 1970. Cancer Death Rates by Site and Sex for Religious and Socioeconomic Groups in New York City. *Environmental Research* 3:234–250.

SIEGEL, M., et al. 1965. Racial Differences in Gamma Globulin Levels: Comparative Data for Negroes, Puerto Ricans, and Other Caucasians. *Journal of Laboratory and Clinical Medicine* 66:715–720.

SNARR, RICHARD, and JOHN C. BALL. 1974. Involvement in a Drug Subculture and Abstinence Following Treatment among Puerto Rican Narcotic Addicts. *British Journal of Addiction* 69:243–248.

STEWART, HAROLD L., et al. 1966. Epidemiology of Cancers of Uterine Cervix and Corpus, Breast and Ovary in Israel and New York City. *Journal of the National Cancer Institute* 37:1–95.

STRAUSS, ANSELM L. 1969. Medical Organization, Medical Care and Lower Income Groups. *Social Science and Medicine* 3:143–177.

SUCHMAN, EDWARD A. 1964. Sociomedical Variations among Ethnic Groups. *American Journal of Sociology* 70:319–331.

SUCHMAN, EDWARD A., and BERNARD S. PHILLIPS. 1958. An analysis of the Validity of Health Questionnaires. *Social Forces* 36:223–232.

SVARSTAD, BONNIE L. 1976. Physician-Patient Communication and Patient Conformity with Medical Advice. In *The Growth of Bureaucratic Medicine,* ed. David Mechanic. New York: Wiley.

SWEET, JAMES A. 1974. Differentials in the Rate of Fertility Decline: 1960–1970. *Family Planning Perspectives* 6:103–107.

TALLMER, MARGOT. 1977. Some Factors in the Education of Older Members of Minority Groups. *Journal of Geriatric Psychiatry* 10.1:89–98.

TEIRSTEIN, ALVIN S., LOUIS E. SILTZEACH, and HERBERT BERGER. 1976. Patterns of Sarcoidosis in Three Population Groups in New York City. *Annals of the New York Academy of Sciences* 278:371–376.

TORRES, ROSA MARINA. 1959. Dietary Patterns of the Puerto Rican People. *American Journal of Clinical Nutrition* 7:349–355.

TORRES-MATRULLO, CHRISTINE. 1976. Acculturation and Psychopathology among Puerto Rican Women in Mainland United States. *American Journal of Orthopsychiatry* 46:710–719.

TRAUTMAN, EDGAR C. 1961. The Suicidal Fit: A Psychobiologic Study on Puerto Rican Immigrants. *Archives of General Psychiatry* 5:76–83.

U.S. BUREAU OF THE CENSUS. 1978. *Current Population Reports.* Series P–20, no. 328, Persons of Spanish Origin in the United States: March 1978 (Advance Report). Washington, D.C.: U.S. Government Printing Office.

U.S. COMMISSION ON CIVIL RIGHTS. 1976. *Puertorriqueños en los Estados Unidos continentales: un futuro incierto.* Washington, D.C.

U.S. DEPARTMENT OF HEALTH, EDUCATION, and WELFARE. 1978. Acute Conditions: Incidence and Associated Disability, United States, July 1976– June 1977. Vital and Health Statistics, series 10, no. 125. DHEW Publication no. (PHS) 78–1553. Washington, D.C.: U.S. Government Printing Office.

VAETH, STEPHEN. 1974. Rubella among Puerto Rican Basic Trainees. *Military Medicine* 142:539–541.

WAGENHEIM, KAL. 1975. *A Survey of Puerto Ricans on the U.S. Mainland in the 1970s.* New York: Praeger.

WEIDMAN, HAZEL H. 1978. Miami Health Ecology Project Report: A Statement on Ethnicity and Health, vol. 1. Department of Psychiatry, University of Miami School of Medicine (manuscript).

WEISENBERG, MATISYOHU, et al. 1975. Pain: Anxiety and Attitudes in

Black, White, and Puerto Rican Patients. *Psychosomatic Medicine* 37:123–135.

WHITBY, L. G., et al. 1974. Screening for Disease. *Lancet* 2:7884–7895 (9 parts).

WHITE, KERR L. 1967. Improved Medical Care Statistics and the Health Services System. *Public Health Reports* 82:847–854.

WINSBERG, GWYNNE ROESELER, et al. 1974. Schistosomiasis in Chicago: A Study of the Westown Puerto Rican Population. *American Journal of Epidemiology* 100:324–332.

―――. 1975. Prevalence of Intestinal Parasites in Latino Residents of Chicago. *American Journal of Epidemiology* 102:526–532.

WISE, HAROLD B. 1968. Montefiore Hospital Neighborhood Medical Care Demonstration: A Case Study. *Milbank Memorial Fund Quarterly* 46.3 (Part 1):297–307.

YOHAI, FANNY. 1977. Dietary Patterns of Spanish-speaking People Living in the Boston Area. *Journal of the American Dietetic Association* 71:273–275.

ZOLA, IRVING KENNETH. 1964. Illness Behavior in the Working Class. In *Blue Collar World,* ed. Arthur B. Shostak and William Gomberg. Englewood Cliffs, N.J.: Prentice-Hall.

―――. 1966. Culture and Symptoms An Analysis of Patients' Presenting Complaints. *American Sociological Review* 31:615–630.

―――. 1973. Pathways to the Doctor—From Person to Patient. *Social Science and Medicine* 7:677–689.

8
Guidelines for Culturally Appropriate Health Care

ALAN HARWOOD

THE FOREGOING CHAPTERS have provided detailed information on the health beliefs and behaviors of seven American ethnic groups. Clinicians who routinely treat members of one or more of these groups should, of course, read the specific chapters on those groups. However, comparison of the information contained in the seven chapters also reveals a number of key issues that arise in the health care of patients and their families from all seven groups. These recurrent issues allow for the development of general guidelines for the delivery of health services to ethnic groups. The guidelines thus supplement the discussion on practical applications included in the Introduction (pp. 20–27). The prescriptions presented in this chapter will be useful both to clinicians who treat people from ethnic categories that are not specifically included in this volume and, as a recapitulation of major issues, to practitioners who deliver care to the seven groups discussed previously in greater detail.

The health-care issues that will be covered in this concluding chapter focus specifically on illness rather than disease. Consequently, no comparative statements about epidemiology will be provided, largely because the data on different ethnic groups have been collected using different categories and measures of health status. The discussion will follow the major headings that have been used for structuring information throughout this book. It will begin with a consideration of sources of variation *within* ethnic groups and suggest a set of predictors that will assist clinicians in identifying individual patients whose behavior in health-care contexts is likely to be influenced by ethnic norms.

Recognizing Intraethnic Variation in Clinical Care

Though standards for health behavior may be shared among people of an ethnic category, each patient remains, nonetheless, an individual who may subscribe to the standards of his group to varying degrees and in varying situations. Five major factors may be identified that contribute to variation in the health beliefs and behaviors of members of ethnic categories, and the alert clinician should evaluate each patient individually in terms of these factors in order to determine the needs of the particular patient and the degree to which ethnic health standards and behaviors are likely to be relevant to his care.

Since many factors that are typically listed as sources of intraethnic variation are highly intercorrelated (for example, education and level of acculturation, income and previous experience with biomedical services), the following sections focus on five major factors that may be viewed as contributing relatively independent effects on health behavior.

Exposure to Biomedical and Popular Standards of Health Care

The degree to which patients adhere to ethnic standards of health behavior is related to the amount and kind of exposure they have had to biomedical and popular American standards and behaviors—in short, the extent to which they have been acculturated to more pervasive American norms of health behavior. A number of specific (often intercorrelated) determinants of this exposure or acculturation can be enumerated:

1. A relatively high level of formal education (probably a minimum of several years of secondary school).
2. Greater generational removal from immigrant status.
3. A low degree of encapsulation within an ethnic and family social network.
4. Experience with medical services that incorporate patient education and personalized care into treatment.
5. Previous experience with particular diseases in the immediate family.
6. For immigrants, immigration to this country at an early age.
7. Urban, as opposed to rural, origin.
8. Limited migration back and forth to the mother country.

In the absence of any highly predictive single indicator of adherence to ethnic health standards or behaviors, the clinician should, as part of his early interaction with patients, determine their status on these eight dimensions to assess the importance that ethnic health culture may assume in their ongoing care. It is necessary to recognize, however, that even patients who are predicted to display low adherence to an ethnic health culture on the basis of these indicators may nevertheless resort to ethnically derived, nonmainstream modes of behavior in certain situations (for example, in cases of terminal illness, or when symptoms have been dismissed by a biomedical practitioner as being of unknown or psychological origin). Therefore, although the factors enumerated above will differentiate with reasonable accuracy those patients who are most likely to follow ethnically based norms of health behavior, treatment of individual patients may in certain situations necessitate knowledge of ethnic health standards and behaviors on the part of the clinician.

Income

Though evidence indicates that changes in the medical delivery system instituted in this country during the past decade or so have generally reduced the effect of income differentials on health-care utilization (Wolinsky 1978), this factor still continues to produce important variations in other health behaviors. From the sources of care actually used and the sequence in which different types of care are resorted to, to the ability to carry through on expensive treatment regimens and the support systems available for long-term care, income differences contribute markedly to variations in patients' behavior within ethnic groups.

Occupation

A person's occupation particularly influences the kinds of health hazards to which he is exposed, the point at which he may be willing to discontinue work and adopt the sick role, and compliance with activity, diet, or other restrictions of a treatment regimen. The principal kinds of occupational differences that assume importance for these health behaviors are as follows: migrant as opposed to fixed occupation, manual in contrast to clerical or other more sedentary work, and of course regularity of employment. All these occupational variables may result in intraethnic variation in health behavior.

Area of Origin in the Mother Country

Because the ethnic categories recognized in this country are a product of our own social and cultural history, one cannot assume that the health beliefs and practices of immigrants who are placed together within these categories are necessarily shared. In this volume, for example, Ragucci discusses internal variation among Italian Americans coming from different provinces of Italy, and Laguerre also speaks of regional variation in so small a country as Haiti. Though area of origin undoubtedly contributes less to intraethnic variation than factors such as income and acculturation, it cannot be entirely ignored.

Religion

Though members of a single ethnic group often profess the same religion, this is not always the case, and religious differences can produce intraethnic variations in health behavior. Of the groups covered in this volume, for example, intraethnic religious variation has been singled out among urban blacks, Haitians, Navajos, and Puerto Ricans as having important effects on adherence to certain treatment regimens and on reactions to chronic and terminal disease.

Implications for the Clinician

Of major importance to the clinician with regard to intraethnic variation is a way of identifying those patients who are most likely to adhere to ethnic standards of health behavior—that is, "behavioral ethnics."[1] The eight factors specified earlier in this section can serve this function by screening out those people who are most acculturated to general American health norms and are thus least likely to operate as behavioral ethnics in health-care situations. However, one must recognize that even the behavior of behavioral ethnics will not necessarily be uniform and will vary according to income, occupation, and the other major factors enumerated above.

Ethnic Concepts of Disease and Illness in Clinical Care

In the past decade or so both the increase of medical services to low-income and rural Americans and the educational effects of the mass media (particularly television) have caused biomedical ideas to be disseminated to increasing numbers of people. As a result, the ignorance of biomedical categories of disease, their symptoms, and their possible causes, which was frequently demonstrated in the literature of the 1960s (see, for example, Samora, Saunders, and Larson 1961; Suchman 1964; Jenkins 1966; and Plaja, Cohen, and Samora 1968), appears to have diminished considerably. In addition, as the foregoing chapters reveal, more and more people of every ethnic background turn in most instances today to biomedical sources as the first and preferred mode of care outside the home.

In spite of this more widespread dissemination of biomedical knowledge and greater utilization of mainstream health services, ethnic conceptions of illness and disease still affect health care, with particular regard to patient compliance, the effects of simultaneously using biomedical and alternative sources of care, and the management of culture-specific syndromes. Moreover, as Schreiber and Homiak point out in this volume, greater utilization of mainstream medicine may extend people's knowledge of the more observable aspects of biomedicine, but it cannot lead to greater lay knowledge of biomedical ideas unless special educational efforts are made by health-care personnel. To assist the clinician in responding to these various factors that make folk and popular concepts of disease relevant to medical delivery, the general procedures described in the following sections may be found helpful.

Patient Assessment

Applying the information on sources of intraethnic variation enumerated above, the clinician should assess each patient in terms of the probability that he espouses ethnic concepts of disease. Because individuals not so identified may nonetheless utilize ethnic concepts under particular circumstances, it is also advisable for the clinician to question patients concerning their ideas about their diseases under the following circumstances: (1) in treating chronic disease, where good patient-practitioner communication is demonstrably important; (2) in diagnosing and treating diseases that relate specifically to known folk etiological notions; (3) in treating conditions whose symptoms overlap in whole or in part with a culture-specific syndrome; and (4) in life-threatening situations— for example, serious acute or chronic disease. These four circumstances have been singled out for special attention because they are ones in which cultural beliefs about disease are most likely to affect patient attitudes and adherence to prescribed regimens. Circumstances (2) and (3) will be discussed in greater detail later in this section.

Eliciting the Patient's Concept of Disease

The issue of eliciting the patient's concept of disease was discussed at some length in the Introduction (pp. 23–24); however, it may be useful here to expand a point made in that context—namely, that the clinician should take particular care to elicit the patient's concept of his problem in a way that is nonjudgmental and that communicates genuine interest in the response. This might be accomplished by the following kind of preliminary explanation: "I know that patients and doctors sometimes have different ideas about diseases and what causes them. So it's often important in treating a disease to get clear on how both the doctor and the patient think about it. That's why I'd like to know more about your ideas on [whatever disease or symptom is relevant to the situation]. That way I can know what your concerns are, and we can work together in treating your sickness." (Of course, clarification of patients' disease concepts may also be relevant to other clinical tasks, such as eliciting a history or explaining a diagnostic procedure, and the wording of the introductory comment would have to be modified accordingly.) Following such an introductory statement, a patient's concepts of his disease might then be elicited according to the format proposed by Kleinman, Eisenberg, and Good (1978) and discussed in note 6 to the Introduction.

Identifying Sources of Discrepancy between Patients' and Practitioners' Concepts of Disease or Illness

Although the elicitation procedure suggested above adequately serves to reveal discrepancies between patients' and practitioners' concepts, specifying the kinds of discrepancies that are likely to occur can alert the clinician to the most frequent sources of confusion or "noise" in communication with patients. In this way the provider can be sure that his questions have tapped most potential areas of miscommunication.

A frequent source of poor communication between clinicians and patients occurs when one party uses a term that is unfamiliar to the other in labeling a disease or symptom. However, this kind of miscommunication is readily perceived and easily rectified by a request for an explanation of the unknown term, and patients should be encouraged to ask for such clarification from health-care practitioners. A more insidious source of poor communication in medical encounters occurs when patients and biomedically trained providers use the same term but mean different things by it. In this situation the lack of accurate communication may go undetected because both speakers are using the same term. Variations in the speakers' meanings commonly arise from the following sources:

1. The same term for a disease or symptom may be applied to different pathological states, to different bodily organs, and so forth—in other words, the objects to which a term refers may differ for the two speakers.
2. Ideas about the etiology of the disease or symptom may differ.
3. Concepts of how the disease is thought to relate to other diseases or bodily conditions may be dissimilar.
4. The emotional connotation of a term for a disease or symptom may be different for the patient and the practitioner. This situation is most likely to influence the therapeutic outcome when the two parties differ over their estimation of the severity of the condition.

To lessen the chance of miscommunication about diseases or symptoms, the clinician can check with the patient to see whether any of these likely sources of conceptual discrepancy is operative.

Working with Common Ethnic Concepts of Disease Etiology

Although specific conceptual differences clearly exist among the various ethnic groups discussed in this volume, it is noteworthy that certain general etiological ideas turn up quite consistently across groups. Many of these ideas derive from older traditions of medicine. For the busy clinician who treats members of various ethnic categories, awareness of the following more pervasive etiological concepts can obviate the necessity of remembering details for specific groups and yet provide sufficient background to recognize issues that may require special inquiry with patients.

BLOOD BELIEFS Ideas concerning the quantity or quality of blood (for example, too much, too little; too thick, too thin; dirty; high, low) appear in almost all ethnic traditions. As a result, any disease or diagnostic procedure involving the blood should elicit special concern, discussion, and explanation from the clinician.

"Hot"/"cold" beliefs   Still operative among a variety of ethnics (for example, Chinese, Haitians, Mexicans, and Puerto Ricans in this volume) is the notion that disease constitutes a bodily imbalance that may be precipitated by a variety of situations or foods that can throw the body into an abnormally "hot" or "cold" state. Since such an imbalanced condition is thought to be cured by administering specific foods or medications having compensatory effects, these ideas may influence adherence to prescribed treatment regimens and should therefore be explored.

Drafts   Often, but not necessarily, related to "hot"/"cold" beliefs is the idea that respiratory infections, muscular and articular aches and pains, or muscular spasms are caused by air currents, to which the body is particularly susceptible while "the pores are open" (that is, when perspiring or after childbirth or surgery). Attention to this belief may be particularly warranted with patients suffering from any of the aforementioned conditions or from a fever. It may also be important in enhancing the comfort of patients during hospitalization, when they are likely to consider themselves particularly susceptible to drafts.

Psychosomatic causation   Psychological states (stress, worry, grief) and situational factors (poor housing, loss of work, family disputes, and so on) are seen as either causing or contributing to disease by nearly all the ethnic groups surveyed in this volume, and further ethnographic evidence on theories of disease indicates widespread concurrence in this view. Thus with patients of varying ethnic backgrounds, discussion of and therapeutic attention to consciously perceived psychosocial factors is particularly important in the treatment of illness. Pursuit of unconscious motivation may be perceived as blame, however, and could be counterproductive.

Treating Culture-Specific Syndromes

All labeled syndromes are in a sense "culture-specific"—that is, part of a larger, shared classification of symptom or problem clusters. Therefore, the term "culture-specific syndrome" is in fact "medicocentric" and refers to a labeled set of symptoms or problems that does not overlap sufficiently with a biomedical category to translate readily to it. Thus a culture-specific syndrome may involve either an assemblage of symptoms that is not found among most patients treated by Western biomedical professionals and is therefore not part of the standard biomedical nosology, or a set of symptoms that only partially overlaps with a standard biomedical designation. In the present volume a number of these syndromes have been described (for example, "evil eye" among Italian Americans, Mexican Americans, and Puerto Ricans; *susto* and *mollera caída* among Mexican Americans; *sézisman* among Haitians; "fright" among Chinese).

Knowledge of culture-specific syndromes is important to the clinician when he is treating symptoms that are included as part of such a syndrome, since such symptoms may be treated with folk or popular remedies either prior to or simultaneously with biomedical procedures. In such cases questioning the patient on the treatment instituted for the syndrome will enable the clinician to judge the potential effects of the dual regimens. Knowledge of culture-specific syndromes may also help the clinician understand patients' anxieties over experiencing certain symptoms that are viewed as part of or prodromal to a serious culture-specific condition.

The clinician can often learn about the culture-specific syndromes of a group that is not covered in this volume by discussing the concept with members of the ethnic group or with health professionals or paraprofessionals who have had extensive experience in treating members of the group.

Managing Discrepancies between Practitioners' and Patients' Concepts of Disease

After eliciting a patient's disease model, the clinician should clearly and thoroughly explain his own view of the patient's problem in nonjargonistic terms. Discrepancies between the clinician's and patient's models will then become apparent and should be discussed overtly.

Three general methods of handling such discrepancies are available: (1) *patient education,* in which the knowledge and authority of the biomedical practitioner are employed to change the ideas and perceptions of the patient; (2) *working within the patient's conceptual system,* in which a treatment plan is instituted which is considered effective by the clinician and which does not violate (or is at least not contraindicated by) the patient's conceptual system; or (3) *negotiating a compromise,* by which the patient and clinician agree to a treatment plan that accommodates each party's view of the situation to some degree but does not require either one to accept the other's model of the disease.

Becoming Ill: How Patients' Evaluations of Symptoms Affect Treatment

Although the decision that one is ill occurs for the most part before medical treatment is undertaken, many of the factors that contribute to that decision have implications for clinical practice. For one thing, the social or psychological concerns that lead a person to decide that he is ill often bear little perceptible relationship to the deviations in somatic variables that determine a biomedical diagnosis of disease. Thus, a clinician may cure a patient's somatic problem but fail to treat the concerns that have led him to seek treatment; or conversely, the clinician may remove the patient's concern but fail to cure the disease. Because of this frequent disjunction between illness and disease, it is important for the clinician to consider the specific experiences that have led patients to decide that they are ill so that these factors may also receive attention in the overall treatment plan.

The foregoing chapters on individual ethnic groups suggest certain general issues concerning the illness experience of behavioral ethnics that are relevant to their clinical care. These issues will be reviewed here, followed by specific suggestions for developing treatment plans.

General Observations on the Illness Experience

VARIABLES PRECIPITATING THE ILLNESS EXPERIENCE   A comparison of the ethnic groups included in this volume reveals that two factors recur consistently as determinants of people's sense that they are ill: (1) the duration, location, and intensity of symptoms, and (2) the social effects of the symptoms in terms of interference with either valued social activities or the fulfillment of role responsibilities. Though this finding is by no means new or unexpected (see Zola 1964; Mechanic 1969: 195), it does suggest a greater salience of these factors over other ones that have also been observed to determine people's perceptions that they are ill (for example, availability of treatment resources, variable tolerance thresholds for particular signs and symptoms, availability of information).

The data in this book further show that ethnicity influences these two preeminent determinants of people's experience of illness in ways that are particularly pertinent for the clinician. Specifically, different symptoms stand out as more salient signals of illness in different ethnic groups, and the particular social activities or important role responsibilities that are likely to precipitate a sense of illness when they are interfered with also vary across ethnic groups. As reported in specific chapters, for example, "pain" appears to be a particularly salient symptom for urban black Americans, Haitians, and Navajos; impotence for Chinese males; gastrointestinal and "liver" problems for Italian Americans; weight loss and fever for both Hispanic groups included in this book and, in addition, gastrointestinal symptoms for Mexican Americans and respiratory problems for Puerto Ricans. A similar phenomenon of differing importance of symptoms may obtain in other ethnic groups as well and should be kept in mind by clinicians.

WOMEN AS INTERPRETERS OF SYMPTOMS   An additional and not un-expected generalization deriving from the material presented in this book is that women constitute the principal evaluators of illness not only for children but generally also for other adults. (For the ethnic groups surveyed here, literate members of the family may also be specially enlisted in this activity.) It therefore seems reasonable to suggest that preventive health campaigns be directed particularly toward women through a variety of media and especially through audiovisual forms.

Clinical Issues Concerning the Illness Experience

The various factors that influence a patient's decision that he is ill suggest the following five issues which should be handled in clinical care in order to ensure more effective therapy.

RELIEF OF PAIN OR OTHER SYMPTOMS   Since experiencing pain or certain specific symptoms is likely to precipitate the perception of illness, patients often regard an illness as terminated when relief of symptoms has been achieved. As a result, it is particularly important for the clinician to decide whether continuation of therapy is necessary beyond the point at which symptoms have abated. If so, it is advisable to discuss with the patient both the reasons for continuation and possible consequences of noncompliance.

ANXIETY-PROVOKING SYMPTOMS   The information on illness behavior reviewed in this book indicates that certain symptoms appear to be not only more salient but also more anxiety-provoking for members of different ethnic groups. For example, fever and respiratory problems evoke particular concern for Puerto Ricans; "mind loss" (fainting or seizures) for Navajos; weakness for Haitian Americans. In view of these differences, it is important for the clinician to learn which symptoms tend to evoke unusual anxiety for the ethnic groups he may see most frequently in practice and to take the time to discuss those symptoms with patients in some depth—specifically with regard to their causes, severity, and the ways in which the treatment regimen will affect them.

FEAR OF TREATMENT   Since fear of certain forms of medical treatment may influence patients' decisions to consider themselves as ill, it is important for the clinician to know which forms of treatment are most likely to provoke anxiety in order to work with patients about such feelings. To some extent, ethnicity can serve as a predictor of specific feared treatments (for example, procedures involving blood loss among Chinese). In addition, although surgery and hospitalization provoke anxiety whatever the patient's ethnic affiliation, these procedures are likely to be more traumatic for non-English speakers, particularly when hospital personnel who speak the patient's language are not readily available. (For further discussion of this topic, see the section on language use in the clinical encounter later in the chapter.)

INTERFERENCE WITH ROLE RESPONSIBILITIES   Since the experience of being ill may well be precipitated by a person's inability to carry out normal role responsibilities, it is often important for the clinician to determine the areas of the patient's life that have been affected in this way. Whether the role be that of family provider, parent, or homemaker, the clinician may be called upon to sanction the patient's discontinuance of role performance and should also be prepared to discuss with the patient and family alternative ways of fulfilling the sick person's duties.

INTERFERENCE WITH VALUED ACTIVITIES   In narratives of illness episodes, patients often indicate valued activities that have been disturbed as a result of their symptoms. Because certain activity patterns are more common in particular ethnic groups (for example, visiting and sharing sweet foods with neighbors and kin among Italian Americans), specific activities may be mentioned more frequently by patients of different ethnic categories. The alert clinician should discuss any limitations on such activities that are occasioned by a particular regimen and help patients devise ways of coping with these limitations.

Coping with Illness outside the Mainstream Medical System

The vast majority of illness is treated either at home or by non-biomedically trained practitioners (Zola 1972). In addition to taking a considerable burden off the mainstream medical delivery system, these two sources of care have an impact on mainstream health care in other ways as well. Moreover, both are influenced by ethnic traditions.

Home Treatment: Implications for Mainstream Health Care

On the basis of the admittedly limited evidence presented in earlier chapters, it seems fair to conclude that the conditions treated at home by members of all ethnic groups are by and large the minor and self-limiting problems that mainstream medicine is not specialized to deal with anyway (for example, occasional headaches, minor upper respiratory infections and digestive problems, trivial burns and cuts, muscular aches). Moreover, delay in presentation for treatment of serious diseases seems to be motivated in all ethnic groups principally by an unwillingness to miss work, fear of a grave diagnosis, fear of a drastic treatment procedure (like surgery), and the stigma attached to certain symptoms. Although the relative influence of these various factors and the particular motivating fears or stigmata vary somewhat among ethnic groups, delay in seeking medical treatment seems more a function of individual social and psychological circumstances than ethnically shared standards of behavior.

The data on home treatment do, however, suggest two important implications for mainstream health care, which are discussed in the following subsections.

INCORPORATING PREFERRED MODES OF TREATMENT INTO STANDARD REGIMENS   Although diet therapy and herbal remedies are quite widely used across different ethnic groups, certain less common modes of treatment assume particular importance for specific groups (for example, massage among Puerto Ricans and Mexican Americans; sweat baths and heat treatments among Navajos). In addition, diet therapy plays a more important role in some ethnic groups than others, specifically in those groups which espouse a theory of disease that contains specific postulates about diet (for example, "hot"/"cold" theories among Chinese, Mexican, Haitian, and Puerto Rican Americans). Furthermore, although herbal remedies are widely giving way to patent medicines, they tend to be retained in groups in which the wider theoretical justification for herbal treatment is retained as well.

These cultural preferences for certain modes of treatment suggest that biomedical regimens may be more effectively administered if they incorporate ethnically preferred therapeutic modes. For example, dietary control of diabetes or hypertension, when practicable, may be more effective with Chinese or Haitian patients, who tend to see dietary changes as integral to good medical care. Or when increased intake of liquids is important to biomedical therapy, herbal teas might be recommended in addition to the usual prescription of water or juice. In short, awareness of culturally preferred modes of treatment, as evidenced in forms of therapy used in the home, and inclusion of such preferences in standard regimens may promote compliance.

SELF-MEDICATION AS A POSSIBLE HEALTH HAZARD   Most herbal and over-the-counter preparations commonly used in the home probably have no injurious effects either in and of themselves or in combination with prescription medications. However, some herbs and over the counter drugs may be contraindicated for specific diseases or when taken in conjunction with certain other medications. Because our data indicate that many patients of varying ethnic backgrounds take home remedies simultaneously with prescription medicines, it may behoove the clinician to question patients about the kinds of home remedies they may be taking, as well as the quantity and frequency of dosages. Since our data also show that certain herbs and over-the-counter preparations are more popular among different ethnic groups, it is important for the clinician to learn what the pharmacological properties are of the most popular preparations used by members of an ethnic group she commonly sees in practice.

Alternative Healers: Implications for Mainstream Health Care

People turn to nonmainstream health practitioners for a number of reasons. Our data indicate that some of these reasons apply universally across ethnic groups, whereas others seem limited to a few groups. Three sets of general reasons for utilizing alternative healers apply across ethnic groups. The first of these reasons has to do with the availability of mainstream health services—namely, and not surprisingly, people turn to alternative healers when mainstream care is, for one reason or another, unobtainable. The major causes for this unavailability are the expense and the distance in time or space from a source of care. Members of specific ethnic groups may also experience special circumstances that make mainstream services unavailable (for example, the risk of discovery and deportation for illegal immigrants among Mexicans and Haitians).

The second reason for patronizing alternative healers is to secure treatment for conditions that mainstream medicine has not treated to the patient's satisfaction. Thus, many patients turn to alternative sources of care only after they have tried the mainstream system. Specific situations that may lead to this form of behavior include instances when a mode of treatment has been recommended that is considered too drastic (often surgery); when a chronic ailment is refractory to standard therapy; or when a medical practitioner has communicated to a patient either that he "doesn't know what's wrong," or that in his professional judgment nothing is wrong.

The third general reason for consulting alternative healers is for treatment of psychosocial problems. Each of the ethnic groups discussed sustains various kinds of healers who primarily treat problems of living—from the less formally organized "therapeutic women" among Italian Americans and the root workers patronized by some urban blacks to the more formally organized Haitian Voodoo priests, Mexican *curanderos,* Navajo singers, and Puerto Rican *espiritistas.* To some extent, use of these healers can be construed as reflecting a problem of access to mainstream medical care, which has failed by and large to provide inexpensive, appropriate psychosocial counseling to low-income populations (particularly when they are non-English-speaking). Whether the medical system should undertake this task on a wide scale is not at issue here; the point is simply that this need is being met partly through specialists from ethnic subcultures.

In addition to these general reasons for consulting alternative healers, there are further grounds for their use that obtain only within particular ethnic subcultures. In certain ethnic groups people turn to lay specialists for treatment of culture-specific syndromes or for treatment of conditions thought to be caused by etiological agents not recognized in biomedical theory (for example, spirits, sorcery, "wind"). In the latter case people may use mainstream medicine for relief of symptoms while they concurrently consult an ethnic healer for removal of the cause; such practices are reported in this volume among Chinese Americans and Navajos.

IMPLICATIONS FOR MAINSTREAM HEALTH CARE The use of alternative healers suggests three points that mainstream clinicians might bear in mind.

1. In some cases alternative forms of therapy may render biomedical diagnosis and treatment difficult. The same issues raised earlier with regard to herbal remedies in home treatment may be relevant here. In addition, our data reveal that lay healers occasionally, though apparently rarely, forbid the use of prescription drugs. Therefore, in cases where a patient may be receiving therapy jointly from a lay healer, the clinician might verify whether this is so and question nonjudgmentally the nature of the therapy that is being followed. If any contraindicated procedures should be revealed in this way, changes in either one or both modes of therapy might then have to be negotiated with the patient and perhaps also with the healer.

2. More often than not, however, alternative healers appear to complement the delivery of mainstream medical services. Indeed, our data indicate that many of these healers refer clients to mainstream sources of care. In such cases, and when patients seek help from lay healers for psychosocial problems that are concomitant with chronic ailments, therapy may be improved by consultation and overt cooperation between the two sources of care. (Several models for the articulation of lay and biomedical services have been discussed earlier in the Introduction; see p. 26.)

3. Mainstream medical practitioners may also incorporate elements of the interpersonal style of alternative healers in order to enhance rapport with patients and potentially improve compliance. Knowledge of the style in which nonmainstream practitioners deliver care can often provide the clinician with a clue to culturally expected behaviors in therapeutic encounters. For example, lay healers typically establish a warm, intimate relationship with clients and their families and this practice might usefully be applied to mainstream settings particularly for the care of chronic disease.

Ethnic Factors in Encounters with Mainstream Medicine

Many issues that are pertinent to health-care encounters have already been discussed in previous sections. In this section the focus will be on face-to-face interaction between health personnel and members of ethnic groups, since it is probably in this area that ethnic factors are most central to the delivery of care.

Sources of Mainstream Care

Although members of most ethnic groups express a preference for office-based private practitioners, the sources of care people actually use vary considerably both between and within ethnic groups. (See the sections on medical-care settings in the foregoing chapters for reviews of the data on specific ethnic groups.)

Regardless of where a particular behavioral ethnic receives care, however, the essential issue for the clinician is that the treatment of such a patient will typically require more time than the treatment of other patients. Extra time may be required for translation, for discussion and clarification of biomedical concepts, for explanation of the diagnosis and negotiation of the treatment regimen, and for the important task of socializing the patient (whose experience of medical care has often been in another country) to the health-care delivery system of this country. (Patients from other societies often need to be instructed on issues such as the distinction between general practitioners and specialists, how outpatient clinics are structured, what services are provided for hospitalized patients, what kinds of services various health-care personnel can be expected to provide for patients, and so on.) Some of this information will be conveyed to patients by their more acculturated kinsmen and friends; however, much of it must be learned in the context of receiving care. Moreover, members of many different ethnic groups themselves express the need for a physician (not another health professional) to spend sufficient time with them to explain a variety of concerns (to be discussed further in the section on patient expectations).

All these time demands imply that behavioral ethnics must frequently be scheduled for longer appointments than are typical in most health-care facilities, a suggestion that contravenes the economics of both private and clinic practice. Nevertheless, physicians working with most first-generation (and often second-generation) ethnic patients, as well as managers of facilities that provide care mainly to behavioral ethnics, must find some way of mitigating the considerable time pressure involved in the delivery of health services without sacrificing the quality and effectiveness of patient care.

Language Use in the Clinical Encounter

The clinician should not assume that a foreign-born patient necessarily wishes to carry on a medical interview in his native language, since the English competence of people of different ethnic backgrounds may vary from nil to that of a native speaker. Therefore, when the patient's language ability is not immediately apparent, the clinician should ask what language he prefers to use.

When the clinician finds it necessary to communicate with patients in another language, an interpreter is in most cases preferable to a phrase book, since the bilingual intermediary allows for clarification and amplification that are impossible with the stock phrases of a manual. Yet the use of an interpreter is not without problems as well, for translators may interpolate their own constructions of what has been said or may fail to convey nuances of meaning implied by the speakers. In addition, the presence of a third person may itself inhibit the patient in communicating about sensitive subjects. In general, however, when a patient brings an adult relative or friend into the consulting room to act as translator, it is usually a sign that the relationship between the two is sufficiently open to permit a free exchange of information. Sometimes children are placed in the role of translator, however, and an awkward situation may develop if subjects should arise in the course of the interview that are considered taboo between parents and children. On the whole, it is best to avoid using nonadult children as translators for their parents.

To improve the quality of translation provided by a patient's companion, the clinician might suggest at the beginning of an interview that the interpreter (1) use the patient's own words as much as possible and (2) request the patient or the practitioner to clarify what they mean if it is not completely plain. In situations where nonbiomedically trained employees of a health-care facility routinely act as translators, a brief training program is often advisable to heighten their skills in translation techniques and medical vocabulary.

Hospitalization, which is apt to provoke anxiety in many people, is a particularly fearful situation for non-English speakers because they cannot ask questions or make their wishes known easily. They therefore tend to feel even more helpless and isolated than Anglophone patients. Two suggestions have been made in this volume for dealing with this problem: (1) to place speakers of the same language in the same room or on the same floor of a hospital, if at all possible; and (2) to provide patients with cards, printed with routine requests in English and the patient's language, which can be shown to nurses or other attendants as necessary. An additional possibility, which may be necessary under certain circumstances, would be to relax visiting rules to allow one bilingual member of the patient's family to remain with him as long as necessary.

Interactional Norms

The usual styles of interaction that people adopt and the standards of performance they use in ordinary interpersonal relations also apply in health-care situations and probably represent the aspect of health care most influenced by specific ethnic subcultures. As a result, few generalizations on interactional norms can be derived from the data presented in this volume. There are, however, several issues about which clinicians should be aware.

GENERAL GUIDELINES   In addition to the suggestion made earlier that mainstream practitioners model some aspects of their behavior after the styles adopted by alternative healers of the same ethnic groups as their patients', three further recommendations can assist the clinician in interacting with people of different ethnic categories.

1. Ethnic groups that derive from kin-based or peasant societies generally accord greater respect to the elderly than is usual in this society. In addition, social interaction between the sexes tends to be more limited in these societies, and standards of modesty between the sexes more rigidly prescribed. As a consequence, the age and sex of the clinician relative to a particular patient should influence the style of interaction he adopts. A younger clinician should therefore adopt toward the elderly of most ethnic groups an attitude of greater respect and seriousness than he might typically display toward older people in this society. Conversely, an older clinician might make special efforts to encourage younger patients to ask questions in order to reduce the reticence the patient may experience in the relationship.

Cross-sex interactions are not quite so easily handled, since nudity or genital examinations, when patient and practitioner are of the opposite sex, may provoke inordinate anxiety and embarrassment for members of many ethnic groups. In many instances patients will simply avoid medical encounters in which a genital examination may be required. When such a procedure is indicated and the involvement of a practitioner of the same sex is not possible, the clinician should carefully explain the purpose of the procedure first as well as the reason why the patient's symptoms indicate that it is necessary. After allowing for questions, the clinician should proceed with the examination with a serious and professional demeanor. Pelvic examinations of virgins violate standards of propriety in many ethnic groups, however, and should be undertaken only when clear indications for the procedure are present.

2. Because the class and professional standing of health-care practitioners tends to make most patients reticent, they need to be encouraged to ask the questions that will help them understand what is wrong and what they can do about it. Encouragement is particularly appropriate with behavioral ethnics, for whom language problems and different perceptions of illness are likely.

3. A patient's reticence can also be reduced by the clinician's listening attentively and unhurriedly to what the patient has to say and conveying

an interest in the patient as a person, either verbally or nonverbally. Since the precise manner in which this interest can most appropriately be communicated may vary for different ethnic groups (direct eye contact, touching, and so on), it may behoove the clinician to discuss this issue with other health-care personnel from the ethnic group.

WORKING WITH ETHNIC VARIATIONS IN PATIENT-PRACTITIONER INTERACTIONS   The style of presenting symptoms seems quite clearly to vary with different ethnic groups. Styles range from the truncated descriptions reported for Haitian Americans in this volume to the florid narratives reported for Italian Americans and the extensive symptom lists observed among Puerto Ricans. Knowing the style of a particular ethnic group allows the clinician to respond in an appropriate manner rather than with impatience or with an ethnocentric perspective. Thus, more restrained patients may be stimulated to report symptoms and other data more fully by consistent probes, accompanied by an explanation as to why the information is important. Furthermore, a lengthy recital of symptoms, with their accompanying emotional and social complications, should lead the clinician neither to ignore some of the symptoms in developing his problem list nor to suspect psychosomatic etiology overhastily. In fact, the clinician who is concerned with treating illness as well as disease may find patients who provide more elaborate histories easier to work with.

The data reported in this volume suggest a number of additional themes that may arise in interactions with members of different ethnic groups: (1) the degree of personalism or impersonality desired in the relationship; (2) whether or not patients feel comfortable with an authoritarian and directive demeanor; (3) the efficacy and appropriateness of assigning blame to the patient for a disease or health behavior; (4) the degree of discomfort occasioned by disagreement between patient and practitioner; (5) the role of touch in establishing rapport; and (6) the degree to which patients are free to decide on a course of action independent of their families. In working with members of different ethnic groups, health practitioners should be aware of these themes and alert to their potential relevance to the medical care of particular ethnic groups. Again, health-care personnel from the same ethnic group as the patient may be able to assist in assessing the relevance of these themes to the care of patients of that group.

Patient Expectations in the Medical Encounter

A pervasive expectation in the clinical encounter, closely related to the interactional issues discussed above, is that the clinician show concern for the patient as a person, rather than as a case. This concern may be displayed through careful listening, politeness, warmth in greeting the patient, and an unhurried manner. The relative importance of these various factors may vary with different ethnic groups.

In addition to personal regard, members of all ethnic groups surveyed in this volume expect to acquire information from health-care personnel, and the physician is generally the preferred source. Specifically, patients want an explanation of the disease—its pathophysiology, the relationship between symptoms and cause, and its severity, possible course, and duration. They often also want to know the relationship between their symptoms and recommended diagnostic and treatment procedures. Since patients' experience of disease is largely through symptoms, explanations relating the biomedical model of disease to patients' symptoms are most relevant to their concerns and often most easily comprehended. Explanations should also be given in nontechnical language, as far as possible, and when a technical term must be used, it should be explained. (The complementary process of eliciting patients' models and explanations of disease has been described both in the Introduction, note 6, and earlier in this chapter.)

Related to patients' desires for an explanation is their frequent sense of exasperation when the practitioner says either that nothing is wrong or that he does not know what is wrong. Such statements imply to some patients of various ethnic traditions that their symptoms are supernaturally caused and may have the effect of referring them to an alternative healer. Depending on a patient's symptoms and the clinical findings, the practitioner may therefore wish to investigate the patient's perception of the illness further in order to discuss his concerns in greater detail and perhaps ultimately to cooperate with an alternative healer on the problem. In some cases the clinician may simply wish to watch the patient for further developments. When a subsequent appointment is scheduled for this purpose, the reason should be explained carefully to avoid heightening the patient's fears while still demonstrating concern for his well-being. For patients from ethnic groups that generally desire a rapid diagnosis (for example, Haitian Americans and Navajos, among the groups reported in this volume), continued surveillance would probably not be useful.

Ethnic Issues in Adherence to Biomedical Treatment

Although various factors that have been observed generally to correlate with patient compliance appear to apply equally to behavioral ethnics, ethnic affiliation does condition some of these factors in ways that mainstream practitioners should bear in mind. For example, enlistment of patients' families in reinforcing treatment regimens for chronic diseases has been widely observed to increase compliance (Heinzelmann and Bagley 1970; Oakes et al. 1970; Gillum and Barsky 1974). Yet because the structure and role allocations of families vary across ethnic groups, the specific relatives a clinician should contact for this purpose differ according to patients' ethnic affiliation. Among the Navajo, for example, matrilineally related women living in close proximity to the patient would be most appropriate; among Mexican Americans, the bilaterally extended family in general should be consulted and, for males in particular, older male relatives; among Puerto Ricans, it might be sufficient to contact the wife/mother or, for elderly patients, their children. As a rule, therefore, clinicians should learn about the family structures of ethnic groups from which their patients come in order to discover which kinsmen are likely to be most influential in medical decisions. In this way these sources of social support can be readily tapped for assisting patients to adhere to treatment regimens.

A second generally observed factor about compliance that is influenced by ethnic membership is the tendency of patients to discontinue medication when symptoms have abated. Although this practice is not unique to behavioral ethnics, a contributing cause for it among ethnics of certain groups is a wariness of overmedication (reported in this volume as a general tendency among Chinese Americans and, with respect to certain forms of medication, among Italian Americans and Puerto Ricans as well). Although this attitude of cautiousness toward the taking of medicines is certainly not harmful as a general rule, its effects on certain chronic conditions are likely to be negative. As a result, clinicians should ascertain whether members of particular ethnic groups whom they frequently treat maintain this attitude, and if so, they should be particularly diligent in explaining the pharmacology of maintenance doses to them.

An additional factor that is generally related to taking routine medications symptomatically is the quality of the doctor-patient relationship—specifically, such aspects as warmth, continuity of care, explanations of both the disease and the treatment regimen, release of tension in the encounter, and feedback from the physician (Marston 1970; Becker, Drachman, and Kirscht 1974; Haynes 1976). As discussed in a number of places earlier, all these aspects of the doctor-patient relationship may be influenced by ethnic factors, and various suggestions for dealing with them have been provided.

Two final influences of ethnicity on adherence to medical regimens, which have also been alluded to previously, bear brief repetition here. First, for many behavioral ethnics compliance with a biomedical regimen does not entail discontinuation of either home remedies or cures prescribed by alternative healers. Occasionally these regimens may be counteractive, and ways of handling such situations have already been described (pp. 493–494). A second ethnic influence on compliance concerns preferences among certain ethnic groups for specific forms of medication or treatment. In addition to a widespread preference for injection over oral administration of medication, different ethnic groups are reported to favor dietary modification or tablets over capsules. Consideration of these preferences in prescribing treatment may promote compliance.

Therapeutic Diets

Since foods are one of the key symbols of ethnic difference in American culture, dietary regimens must incorporate ethnic differences if they are likely to be followed. Thus, the current practice of developing special dietary literature for different ethnic groups should be encouraged. Even with such literature, however, diet is generally one of the most difficult aspects of behavior to change (Sackett and Haynes 1976), although this may be less true among ethnic groups like the Chinese and Haitians whose traditional concepts of therapy lead people to expect dietary modifications.

Ethnically acceptable therapeutic diets should reflect two things: ethnic food preferences and ethnic food beliefs. Therefore, diet lists of admissible and proscribed foods should contain not only items that are typical to a particular ethnic cuisine but also acceptable substitutes for proscribed customary dishes and manners of food preparation. Food beliefs, in their more elaborated forms, generally involve categories of foodstuffs that are thought to be good or bad for certain symptoms or bodily conditions. Among the categories reported in this volume are the "hot"/"cold" classification among Chinese, Haitians, Mexicans, and Puerto Ricans; "wet"/ "dry" among Italians; and "strong"/"weak" among Navajos. Less elaborated beliefs may involve only a few foods that are considered either therapeutic or unhealthy for certain conditions. These kinds of beliefs may in some cases support, and in other cases contravene, standard therapeutic diets. To promote compliance, therefore, particular agreements and contradictions between the two dietary systems should be discussed with patients so that ambiguities can be resolved.

In presenting therapeutic diets to patients, however, it is important to recognize that not all ethnics routinely eat ethnic foods. To prevent stereotyping, the usual practice of taking a diet history to ascertain the food habits of the individual patient is strongly recommended.

A final issue regarding therapeutic diets and ethnicity concerns new immigrants who have previously been placed on a dietary regimen in their country of origin. Since foods that were dietary staples in the home country, particularly if that country is located in the tropics, may be either unavailable or too expensive in the United States, these patients must not only discover foods that are palatable substitutes for their standard fare but also learn whether the substitutes are dietetically acceptable. This information can be assembled by health facilities that have numerous immigrants from tropical areas among their clientele and should be discussed with new patients as needed.

Inpatient Care

In addition to several issues that have already been discussed concerning inpatient care of members of ethnic groups (language problems and the need to orient first-generation ethnics to both hospital procedures and the duties of various staff members concerning patient care), the role of the patient's family in the hospital setting is an important topic for consideration. In many ethnic groups the family plays an important role in patient care and indeed may be required in their countries of origin to provide specific services to hospitalized relatives (for example, feeding or washing). In ethnic groups with strong family organization, sickness is also a time for relatives to display their solidarity, so activities such as visiting the hopsital, preparing food, and otherwise showing a willingness to help all function as important signs of commitment to the kin group. These activities can be important for the psychological state of not only the patient but also family members themselves. Yet hospital rules often hamper the full expression of family concern by restricting the number of visitors or prohibiting patients from eating food brought from outside. Polite explanation of the rationale for the rules to families, relaxation of these rules whenever possible, and other forms of accommodation to this important source of psychological and social support to biomedical therapy are generally desirable.

Helping Families during Recovery, Rehabilitation, and Terminal Illness

Many ethnic groups strongly prefer home care over institutional care for the incapacitated and terminally ill. Among the groups discussed in this volume, Chinese, Haitians, Italians, Mexicans, and Puerto Ricans all manifest this preference, while urban blacks and Navajos do not.

Although there are many reasons for favoring home care, two characteristics of the groups that do so are strong extended-family ties and relatively low participation of women (usually the principal caretakers) in the work force. Indeed, the high percentage of urban black women in the labor force is undoubtedly a major deterrent to home care in that group. (Cultural attitudes—fear of spirit contamination from the dead—largely account for the Navajo viewpoint on this subject, however.) Though the availability of caretakers in certain ethnic groups is important in making home care possible, providers of mainstream health services should nevertheless realize that the burdens imposed on patients' families may be considerable. Therefore, assistance of various kinds (financial, nursing, educational) may be necessary to enable them to carry out what they perceive to be their proper responsibilities.

Access to Biomedical Knowledge: A Crucial Issue for Many Ethnic Patients

This volume has focused on cross-cultural communication as a means of improving the health care of American ethnic populations. Though the information has concentrated on the subcultures of various ethnic groups themselves, it is also important for clinicians to realize where members of ethnic groups acquire their knowledge of the biomedical subculture.[2] In discussing the sources of this information, it will become apparent that both ethnic and class exclusion in this society place considerable limitations on behavioral ethnics' access to this knowledge. The discussion therefore reinforces a point raised earlier in the Introduction—namely, that access to health care and health information are unequally distributed in this society across ethnic and class segments.

The major sources of current information to the American public on the biomedical subculture (its beliefs, premises, methods, and so on) are formal educational institutions, health facilities (both public health and health-care divisions), the mass media, and personal social networks (particularly when these include acquaintances in health-care occupations or professions). Simply listing these sources reveals the limited access to the biomedical subculture that people have who are non-English-speaking, who are encapsulated in an ethnic enclave, or who are of lower socioeconomic class. For both secondary and higher education in this country have either openly discriminated against members of certain ethnic groups or have been unsuccessful in passing knowledge on to members of the lower socioeconomic class. And even though health-care facilities are now much more widely available to behavioral ethnics and the poor, the major sources of health care for lower-class behavioral ethnics are still non-hospital-affiliated private practitioners (many with outmoded knowledge) or emergency rooms, outpatient clinics, and private "Medicaid mills" (where little of the personal rapport that is so necessary to patient education can be developed). Furthermore, the personal networks of behavioral ethnics do not typically include acquaintances with substantial biomedical knowledge. Although the competent training of paraprofessionals and the removal of legal barriers to professional education for minorities have altered this situation somewhat over the past decades, the knowledge that individual patients gain from clinical encounters still provides a major source of information on biomedicine to ethnic social networks.

Of all the sources of biomedical information listed above, the mass media have probably been the most available to behavioral ethnics and members of the lower class. The ethnic press has sometimes been of considerable influence, although, as Jackson has observed in a note following Chapter 1, the need to popularize information in these publications may lead to serious distortions. Television has obviously played a major role in this regard as well, though probably not so much through direct educational efforts as through the medical information that is often contained in more popular programs like soap operas and medical dramas. Here, too, distortions obviously occur. Yet health planners should consider these channels of information seriously in disseminating accurate information on biomedicine to people of all class and ethnic backgrounds.

The Importance of the Clinical Encounter to Behavioral Ethnics

The foregoing discussion makes it clear that the clinical encounter is the most important source of information available to behavioral ethnics on the subculture of biomedicine. For, in addition to being a locus for treatment, it is often the origin of biomedical knowledge that circulates in ethnic social networks. Moreover, unlike the mass media, the clinical situation allows for an exchange of ideas and feelings between patients and health-care providers so that conceptual discrepancies, questions, and personal doubts can be aired and possibly resolved. In short, the clinical encounter is the only area in which the therapeutic strengths and values of both biomedical and ethnic subcultures can be explored and then used for the benefit of patients.

Yet constraints on the time that health-care personnel can actually devote to sharing information and negotiating culturally appropriate therapies in the clinical encounter are manifestly severe. Therefore, a major effort on the part of health-care personnel, planners, and managers needs to be directed toward changing the delivery system so that clinicians are able to spend time in applying ideas and suggestions like the ones discussed in this book. Even without such systemic changes, however, clinicians can improve the efficiency with which they now conduct their work by knowing which aspects of ethnic subcultures are likely to bear most heavily on medical care: namely, ethnic concepts of disease and illness, folk and popular traditions of health care, problems of language and translation, dietary practices, interactional norms, and the role of the family in compliance with long-term treatment. Awareness of these general topics can help the clinician focus on the most important sociocultural issues in the care of individual patients and thus contribute to the delivery of maximally efficient and beneficial service to members of ethnic groups.

Notes

1. As discussed in the Introduction, the term "behavioral ethnic" refers to people who have been raised in a different cultural tradition and whose values, concepts, beliefs, and behavioral norms may therefore differ from those of people who have been socialized into the dominant American culture. They are differentiated from "ideological ethnics," who have been socialized by and large into the dominant American culture of their class but who identify with a particular ethnic group largely for political or economic reasons.

2. The notion of a biomedical subculture and its premises has been discussed in the Introduction.

References

BECKER, MARSHALL H., ROBERT H. DRACHMAN, and JOHN P. KIRSCHT. 1974. A New Approach to Explaining Sick-Role Behavior in Low-Income Populations. *American Journal of Public Health* 64:205–216.

GILLUM, RICHARD F., and ARTHUR J. BARSKY. 1974. Diagnosis and Management of Patient Noncompliance. *Journal of the American Medical Association* 228:1563–1567.

HAYNES, R. BRIAN. 1976. A Critical Review of the "Determinants" of Patient Compliance with Therapeutic Regimens. In *Compliance with Therapeutic Regimens,* ed. David L. Sackett and R. Brian Haynes. Baltimore: Johns Hopkins University Press.

HEINZELMANN, FRED, and RICHARD W. BAGLEY. 1970. Response to Physical Activity Programs and Their Effects on Health Behavior. *Public Health Reports* 85:905–911.

JENKINS, C. DAVID. 1966. Group Differences in Perception: A Study of Community Beliefs and Feelings about Tuberculosis. *American Journal of Sociology* 71:417–429.

KLEINMAN, ARTHUR, LEON EISENBERG, and BYRON GOOD. 1978. Culture, Illness and Care: Clinical Lessons from Anthropologic and Cross-Cultural Research. *Annals of Internal Medicine* 88:251–258.

MARSTON, MARY-VESTA. 1970. Compliance with Medical Regimens: A Review of the Literature. *Nursing Research* 19:312–323.

MECHANIC, DAVID. 1969. Illness and Cure. In *Poverty and Health: A Sociological Analysis,* ed. John Kosa, Aaron Antonovsky, and Irving K. Zola. Cambridge, Mass.: Harvard University Press.

OAKES, THOMAS W., et al. 1970. Family Expectations and Arthritis Patient Compliance to a Hand Resting Splint Regimen. *Journal of Chronic Diseases* 22:757–764.

PLAJA, ANTONIO ORDONEZ, LUCY M. COHEN, and JULIAN SAMORA. 1968. Communication between Physicians and Patients in Outpatient Clinics: Social and Cultural Factors. *Milbank Memorial Fund Quarterly* 46 (Part 1): 161–213.

SACKETT, DAVID L., and R. BRIAN HAYNES, eds. 1976. *Compliance with Therapeutic Regimens.* Baltimore: Johns Hopkins University Press.

Samora, Julian, Lyle Saunders, and Richard F. Larson.   1961.   Medical Vocabulary Knowledge among Hospital Patients. *Journal of Health and Human Behavior* 2:83–92.

Suchman, Edward A.   1964.   Sociomedical Variations among Ethnic Groups. *American Journal of Sociology* 70:319–331.

Wolinsky, Frederic D.   1978.   Assessing the Effects of Predisposing, Enabling, and Illness-Morbidity Characteristics on Health Service Utilization. *Journal of Health and Social Behavior* 19:384–396.

Zola, Irving K.   1964.   Illness Behavior of the Working Class. In *Blue Collar World,* ed. Arthur Shostak and William Gomberg. Englewood Cliffs, N.J.: Prentice-Hall.

———.   1972.   Studying the Decision to See a Doctor: Review, Critique, Corrective. *Advances in Psychosomatic Medicine* 8:216–236.

Index